Manual of Definitive Surgical Trauma Care

Developed for the International Association for Trauma Surgery and Intensive Care (IATSIC), the *Manual of Definitive Surgical Trauma Care* 6e is ideal for training all surgeons and anaesthetists who manage trauma on an infrequent basis.

The Manual is updated every 4 years and reflects the most recent developments in patient management based on new evidence-based information. Its focus is on the importance of the multidisciplinary care of the trauma surgical patient. This sixth edition has evolved, and the all-important section on the Non-Technical Skills which are required has been expanded. A significant number of the original guidelines in trauma have been archived, as they are no longer pertinent or have been superseded. The increasing (and occasionally harmful) role of non-operative management (NOM) has been recognized. The 'Military Environments' and 'Austere Environments' chapters have been substantially revised to reflect current multinational combat experience, and broadened to reflect modern asymmetrical conflicts and the increased need for humanitarian intervention including military peacekeeping in which only one side wears a uniform. Military weapons are used in major cities against the civilian population. More recently, urban, non-military populations have been the targets and victims of heavy military combat including the use of ultra-sophisticated weaponry. Each situation carries its own spectrum of injury and responsibility of care.

Including website access to a selection of videos which provide an anatomic overview of surgical approaches, this resource provides a gold standard educational and training resource to help prepare the relatively fully trained surgeon to manage the difficult injuries that might present to a major trauma centre.

Manual of Definitive Surgical Trauma Care: Incorporating Definitive Anaesthetic Trauma Care

SIXTH EDITION

Edited by Kenneth D Boffard
Jonathan Oliver White

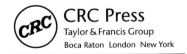

CRC Press
Taylor & Francis Group
Boca Raton London New York

CRC Press is an imprint of the
Taylor & Francis Group, an **informa** business

Sixth edition published 2024
by CRC Press
2385 NW Executive Center Drive, Suite 320, Boca Raton FL 33431

and by CRC Press
4 Park Square, Milton Park, Abingdon, Oxon, OX14 4RN

CRC Press is an imprint of Taylor & Francis Group, LLC

© 2024 selection and editorial matter, Kenneth D Boffard and Jonathan Oliver White; individual chapters, the contributors

First edition published by Arnold 2003

Fifth edition published by CRC Press 2019

ISBN: 9781032192048 (hbk)
ISBN: 9781032157818 (pbk)
ISBN: 9781003258124 (ebk)

DOI: 10.1201/9781003258124

Typeset in LegacySerifStd
by KnowledgeWorks Global Ltd.

Access the Instructor and Student Resources: www.routledge.com/cw/boffard

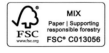

Printed and bound in Great Britain by
TJ Books Limited, Padstow, Cornwall

DEDICATION

This Manual is dedicated to the six surgeons who, in 1993, saw the need for a course in operative trauma surgery and surgical decision-making for those surgeons who would not routinely be involved in the care of the trauma patient, and from whose foresight the course was developed.

Howard Champion	Bethesda, Maryland, USA
Stephen Deane	Sydney, Australia
Abe Fingerhut	Poissy, France
Stenn Lennquist	Linköping, Sweden
David Mulder	Montreal, Canada
Donald Trunkey	Portland, Oregon, USA

**It is also dedicated to all those who serve their country
and place themselves in harm's way for the sake of freedom,
and care of their fellow members of humankind.**

Contents

Video Contents   xxxi

Preface   xxxii

About the Editors   xxxv

Board of Contributors   xxxvi

Contributors Emeritus   xlii

Part 1   TRAUMA SYSTEM AND COMMUNICATION PRINCIPLES   **1**

1   Introduction   **3**

1.1   Injury Prevention   4

1.2   Safe Trauma Care   4

    1.2.1   Individual Factors   4

       1.2.1.1   Individual: Leadership   5

       1.2.1.2   Trauma Team   5

       1.2.1.3   Team: Training   5

    1.2.2   Institutional Factors   5

       1.2.2.1   Dedicated Trauma Service   5

    1.2.3   Performance Improvement Activities   6

    1.2.4   Regional Activities   6

    1.2.5   National Activities   6

    1.2.6   Global Activities   6

1.3   Sustainable Trauma Care   7

    1.3.1   Workforce Training and Development   7

1.4   Surgical Trauma Training Beyond Initial Care   7

    1.4.1   Non-Technical Skills for Surgeons (NOTSS)   7

    1.4.2   The Advanced Trauma Operative Management (ATOM®) Course   8

    1.4.3   The Advanced Surgical Skills for Exposure in Trauma (ASSET®) Course   8

    1.4.4   The Definitive Surgical Trauma Care™ (DSTC) Course   8

    1.4.5   The Definitive Anaesthetic Trauma Care™ (DATC) Course   8

1.5   Conclusion   8

2   Non-Technical Skills in Major Trauma: The Role of Crew Resource Management (CRM) and Communication   **10**

2.1   Overview   10

2.2   The Avoidance of Errors   11

    2.2.1   The 'Swiss Cheese' Theory   11

2.3   Communication in the Trauma Setting   11
        2.3.1   Initial Handover   13
        2.3.2   Communication in Resuscitation and Ongoing Management   13
        2.3.3   Damage Control Decision-Making   13
2.4   Leadership in Trauma Care   14
        2.4.1   Situational Awareness   14
        2.4.2   Role Allocation   15
        2.4.3   Decision-Making   15
        2.4.4   Leadership   16
        2.4.5   Communication   16
2.5   A Six-Step Approach to Perioperative Communication in Trauma   17
2.6   Potential Errors Related to Each Behavioural Theme   19
2.7   Summary   21

Part 2   PHYSIOLOGY AND THE BODY'S RESPONSE TO TRAUMA   **23**

3   Resuscitation Physiology   **25**
3.1   Metabolic Response to Trauma   25
        3.1.1   Definition of Trauma   25
        3.1.2   Initiating Factors   25
                3.1.2.1   Hypovolaemia   26
                3.1.2.2   Inflammation   26
                3.1.2.3   The Consequences of the Pro- and Anti-Inflammatory Responses   28
                3.1.2.4   Coagulation and Inflammation   28
3.2   Hormonal Mediators   29
        3.2.1   Hypothalamus–Pituitary Axis   29
        3.2.2   Adrenal Hormones   30
        3.2.3   Pancreatic Hormones   30
        3.2.4   Renal Hormones   30
        3.2.5   Other Hormones   30
3.3   Effects of the Various Mediators   30
        3.3.1   Hyperdynamic State   30
        3.3.2   Water and Salt Retention   31
        3.3.3   Effects on Substrate Metabolism   31
                3.3.3.1   Carbohydrates   31
                3.3.3.2   Fat   31
                3.3.3.3   Amino Acids   32
                3.3.3.4   The Gut   32
3.4   The Anabolic Phase   32
3.5   Clinical and Therapeutic Relevance   32
3.6   Shock   32
        3.6.1   Definition of Shock   32
        3.6.2   Classification of Shock   33
                3.6.2.1   Hypovolaemic Shock   33
                3.6.2.2   Cardiogenic Shock   34
                3.6.2.3   Decreased LV Filling Pressures   35
        3.6.3   Distributive (Inflammatory) Shock   36
        3.6.4   Neurogenic Shock   36
                3.6.4.1   Clinical Presentation   36

	3.6.5	Measurements in Shock	36
		3.6.5.1 Cardiac Output	36
		3.6.5.2 Indirect Measurement of Flow	37
		3.6.5.3 Direct Measurements	37
		3.6.5.4 Non-Invasive Cardiac Monitoring	38
		3.6.5.5 Invasive Haemodynamic Monitoring	38
3.7	Endpoints in Shock Resuscitation		38
	3.7.1	Post-Shock and Multiple Organ Failure Syndromes	39
	3.7.2	Management of the Shocked Patient	39
		3.7.2.1 Oxygenation	40
		3.7.2.2 Airway Indications for Intubation	40
		3.7.2.3 Breathing Indications for Intubation	40
		3.7.2.4 Breathing Indications for Ventilation	40
		3.7.2.5 Circulatory Indication for Intubation	40
		3.7.2.6 Disability Indications for Intubation	40
		3.7.2.7 Environmental Indication for Intubation	40
	3.7.3	Fluid Therapy for Volume Expansion	40
		3.7.3.1 Hypotensive Resuscitation	40
	3.7.4	Route of Administration	41
		3.7.4.1 Intravenous Devices	41
		3.7.4.2 Intraosseous Devices	41
	3.7.5	Pharmacologic Support of Blood Pressure	41
		3.7.5.1 Norepinephrine (Noradrenaline)	42
		3.7.5.2 Epinephrine (Adrenaline)	42
		3.7.5.3 Dopamine	42
		3.7.5.4 Dobutamine	42
	3.7.6	Prognosis in Shock	42
		3.7.6.1 Recommended Protocol for Shock	42
4	**Transfusion in Trauma**		**46**
4.1	Indications for Transfusion		46
	4.1.1	Oxygen-Carrying Capacity	46
4.2	Transfusion Fluids		46
	4.2.1	Colloids	46
		4.2.1.1 Starches	46
		4.2.1.2 Albumin	46
	4.2.2	Blood	47
		4.2.2.1 Fresh Whole Blood	47
		4.2.2.2 Stored Whole Blood	47
		4.2.2.3 Packed Red Blood Cells	47
		4.2.2.4 Synthetic Blood and Blood Products	48
	4.2.3	Component Therapy (Platelets, Fresh Frozen Plasma [FFP], and Cryoprecipitate)	48
		4.2.3.1 Platelets	48
		4.2.3.2 Plasma: FFP or Freeze-Dried Plasma (FDP)	49
		4.2.3.3 Cryoprecipitate	49
		4.2.3.4 Fibrinogen Concentrate	49
4.3	Effects of Transfusing Blood and Blood Products		49
	4.3.1	Metabolic Effects	49
	4.3.2	Hyperkalaemia	50
	4.3.3	Coagulopathy of Trauma	50

	4.3.4	Other Risks of Transfusion		51
		4.3.4.1	Transfusion-Transmitted Infections	51
		4.3.4.2	Haemolytic Transfusion Reactions	51
		4.3.4.3	Immunological Complications	51
		4.3.4.4	Factors Implicated in Haemostatic Failure	51
4.4	Adjuncts to Enhance Clotting			51
	4.4.1	Prothrombin Complex Concentrate (PCC)		51
	4.4.2	Tranexamic Acid (TXA)		52
	4.4.3	Desmopressin (DDAVP)		52
	4.4.4	Recombinant Activated Factor VIIA		53
4.5	Monitoring the Coagulation Status			53
	4.5.1	Traditional Assays		53
	4.5.2	Viscoelastic Haemostatic Assays (VHAs): Thromboelastography (TEG) and Rotary Thromboelastomerography (RoTEM)		54
4.6	Autotransfusion			57
4.7	Massive Haemorrhage and Massive Transfusion Protocols (MHPS/MTPS)			58
	4.7.1	Definition		58
	4.7.2	Massive Transfusion Protocol		59
4.8	Local Haemostatic Adjuncts			59
	4.8.1	Overview		59
	4.8.2	Tissue Adhesives		59
		4.8.2.1	Fibrin	59
		4.8.2.2	Patches	62
	4.8.3	Local Haemostatic Adjuncts		62
		4.8.3.1	Chitosan (Celox [Meditrade, Crewe, UK]) and Hemcon (Hemcon Medical Technologies, Portland, or, USA)	62
		4.8.3.2	Mineral Zeolyte (Quikclot® [Z-Medical, Wallingford, CT, USA])	63
5	**Pre-Hospital and Emergency Trauma Care**			**66**
5.1	Resuscitation in the Pre-Hospital Setting and Emergency Department			66
5.2	Management of Major Trauma			66
	5.2.1	Resuscitation		68
		5.2.1.1	Civilian Pre-Hospital Tourniquet Use	68
		5.2.1.2	Primary Survey	68
		5.2.1.3	Secondary Survey	73
	5.2.2	Management of Penetrating Trauma		74
5.3	Emergency Department Surgery			74
	5.3.1	Head Trauma		75
	5.3.2	Chest Trauma		75
	5.3.3	Abdominal Trauma		76
	5.3.4	Pelvic Trauma		76
	5.3.5	Long Bone Fractures		77
	5.3.6	Peripheral Vascular Injuries		77
5.4	Summary			77
5.5	Anaesthesiological Considerations			78
6	**Damage Control**			**80**
6.1	Introduction			80
6.2	Damage Control Resuscitation			81
	6.2.1	Overview		81

	6.2.2	Goals		81
		6.2.2.1	Permissive Hypotension	81
		6.2.2.2	Minimize the Use of Crystalloid and Non-Blood Products	81
		6.2.2.3	Blood Product Administration with a Balanced Ratio of Packed Red Blood	
			Cells (PRBCS), Fresh Frozen Plasma (FFP), and Platelets	82
		6.2.2.4	Tranexamic Acid (TXA)	82
		6.2.2.5	Goal-Directed Haemostasis	82
		6.2.2.6	Avoid Hypothermia	82
		6.2.2.7	Restoration of Normocalcaemia	82
	6.2.3	Massive Transfusion/Haemorrhage Protocol (MTP/MHP)	83
6.3	Damage Control Surgery		83
	6.3.1	Overview		83
	6.3.2	Lethal Triad and Deadly Diamond		83
		6.3.2.1	Hypothermia	83
		6.3.2.2	Acidosis	84
		6.3.2.3	Coagulopathy	84
		6.3.2.4	Hypocalcaemia	84
	6.3.3	Damage Control in the Thorax		85
	6.3.4	Damage Control in the Abdomen		85
		6.3.4.1	Stage 1: Patient Selection	85
		6.3.4.2	Stage 2: Operative Haemorrhage and Contamination Control	86
		6.3.4.3	Stage 3: Physiological Restoration in the ICU	89
		6.3.4.4	Stage 4: Definitive Surgery	90
		6.3.4.5	Stage 5: Abdominal Wall Closure	91
	6.3.5	Planned Hernia		92
	6.3.6	Outcomes		92
6.4	Damage Control Orthopaedics (DCO)		92

Part 3 ANATOMICAL AND ORGAN SYSTEM INJURY   **97**

7	**The Neck**		**99**
7.1	Overview		99
7.2	Management Principles: Penetrating Cervical Injury		99
	7.2.1	Initial Assessment and Definitive Airway		99
	7.2.2	Control of Haemorrhage		100
	7.2.3	Injury Location		101
	7.2.4	Mechanism		102
	7.2.5	Frequency of Injury		102
	7.2.6	Use of Diagnostic Studies		102
		7.2.6.1	Computed Tomography Scanning with Contrast:	
			CT Angiography	102
		7.2.6.2	Angiography	102
		7.2.6.3	Other Diagnostic Studies	102
7.3	Management		102
	7.3.1	Mandatory versus Selective Neck Exploration		104
	7.3.2	Management Based on Anatomical Zones		104
7.4	Access to the Neck		104
	7.4.1	Position		105
	7.4.2	Incision		105

7.4.3	Surgical Access		106
	7.4.3.1	Access to the Great Vessels	106
	7.4.3.2	Zone I	107
	7.4.3.3	Zone II	107
	7.4.3.4	Zone III	107
	7.4.3.5	Access to the Aerodigestive Tract	108
7.4.4	Priorities		108
	7.4.4.1	Carotid Artery	108
	7.4.4.2	Tracheal Injuries	109
	7.4.4.3	Pharyngeal and Oesophageal Injuries	109
7.4.5	Midline Visceral Structures		109
7.4.6	Root of the Neck		109
7.4.7	Collar Incisions		109
7.4.8	Vertebral Arteries		110

8	**The Chest**		**114**
8.1	Overview		114
8.2	The Spectrum of Thoracic Injury		114
	8.2.1	Immediately Life-Threatening Injuries	114
	8.2.2	Potentially Life-Threatening Injuries	114
8.3	Pathophysiology of Thoracic Injuries		115
	8.3.1	Paediatric Considerations	115
8.4	Applied Surgical Anatomy of the Chest		116
	8.4.1	The Chest Wall	116
	8.4.2	The Chest Floor	116
	8.4.3	The Chest Contents	116
		8.4.3.1 Tracheobronchial Tree	117
		8.4.3.2 Lungs and Pleurae	117
		8.4.3.3 Heart and Pericardium	118
		8.4.3.4 The Aorta and Great Vessels	118
		8.4.3.5 Oesophagus	118
		8.4.3.6 Thoracic Duct	118
8.5	Diagnosis		118
8.6	Management of Specific Injuries		119
	8.6.1	Damage Control in the Chest	119
	8.6.2	Open Pneumothorax	119
	8.6.3	Tension Pneumothorax (Haemo- or Pneumothorax)	120
	8.6.4	Massive Haemothorax	120
	8.6.5	Retained Haemothorax	121
	8.6.6	Tracheobronchial Injuries	121
	8.6.7	Oesophageal Injuries	121
	8.6.8	Diaphragmatic Injuries	122
	8.6.9	Pulmonary Contusion (PC)	122
	8.6.10	Flail Chest (FC)	122
	8.6.11	Fixation of Multiple Fractures of Ribs,	123
	8.6.12	Pulmonary Laceration	125
		8.6.12.1 Air Embolism	125
	8.6.13	Cardiac Injuries	125
	8.6.14	Injuries to the Great Vessels	126

8.7	Chest Drainage	127
	8.7.1 Drain Insertion	127
	8.7.2 Drain Removal	130
8.8	Surgical Approaches to the Thorax	130
	8.8.1 Anterolateral Thoracotomy	131
	8.8.1.1 Technique	132
	8.8.1.2 Closure	132
	8.8.2 Median Sternotomy	132
	8.8.2.1 Technique	132
	8.8.2.2 Closure	133
	8.8.3 The 'Clamshell' Thoracotomy	133
	8.8.4 Posterolateral Thoracotomy	133
	8.8.5 'Trapdoor' Thoracotomy	133
8.9	Emergency Department Thoracotomy	134
	8.9.1 History	134
	8.9.2 Objectives	134
	8.9.3 Indications and Contraindications	134
	8.9.4 Results	137
	8.9.5 When to Stop an Emergency Department Thoracotomy	137
	8.9.6 Technique	137
	8.9.6.1 Instrument Requirements	137
	8.9.6.2 Approach	137
8.10	Surgical Procedures	138
	8.10.1 Pericardial Tamponade	138
	8.10.2 Cardiac Injury	138
	8.10.3 Pulmonary Haemorrhage	139
	8.10.4 Pulmonary Tractotomy	139
	8.10.5 Lobectomy or Pneumonectomy	139
	8.10.6 Thoracotomy with Aortic Cross-Clamping	139
	8.10.7 Aortic Injury	140
	8.10.8 Tracheobronchial Injury	140
	8.10.9 Oesophageal Injury	140
8.11	Summary	140
8.12	Anaesthesia for Thoracic Trauma	140
	8.12.1 Penetrating Thoracic Injury	140
	8.12.2 Blunt Thoracic Injury	141
	8.12.2.1 Contained Large Vessel Rupture or Aneurysm	141
	8.12.2.2 Pulmonary Contusion	141
	8.12.2.3 Large Airway Disruption	141
	8.12.2.4 Flail Chest	141
	8.12.2.5 Diaphragmatic Injury	142
	8.12.3 Anaesthetic Management of Thoracic Injury	142
9	**Abdomen**	**147**
9.1	The Trauma Laparotomy	147
	9.1.1 Overview	147
	9.1.1.1 Difficult Abdominal Injury Complexes	148
	9.1.1.2 The Retroperitoneum	148
	9.1.1.3 Non-Operative Management OP Penetrating Abdominal Injury	148

9.1.2	The Trauma Laparotomy		149
	9.1.2.1	Preoperative Adjuncts	150
	9.1.2.2	Draping	151
	9.1.2.3	Incision	151
	9.1.2.4	Initial Procedure	152
	9.1.2.5	Perform the Trauma Laparotomy	153
	9.1.2.6	Perform Definitive Packing	155
	9.1.2.7	Specific Routes of Access	155
	9.1.2.8	Specific Organ Techniques	158
9.1.3	Closure of the Abdomen		158
	9.1.3.1	Principles of Abdominal Closure	158
	9.1.3.2	Choosing the Optimal Method of Closure	158
9.1.4	Temporary Closure		159
9.1.5	The Open Abdomen		159
9.1.6	Primary Closure		160
9.1.7	Specific Tips and Tricks		160
	9.1.7.1	Headlight	160
	9.1.7.2	Stirrups and Lithotomy Position	160
	9.1.7.3	Table Tilt	160
	9.1.7.4	Be Flexible – Move!	161
	9.1.7.5	Pericardial Window	161
	9.1.7.6	Washout	161
	9.1.7.7	Drains	161
	9.1.7.8	Stomas	161
9.1.8	Two Catheters: Bladder Injury		162
9.1.9	Early Tracheostomy		162
9.1.10	Briefing for Operating Room Scrub Nurses		163
9.1.11	Summary		163
9.2	Abdominal Vascular Injury		165
9.2.1	Overview		165
9.2.2	Retroperitoneal Haematoma		166
	9.2.2.1	Central Haematoma	166
	9.2.2.2	Lateral Haematoma	166
	9.2.2.3	Pelvic Haematoma	166
9.2.3	Surgical Approach to Major Abdominal Vessels		167
	9.2.3.1	Incision	167
	9.2.3.2	Medial Visceral Rotations	167
	9.2.3.3	Aorta	168
	9.2.3.4	Coeliac Axis	168
	9.2.3.5	Superior Mesenteric Artery	168
	9.2.3.6	Inferior Mesenteric Artery	169
	9.2.3.7	Renal Arteries	169
	9.2.3.8	Iliac Vessels	169
	9.2.3.9	Inferior Vena Cava (IVC)	169
	9.2.3.10	Portal Vein	171
9.2.4	Shunting		171
9.3	Bowel, Rectum, and Diaphragm		172
9.3.1	Overview		172
9.3.2	Diaphragm		173
9.3.3	Stomach		175

9.3.4	The Duodenum		175
9.3.5	Small Bowel		175
	9.3.5.1	The Stable Patient	175
	9.3.5.2	The Unstable Patient	176
9.3.6	Large Bowel		176
	9.3.6.1	The Stable Patient	176
	9.3.6.2	The Unstable Patient	177
9.3.7	Rectum		177
9.3.8	Mesentery		177
9.3.9	Adjuncts		177
	9.3.9.1	Antibiotics	177
9.4	The Duodenum		179
9.4.1	Overview		179
9.4.2	Mechanism of Injury		179
	9.4.2.1	Penetrating Trauma	179
	9.4.2.2	Blunt Trauma	179
	9.4.2.3	Paediatric Considerations	179
9.4.3	Diagnosis		179
	9.4.3.1	Clinical Presentation	179
	9.4.3.2	Serum Amylase and Serum Lipase	180
	9.4.3.3	Diagnostic Peritoneal Lavage/Ultrasound	180
	9.4.3.4	Radiological Investigation	180
	9.4.3.5	Diagnostic Laparoscopy	180
9.4.4	Duodenal Injury Scale		180
9.4.5	Management		180
9.4.6	Surgical Approach		181
	9.4.6.1	Intramural Haematoma	181
	9.4.6.2	Duodenal Laceration	183
	9.4.6.3	Repair of the Perforation	183
	9.4.6.4	Complete Transection of the Duodenum	183
	9.4.6.5	Duodenal Diversion	184
	9.4.6.6	Duodenal Diverticulation	184
	9.4.6.7	Pyloric Exclusion	184
	9.4.6.8	Pancreaticoduodenectomy (Whipple's Procedure)	184
9.5	The Liver and Biliary System		185
9.5.1	Overview		185
9.5.2	Resuscitation		187
9.5.3	Diagnosis		188
9.5.4	Liver Injury Scale		188
9.5.5	Management		190
	9.5.5.1	Non-Operative Management (NOM)	190
	9.5.5.2	Subcapsular Haematoma	193
	9.5.5.3	Operative (Surgical) Management	193
9.5.6	Surgical Approach		193
	9.5.6.1	Incision	194
	9.5.6.2	Initial Actions	195
	9.5.6.3	Techniques for Temporary Control of Haemorrhage	195
	9.5.6.4	Mobilization of the Liver	199
	9.5.6.5	Hepatic Isolation	199

	9.5.7	Perihepatic Drainage	200
	9.5.8	Complications	200
	9.5.9	Injury to the Retrohepatic Vena Cava	201
	9.5.10	Injury to the Porta Hepatis	201
	9.5.11	Removal of Packs (Aim for 36–49 Hours)	202
	9.5.12	Injury to the Bile Ducts and Gallbladder	202
9.6	Pancreas		204
	9.6.1	Overview	204
	9.6.2	Anatomy	204
	9.6.3	Mechanisms of Injury	205
		9.6.3.1 Blunt Trauma	205
		9.6.3.2 Penetrating Trauma	205
	9.6.4	Diagnosis	205
		9.6.4.1 Clinical Evaluation	205
		9.6.4.2 Serum Amylase and Serum Lipase	205
		9.6.4.3 Ultrasound	205
		9.6.4.4 Diagnostic Peritoneal Lavage (DPL)	205
		9.6.4.5 Computed Tomography (CT)	205
		9.6.4.6 Endoscopic Retrograde Cholangiopancreatography (ERCP)	206
		9.6.4.7 Magnetic Resonance Cholangiopancreatography (MRCP)	206
		9.6.4.8 Intraoperative Pancreatography	206
		9.6.4.9 Operative Evaluation	206
	9.6.5	Pancreas Injury Scale	207
	9.6.6	Management	207
		9.6.6.1 Non-Operative Management	207
		9.6.6.2 Operative Management	207
	9.6.7	Surgical Approach	208
		9.6.7.1 Incision and Exploration	208
		9.6.7.2 Pancreatic Injury: Surgical Decision-Making	208
	9.6.8	Adjuncts	211
		9.6.8.1 Somatostatin and its Analogues	211
		9.6.8.2 Nutritional Support	211
	9.6.9	Pancreatic Injury in Children	211
	9.6.10	Complications	211
		9.6.10.1 Early Complications	212
		9.6.10.2 Late Complications	212
	9.6.11	Summary of Evidence-Based Guidelines	212
9.7	Spleen		215
	9.7.1	Overview	215
	9.7.2	Anatomy	216
	9.7.3	Diagnosis	216
		9.7.3.1 Clinical	216
		9.7.3.2 Ultrasound	216
		9.7.3.3 Computed Tomography (CT) Scan	216
	9.7.4	Splenic Injury Scale	216
	9.7.5	Management	218
		9.7.5.1 Non-Operative Management (NOM)	218
		9.7.5.2 Operative Management	218
	9.7.6	Surgical Approach	219
		9.7.6.1 Spleen Not Actively Bleeding	220

		9.7.6.2	Splenic Surface Bleed Only	220
		9.7.6.3	Minor Lacerations	220
		9.7.6.4	Mesh Splenorrhaphy and Partial Splenectomy	220
		9.7.6.5	Splenectomy	220
		9.7.6.6	Drainage	221
	9.7.7	Perioperative Considerations		221
		9.7.7.1	Haemostatic Resuscitation	221
		9.7.7.2	Repeat Imaging	221
		9.7.7.3	Mobilization	221
		9.7.7.4	Return to Normal Activities	221
		9.7.7.5	Venous Thromboembolism (VTE) Prophylaxis	221
	9.7.8	Outcomes		221
	9.7.9	Vaccination and Prevention of OPSI		222
9.8	The Urogenital System			223
	9.8.1	Overview		223
	9.8.2	Renal Injuries		223
		9.8.2.1	Diagnosis	224
		9.8.2.2	Renal Injury Scale	224
		9.8.2.3	Management	224
		9.8.2.4	Surgical Approach	230
		9.8.2.5	Adjuncts	232
		9.8.2.6	Postoperative Care	232
	9.8.3	Ureteric Injuries		233
		9.8.3.1	Diagnosis	233
		9.8.3.2	Surgical Approach	233
		9.8.3.3	Complications	234
	9.8.4	Bladder Injuries		234
		9.8.4.1	Diagnosis	234
		9.8.4.2	Management	234
		9.8.4.3	Surgical Approach	234
	9.8.5	Urethral Injuries		235
		9.8.5.1	Diagnosis	235
		9.8.5.2	Management	235
		9.8.5.3	Ruptured Urethra	235
	9.8.6	Injury to the Scrotum		236
		9.8.6.1	Diagnosis	236
		9.8.6.2	Management	236
	9.8.7	Gynaecological Injury and Sexual Assault		236
		9.8.7.1	Management	236
		9.8.7.2	Guideline	236
	9.8.8	Injury of the Pregnant Uterus		236
10	**The Pelvis**			**238**
10.1	Anatomy			238
10.2	Classification			239
	10.2.1	Tile's Classification		239
		10.2.1.1	Type A: Completely Stable	239
		10.2.1.2	Type B: Vertically Stable but Rotationally Unstable	239
		10.2.1.3	Type C: Wholly Unstable in Rotational and Vertical Planes	239
		10.2.1.4	A Jumper's Fracture	241

	10.2.1.5 Acetabular Fractures	241
	10.2.1.6 Fracture Combinations	241
10.2.2	Young and Burgess Classification	241
	10.2.2.1 Anteroposterior Compression (APC) (Types 1, 2, and 3)	243
	10.2.2.2 Lateral Compression (LC) (Types 1, 2, and 3)	243
	10.2.2.3 Vertical Shear (VS)	243
	10.2.2.4 Combined Mechanism (CM)	243
10.3	Clinical Examination and Diagnosis	243
10.4	Resuscitation	244
10.4.1	Haemodynamically Normal Patients	244
10.4.2	Haemodynamically Stable Patients (Transient Responders)	244
10.4.3	Haemodynamically Unstable Patients (Non-Responders)	244
10.5	External Fixation	246
10.5.1	Iliac-Crest Route	246
10.5.2	Supra-Acetabular Route	246
10.5.3	Pelvic C-Clamp	246
10.6	Laparotomy	246
10.7	Extraperitoneal Pelvic (EPP) Packing	247
10.7.1	Technique of Extraperitoneal Packing	247
10.8	Associated Injuries	250
10.8.1	Head Injuries	250
10.8.2	Intra-abdominal Injuries	250
10.8.3	Bladder and Urethral Injuries	250
10.8.4	Urethral Injuries	250
10.8.5	Anorectal Injuries	250
10.8.6	Vaginal Injuries	251
10.9	Open Pelvic Fractures	251
10.9.1	Diagnosis	251
10.9.2	Surgery	251
10.10	Summary	251
11	**Extremity Trauma**	**254**
11.1	Overview	254
11.2	Management of Severe Injury to the Extremity	254
11.2.1	Life-Saving	254
11.2.2	Limb-Saving	254
11.3	Management of Vascular Injury of the Extremity	255
11.3.1	Shunts	256
11.3.2	Chemical Vascular Injuries	258
11.4	Crush Syndrome	258
11.5	Management of Open Fractures	258
11.5.1	Severity of Injury (Gustilo Classification)	258
11.5.2	Sepsis and Antibiotics	259
11.5.3	Venous Thromboembolism	259
11.5.4	Timing of Skeletal Fixation in Polytrauma Patients	259
	11.5.4.1 Respiratory Insufficiency	259
	11.5.4.2 Head Injury	259
11.6	Life-Threatening Limb Trauma: Life Versus Limb	260
11.6.1	Scoring Systems	260
	11.6.1.1 Mangled Extremity Syndrome Index (MESI)	260

	11.6.1.2	Predictive Salvage Index System	261
	11.6.1.3	Mangled Extremity Severity Score (MESS)	261
	11.6.1.4	Nisssa Scoring System	261
11.7	Compartment Syndrome		262
11.8	Fasciotomy		263
	11.8.1	Lower Leg Fasciotomy	264
	11.8.1.1	Two-Incision, Four-Compartment Fasciotomy	264
	11.8.1.2	Single-Incision Fasciotomy	265
	11.8.1.3	Fibulectomy	265
	11.8.1.4	Subcutaneous Fasciotomy	266
	11.8.2	Upper Leg	266
	11.8.3	Upper and Lower Arm	266
11.9	Complications of Major Limb Injury		267
11.10	Summary		267

12	**Head Trauma**		**270**
12.1	Introduction		270
12.2	Injury Patterns and Classification		270
	12.2.1	Severity	270
	12.2.2	Pathological Classification of TBI	270
	12.2.2.1	Blunt Head Trauma	271
	12.2.2.2	Penetrating Head Trauma	271
	12.2.2.3	Blunt Cerebrovascular Injury (BCVI)	271
12.3	Physiological Parameters in TBI		272
	12.3.1	Mean Arterial Pressure (MAP)	272
	12.3.2	Intracranial Pressure	272
	12.3.3	Cerebral Perfusion Pressure	274
	12.3.4	Cerebral Blood Flow	274
12.4	Pathophysiology of TBI		274
12.5	Management of TBI		274
12.6	CPP Threshold		274
12.7	ICP Monitoring		275
	12.7.1	ICP Monitoring Devices	275
	12.7.1.1	CSF Drainage	275
	12.7.2	ICP Management: Do's and Don't's	275
	12.7.2.1	Hyperventilation	275
	12.7.2.2	Osmotherapy (Mannitol and Hypertonic Saline)	275
	12.7.2.3	Barbiturates and Propofol	275
	12.7.2.4	Steroids	276
12.8	Imaging		276
12.9	Indications for Surgery		276
	12.9.1	Burr Holes and Emergency Craniotomy	276
	12.9.1.1	Emergency Burr Hole Craniotomy	276
	12.9.1.2	Emergency Craniotomy	278
12.10	Adjuncts to Care		278
	12.10.1	Infection Prophylaxis	278
	12.10.2	Seizure Prophylaxis	278
	12.10.3	Nutrition	279
	12.10.4	Deep Vein Thrombosis (DVT) Prophylaxis	279
	12.10.5	Steroids	279

12.11 Paediatric Considerations   279
12.12 Pearls and Pitfalls   279
12.13 Summary   279

13   Burns   282
13.1   Overview   282
13.2   Burns Pathophysiology   282
13.3   Anatomy   283
13.4   Special Types of Burn   284
       13.4.1   Chemical Burns   284
       13.4.2   Electrical Injury   285
13.5   Depth of the Burn   286
       13.5.1   Superficial Burn (Erythema)   286
       13.5.2   Superficial Partial Thickness   286
       13.5.3   Deep Partial Thickness   286
       13.5.4   'Indeterminate' Partial-Thickness Burns   287
       13.5.5   Full Thickness   287
13.6   Total Body Surface Area Burned (TBSA)   287
13.7   Management   288
       13.7.1   Safe Retrieval   288
       13.7.2   First Aid   288
       13.7.3   Initial Management   288
                13.7.3.1   Airway   288
                13.7.3.2   Inhalational Toxicity   288
                13.7.3.3   Analgesia   289
                13.7.3.4   Intravenous Access   289
                13.7.3.5   Emergency Management of the Burn Wound   289
                13.7.3.6   Fluid Resuscitation   289
                13.7.3.7   Associated Injuries   290
       13.7.4   Escharotomy and Fasciotomy   290
       13.7.5   Definitive Management   291
                13.7.5.1   'Closing' the Burn Wound   291
                13.7.5.2   Technique of Excision and Split-Skin
                           Grafting (SSG)   292
                13.7.5.3   Tumescent Technique   292
                13.7.5.4   Wound Coverage   292
                13.7.5.5   Burn Wound Excision and Closure   295
       13.7.6   Assessing and Managing Airway Burns   296
                13.7.6.1   Upper Airway   296
                13.7.6.2   Lower Airway   296
       13.7.7   Tracheostomy   296
13.8   Special Areas   296
       13.8.1   Face   296
       13.8.2   Hands   296
       13.8.3   Perineum   297
       13.8.4   Feet   297
13.9   Adjuncts in Burn Care   297
       13.9.1   Nutrition in the Burned Patient   297
                13.9.1.1   Paediatric Burn Nutrition   298

	13.9.2	Ulcer Prophylaxis	298
	13.9.3	Venous Thromboembolism Prophylaxis	298
	13.9.4	Vitamin C	298
	13.9.5	Anabolic Steroids	298
	13.9.6	Antibiotics	298
	13.9.7	Other Adjuncts	299
13.10	Palliative Care for Burns		299
13.11	Summary		299

14   Special Patient Situations   301

14.1	Paediatric Trauma		301
	14.1.1	Introduction	301
	14.1.2	Injury Patterns	301
	14.1.3	Pre-Hospital	302
	14.1.4	Resuscitation Room	302
		14.1.4.1 Airway	302
		14.1.4.2 Breathing	303
		14.1.4.3 Circulation	303
		14.1.4.4 Disability	303
		14.1.4.5 Cardiac Arrest	304
	14.1.5	Specific Organ Injury	304
		14.1.5.1 Head Injury	304
		14.1.5.2 Thoracic Injury	307
		14.1.5.3 Abdominal Injury	307
		14.1.5.4 Genitourinary Injury	308
		14.1.5.5 Pelvic Injury	308
		14.1.5.6 Spine Injury	308
		14.1.5.7 Suspected Non-Accidental Injury (NAI)	308
	14.1.6	Analgesia	308
	14.1.7	Anaesthesiology in Children	310
14.2	Trauma in the Elderly		310
	14.2.1	Definition of 'Older' and Susceptibility to Trauma	310
	14.2.2	Access to Trauma Care	310
	14.2.3	Physiology	310
		14.2.3.1 Respiratory System	311
		14.2.3.2 Cardiovascular System	311
		14.2.3.3 Nervous System	311
		14.2.3.4 Renal	311
		14.2.3.5 Musculoskeletal	311
		14.2.3.6 Influence of Comorbid Conditions	311
	14.2.4	Multiple Medications: Polypharmacy	311
	14.2.5	Analgesia	312
	14.2.6	Anticoagulants	312
	14.2.7	Decision to Operate	312
	14.2.8	Outcome	312
	14.2.9	Anaesthetic Considerations in the Elderly	313
14.3	Trauma in Pregnancy		313
	14.3.1	Evaluation	314
14.4	Non-Beneficial (Futile) Care		314

Part 4   MODERN THERAPEUTIC AND DIAGNOSTIC TECHNOLOGY   **319**

15   **Minimal Access Surgery in Trauma**   **321**
        15.1   Laparoscopy   321
                15.1.1   Screening/Diagnostic Laparoscopy   321
                        15.1.1.1   Blunt Trauma   321
                        15.1.1.2   Penetrating Trauma – Stab Wounds   321
                        15.1.1.3   Penetrating Trauma – Gunshot Wounds   321
                15.1.2   Diagnostic Laparoscopy   321
                15.1.3   Non-Therapeutic Laparoscopy   322
                15.1.4   Therapeutic Laparoscopy   322
                15.1.5   Technique   322
                15.1.6   Risks   322
                15.1.7   Applications   323
                        15.1.7.1   Bowel Injury   323
                        15.1.7.2   Splenic Injury   323
                        15.1.7.3   Liver Injury   323
                        15.1.7.4   Diaphragmatic Injury   323
                        15.1.7.5   Bladder Injury   324
        15.2   Video-Assisted Thoracoscopic Surgery   324
                15.2.1   Technique   324
                15.2.2   Applications   324
                15.2.3   Summary   324
        15.3   Resuscitative Endovascular Balloon Occlusion of the Aorta (Reboa)   324
                15.3.1   Anatomy   325
                15.3.2   Physiology   326
                15.3.3   Insertion Technique   326
                15.3.4   Monitoring   328
                15.3.5   Total, Partial, and Intermittent Occlusion, and Targeted Blood Pressure   328
                15.3.6   Perioperative and Postoperative Care   328
                15.3.7   Indications   328
                15.3.8   Contraindications   329
                15.3.9   Complications   329
                15.3.10 Summary   329

16   **Imaging in Trauma**   **334**
        16.1   Radiation Doses and Protection from Radiation   334
        16.2   Principles of Trauma Imaging   335
                16.2.1   Extended Focused Assessment by Sonography for Trauma (eFAST)   336
                16.2.2   Indications and Results   337
                        16.2.2.1   Penetrating Thoracic Trauma   337
                        16.2.2.2   Blunt Thoracic Trauma   337
                        16.2.2.3   Penetrating Abdominal Trauma   337
                        16.2.2.4   Blunt Abdominal Trauma   337
                        16.2.2.5   Pelvic Trauma   337
                16.2.3   Other Applications of Ultrasound in Trauma   337
                16.2.4   Training   338
        16.3   Pitfalls and Pearls   338
        16.4   Low-Dose X-Ray (Lodox®)   338

16.5	CT in Trauma	339
	16.5.1 Pan CT	339
	16.5.2 CT Angiography	339
	16.5.3 CT in Specific Body Regions	339
	16.5.3.1 CT of the Neck	339
	16.5.3.2 CT of the Chest	339
	16.5.3.3 CT of the Abdomen	341
	16.5.3.4 CT Angiography of the Limbs	342
16.6	Catheter-Directed Angiography (CDA)	343
	16.6.1 Diagnostic	343
	16.6.2 Therapeutic	343
16.7	Retained Weapons	343
16.8	Summary	343

Part 5 SPECIALIZED ASPECTS OF TOTAL TRAUMA CARE   **345**

17	**Critical Care of the Trauma Patient 2024**	**347**
17.1	Introduction	347
17.2	Phases of ICU Care	347
	17.2.1 Resuscitative Phase (First 24 Hours Post-Injury)	347
	17.2.1.1 'Traditional' Endpoints of Resuscitation	347
	17.2.1.2 Post-Traumatic Acute Lung Injury	348
	17.2.1.3 Respiratory Assessment and Monitoring	348
	17.2.1.4 Mechanical Ventilation (MV)	348
	17.2.1.5 Ventilatory Mode (Actual Mode Is Unimportant)	349
	17.2.2 Early Life Support Phase (24–72 Hours Post-Injury)	349
	17.2.2.1 Priorities	349
	17.2.3 Prolonged Life Support (> 72 Hours Post-Injury)	349
	17.2.3.1 Respiratory Failure	349
	17.2.3.2 Infectious Complications	350
	17.2.3.3 Non-Infectious Causes of Fever	350
	17.2.3.4 Percutaneous Tracheostomy	350
	17.2.3.5 Weaning From Ventilatory Support	350
	17.2.3.6 Extubation Criteria ('SOA2P')	350
	17.2.4 Recovery Phase (Transition from the ICU)	350
17.3	Extracorporeal Membrane Oxygenation (ECMO)	351
	17.3.1 Overview	351
	17.3.2 Modes of ECMO	351
	17.3.2.1 Veno-Venous ECMO (VV-ECMO)	351
	17.3.2.2 Veno-Arterial ECMO (VA-ECMO)	352
	17.3.2.3 Arteriovenous ECMO (AV-ECMO), More Commonly Termed Extracorporeal Carbon Dioxide Removal (ECCO2R)	352
	17.3.3 ECMO Exclusion Criteria	352
17.4	Coagulopathy of Major Trauma	353
	17.4.1 Management	353
17.5	Hypothermia	354
17.6	Multisystem Organ Dysfunction Syndrome	355
17.7	Systemic Inflammatory Response Syndrome (SIRS)	355

17.8 Sepsis 355
  17.8.1 Definitions 355
    17.8.1.1 Sepsis 356
    17.8.1.2 Septic Shock 356
  17.8.2 'Surviving Sepsis' Guidelines 357
17.9 Antibiotics 370
  17.9.1 Criteria 371
17.10 Abdominal Compartment Syndrome (ACS) 372
  17.10.1 Introduction 372
  17.10.2 Definition 372
  17.10.3 Pathophysiology 372
  17.10.4 Effect of Raised IAP on Individual Organ Function 372
    17.10.4.1 Cardiovascular 372
    17.10.4.2 Respiratory 374
    17.10.4.3 Visceral Perfusion 374
    17.10.4.4 Renal 374
    17.10.4.5 Intracranial Pressure 374
  17.10.5 Measurement of IAP 374
    17.10.5.1 Measurement of Abdominal Perfusion Pressure (APP) 374
  17.10.6 Management 375
    17.10.6.1 Prevention 375
    17.10.6.2 Treatment 375
    17.10.6.3 Reversible Factors 375
  17.10.7 Surgery for Raised IAP 375
    17.10.7.1 Tips for Surgical Decompression for Raised IAP 375
  17.10.8 Management Algorithm 375
17.11 Acute Kidney Injury 378
17.12 Rhabdomyolysis 378
17.13 Metabolic Disturbances 379
17.14 Nutritional Support 380
  17.14.1 Access for Enteral Nutrition 381
    17.14.1.1 Simple 381
    17.14.1.2 More Complicated, Longer Term 381
  17.14.2 Monitoring Nutritional Support 381
17.15 Prophylaxis in the ICU 381
  17.15.1 Stress Ulceration 381
  17.15.2 Deep Venous Thrombosis and Pulmonary Embolus 382
  17.15.3 Tetanus Prophylaxis 383
  17.15.4 Line Sepsis 383
17.16 Pain and Delirium Control 383
  17.16.1 Pain Control 383
  17.16.2 Delirium 384
17.17 ICU Tertiary Survey 384
  17.17.1 Evaluation for Occult Injuries 384
  17.17.2 Assess Comorbid Conditions 384
  17.17.3 ICU Summary 384
17.18 Family Contact and Support 384

18 Trauma Anaesthesia **389**
18.1 Introduction 389
18.2 Planning and Communicating 389

18.3   Damage Control Resuscitation (DCR)   390
    18.3.1   Limited Fluid Administration   390
    18.3.2   Targeting Coagulopathy   391
    18.3.3   Prevent and Treat Hypothermia   392
18.4   Damage Control Surgery   392
    18.4.1   Anaesthetic Procedures   392
        18.4.1.1   Airway   392
        18.4.1.2   Breathing   393
        18.4.1.3   Circulation   394
        18.4.1.4   Vascular Access   394
    18.4.2   Monitoring   395
18.5   Anaesthesia Induction in Hypovolaemic Shock   395
    18.5.1   Introduction   395
    18.5.2   Drugs for Anaesthesia Induction   396
        18.5.2.1   Ketamine   397
        18.5.2.2   Propofol   397
        18.5.2.3   Etomidate   397
        18.5.2.4   Thiopental   398
        18.5.2.5   Midazolam   398
18.6   Battlefield Anaesthesia   398
    18.6.1   Damage Control Anaesthesia in the Military Setting   399
    18.6.2   Battlefield Analgesia   399

19   Austere Environments   401
19.1   Definition   401
19.2   Overview   401
19.3   Infrastructure and Team Composition   402
    19.3.1   Location   402
    19.3.2   Hospital Structures   402
        19.3.2.1   Water Supply   402
        19.3.2.2   Energy   402
        19.3.2.3   Waste Disposal   402
        19.3.2.4   Sterilization Department   402
        19.3.2.5   Surgical Equipment   402
        19.3.2.6   Blood Bank   403
    19.3.3   Health Protection of the Deployed Surgical Team   403
        19.3.3.1   Vector-Borne Disease   403
        19.3.3.2   Enteric Illness   403
        19.3.3.3   Road Trauma   403
        19.3.3.4   Physical, Sexual, and Mental Health   403
19.4   Caseload and Surgical Techniques to Have in Mind   403
    19.4.1   Caseload   403
    19.4.2   Bleeding Control   404
    19.4.3   Control of Contamination   404
    19.4.4   Treatment of Wounds   404
        19.4.4.1   Delayed/Neglected Wounds   404
        19.4.4.2   War Wounds   404
    19.4.5   Amputations   404
    19.4.6   Stabilization of Fractures   404
    19.4.7   Obstetrics   404
    19.4.8   Anaesthesia   405

19.5   Postoperative Care and Documentation   405
19.6   Summary   405

20   Military Environments   **408**
20.1   Introduction   408
20.2   Injury Patterns   409
20.3   Military Trauma Systems   411
         20.3.1   The Echelons of Medical Care   411
                    20.3.1.1   Role 1   411
                    20.3.1.2   Role 2   411
                    20.3.1.3   Role 3   411
                    20.3.1.4   Role 4   412
         20.3.2   Incident Management and Multiple Casualties   412
                    20.3.2.1   Confirm   412
                    20.3.2.2   Clear   412
                    20.3.2.3   Cordon   412
                    20.3.2.4   Control   412
         20.3.3   Incident Command and Control   412
                    20.3.3.1   Safety   413
                    20.3.3.2   Communication   413
                    20.3.3.3   Assessment   413
                    20.3.3.4   Triage   413
                    20.3.3.5   Treatment   414
                    20.3.3.6   Transport   414
20.4   Triage   414
         20.4.1   Source and Aim of Triage   414
         20.4.2   Forward Surgical Teams and Triage   415
         20.4.3   Forward Surgical Team Decision-Making   415
         20.4.4   Selection of Patients for Surgery   416
20.5   Mass Casualties   416
20.6   Evacuation   417
20.7   Resuscitation   417
         20.7.1   Overview   417
         20.7.2   Damage Control Resuscitation (DCR)   419
         20.7.3   Damage Control Surgery (DCS) in the
                    Military Setting   419
20.8   Battlefield Analgesia   420
20.9   Battlefield Anaesthesia   420
         20.9.1   Induction of Anaesthesia   421
         20.9.2   Maintenance of Anaesthesia   422
20.10 Critical Care   422
20.11 Translating Military Experience to Civilian Trauma Care   422
         20.11.1 Leadership   422
         20.11.2 Front-End Processes   422
         20.11.3 Common Training   423
         20.11.4 Governance   423
         20.11.5 Rehabilitation Services   423
         20.11.6 Translational Research   423
20.12 Summary   423

21   Ballistics and Blast Injuries   **426**

21.1   Definition   426

21.2   The Science   426

    21.2.1   Kinetic Energy   426

    21.2.2   Wounding Energy   427

21.3   Bullets   427

    21.3.1   Internal Ballistics   427

    21.3.2   External Ballistics   428

    21.3.3   Terminal Ballistics   428

    21.3.4   Wound Ballistics   428

        21.3.4.1   Pistol/Low-Energy Bullets   428

        21.3.4.2   Rifle/High-Energy Bullets   430

    21.3.5   Antibiotics   430

        21.3.5.1   Bacterial Contamination – General: Gram-Negative Cover   430

        21.3.5.2   Bacterial Contamination – Abdominal Cavity   431

        21.3.5.3   Tetanus Toxoid If Not Previously Received   431

    21.3.6   General Treatment Principles   431

21.4   Shotgun Injuries   431

21.5   Blast Injury   433

    21.5.1   Primary Blast Injury   433

    21.5.2   Secondary Blast Injury   434

    21.5.3   Tertiary Blast Injury   434

    21.5.4   Quaternary Blast Injury   434

    21.5.5   Quinary Blast Injury   434

    21.5.6   Diagnosis and Management of Blast Injuries   434

        21.5.6.1   Rupture of the Tympanic Membrane   434

        21.5.6.2   Blast Lung Injury (BLI)   435

        21.5.6.3   Intra-abdominal Injuries   435

        21.5.6.4   Other Injuries   436

        21.5.6.5   Extremity Injuries   436

        21.5.6.6   White Phosphorus   437

    21.5.7   Summary   437

22   Psychology of Trauma   **439**

22.1   Definition   439

22.2   Reactions to Trauma   439

    22.2.1   Biological: The Physiological Impact   439

    22.2.2   Psychological: The Mental, Emotional, and Behavioural
             Impact   440

    22.2.3   Social   440

22.3   Post-Traumatic Stress Disorder   441

22.4   Trauma and the Intensive Care Unit (ICU)   442

22.5   The Clinical Psychologist   442

    22.5.1   The Role of the Clinical Psychologist in Trauma   442

        22.5.1.1   For the Patient   442

        22.5.1.2   For the Support System   443

        22.5.1.3   For the Team   443

22.6   When to Call the Clinical Psychologist   443

22.7   Summary   444

23	**Physical and Rehabilitation Medicine (P&RM)**	**445**
	23.1 Definition	445
	23.2 The Rehabilitation 'Team'	445
	23.3 Rehabilitation Starts in the ICU	445
	23.4 Outcomes-Based Rehabilitation (OBR)	446
	23.4.1 FIM/FAM Assessment	446
	23.4.2 Glasgow Outcome Scale	446
	23.4.3 Rancho Los Amigos Scale	448
	23.4.4 International Classification of Functioning, Disability and Health (ICF)	448
	23.5 World Health Organisation Initiatives	448
	23.5.1 World Rehabilitation Alliance	448
	23.5.2 Rehabilitation 2030	448
	23.6 Summary	449
Appendix A	**Trauma Systems**	**451**
	A.1 Introduction	451
	A.2 The Inclusive Trauma System	451
	A.3 Components of an Inclusive Trauma System	451
	A.3.1 Administration	452
	A.3.2 Prevention	452
	A.3.3 Public Education	453
	A.3.4 The Healthcare System	453
	A.4 Management of the Injured Patient Within a System	453
	A.5 Steps in Organizing a System	453
	A.5.1 Public Support	453
	A.5.2 Legal Authority	453
	A.5.3 Establish Criteria for Optimal Care	454
	A.5.4 Designation of Trauma Centres	454
	A.5.5 System Evaluation	454
	A.6 Results and Studies	454
	A.6.1 Panel Review	454
	A.6.2 Registry Study	454
	A.6.3 Population-Based Studies	454
	A.7 Summary	455
Appendix B	**Trauma Scores and Scoring Systems**	**457**
	B.1 Introduction	457
	B.2 Physiological Scoring Systems	457
	B.2.1 Glasgow Coma Scale (GCS)	457
	B.2.2 Paediatric Trauma Score (PTS)	457
	B.2.3 Revised Trauma Score (RTS)	457
	B.2.4 Acute Physiologic and Chronic Health Evaluation II (APACHE II)	458
	B.3 Anatomical Scoring Systems	458
	B.3.1 Abbreviated Injury Scale (AIS)	458
	B.3.2 The Injury Severity Score (ISS)	460
	B.3.3 The New Injury Severity Score (NISS)	460
	B.3.4 Anatomic Profile Score (APS)	460
	B.3.5 ICD-Based Injury Severity Score (ICISS)	461
	B.3.6 Organ Injury Scaling System	461

	B.3.7	Penetrating Abdominal Trauma Index (PATI)	461
	B.3.8	Revised Injury Severity Classification (RISC) II	461
B.4	Comorbidity Scoring Systems		462
B.5	Outcome Analysis		462
	B.5.1	Functional Independence Measure (FIM) and Functional Assessment Measure (FAM) (FIM + FAM)	462
	B.5.2	Glasgow Outcome Scale (GOS)	463
	B.5.3	Major Trauma Outcome Study (MTOS)	464
	B.5.4	A Severity Characterization Of Trauma (ASCOT)	465
B.6	Comparison of Trauma Scoring Systems		465
B.7	Scaling System for Organ-Specific Injuries		470
B.8	Summary		485

Appendix C   Trauma Guidelines   **487**
C.1	Eastern Association for the Surgery of Trauma (East)		487
	C.1.1	Archived Guidelines	487
	C.1.2	Current Guidelines: Trauma	488
	C.1.3	Current Guidelines: Critical Care	489
	C.1.4	Injury Prevention	489
C.2	Western Trauma Association (WTA) Algorithms		490
	C.2.1	Additional Algorithms	492
C.3	Surgical Critical Care.Net		492
C.4	American College of Surgeons (ACS)		494
C.5	American Association for the Surgery of Trauma (AAST)		494
C.6	Brain Trauma Foundation Guidelines		495
C.7	European Society of Trauma and Emergency Surgery (ESTES)		495
C.8	World Society of Emergency Surgery (WSES) Guidelines		495

Appendix D   The Definitive Surgical Trauma Care Course: The Definitive Anaesthetic Trauma Care Course: Course Requirements and Syllabus   **497**
D.1	Background		497
D.2	Course Development and Testing		498
D.3	Course Details		498
	D.3.1	Ownership	498
	D.3.2	Mission Statement	498
	D.3.3	Application to Hold a Course	498
	D.3.4	Eligibility to Present	498
		D.3.4.1 Local Organizations	498
		D.3.4.2 National Organizations	498
	D.3.5	Course Materials and Overview	498
	D.3.6	Course Director	499
	D.3.7	Course Faculty	499
	D.3.8	Course Participants	499
	D.3.9	Practical Skill Stations	499
	D.3.10	Course Syllabus	499
	D.3.11	Course Certification	499
D.4	Iatsic Recognition		500
D.5	Course Information		500
	D.5.1	The DSTC Course	500
		D.5.1.1 Course Objectives	500

D.5.2	The DATC Course	500
D.5.2.1	Course Objectives	500
D.5.2.2	Description of the Course	500
D.5.1.3	Summary	501

Appendix E Definitive Surgical Trauma Care™ Course: Core Surgical Skills — **503**

E.1	The Neck	503
E.2	The Chest	503
E.3	The Abdominal Cavity	503
E.4	The Liver	504
E.5	The Spleen	504
E.6	The Pancreas	504
E.7	The Duodenum	504
E.8	The Genitourinary System	504
E.9	Abdominal Vascular Injuries	504
E.10	Peripheral Vascular Injuries	505
E.11	Insertion of Resuscitative Balloon Catheter (Reboa)	505
E.12	Insertion and Use of Vacuum Wound Dressing	505

Appendix F Briefing for Operating Room Scrub Nurses — **507**

F.1	Introduction	507
F.2	Preparing the Operating Room	507
F.2.1	Environment	507
F.2.2	Blood Loss	507
F.2.3	Instruments	508
F.2.4	Cleaning	508
F.2.5	Draping	508
F.2.6	Adjuncts	508
F.3	Surgical Procedure	509
F.3.1	Instruments	509
F.3.2	Special Instruments and Improvised Gadgets	510
F.4	Abdominal Closure	510
F.5	Instrument and Swab Count	511
F.6	Medicolegal Aspects and Communication Skills	511
F.7	Critical Incident Stress Issues	512
F.8	Conclusion	512

Index — **513**

Video Contents

For access to the videos listed below, please go to www.routledge.com/cw/boffard

- Access to the anterior mediastinum
- Access to the axilla
- Access to the neck
- Aorta
- Bleeding control
- Craniotomy
- Fasciotomy
- Heart
- Heart and lung
- Iliac shunting
- Kidney
- Laparotomy

- Liver
- Pancreas
- Pelvic packing
- Small bowel
- Spleen
- Sternotomy
- Stomach
- Thoracic
- Ureteric repair
- Excision and grafting of major burns
- Application of the vacuum dressing

Preface

He who desires to practice Surgery must go to war.
Corpus Hippocraticum
Hippocrates (460–377 BCE)

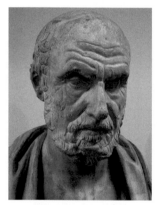

'Related to this is the surgery of wounds arising in military service, which concerns the extraction of missiles. In city practice experience of these is but little, for very rarely even in a whole lifetime are there civil or military combats. In fact such things occur most frequently and continuously in armies abroad. Thus, the person intending to practice this kind of surgery must serve in the army and accompany it on expeditions abroad; for in this way he would become experienced in this practice'.

Hippocrates – The Physician 14, as translated by Paul Potter
Loeb Classical Library, Hippocrates, *Volume VIII*

In years past, many surgeons honed their skills in war and translated them into the techniques required in peace. In the 21st century, this has changed, and most surgeons work in an environment of peace. In many countries, the incidence of injury, particularly from vehicle-related trauma, has fallen below the numbers recorded when records were first kept.

Many injuries are now treated non-operatively, so operative exposure and the skills required are reduced. For this reason, the decision *not* to operate may be based on inexperience or insecurity, rather than on good clinical judgement. Unless dealing with major trauma on a frequent basis, few surgeons, anaesthesiologists, intensive care specialists, or allied medical and nursing staff can attain, let alone sustain, the level of skill necessary for decision-making in the care of a patient with multiple injuries.

Good judgement comes from experience.
Experience comes from bad judgement.

Planning the response requires a clear understanding of:

- The causation including mechanism of injury.
- The initial, pre-hospital, and emergency department care of the patient.
- The physiological condition in which the patient is delivered to the hospital and subsequently to the operating theatre will be determined by the initial response, which itself may determine outcome.
- The resources, both physical and intellectual, within the hospital, and the ability to anticipate and identify the specific problems associated with patients with multiple injuries.
- The limitations in providing specialist expertise within the time frame required.

In 1993, five surgeons (Don Trunkey, and Howard Champion, United States; Stephen Deane, Australia; Abe Fingerhut, France; and David Mulder, Canada), all members of the International Society of Surgery – Société Internationale de Chirugie (ISS-SIC) and the International Association for Trauma Surgery and Intensive Care (IATSIC), met in San Francisco during the meeting of the American College of Surgeons. The experience that Sten Lennquist, from Sweden, had gained offering 5-day courses for surgeons in Sweden was integrated into the programme development, and prototype courses were offered in Paris, Washington, and Sydney. It was apparent that there was a specific need for further training in the technical aspects of surgical care of the trauma patient, and that routine surgical training was too organ-specific or area-specific to allow the development of appropriate judgement and decision-making skills in traumatized patients with multiple injuries.

They suggested that a short course focussing on the life-saving surgical techniques and surgical decision-making was required for surgeons, in order to further train the surgeon who dealt with major surgical trauma on an infrequent basis. This course would meet a worldwide need and be the next step after the well-recognized and accepted American College of Surgeon Advanced Trauma Life Support (ATLS®) course. The material presented in these courses has been refined, a system of training developed using professional education expertise, and the result forms the basis of the standardized Definitive Surgical Trauma Care (DSTC™) course that now takes place.

The DSTC course uses a mixture of education (to modify the 'mind-set' of the participating learners) and training (to modify the 'skill set' of those learners). A unique feature of the course is that while the principles are standardized, once the course has been established nationally in a country, it can then be modified to suit the needs and circumstances of the environment in which the care takes place. The Education Committee of IATSIC oversees the quality and content of the courses. In addition to the initial 'founding' countries (Australia, Austria, South Africa, and Sweden), courses have been delivered in more than 32 countries across the world, with the new participants joining the IATSIC programme each year.

The course has been the 'gold standard' for trauma and trauma critical care since 1999. By 2014, the indispensable contribution made by anaesthesiology was recognized, and with enthusiastic inputs of anaesthetic faculty in the Netherlands, Portugal, Scandinavia, Spain, Sweden, Switzerland, and the United Kingdom, the Definitive Anaesthetic Trauma Care (DATC™) course was added as a critically important option in 2015. The course is fully integrated into DSTC and enhances the concept of the multidisciplinary care of the trauma surgical patient.

This Manual is updated approximately every 4 years. It was first published in 2003; subsequently in 2007, 2011, 2015, and 2019; and this sixth edition in 2024. To date, 700 courses have been held, and 11,000 professionals trained. The annual number of courses presented is now comparable to those presented before COVID. The course and its Manuals are presented in Japanese, French, Hebrew, Portuguese, and Spanish, as well as English.

Because of the immediate, uncontrolled circumstances of the injury, it is not, in itself, enough to treat well; it is essential to learn from others, both from their triumphs and from their errors. In parallel with the aviation industry, integrated simultaneous care, working as a team around the patient, is the ultimate goal.

Error is normal. Do not blame error.
Learn from the error and
prevent it happening again.

This sixth edition has evolved, and care information has been revised and updated, considering new evidence-based information. The all-important section on the non-technical skills which are required has been expanded. A significant number of the original guidelines in trauma have been archived, as they are no longer pertinent or have been superseded. The increasing (and occasionally harmful) role of non-operative management (NOM) has been recognized.

With support from our helpful publishers, we are now able to use colours to enhance the Manual and the way specific information is displayed.

The 'Military Environments' and 'Austere Environments' chapters have been substantially revised to reflect current multinational combat experience, and broadened to reflect modern asymmetrical conflicts and the increased need for humanitarian intervention including military peacekeeping in which only one side wears a uniform. Military weapons are used in major cities against the civilian population. More recently, urban, non-military populations have been the targets and victims of heavy military including ultra-sophisticated combat weapons. Each situation carries its own spectrum of injury and responsibility of care.

The Board of Contributors, responsible for this Manual, is made up of those who have contributed to global trauma care and the DSTC and DATC programme. About 50% of the Board is new blood, bringing diverse new expertise into this established resource. They are warmly welcomed. At the same time, a number of long-term contributors have stood down. We salute them for their commitment over the years and wish them well. The Board Members' support, knowledge, and practical expertise are unrivalled. We would like to thank them for their very great efforts put into the preparation, editing, dissection, re-dissection, and assembly of the Manual and the course.

The book is divided into sections:

- Trauma systems and crew resource management (CRM) communication principles, including non-technical skills
- Physiology and the body's response to trauma
  - Resuscitation physiology
  - Transfusion
  - Damage control
- Chapters on each anatomical area or organ system, divided into both an overview of the problems and pitfalls specific to that system, and the surgical techniques required to deal with major injury in that area including burns, brain injury, and extremes of age
- Chapters on modern diagnostic and therapeutic technology:
  - Imaging
  - The role of minimally invasive resuscitation and surgery
- Additional modules which cover specific aspects of specialized care:
  - Increased importance for care of children and the elderly
  - Trauma anaesthesia, with specific organ system support in many chapters
  - Critical care

- Work in the austere environment
- Military conditions
- Ballistics and blast injuries
- It is recognized that true trauma care extends far beyond the care of the patient's physical injuries only:
  - Trauma support services – for the patient and those caring for the patient
  - Psychological support
  - Physical rehabilitation after trauma
  - Dealing with disability
- A separate appendix for the use of operating room scrub nurses is included.
- As before, the Manual contains all the resources for trauma scoring and injury assessment, and a summary of currently accepted trauma guidelines.

It is not enough to be a good operator.
The effective practitioner is part of a multidisci-
plinary team that plans for and is trained to provide
the essential medical and surgical response required
in the management of the injured patient.

This Manual remains dedicated to all those who care for the injured patient and whose passion is to do it well.

Ken Boffard and Jonathan Oliver White

About the Editors

Ken Boffard is Emeritus Professor of Surgery at the University of the Witwatersrand, Trauma Director at Milpark Hospital, Johannesburg, and previously Head of the Department of Surgery at Johannesburg Hospital and Head of the Johannesburg Hospital Trauma Unit, at the University of the Witwatersrand. He qualified in Johannesburg and trained in Surgery at the Birmingham Accident Hospital and Guy's Hospital.

He is Past President of the International Society of Surgery (ISS) in Switzerland, and currently serves as Secretary-General of the Society; he is also past President of the International Association for Trauma Surgery and Intensive Care (IATSIC). He is a Fellow of six surgical colleges and has received Honorary Fellowships from the American College of Surgeons, Royal College of Surgeons of Thailand, College of Surgeons of Sri Lanka, Deutsche Gesellschaft für Orthopädie und Unfallchirurgie, Japanese Association for the Surgery of Trauma, and Association of Surgeons of Great Britain and Ireland. He is an elected Member of the Academy of Master Surgical Educators of the American College of Surgeons.

His passion is surgical education, and various aspects of trauma resuscitation, intensive care, and regional planning of trauma systems. His interests include flying (he is a licenced fixed-wing and helicopter pilot), scuba diving, and aeromedical care. His research interests include coagulation, haemostasis, and critical bleeding.

He is a Colonel in the South African Military Health Service.

He is a Freeman of the City of London by redemption, and an elected Liveryman of the Guild of Air Pilots of London.

He is married with two children.

Jonathan Oliver White is a Consultant Anaesthetist and Intensivist working in Denmark. He studied at Cambridge University, UK, qualifying in 1998, and trained as an anaesthetist and intensivist at Copenhagen University Hospital, becoming a specialist in Denmark in 2003. He has been affiliated to DSTC / DATC for 12 years and has held the post as Chairman of the DATC organization.

He is head of education and simulation on the ICU and has responsibility for trauma and airway management.

He has four children and a lot of energy.

Board of Contributors

(A) Anaesthetics
(IC) Intensive/Critical Care
(S) Surgery

EDITORS

Ken Boffard (S/IC)
Col (Res) SA Military Health Service
Subspecialist Trauma and Critical Care Surgeon
Trauma Director and Academic Head
Netcare Milpark Hospital Academic Trauma Centre
Professor Emeritus
Department of Surgery
Faculty of Health Sciences
University of the Witwatersrand
Johannesburg, South Africa

Jonathan Oliver White (A/IC)
Consultant ICU and Anaesthesiologist
Intensive Care Unit
Rigshospitalet
Copenhagen University Hospital
Copenhagen, Denmark

BOARD OF CONTRIBUTORS

Henrique Alexandrino (S)
Consultant in Trauma and Emergency Surgery
Coimbra University Hospital Centre
Professor of Surgery
Faculty of Medicine
University of Coimbra
Coimbra, Portugal

Miklosh Bala (S)
Director of Trauma and Emergency Surgery
Hadassah Medical Center
Associate Professor, General Surgery
Faculty of Medicine
Hebrew University in Jerusalem
Jerusalem, Israel

Zsolt J Balogh (S)
Director of Trauma
John Hunter Hospital
Professor, Surgery and Traumatology
Discipline of Surgery
School of Medicine and Public Health
University of Newcastle
Newcastle, NSW, Australia

Sérgio Faria Baptista (A)
Consultant Anaesthesiologist
Anaesthesiology Department
Centro Hospitalar do Médio Tejo, E.P.E.
Abrantes, Tomar, Portugal

Adam Brooks (S)
LTC (Res) Royal Army Medical Corps
Director East Midlands Major Trauma Centre
Consultant Surgeon
Queens Medical Centre
Honorary Assistant Professor
Department of Surgery
Nottingham University Hospital
Nottingham, United Kingdom

Jeremy Cannon (S/IC)
COL (Ret) USAF Reserve, Medical Corps
Trauma Program Medical Director
Penn Presbyterian Medical Center
Adjunct Professor of Surgery, Uniformed Services
    University of the Health Sciences, Bethesda, Maryland
Professor of Surgery
Division of Traumatology, Surgical Critical Care and
    Emergency Surgery
Department of Surgery
Perelman School of Medicine at the University of
    Pennsylvania
Philadelphia, USA

Kate Martin (S)
General and Trauma Surgeon
Royal Melbourne Hospital
Clinical Senior Lecturer
Department of Surgery
University of Melbourne
Melbourne, Vic, Australia

Tascha Meredith
Clinical Psychologist
Netcare Milpark Academic Trauma Centre
University of the Witwatersrand
Johannesburg, South Africa

Yasumitsu Mizobata (S)
Professor, Department of Traumatology and Critical
    Care Medicine
School of Medicine
Osaka Metropolitan University
Osaka, Japan

Maeyane S Moeng (S/IC)
Subspecialist Trauma and Critical Care Surgeon
Head of Trauma
Charlotte Maxeke Johannesburg Academic Hospital
Netcare Milpark Hospital Academic Trauma Centre
Adjunct Professor and Head Academic Division of
    Trauma Surgery
University of the Witwatersrand
Johannesburg, South Africa

Michael Mölmer (S)
Major, Danish Armed Forces Health Command
Orthopaedic and Trauma Surgeon
Senior Consultant, Trauma Subsection
Orthopaedic Department
Nordsjællands Hospital
Hillerød, Denmark

Michael Muller (S)
General Surgeon (Burns and Trauma)
Royal Brisbane and Women's Hospital
Professor, Department of Surgery
University of Queensland
Surgeon/Education Lead
Jamieson Trauma Institute
Brisbane, Australia

Pål Aksel Næss (S)
Senior Consultant in Trauma and Paediatric Surgery
Oslo University Hospital
Professor of Trauma Surgery
Institute of Clinical Medicine
University of Oslo
Oslo, Norway

Dan Nevin (A)
Consultant Anaesthesiologist and Consultant in
    Prehospital Care
HEMS and Trauma Anaesthetist
Royal London Hospital and London's Air Ambulance
Barts Health NHS Trust
London School of Medicine
London, England

George V Oosthuizen (S)
Subspecialist Trauma and Critical Care Surgeon
Head of Trauma
Tygerberg Hospital
Associate Professor
Executive Head: Department of Surgery
Faculty of Medicine and Health Sciences
Stellenbosch University Tygerberg Campus
Cape Town, South Africa

Maria del C. Ortega-Gonzalez (A)
Specialist Anaesthesiologist
Milpark Hospital Academic Trauma Centre
Johannesburg, South Africa

Per Őrtenwall (S)
Consultant Surgeon
Sahlgrenska University Hospital
Associate Professor
Department of Surgery
University of Gothenburg
Gothenburg, Sweden

Hussein Pahad (IC)
Consultant Pulmonologist/Intensivist
Netcare Milpark Academic Trauma Centre
University of the Witwatersrand
Johannesburg, South Africa

Martin Schreiber (S/IC)
COL. MC, USAR
Chief Division of Trauma, Critical Care, and Acute Care
    Surgery
Director, Donald D. Trunkey Center for Civilian and
    Combat Casualty Care
Adjunct Professor of Surgery, Uniformed Services
University of the Health Sciences
Professor of Surgery
Oregon Health and Sciences University
Portland, Oregon, USA

David M Scott (A)
Group Captain: Royal Australian Air Force
Trauma Lead/Clinical Director Anaesthesia and
    Intensive Care Royal Australian Air Force
Associate Professor
Department of Anaesthesia and Pain Medicine
Lismore Base Hospital
Lismore, Australia

Mark Seamon (S/IC)
Division of Trauma, Surgical Critical Care, and
    Emergency Surgery
Penn Presbyterian Medical Center
Professor of Surgery
Director of Education, Director of Research
Perelman School of Medicine at the University of
    Pennsylvania
Philadelphia, USA

Rezvaneh Rose Shakerian (S)
Consultant General and Trauma Surgeon
Royal Melbourne Hospital
Melbourne, Australia

Oliver Smith (A/IC)
Consultant Anaesthesiologist and Intensivist
Charlotte Maxeke Johannesburg Academic Hospital
Department of Anaesthesia and Critical Care
Faculty of Health Sciences
University of the Witwatersrand
Johannesburg, South Africa

Jacob Steinmetz (A)
Consultant Anaesthesiologist
Danish Air Ambulance
University of Aarhus
Aarhus, Denmark
Professor
Department of Anaesthesiology
Trauma Centre and Department of Anaesthesia
Rigshospitalet
University of Copenhagen
Copenhagen, Denmark

Jakob Stensballe (A)
Consultant Anaesthesiology and Transfusion Medicine
Department of Anaesthesiology, Surgery, Trauma Center
Capital Region Blood Bank
Rigshospitalet
Center for Endotheliomics
Clinical Academic Group
Greater Copenhagen Health Science Partners
Copenhagen University Hospital
Copenhagen, Denmark

Elmin Steyn (S)
Head of Surgery: Tygerberg Hospital
Associate Professor of Surgery
University of Stellenbosch
Cape Town, South Africa

Nigel Tai (S)
16 Medical Regiment
Consultant Surgeon
Air Assault Brigade
United Kingdom
Consultant in Trauma and Vascular Surgery, Barts
    Health NHS Trust & London School of Medicine
Honorary Clinical Professor of Trauma Surgery and
    Innovation
Barts and the London School of Medicine and Dentistry
London, United Kingdom

Edward C T H Tan (S)
Consultant Trauma Surgeon
HEMS Physician
Associate Professor
Department of Surgery
Radboud University Medical Center
Nijmegen, the Netherlands

B Ignacio Monzon Torres (S)
Trauma Director
Subspecialist Trauma Surgeon
Ahmed Kathrada Private Hospital
Lenmed Health Hospital Group
Johannesburg, South Africa

Fernando Turégano (S)
Head of Division of Emergency Surgery
University General Hospital Gregorio Marañón
Associate Professor
Department of Surgery
Complutense University of Madrid
Madrid, Spain

Selman Uranues (S)
Head of Center for Minimally Invasive Surgery
Professor of Surgery
Section for Surgical Research
Department of Surgery
Medical University of Graz
Graz, Austria

Pantelis Vassiliu (S)
Professor of Surgery
National and Kapodistrian University of Athens
    (NKUA)
4th Surgical Clinic
Attikon Hospital
Athens, Greece

Adrian O Wilson
Specialist, Internal Medicine and Gerontology
Professor Emeritus
Dunsmore, UK

Virginia S Wilson
Physiatrist
Physical and Rehabilitation Medicine Physician
Netcare Rehabilitation Hospital
Johannesburg, South Africa

David Zonies (S/IC)
COL. (Ret) USAFR
Associate Chief Medical Officer
OHSU Health System
Adjunct Professor of Surgery
Uniformed Services University of the Health Sciences
Professor of Surgery
Oregon Health and Sciences University
Portland, Oregon, USA

Contributors Emeritus

FROM THE FIFTH EDITION

Philip Barker (S)

Chris Bleeker (A)

Ian Civil (S)

Joe Dawson (S)

Elias Degiannis (S/IC)

Dietrich Doll (S)

Abe Fingerhut (S)

Sache Flohé (S)

Georgios Gemenetzis (S)

Lauri Handolin (S)

Gareth Hide (S)

Anders Holtan (A)

Ilja Laesser (Rad)

Rifat Latifi (S)

Gilberto Leung (S)

Ron Maier (S/IC)

Carlos Mesquita (S)

Ernest E Moore (S/IC)

Michael Parr (A)

Andrew Peitzman (S/IC)

Louis Riddez (S)

Jeffrey V Rosenfeld (S)

Katharina Heim Schoettker (A)

Patrick Schoettker (S)

C William Schwab (S/IC)

Arie B van Vugt (S)

Part 1

Trauma system and communication principles

Introduction 1

Globally, injury is the third leading cause of death for all ages and the leading cause of death from age 1 to 44 years. More than 50% of all deaths occur minutes after injury, and most immediate deaths are due to massive haemorrhage or neurological injury. Autopsy data demonstrate that central nervous system injuries account for 50%–70% of all injury deaths, and haemorrhage accounts for 15%–30%. It is within this latter group of haemorrhage-related deaths where prompt decision-making and effective use of surgical techniques have the greatest opportunity to save lives.

With improving pre-hospital care across the world, patients who would previously have died at the scene are reaching hospital alive. In many situations, their airway and ventilation are already controlled, but the deaths occur in hospital from uncontrolled bleeding. Whilst there are surgical techniques for the control of bleeding, the timing and appropriateness of their use and a clear understanding of the physiology of trauma are essential for a successful outcome.

Modern military conflicts are in general asymmetric (with only one side in uniform), are generally local and well contained, and do not produce casualties in large numbers nor on a frequent basis. For this reason, it is difficult to maintain the number of military specialists required who can be deployed immediately to perform highly technical surgical or resuscitative procedures required in the battlefield arena or under austere conditions. Simultaneously, more military weapons and munitions are being deployed, especially with the new event of "drone-based warfare" in the civilian environment, either isolated or widely targeted. It is also difficult for career military surgeons to gain adequate exposure to battlefield casualties, or indeed penetrating trauma in general, and many military training programmes are now looking to their civilian counterparts for assistance.

It is critical that surgical teams responsible for the management of injured patients, whether military or civilian, are adequately skilled in the assessment, diagnosis, and operative and resuscitative management of life-threatening injuries. There remains a poorly developed appreciation of the potential impact that timely and appropriate surgical intervention can have on the outcome of a severely injured patient. Partly through lack of exposure, difficulty in time availability, or release from hospital duties, and partly because of other interests, many specialists quite simply no longer have the expertise to deal with such life-threatening situations.

From the point of view of the injured patient, there is *double jeopardy*: the risks to health due to the traumatic insult to tissue and physiology; and the risk posed by the therapy required to restore health – both from the *injury* and from the *treatment*. Minimizing the potential for iatrogenic harm through the provision of safe care is especially challenging in major trauma due to the complexity and urgency of the disease. The aim of this chapter is to iterate the minimal essential components of individual, hospital, and system practice to deliver safe care.

In many countries, trauma continues to be a major public health problem and financial burden, both in the pre-hospital setting and within the hospital system, claiming more than 5 million lives every year. In addition to increasing political and social unrest in many countries, and an increasing use of firearms for interpersonal violence, the motor vehicle has become a substantial cause of trauma worldwide. In higher-income countries, there are changing demographics; the average age of major trauma is 50, with more frequent low-energy severe injuries in patients with multiple comorbidities. These socio-economic determinants result in large numbers of injured patients. Injury prevention is a key element in limiting the societal impact of trauma, but, once a patient is injured, effective acute care and rehabilitation are essential for optimal patient outcomes. Improving all aspects of emergency care is important; however, improved surgical and resuscitation skills have particular roles in saving lives and minimizing disability.

DOI: 10.1201/9781003258124-2

In many industrialized high-income countries (HICs) or upper-middle-income countries (UMICs), there is limited exposure to the full range of trauma care due to a lower incidence of major trauma and more hospitals and doctors per capita. Many surgical and anaesthetic colleagues may have very limited trauma experience, both from their training and from reduced case exposure. There is a crisis in obtaining operative experience on trauma patients where the injury mechanism is predominantly blunt. In these centres, the trauma laparotomy rate is about 1 per every 20–30 major trauma activations due to the primarily non-operative management of blunt abdominal parenchymal organ injuries. This means it is difficult to develop and maintain experience in trauma resuscitation and trauma surgery.

The question of safe trauma care also requires an examination of the sustainability of trauma care within the workforce and training, and the role of innovative simulation models, research and innovation, translation from civilian to military experience, and *vice versa* as means to ensure that healthcare professionals working with trauma patients can continue to offer the very best care available, using reliable existing data.

Standard surgical training is increasingly organ-specific, reducing even further the broad skills required for trauma management. Laparoscopic surgery, microsurgery, robotics, interventional radiographic procedures, and other sophisticated operating techniques may improve outcomes pertaining to elective surgery but have a negative impact on acquisition of the complex skill set needed to manage a severely injured trauma patient.

Many less industrialized developing countries – lower-middle-income countries (LMICs) and low-income countries (LICs) – have a less developed infrastructure, both pre-hospital and in-hospital; a higher load of severely injured patients; and significantly fewer resources.

1.1 INJURY PREVENTION

Injury prevention can be divided into three parts:

- *Primary prevention* (*prevent the injury from happening*): Education and legislation are used to reduce the incidence of injury (e.g., driving under the influence of alcohol).
- *Secondary prevention* (*minimize the chance of injury from a traumatic event*): Minimizing the incidence of injury through design (e.g., seatbelts and helmets).

- *Tertiary prevention* (*minimizing the severity and physiological impact of the effects of that injury once it has occurred*): By better and earlier care, preferably evidence based.

Although primary and secondary prevention of injury will undoubtedly play the major role in reducing the incidence of trauma, they will not be eliminated, and therefore there is a need to maintain effective tertiary prevention. This requires training within complex multidisciplinary teams, and a focus on both the decision-making and the medical and surgical procedures required, for the advanced management of patients with multiple injuries and the correction of any associated deranged physiology.

1.2 SAFE TRAUMA CARE

1.2.1 Individual Factors

It is accepted that to safely practice trauma surgery, the trauma surgeon and trauma anaesthesiologist must have undergone a validated general training pathway culminating in exposure to a period of specific trauma training. Lexical knowledge (education, or the 'when') and technical expertise (skills, or the 'how') represent the foundational aspects but by themselves are insufficient unless they are linked. Professionalism is also characterized by rigorous adherence to personal and team safety. However, the reality is that a significant amount of trauma care in the world is delivered by individuals who may not have had the requisite training, nor the resources required.

Over the past decades, the importance of non-technical skills (see Chapter 2) has become increasingly well recognized. The nomenclature for such skills differs from sector to sector (e.g., medicine = *non-technical skills*; aviation = *Crew Resource Management [CRM] skills*; social science = *interpersonal skills*; psychology = *emotional intelligence*; US Army = *soft skills*), but the competencies are broadly the same: teamwork, communication, leadership, decision-making, conflict resolution, assertiveness, management of stress and fatigue, workload management, prioritization of tasks, and situational awareness.[1] Consistent delivery of non-technical skills is very important in minimizing error, as very few preventable trauma deaths are attributable to purely technical mistakes (see Chapter 2).

Filtering out information regarded as useless may also discard information that is important. Assessment without all available information may cause false assumptions to be made and false narratives to be laid down. Rapidity of decision-making increases the risk of error, and relying on experience does not always map on to the present, particularly if post-hoc processing leads to overly optimistic interpretation of the success of a previous strategy and thus reinforcement error.

1.2.1.1 INDIVIDUAL: LEADERSHIP

The classical *leader–follower model* may not be ideal for trauma practice settings.[1] Expertise is distributed among various members of the trauma team, and the leadership function may flux between different team members according to the phase of trauma resuscitation and the need to respond dynamically to changes in patient condition (the *hierarchical-but-fluid model*).[2] Leadership demands accurate assessment of the situation and the ability to continually monitor progress and reappraise the array of options for each decision node – a characteristic formulated as the '3D trauma surgeon' by Hirshberg and Mattox.[3] Elements that the 3D surgeon should be able to deliver include:

- *Tactics*: Technical aspects of the operation.
- *Strategy*: A 'big-picture' appreciation of the risks that the patient faces immediately and in the near- and medium-term elements of operation.
- *Team*: Clear communication to coordinate efforts to ensure working towards the same goals.

Mishandling the team dimension during a trauma operation is one of the worst mistakes you can make.[3]

1.2.1.2 TRAUMA TEAM

Trauma care faces several challenges in performing at a consistent level. It is rarely the same team that manages the patient: shift work introduces different leaders, different specialists, and different levels of expertise. Given the fact that they may face the requirement to deliver critical resuscitative functions within moments of meeting each other, there is ample opportunity for error due to an inappropriate skill mix, unfamiliarity with each other's styles or even names, with significant potential for excess morbidity and mortality.

Dysfunctional teams are usually obvious to external observers but not necessarily so from within when poor behaviours (e.g., lack of communication leading to failure to establish a shared mental model) may become habitual and normalized. Conversely, high-performing teams talk to each other and are safer.

High-performing teams better demonstrate the following behaviours:

- Situational awareness (SA)-seeking behaviour.
- Clear leadership and followership with the facility to model adaptive behaviours when needed, with appropriate distribution of workload and monitoring/support of team members.
- Closed-loop communication (seeking confirmation that intended messages are understood by the recipient) with clear means of escalating urgency (standardized prompts) and facilitation of calm assertiveness.
- Low-gradient or flat hierarchy of communication, such that team members are empowered to speak up and relay concerns as they see fit.
- Readiness to participate in open *team debriefs* to review performance, learn why things went well or less well, and adopt change if required.

1.2.1.3 TEAM: TRAINING

Specific courses designed to deliver non-technical competencies (situational awareness, decision-making, communication, teamwork, and leadership) are increasingly available (e.g., the Non-Technical Skills for Surgeons [NOTSS] course;[4] see also Chapter 2), and they contain lessons derived from other safety-critical industries, such as CRM in aviation,[5] where failure may lead to catastrophe, and the US Department of Defense's Team STEPPS programme.[6]

1.2.2 Institutional Factors

1.2.2.1 DEDICATED TRAUMA SERVICE

A dedicated trauma admitting service is responsible for the polytrauma patient from admission to discharge. This involves acute and ongoing leadership in comprehensive inpatient care, daily ward rounds and identification of ongoing care needs, liaison with other surgical and non-surgical services, safe discharge, and follow-up.

1.2.3 **Performance Improvement Activities**

Institutional performance improvement or a Quality Improvement Programme (QIP) encompasses:

1. The identification of preventable death and contributory factors[1] (such a peer-review endeavour may be more effective than the use of the Trauma and Injury Severity Score [TRISS] for the identification of potentially preventable death)[7].
2. Tracking of trends via long-term mortality monitoring (which allows for institution of corrective action plans and is associated with improvement in patient outcome in level 1 trauma centres)[8,9].
3. Improvement in patient pathways, development of evidence-based standard operating procedures designed to reduce variation in care, teamworking, decision-making, and interprofessional dynamics[7].

One of the most effective methods to improve patient safety at a hospital level is a robust, respectful, and constructive mortality and morbidity review process. The purpose of this process is to review and discuss all trauma management errors in a non-blame environment and to peer review all trauma deaths. Causes of death or severe complications are stratified into the following:

- *Anticipated*: Not preventable.
- *Unanticipated but without room for improvement*: Potentially preventable.
- *Unanticipated with room for improvement*: Preventable; allows further in-depth discussion where issues are discussed, and action plans are made and, most importantly, implemented and audited. Errors need to be highlighted and addressed with loop closure mechanisms even from non-preventable death situations. Areas for improvement are:
  - *System related*
  - *Professional staff related*
  - *Patient related*
  - *Resource related*

Errors and omissions are often related to:[1,7,8]

- Resuscitation issues
- Airway management
- Massive transfusion
- Pelvic fracture management
- Venous thromboembolism (VTE) prophylaxis
- Missed injuries
- Excessive dwell time in the emergency department

Within this framework, 'near-misses' are just as important to discuss as deaths. In the United States, this process is required for trauma centre verification, and in the British Major Trauma System, such activity is required to be formally resourced and evidenced during peer review to retain its designated status.

1.2.4 **Regional Activities**

Remote and rural communities are particularly vulnerable, as they have four times higher trauma mortality than metropolitan areas.[10] Strong regional trauma systems can thus have additional benefit over and above their expected impact in rural communities.

1.2.5 **National Activities**

The benefit of audit and quality improvement initiatives can be followed from the team level all the way up to the national level.

National trauma registries involve the collection of data of trauma patients including the mechanism of injury, injuries sustained including injury severity scores, treatments received, and outcomes. Such national registries are valuable for research, audit and peer comparison, and institution of national quality improvement initiatives.

Several non-government, non-profit organizations exist to audit, research, educate, and implement national initiatives in injury prevention. As road traffic collisions comprise the majority of trauma in Australasia and Western Europe, the majority are based on road safety. These include the Australasian College of Road Safety, the Australian Road Safety Conference, and Sweden's impressive Vision Zero campaign which led to a 30% drop in traffic fatalities since its inception in 1997, despite a significant increase in traffic volume during the same period.[11] The Vision Zero initiative has since spread globally, including to the United States and Canada.

1.2.6 **Global Activities**

A massive disparity exists in the likelihood of survival of a person sustaining a life-threatening but salvageable injury in a LIC (36% mortality) compared to a HIC (6%).[12] Consequently, 90% of trauma deaths occur in LICs and middle-income countries (MICs) and comprise the leading cause of death globally, killing more people than

HIV, malaria, and tuberculosis combined. Road traffic accidents are the eighth leading cause of death globally, and international meetings such as the World Innovation Summit for Health (WISH) Forum for Road Traffic and Trauma Care focus on the global impact of such trauma, a large majority of which occurs in LICs and MICs. The World Health Organisation (WHO) has produced *Guidelines for Essential Trauma Care*, a set of minimum standards for worldwide trauma care.[12] These were based on low-cost improvements that are achievable in virtually every setting across the globe. In 2008, WHO produced the Safe Surgery Checklist, and whilst it is not specific to trauma, it certainly has application and utility.

With the success of the standard WHO checklist now firmly embedded into routine surgical practice, WHO produced a Trauma Care Checklist which has subsequently been tested in 11 centres around the world, nine of which are in LICs and MICs.[13] The 18-point checklist covers history, examination, investigations, and monitoring; it has improved the processes measured and may improve outcomes.

There is global recognition of polytrauma as a disease by WHO's inclusion of it in the International Classification of Diseases, eleventh revision (ICD-11).[14] Charitable organizations can play an important global role, particularly in trauma education such as advanced trauma life support (ATLS)-like courses in developing countries. The largest programme for developing countries is the International Association for Trauma Surgery and Intensive Care (IATSIC) National Trauma Management Course (NTMC™), which is taught across India, Sri Lanka, and 12 other developing countries.

Delivery of safe trauma care in the model generated by HICs is typified by complexity and expense. In developing countries with more limited resources, the focus needs to be on strengthening local processes preferentially, by using existing resources to ensure solutions are locally relevant.

1.3 SUSTAINABLE TRAUMA CARE

There is a need to provide training in the skills and techniques necessary to resuscitate and manage seriously injured patients surgically beyond the emergency department, operative techniques, surgical decision-making, intensive care, and continued care until rehabilitation. The course that is needed must be flexible so that it meets the local needs of the country and circumstances in which it is being taught.

1.3.1 Workforce Training and Development

For all development, the process is a mixture of education (to modify the mind-set of the participating learners – the 'what to do') and training (to modify the skill set of those learners – the 'how to do').

Specific technical competence can be facilitated through simulation, and advanced human patient simulators have been developed to allow simulation training in trauma skills, ranging from low-fidelity rigs to highly sophisticated mannequins. Examples include Trauma Man and Synman® (intercostal drain insertion, pericardiocentesis, peritoneal lavage, cricothyroidotomy, and tracheostomy), Air-Man® (airway complications), VIRGIL® (chest trauma), and UltraSim® (Focused Assessment with Sonography for Trauma [FAST] scan training).[7] The novel use of cadavers, such as a pulsatile cadaveric model (perfused cadaver), allows very realistic training in cardiac-penetrating injuries, lung lacerations, liver and retrohepatic vena cava injuries, cricothyroidotomy, tracheostomy, open fractures, and carotid and extremity vessel injuries.

However, simulation is still inadequate when it comes to mimicking physiological dynamic changes, coagulation, haemostasis, packing, and anatomical reconstruction. The mere fact that it is a simulation removes some credibility. The more sophisticated a simulator, often the more expensive it is, making expensive courses more expensive, and sometimes unaffordable.

For trainee surgeons, there are several opportunities that can be pursued to address deficiencies in standard training programmes. These are short courses, designed to highlight these needs; informal fellowships at high-volume centres with a large proportion of penetrating trauma cases (typically, in the United States and South Africa); and dedicated trauma/critical care fellowships in the United States and South Africa.

1.4 SURGICAL TRAUMA TRAINING BEYOND INITIAL CARE

1.4.1 Non-Technical Skills for Surgeons (NOTSS)[4]

NOTSS is a behaviour rating system based on a skills taxonomy. It is from the Royal College of Surgeons of Edinburgh, and it plays a significant role in patient safety.

The aim of the NOTSS project was to develop and test an educational system for assessment and training of non-technical skills in the intraoperative phase of surgery. NOTSS is a behaviour rating system based on a skills taxonomy that allows valid and reliable observation and assessment of four categories of surgeons' non-technical skill: situation awareness, decision-making, communication and teamwork, and leadership.

These are the essential non-technical skills that surgeons need to perform safely in the operating room, and NOTSS allows measurement of several ACGME (Accreditation Council for Graduate Medical Education) competencies, including professionalism, interpersonal and communication skills, and systems-based practice. The skills taxonomy can be used to structure training and assessment in this important area of surgical competence.

1.4.2 The Advanced Trauma Operative Management (ATOM®) Course[15]

This American College of Surgeons course was originally developed by Lenworth M. Jacobs about 15 years ago. It is a one-day course comprising a didactic lecture series followed by exercises on live-tissue models. It is an effective method of increasing surgical competence and confidence in the operative management of penetrating injuries to the chest and abdomen.

1.4.3 The Advanced Surgical Skills for Exposure in Trauma (ASSET®) Course[16]

Another programme developed by the American College of Surgeons, this one-day cadaver-based course is designed to teach the anatomical exposures necessary for control of haemorrhage in the trunk, neck, extremities, and junctional areas, based on case presentations requiring surgical access.

1.4.4 The Definitive Surgical Trauma Care™ (DSTC) Course[17]

This was developed in 1993 through an international collaboration of six surgeons, and it is controlled by IATSIC, an Integrated Society of the International Society of Surgery–Société Internationale de Chirugie (ISS-SIC) in Zurich, Switzerland. It comprises a 3-day course with short interactive presentations, group discussions, case discussions, and operative exercises on a live-tissue model. The emphasis teaches learners the critical decision-making processes required through both advanced *education* (modification of mind-set) and *training* in the surgical techniques required (modification of skill set) to choose the best method of management. The course has taken place in 32 countries and in several languages (English, French, Hebrew, Japanese, Portuguese, and Spanish). Additional 'modules' such as Critical Care, Military Care, Austere Conditions, and one emphasizing team interaction – Non-Technical Skills in Trauma (Chapter 2) – have been added, allowing the course to be tailored to its audience. To date, 700 courses have been held, with over 11,000 surgeons and anaesthesiologists trained.

1.4.5 The Definitive Anaesthetic Trauma Care™ (DATC) Course[17]

The DATC™ course was established in 2006 as predeployment training for military anaesthesiologists. It developed as an add-on module to the DSTC™ course to enhance understanding of trauma management. In 2015, anaesthesiology was introduced into IATSIC as a module of DSTC™. Cooperation between the two specialities allows the complex teamwork required in the management of a major trauma patient to be simulated and practiced. The integration of the DATC™ module into the DSTC™ course program, including the aspects of the critical care required, highlights the importance of modern-day trauma management techniques with the focus on the multidisciplinary nature of trauma care by a trauma team. The current DATC™ and DSTC™ courses have participants from interventional radiology, medical and surgical specialities including critical care, as well as nursing scrub staff, thus making the course unique in its team approach.

Details of the course appear in Appendix D of this manual.

1.5 CONCLUSION

There are numerous opportunities for safer trauma care at every level. At the individual and team levels, this is predominantly in the reduction of human error by understanding cognitive biases and improving communication and teamwork. At the institutional level, scrupulous audit and peer review identifies not only individual and team errors but, more importantly, institutional systemic failures, and it ensures constant performance improvement. At a regional level, the implementation and governance of trauma networks ensure the best trauma care to a whole population or geographical area, taking into consideration its individual requirements and needs. Injury prevention initiatives at a national level have been shown to have tremendous impact on mortality; and, finally, to redress the imbalance of trauma outcomes between LICs and HICs, numerous initiatives are in place.

REFERENCES

1. Klein KJ, Ziegert JC, Knight A, Xiao Y. A Leadership System for Emergency Action Teams: Rigid Hierarchy and Dynamic Flexibility. In: *Team Leadership System.* University of Pennsylvania and University of Maryland, Baltimore. *Academy of Management Journal.* 2004 **47(6)**, 1–55. https://www.researchgate.net/publication/242315366_A_LEADERSHIP_SYSTEM_FOR_EMERGENCY_ACTION_TEAMS_RIGID_HIERARCHY_AND_DYNAMIC_FLEXIBILITY. (accessed online February 2024.)

2. Heuristics and Cognitive Biases. Available from: https://betterhumans.coach.me/cognitive-bias-cheat-sheet-55a472476b18 (accessed online July 2023).

3. *Top Knife – The Art & Craft of Trauma Surgery.* Hirshberg & Mattox. TFM Publishing Ltd, 2005 (Reprinted 2018).

4. *The Non-Technical Skills for Surgeons (NOTSS) System Handbook V2.0.* Royal College of Surgeons of Edinburgh, Scotland. 2020. Available from https://www.rcsed.ac.uk/media/682516/notss-system-handbook-v20.pdf (accessed online July 2023).

5. Physicians will Learn Assertiveness. Human Resources. Healthcare-in-Europe.com. 2016. Available from: https://healthcare-in-europe.com/en/news/physicians-will-learn-assertiveness.html (accessed online July 2023).

6. King HB, Battles J, Baker DP, Alonso A, Salas E, Webster J, et al. TeamSTEPPS: Team Strategies and Tools to Enhance Performance and Patient Safety. In: *Advances in Patient Safety: New Directions and Alternative Approaches,* Vol 3, Performance and Tools. https://www.ahrq.gov/teamstepps-program/index.html (accessed online August 2023)

7. Fallon WF Jr, Barnoski AL, Mancuso CL, Tinnell CA, Malangoni MA. Benchmarking the quality-monitoring process: a comparison of outcomes analysis by trauma and injury severity score (TRISS) methodology with the peer-review process. *J Trauma.* 1997 May;**42(5)**:810–5; discussion 815–7. doi: 10.1097/00005373-199705000-00010.

8. Sarkar B, Brunsvold ME, Cherry-Bukoweic JR, Hemmila MR, Park PK, et al. American college of surgeons' committee on trauma performance improvement and patient safety program: maximal impact in a mature trauma center. *J Trauma.* 2011 Nov;**71(5)**:1447–53; discussion 1453–4. doi: 10.1097/TA.0b013e3182325d32.

9. Hoyt DB, Coimbra R, Potenza B, Doucet J, Fortlage D, Holingsworth et al. A twelve-year analysis of disease and provider complications on an organized Level I trauma service: as good as it gets? *J Trauma.* 2003 Jan;**54(1)**:26–36; discussion 36–7.

10. Fatovich DM, Jacobs IG. The relationship between remoteness and trauma deaths in Western Australia. *J Trauma.* 2009 Nov;**67(5)**:910–4. doi: 10.1097/TA.0b013e3181815a26.

11. Vision Zero Initiative Sweden. 1997. Available from: https://visionzeronetwork.org/about/what-is-vision-zero/ (accessed online July 2023).

12. *Guidelines for Essential Trauma Care.* World Health Organisation, International Society of Surgery, (ISS) and International Association for the Surgery of Trauma and Surgical Intensive Care (IATSIC), 2012. Available from: https://www.who.int/publications/i/item/guidelines-for-essential-trauma-care/ (accessed online July 2023).

13. Lashoher A, Schneider EB, Juillard C, Stevens K, Colantuoni E, Berry WR et al. Implementation of the world health organisation trauma care checklist programme in 11 centres across multiple economic strata: effect on care process measures. *World J Surg.* 2017 Apr;**41(4)**:954–62. doi: 10.1007/s00268-016-3759-8.

14. World Health Organisation International Classification of Disease ICD-11. https://www.who.int/standards/classifications/classification-of-diseases (accessed August 2023).

15. Advanced Trauma Operative Skills (ATOM). https://www.facs.org/quality-programs/trauma/education/advanced-trauma-operative-management/ (accessed August 2023).

16. Advanced Surgical Skills for Exposure in Trauma (ASSET®) Course. https://www.facs.org/quality-programs/trauma/education/asset/

17. Definitive Surgery of Trauma Care (DSTC™) Course. https://www.iatsic.org/DSTC-Introduction/

Non-Technical Skills in Major Trauma: The Role of Crew Resource Management (CRM) and Communication

2

2.1 OVERVIEW

Management of a trauma patient is a challenging process. Swift and accurate clinical assessment is required, and time-sensitive decisions and life-saving procedures have to be performed in an unstable patient under a great deal of uncertainty. The ABCDE approach (airway, breathing, circulation, disability, and exposure) provides a useful framework for emergency room (ER) management, and the principles of surgical management include early transfer to the operating room (OR) and quick control of bleeding and contamination. This requires a coordinated response by the ER and OR teams, usually composed of surgeons, anaesthesiologists, other medical specialties, and nurses. All these providers are self-motivated to excel as individuals at their technical and decision-making skills.

Non-technical skills are social and cognitive skills that improve task performance and completion. There is compelling evidence to support the incorporation of Non-Technical Skills for Surgeons (NOTSS) training into undergraduate and postgraduate settings, particularly in trauma. For proper team function, not only should all team members be knowledgeable and proficient in their particular technical skills, but it is self-explanatory that when training these principles of crew resource management (CRM), the participation of the whole trauma team is mandatory.

A team of experts does not necessarily make an expert team.

Root cause analysis of adverse events in surgery has shown that failures in coordination, planning, task management, and particularly communication are the main causes of medical errors.[1] Trauma teams are particularly exposed to medical errors.

The airline industry has long recognized the role of team training and non-technical skills in reducing hazards. The recognition that human factors, and not mechanical failure, were a recurring theme in many aviation disasters (65%) led to an increased focus on non-technical skill training in the training programme of pilots, referred to in aviation as CRM. This is a concept in which effective use is made of all available resources needed to complete a safe and efficient operation. CRM implementation has made airline travel significantly safer, and the transposition to the medical context, with specific training in non-technical skills, has also brought great benefits.

Other high-risk industries subsequently followed suit, and 40 years ago the medical community adopted CRM as a component in the training of critical clinical situations. The subsequent years have seen implementation of

DOI: 10.1201/9781003258124-3

CRM in numerous surgical and medical subspecialities, of which the setting of traumatology has been no exception. Trauma team training based upon the principles of CRM has become an integral part in the daily practice in trauma centres worldwide.

The principles of CRM are built upon a concept of training in human factors with the aim of optimizing communication dynamics in the setting of the multidisciplinary team. The goal is to reduce medical errors and improve decision-making and outcome in trauma care. What makes trauma care so special is that the decision-making must take place and the interventions must be executed in a very condensed period (e.g., minutes or even seconds, compared to hours or even days/weeks in other, less urgent forms of surgery). This underlines the need for teamwork based on the correct non-technical skills and CRM.

The most important aspects of CRM include:

- Situational awareness
- Preparation and planning
- Calling for help early
- Displaying effective leadership
- Allocating attention wisely with use of all available resources
- Prioritizing and distributing the workload
- Communicating effectively

The Definitive Surgical Trauma Care (DSTC) course, and the associated Definitive Anaesthetic Trauma Care (DATC) and Definitive Perioperative Nurse Trauma Care (DPNTC) courses when available, provide an excellent opportunity to demonstrate the importance of NOTSS.[2]

2.2 THE AVOIDANCE OF ERRORS

Errors may be of several origins:

- *Errors of omission*: Omitting to do 'something'.
- *Errors of commission*: The 'something' is the wrong thing.
- *Errors of interpretation*: Not registering the key messages, or focussing on only one aspect of the problem.
- *Errors of communication*: Members of the team are not involved in the decision-making.
- *Errors of judgement*: A mix of any of the above.

2.2.1 The 'Swiss Cheese' Theory

Described initially in 2001 by James T. Reason,[3,4] a British psychologist at the University of Manchester, the *Swiss cheese model* has become the standard for assessing patient security to expose the failure of systems, like medical mishap. It has been used by the healthcare industry, emergency services organizations, the aviation industry, and the safety industry since it was developed. It is also known as the *cumulative act effect*. Reason's Swiss cheese model has become the dominant paradigm for analysing medical errors and patient safety incidents.

In a complicated system, prevention of hazards is done by analysis of a chain of barriers. All barriers contain unplanned holes, or weaknesses; thus, they resemble Swiss cheese. The holes in the Swiss cheese model randomly close and open due to inconsistent weaknesses. The defences of an organization against the failure are represented like barriers in slices of Swiss cheese, and individual weaknesses are shown by the holes in the slices as part of the system; all holes are different in position and size in those slices. The hazard reaches the patient only when all the holes simultaneously align. In most of the cases, there can be four levels of failure for an accident:

- Unsafe supervision
- Unsafe acts
- Organizational influence
- Preconditions for unsafe acts

The failure of the system occurs when holes in slices simultaneously align in aggregate, giving permission, or what James Reason called 'a trajectory of accident opportunity', so that in all the defences, jeopardy passes through all holes, which causes failure.

2.3 COMMUNICATION IN THE TRAUMA SETTING

The complex task of managing a severely injured trauma patient arriving in the hospital requires both highly specialized surgical and medical skills as well as an ability to master the core concepts of CRM.

For trauma care to be effective, there needs to be open communication between all members of the trauma team. At the centre of this process are the surgeon and

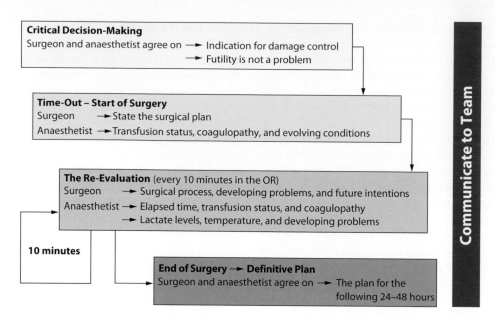

Figure 2.1 The decision-making process in stages.

the anaesthetist, who in collaboration have the responsibility of prioritizing interventions and management. The team leader must keep the entire team constantly orientated regarding the management of a patient whose physiology and subsequent treatment plans are under constant evolution. The deliverance of optimal care in a trauma patient undergoing damage control surgery is a complex process whereby a group of individuals with differing skill sets need to function with a common purpose; all members are listened to (not just heard) and their individual skills utilized to deliver the most appropriate medical care. The communication is divided into phases (see **Figure 2.1**).

Human factors are vital to the timely assessment and treatment of the complex trauma patient.[5] In the stressful and sometimes highly charged environment of the trauma bay or the OR, surgeons and anaesthetists can be tempted to focus on immediate individual tasks with the potential of developing what is commonly termed *tunnel vision* or *task fixation*. This can lead to a situation where focus on single problems is potentially prioritized over other life-threatening issues, thereby leading to loss of control of the situation. The loss of situational awareness described, and the evolution of fixation errors, may prove fatal to the outcome of the severely injured trauma patient. In trauma care, as in other disciplines, inadequate communication, poor teamwork and lack of leadership, and consequent poor task prioritization

have been shown to have a profound impact on patient outcome.

The 'cone in the cube' analogy is used (see **Figure 2.2**).[6] Two groups of people are assigned the task of describing a shape inside an opaque cube. One group looks through peephole A on the side of the box. They see a triangle. The other looks through peephole B on the top of the box. They see a circle. The two groups fall into conflict about what is in the cube, and each substantiates the validity of its claims based on professed superior experience, values, intelligence, or power.

The Cone-in-the-Cube

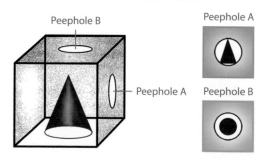

Figure 2.2 Interpretation of information in trauma.

Source: © *You're It: Crisis, Change, and How to Lead When It Matters Most*. Leadership Now. 2019. With permission.

It is critically important to incorporate multiple per-spectives in the care of the trauma patient, including observations and cues from both the surgical and anaes-thetic teams. In critical situations, it is easy to fall into pre-established ideas and, once triggered, difficult for your brain to be convinced otherwise. Intentionally tak-ing brief intervals (e.g., every 20–30 minutes during the case) before moving on to the next phase or procedure, to step back and openly communicate between teams, pro-vides an optimal approach to surgical care of the injured patient, even (especially) in situations of severe stress.

2.3.1 Initial Handover

The handover is a critical phase during patient manage-ment; many medical errors arise here, and thus it has been the focus of intense evaluation regarding which strategies to optimize. It is important that the hando-ver is conducted in silence unless there is an imminent threat to the patient's survival. The most commonly used acronym, (AT)MIST, is used to describe in a short and concise manner the salient aspects of a traumatized patient. The importance of a structured approach to handover ensures that essential information is provided in a concise and reproducible format without distracting superfluous information.

- **A**ge
- **T**ime of injury
- **M**echanism of injury
- **I**njuries sustained
- **S**igns and symptoms
- **T**reatment

2.3.2 Communication in Resuscitation and Ongoing Management

Communication during the resuscitation and ongo-ing management of the unstable trauma patient, from an operational perspective, can be described in four phases:

- Initial decision-making process prior to resuscitation in the emergency department
- Before commencement of surgery
- Re-evaluation during surgery
- Completion of surgery, and before transfer to the critical care environment

The critical decision-making process is typically started in the emergency department/trauma bay, and the surgeon together with the anaesthetist agree on a management plan for resuscitation, damage control sur-gery, and critical care. At this early start, evaluation of the futility of care is also a legitimate consideration.

In the OR, or shortly before the commencement of sur-gery, the surgeon states the surgical plan based on the clinical, laboratory, and imaging findings (if present). The anaesthesiologist summarizes the physiological status of the patient including blood volume/transfusion status, the presence of coagulopathy, and any other evolving conditions that will affect immediate management. This is often a moment when the decision regarding damage control needs to be considered/raised based on available information.

During damage control surgery and resuscitation, re-eval-uation is performed around every 10 minutes to maintain team situational awareness and allow effective anticipation and planning of all aspects of the care of the patient. During the re-evaluation, the surgeon states the surgical progress, developing problems, and future intentions, whilst the anaesthetist reports the elapsed time, transfusion status, developing coagulopathy, lactate levels, temperature, and other relevant established or developing problems.

Upon completion of surgery, the anaesthetist and surgeon recapitulate the patient's condition, the pro-cedures performed, and an action plan for the follow-ing 24–48 hours. They are responsible for ensuring the transfer of relevant information within the team and externally with collaborators, such as the intensive care unit (ICU), blood bank, radiology, and so on. The trauma leader plans the tertiary survey within the following 24 hours. The process is summarized in **Figure 2.1**.

2.3.3 Damage Control Decision-Making[7]

Communication in damage control surgery and during resuscitation efforts, from an operational perspective, can be described in four phases (see **Figure 2.1**).

The critical decision-making process is typically started in the emergency department/trauma bay on arrival, and the surgeon together with the anaesthe-tist agree on, and plan for, damage control surgery and resuscitation. At this early start, evaluation of the futil-ity of care is also a legitimate consideration.

In the OR, or shortly before the commencement of surgery, the surgeon states the surgical plan based on the clinical and imaging findings (if present). The anaes-thesiologist states the transfusion status, the presence of coagulopathy, and any other evolving conditions that should be considered. During the damage control surgery and resuscitation, re-evaluation is performed every 10 minutes for the entire trauma or theatre team to maintain team situational awareness and allow effective anticipation and planning of all aspects of the care of the patient. In the re-evaluation, the surgeon states the surgical progress, developing problems, and future intentions, whilst the anaesthetist reports the elapsed time, transfusion status, developing coagulopathy, lactate levels, temperature, and other relevant developing problems.

It is critically important to incorporate multiple perspectives in the care of the trauma patient, including observations and cues from both the surgical and anaesthetic teams. In critical situations, it is easy to fall into pre-established ideas and, once triggered, difficult for your brain to be convinced otherwise. Intentionally taking brief intervals (e.g., every 20–30 minutes during the case) to step back and openly communicate between teams provides an optimal approach to surgical care of the injured patient.

Upon completion of surgery, the anaesthetist and surgeon recapitulate the patient's condition and the procedures performed and agree on the plan for the following 24–48 hours. They are responsible for ensuring transfer of relevant information internally in the team and externally with collaborators such as the blood bank, ICU, and so on. The trauma leader plans the tertiary survey within the following 24 hours.

2.4 LEADERSHIP IN TRAUMA CARE

Leadership is the key to effective trauma care. A good team leader should possess the ability to make quick decisions under pressure based on available information, plan and execute treatment strategies in cooperation with team members, regularly review the patient's response to treatment, and maintain an overview of the plan to follow including possible pitfalls to avoid. Communication should be concise and unambiguous, but at the same time the team leader should be open and responsive to input from *all* team members – medical, nursing, and allied disciplines. There are several ways of describing successful leadership; one is the NOTSS taxonomy identified by University of Aberdeen Industrial Psychology Research and the Royal College of Surgeons of Edinburgh, both in Scotland.[8] NOTSS can also be used for behavioural scoring and research. A multilevel assessment that is simulation based has been described (see **Table 2.1**).[9–12]

Table 2.1 Non-Technical Skills for Surgeons (NOTSS) Taxonomy

Category	Element
Situation awareness	• Gathering information • Understanding information • Projecting and anticipating future state
Decision-making	• Considering options • Selecting and communicating options • Implementing and reviewing decisions
Task management	• Planning and preparation • Flexibility/Responding to change
Leadership	• Setting and maintaining standards • Supporting others • Coping with pressure
Communication and teamwork	• Exchanging information • Establishing a shared understanding • Coordinating team activities

These non-technical skills are not learnt from a textbook; they are acquired and reinforced through training in simulated environments with professional instructors who have expertise in both the principles of CRM as well as briefing and debriefing.

Several NOTSS are particularly relevant for trauma management:

• Situational awareness
• Role allocation
• Decision-making
• Leadership
• Communication

2.4.1 Situational Awareness

Situational awareness is defined as 'the perception of elements in the environment within a volume of time and space, the comprehension of their meaning and the projection of their status in the near future'.[13]

This means that both the surgeon and anaesthesiologist should go beyond the information provided by the senses, integrate all available information with previous knowledge, and expand the consciousness both in physical space and in time. This is considered one of the most important NOTSS and usually requires some degree of clinical experience and previous exposure to similar situations. However, it can also be acquired and developed by the junior trainee.

Situational awareness starts immediately with pre-hospital notification. The AT-MIST information, although only indicative, can provide a glimpse of the potential clinical status of the patient and likely needs. A trigger for damage control surgery can start at this stage. After patient arrival and during initial assessment, situation awareness goes well beyond the patient's response to resuscitation. Both the resources, physical and human, and the environment come into play when deciding the predicted course of action. Intraoperatively, it can be difficult for all team members to attain and maintain situational awareness. During the operation, the surgeon, and sometimes the anaesthesiologist, will have to perform delicate procedures requiring *focus vision*, causing a decrease in situational awareness. Since there may be many and unexpected intraoperative adverse events, it is paramount that situational awareness be shared between the leaders of the trauma team – the surgeon and anaesthesiologist. A tool to prevent this is the use of routine timeouts and situation reports ('sit reps').[7] During these, provided there is temporary control of bleeding, the entire team briefs with a concise update. A useful structure for this is the TBCS (time/temperature, blood pressure/volume/gases, clotting, and surgical progress) mnemonic, a tool first developed in military advanced surgical hospitals but easily transferable to the civilian setting (see **Table 2.2**). By using this tool, the entire team can maintain situational awareness and avoid tunnel vision.

Table 2.2 TBCS Mnemonic for Intraoperative Timeouts

Periodic: 10 Seconds Every 10–30 Minutes	
T	**T**ime since the start of the procedure
	Temperature
B	**B**lood pressure
	Blood volume given so far
	Blood gases
C	**C**lotting (e.g., TEG or RoTEM)
S	**S**urgical progress

When a senior surgeon is available to scrub in, it is helpful that the assistant second surgeon maintains situational awareness, especially when the lead surgeon is on focus vision. Nonetheless, both surgeons' attention may be required in the operative field at times, making the use of intraoperative timeouts essential to keep situational awareness.

Finally, situational awareness not only should be about the patient, the resources, and the context, but also should contemplate the team members. Some team members may be overwhelmed, whilst others may be unused. The team leaders should use situational awareness to recognize and manage this.

2.4.2 Role Allocation

Whilst role allocation is flexible in the ER, with some members able to perform multiple tasks, it is usually obvious in the OR: the surgeons will perform the operation, and the anaesthesiologist will manage general anaesthesia and resuscitation. However, some degree of role allocation is required in the trauma OR, for instance for contacting the blood bank, placing lines, and bringing extra equipment. A good moment to do this is during patient handover from the ER to the OR, when all the team should brief. The scrub and anaesthesia nurses should have their role clearly defined, and all team members' names should be clearly identified. After this initial OR team briefing, the surgeon and anaesthesiologist can brief their respective nursing staff with more detail.

The surgeon's role during induction also requires allocation, particularly because the patient may require a surgical airway, or a chest decompression for a tension pneumothorax after positive pressure ventilation. A member of the surgical team should be clearly designated for these roles. Role allocation, like most NOTSS, requires excellent communication between the team members.

2.4.3 Decision-Making

The thought process used in decision-making can have two distinct pathways:[14]

- *Type 1 decisions* are based on pattern recognition, are intuitive, and require little mental effort. They are used for simple, daily tasks.
- *Type 2 decisions* use deductive processes, are logical and concept based, require mental work, and are thus slower.

In our daily life, we use them interchangeably.

In stressful scenarios, our brain is prompted to use type 1 decisions. A good example of knowing this thought process is the management of the bleeding patient. Both the experienced and the inexperienced surgeon will initially control bleeding with simple manoeuvres, for instance digital or manual compression of a bleeding artery. A less experienced surgeon will likely proceed to immediately clamp or obtain proximal and distal control, sometimes without proper exposure (type 1 decision). However, the experienced surgeon will more likely pause and assess his/her options, communicate with the anaesthesiologist to check on the patient status, and report the findings and the plan (type 2 decision).

Whilst training and experience may attenuate this trend towards repetitive type 1 use, a helpful tool is the intraoperative timeouts. By forcing a stop, they redirect the focus and can help the team members to weigh the options. Good team communication is paramount to proper information sharing and good decision-making.

2.4.4 Leadership

The leadership in a trauma OR must be shared. Whilst the indication for surgery (i.e., the decision to operate) rests on the surgeon, the actual conduct of the operation requires shared decisions with the anaesthesiologist. At critical moments, particularly during induction, cardiocirculatory arrest, or other severe unexpected events, it is desirable that the anaesthesiologist assumes a leadership role. Another time is when the surgeon's focus is too narrow to allow for a comprehensive view of the case, for instance during a procedure requiring focus, such as placing an intra-arterial shunt. Another example is during direct heart compressions, through a thoracotomy. The surgeon's attention is inevitably on making sure the field is dry and the aortic clamp is not slipping, and on the bimanual compressions. Thus, at this stage, it is the anaesthesiologist who is the team leader, deciding on drugs and timing of internal paddle defibrillation.

> *Good communication between the surgeon and anaesthesiologist is mandatory in order for this 'two-headed brain' to work.*

2.4.5 Communication

As is obvious from the previous sections, communication is, by far, the most important non-technical skill. Good communication is a team's greatest asset or its greatest drawback. In fact, it is estimated that 70%–80% of healthcare errors are due to poor communication.[15] Fortunately, there are rules for proper communication in emergency scenarios.

Good perioperative communication should use the principles of closed-loop communication, which are:

- Direct communication, using name
  - Preoperative OR team briefing should serve to know names and allocate roles.
- Visual contact, if possible
  - Obviously, the surgeon may not be able to do this if the surgical field requires attention.
- The recipient acknowledges the message and confirms that the message was clearly understood, and the task completed.

Closed-loop communication is associated with increased speed and efficiency of tasks in the resuscitation setting.[16]

Communication starts well before the operation starts, and it is mandatory during and essential after the operation is concluded. Nonetheless, there should be safeguards to avoid overcommunication. A good rule of thumb is to see communication as a drug or as a surgical instrument. It should be used in the proper timing and dosing. Interrupting the anaesthesiologist during a difficult airway, or the surgeon during a difficult supracoeliac aortic clamping, can be disturbing. During these moments, only game-changing information should be provided, such as sudden patient deterioration or severe, unexpected intraoperative events.

Trauma leaders should work towards 'meta-leadership', the ability to weave together multiple data inputs and teams to optimally care for the trauma patient. This includes having self-awareness of the situation, identifying the complexity in unknown situations, and being 'capable of influencing other team members (e.g., services) to collaborate in patient care'.[17] This is exemplified in an adaptation of the VUCA acronym:

- *Volatile*: The trauma patient is unstable and may have dynamic physiology.
- *Uncertain*: The sources of bleeding or injury may not be completely understood early during surgical care.
- *Complex*: Multisystem injury requires the input of multiple specialists (e.g., polytrauma patient with concomitant brain, hollow-viscous, vascular, and orthopaedic injuries).

• *Ambiguous*: Unclear diagnoses and best next treatment options may exist (e.g., when initially unknown in a polytrauma patient, hypotension may be secondary to haemorrhage, cardiac blunting, or neurogenic shock).

2.5 A SIX-STEP APPROACH TO PERIOPERATIVE COMMUNICATION IN TRAUMA

There are key moments in the patient's path through the OR, including immediately before and after, that mandate that the whole team is coordinated. Relevant data, such as the patient's physiology, suspected injuries, resources that are needed, and potential hazards, should be shared.

This can be achieved with proper communication, which can be divided into six distinct stages (see **Table 2.3** below):

Step 1 – Before patient arrival: OR team notice

• A pre hospital notification of the ER of a severely injured patient should prompt immediate preparations in the OR for a damage control procedure.
• Although precise information is rarely obtained at this stage, several key data from the AT-MIST should alert the OR team to ensure surgical material and anaesthetic equipment are ready.
• It is desirable that both the surgeon and anaesthesiologist are part of the ER team in the preparation for the patient's arrival; if not, step 3 becomes even more relevant.

Step 2 – After patient arrival in ED: Decision and preparation for emergency surgery

• Decision for emergency surgery should be swiftly communicated to the remaining OR team, including OR nurses as well as assistant surgeons and the anaesthetic team (if not already present in the ER), in order to ensure that everything is ready to receive the patient in the OR and start the damage control surgery.
• Whilst this turns a potential activation into a real one, the preliminary steps taken in step 1 have made this stage easier.
• In some hospital settings, steps 1 and 2 are done together.

Step 3 – Before surgery: Preoperative communication

• This is a key moment in the OR and a potentially hazardous one. It requires a handover of information from the ER to the OR team, particularly if the anaesthesiologist was not already present in the ER resuscitation. OR nurses should be briefed on the status, potential injuries, and required resources. It is useful that the OR nursing team be allocated to positions – anaesthesiology assistant, scrub, and circulation – and quickly receive further information; all the team members' names should be known.
• A key moment is anaesthetic induction, and there is real potential for patient deterioration. Loss of airway ('can't intubate, can't ventilate' scenario), tension pneumothorax, and immediate cardiovascular collapse (due to loss of muscle tone and cardiovascular depression from anaesthetic drugs) require that anaesthesiology and surgical teams coordinate their action. The surgical team should be scrubbed and gowned, and the patient prepped, before induction. Good role allocation and shared leadership are required, besides optimal communication.
• Just before the incision, there should be a brief pause in which the entire OR team participates to present the surgical plan and the patient's clinical status, and to confirm that all materials, drugs, and blood products are available.

Step 4 – During surgery: Intraoperative communication

• During surgery, immediate control of bleeding is the priority, and once this is achieved the surgeon should request a short timeout. This will allow the team to pause, update status, and reassess, avoiding spiralling into repeated type 1 decisions. This timeout, using the TBCS tool, will be useful to grasp the physiology, which is dynamic, and plan the next move.
• The decision to perform a damage control procedure should be clearly announced to the whole team.
• Regular intraoperative communication at intervals, again using the TBCS, will allow the team to 'steer' the patient's status more accurately; indeed, a patient initially planned to have a damage control procedure who recovers well with damage control resuscitation may be treated with definitive surgery; in these cases, the decision for definitive surgery should be clearly stated.

Table 2.3 Six-Step Approach to Perioperative Communication in Trauma Surgery

- Keep it clear, concise, and objective.
- Avoid information overflow.
- Use direct and closed-loop communication.
- Keep a calm and collected attitude: 'It's just another day at the job'.

STEP 1 – BEFORE Patient arrives at the hospital / OR	STEP 2 – PREPARE Everything before the patient arrives at the hospital / OR
• A – Age of patient • T – Time • M – Mechanism of injury • I – Injuries found • S – Signs • T – Treatment administered	Surgeon ← → Scrub nurse Anaesthetist ← → Anaesthesia nurse Contact: Blood bank ICU Angiography

STEP 3 – BEFORE Surgery	STEP 4 – DURING Surgery

Surgeon
 	
• Correct patient
• Clinical and imaging findings
• Surgical plan
 	
Anaesthesiologist
 	
• T: Temperature (patient and OR)
• C: Clotting (TEG or RoTEM)
• Confirm: Antibiotics / TXA / Blood.
• Communicate plan for induction.
 	
Nurses
 	
• Needs for damage control surgery
• Needs for damage control anaesthesia
	AFTER INITIAL CONTROL OF SURGICAL BLEEDING
	
	• What was found?
	• What is the initial plan?
	• Damage control surgery vs. definitive surgery.
	
	PERIODIC: 10 SECONDS EVERY 10–30 MINUTES
	
	• T Time since the start of the procedure
	   Temperature
	
	• B Blood pressure
	   Blood volume given
	   Blood gases
	
	• C Clotting (e.g., TEG or RoTEM)
	• S Surgical process and plan
	
	DURING CRITICAL MANOEUVRES
	
	• Packing, rotation, clamping, and unclamping

STEP 5 – SIGN-OUT	STEP 6 – TEAM DEBRIEF

• Summarize the patient's injuries/physiology.
• What has been done? Surgeon/anaesthesiologist?
• What has been left untreated?
• Document number of packs and/or instruments left inside.
• What is the plan now?
• Where is the patient going? ICU/angiography?
• Plan for pharmacological support.
   ◦ Antibiotic
   ◦ Thromboprophylaxis
	• Immediately after the sign-out
	• What went well?
	• What could be improved?
	• Technical skills
	• Non-technical skills
	• What did we learn for the next case?

- Intraoperative communication is also critical during key surgical manoeuvres that have significant physiologic impact, such as liver rotation, major vessel clamping and unclamping, hepatic or renal hilar clamping, or heart mobilization. This requires closed-loop communication in order to properly coordinate the team.

Step 5 – Sign-out: Before patient leaves the OR

- This is another critical moment. Both the surgical (swab and instrument count, injuries found, procedures performed, and timing of expected second-look) and anaesthetic records (blood products, venous accesses, drugs, physiological status, and past medical history from records) should be summarized and known by both the surgical and anaesthetic teams.
- The probabilities of other associated injuries being present should be addressed at this stage, and the patient's status reviewed, in order to decide between immediate transfer to CT or to the ICU.
- Again, the TBCS tool is helpful to summarize what was done and what the response was.
- Contact with the ICU team, ideally performed at step 2, is mandatory at this stage to update the patient's status and define a plan (e.g., timing of second-look or definitive abdominal closure).

Stage 6 – Team debriefing[18]

- A trauma damage control room can be an intense and at times off-putting experience, causing moral damage to the team members and potentially contributing to feelings of helplessness and burnout; this is particularly true when there was significant interpersonal tension or communication issues, or when the patient died in the OR.
- It is difficult to gather the whole team after the operation for a number of reasons (reallocation to other clinical tasks, shifts ending, lack of belief in debriefing, and fear of accusation of misconduct). However, it is desirable to assemble the team, particularly after a challenging case.
- There are several strategies to conduct a postcritical debriefing. One way to start is to have the facilitator clearly state that every team member performed at the best of their individual skills and that the debriefing will only focus on the teamwork. This may help in taking down some barriers to a frank discussion.
- Every trauma case is a learning opportunity to improve. Debriefing will help in this and may improve team cohesion. Good judgement is mandatory.

2.6 POTENTIAL ERRORS RELATED TO EACH BEHAVIOURAL THEME

Error is normal,
Therefore, do not blame error,
but anticipate it and prevent it.

Errors will occur. By understanding the potential pitfalls, and with a mind-set like that in the aviation environment, they can be minimized (see **Table 2.4**).

Table 2.4 Potential Errors Related to Each Behavioural Theme

Themes	Potential Errors
Cognitive Skills – Situational Awareness	
Mechanism	• Failure to obtain data from the pre-hospital setting • Failure to incorporate knowledge of mechanism into understanding of potential forces that the patient has been subjected to, or which structures may potentially have been injured
Physiologic burden	• Failure to obtain vital signs from pre-hospital setting • Failure to evaluate for neurological status • Failure to assess need for airway control • Failure to evaluate for respiratory status • Failure to evaluate for haemodynamic status • Failure to take into consideration trend in physiologic parameters • Failure to take into consideration timing of physiologic parameters

(Continued)

Table 2.4 (*Continued*) Potential Errors Related to Each Behavioural Theme

Themes	Potential Errors
Cognitive Skills – Situational Awareness	
Injury and pattern recognition	• Failure to recognize a critical/unstable patient and lacking awareness of the overall trauma burden • Failure to pick up on the subtle cues that suggest severe injury
Active and confirmatory reconciliation	• Failure to evaluate response to treatment • Failure to consistently reassess diagnoses and management plans
Data processing and metacognition	• Losing sight of the bigger picture by focusing too much on irrelevant details (inattentional blindness or tunnel vision) • Allowing nonempirical data and biases to influence judgement
Environmental limitations	• Lacking awareness of the resources of the institution, thereby leading to delays • Failure to call for additional resources and personnel when necessary • Transferring the patient without rendering the patient safe for transfer
Self-limitations	• Failure to recognize when a given situation surpasses one's abilities (e.g., due to skill set, experience, comfort level, and/or fatigue) • Failure to call for additional personnel when help is needed
Cognitive Skills – Decision-Making	
Forward planning	• Minimizing severity of injuries • Failure to mobilize the proper resources in a timely fashion • Failure to plan for worst-case scenarios and potential patient deterioration
Managing the injury	• Failure to follow ATLS protocols • Failure to follow best-practice guidelines and established management algorithms • Failure to investigate all body cavities to determine site of injury
Prioritizing	• Under-triaging patients • Failure to address life-threatening injuries before nonurgent injuries
Escalation of aggressiveness	• Devising and implementing a management plan that is not aggressive enough • Devising and implementing a management plan that is inappropriately aggressive
Interpersonal Skills – Leadership	
	• Failure to introduce yourself as team leader • Ineffective coordination of team members (e.g., losing control of team members) • Overly micromanaging specific tasks instead of acting as the leader • Inability to cope under pressure in a chaotic environment • Failure to provide feedback to team members on performance
Interpersonal Skills – Teamwork and Communication	
	• Failure to establish team member roles ahead of time • Failure to listen to other team members • Failure to obtain confirmation of task delegation (closed-loop communication) • Failure to effectively share management plan with other team members • Failure to limit the physical environment to necessary personnel only

Source: Reproduced with permission: Madani A et al. *J Surg Educ.* 2018; 75(2):365.

2.7 SUMMARY

Trauma care is particularly challenging, in that decisions and interventions are extremely time sensitive. Factors such as injury severity, physiology, and interdisciplinary specialist interactions combine to compound the risk of error in high-stress situations, and elicit the same responses as in the aviation environment. Advance planning, good leadership, effective teamwork, clear communication, and the timeous anticipation of problems when possible will minimize risks to the patient.

In the trauma OR, the patient is usually in a critical condition. This requires that every team member is at the best of their individual, technical skills. But this is not enough, as excellent individual performance does not guarantee excellent team performance. Proper knowledge of non-technical skills, particularly excellent communication, is paramount to a good outcome. Fortunately, undergraduate curricula are becoming increasingly aware of this, and NOTSS is becoming routine in many medical schools. The opportunity that the DSTC and joint DATC–DSTC courses provide for a realistic, immersive simulation training in a bleeding model should be used to also promote team training.

Pearls and pitfalls

- Failure to properly address the non-technical aspects of a trauma operation can jeopardize the patient's management, increase the likelihood of hazards and errors, and lead to worse outcomes.
- Intraoperative timeouts, or sit reps, can help maintain proper team situational awareness and assist with decision-making. Closed-loop communication should be used.
- Communication can be a team's greatest asset or its greatest flaw. A stepwise approach to perioperative communication, emphasizing key pre-, intra-, and postoperative moments, is paramount to ensure smooth teamwork.

REFERENCES AND RECOMMENDED READING

References

1. Cohen TN, Cabrera JS, Litzinger TL, Captain KA, Fabian MA, Miles SG, et al. Proactive safety management in trauma care: applying the human factors analysis and classification system. *J Healthc Qual.* 2018 Mar/Apr;**40(2)**:89–96. doi: 10.1097/JHQ.0000000000000094.

2. Alexandrino H, Baptista S, Vale L, Júnior JHZ, Espada PC, Junior DS, et al. Improving intraoperative communication in trauma: the educational effect of the joint DSTC™–DATC™ courses. *World J Surg.* 2020 Jun;**44(6)**:1856–62. doi: 10.1007/s00268-020-05421-5.

3. 'James Reason's Swiss Cheese Theory'. Available from: http://www.researchomatic.com/James-Reasons-Swiss-Cheese-Theory-129350.html (accessed 27 online July 2023).

4. Reason JT, Carthey J, de Leval MR. Diagnosing "vulnerable system syndrome": an essential prerequisite to effective risk management. *Qual Health Care.* 2001 Dec;**10(Suppl 2)**:ii21–5. doi: 10.1136/qhc.0100021.

5. Catchpole K, Ley E, Wiegmann D, Blaha J, Shouhed D, Gangi A, et al. A human factors subsystems approach to trauma care. *JAMA Surg.* 2014 Sep;**149(9)**:962–8. doi: 10.1001/jamasurg.2014.1208.

6. Marcus L, McNulty E, Henderson JM, Dorn BC. You're It: Crisis, Change, and How to Lead When It Matters most. 2019. https://www.leadershipnow.com/leading-blog/2020/06/youre_it_the_call_for_metalead.html (accessed online August 2023).

7. Arul GS, Pugh HE, Mercer SJ, Midwinter MJ. Optimising communication in the damage control resuscitation: damage control surgery sequence in major trauma management. *J Roy Army Med Corps.* 2012 Jun;**158(2)**:82–4. doi: 10.1136/jramc-158-02-03.

8. Non-Technical Skills for Surgeons (NOTSSS) System Handbook V2.0 University of Aberdeen and Royal College of Surgeons of Edinburgh, Scotland. 2019. Available from: efaidnbmnnnibpcajpcglclefindmkaj/https://www.rcsed.ac.uk/media/682516/notss-system-handbook-v20.pdf

9. Doumouras AG, Keshet I, Nathens AB, Ahmed N, Hicks CM. Trauma Non-Technical Training (TNT-2): the development, piloting, and multilevel assessment of a simulation-based, interprofessional curriculum for team-based trauma resuscitation. *Can J Surg.* 2014 Oct;**57(5)**:354–5. doi: 10.1503/cjs.000814.

10. Hicks C, Petrosoniak A. The human factor: optimizing trauma team performance in dynamic clinical environments. *Emerg Med Clin North Am.* 2018 Feb;**36(1)**:1–17. doi: 10.1016/j.emc.2017.08.003.

11. Hughes KM, Benenson RS, Krichten AE, Clancy KD, Ryan JP, Hammond C. A crew resource management program tailored to trauma resuscitation improves team behaviour and communication. *J Am Coll Surg.* 2014 Sept;**219(3)**:545–51. doi: 10.1016/j.jamcollsurg.2014.03.049.

12. McCulloch P, Rathbone J, Catchpole K. Interventions to improve teamwork and communications among health care staff. *Br J Surg.* 2011 Apr;**98(4)**:469–79. doi: 10.1002/bjs.7434.

13. Endsley MR. Measurement of situation awareness in dynamic systems. *Human Factors.* 1995;**37(1)**:65–84. doi: 10.1518/001872095779049499.

14. Yu R. Stress potentiates decision biases: a stress induced deliberation-to-intuition (SIDI) model. *Neurobiol Stress.* 2016 Feb;**12(3)**:83–95. doi: 10.1016/j.ynstr.2015.12.006. eCollection 2016 Jun.

15. Hayden EM, Wong AH, Ackerman J, Sande MK, Lei C, Kobayashi L, et al. Human factors and simulation in emergency medicine. *Acad Emerg Med.* 2018 Feb;**25(2)**:221–9. doi: 10.1111/acem.13315. Epub 2017 Nov 15.

16. El-Shafy IA, Delgado J, Akerman M, Bullaro F, Christopherson NAM, Prince JM. Closed-loop communication improves task completion in pediatric trauma resuscitation. *J Surg Educ.* 2018 Jan-Feb;**75(1)**:58–64. doi: 10.1016/j.jsurg.2017.06.025.

17. Alkhaldi KH, Austin ML, Cura BA, Dantzler D, Holland L, Maples DL, et al. Are you ready? crisis leadership in a hyper-VUCA environment. *Am J Disaster Med.* 2017 Spring;**12(2)**:107–34. doi: 10.5055/ajdm.2017.0265.

18. Madani A, Gips A, Razek T, Deckelbaum DL, Mulder DS, Grushka JR. Defining and measuring decision-making for the management of trauma patients. *J Surg Educ.* 2018 Mar - Apr;**75(2)**:358–69. doi: 10.1016/j.jsurg.2017.t07.012.

Recommended Reading

The Non-Technical Skills for Surgeons (NOTSS) System Handbook V2.0 University of Aberdeen and Royal College of Surgeons of Edinburgh, Scotland. 2019. Available from: efaidnbmnnnibpcajpcglclefindmkaj/https://www.rcsed.ac.uk/media/682516/notss-system-handbook-v20.pdf

Hughes KM, Benenson RS, Kritchten AE, Clancy KD, Ryan JP, Hammond C. A crew resource management program tailored to trauma resuscitation improves team behaviour and communication. *J Am Coll Surg.* 2014 Sep;**219(3)**:545–51. doi: 10.1016/j.jamcollsurg.2014.03.049. Epub 2014 May 2.

Marcus LJ, McNulty EJ, Henderson JM, Dorn BC, et al. *You're It: Crisis, Change, and How to Lead When it Matters Most.* Public Affairs, New York. 2019.

Part 2

Physiology and the body's response to trauma

___

Resuscitation Physiology **3**

3.1 METABOLIC RESPONSE TO TRAUMA

3.1.1 Definition of Trauma

Physical injury is accompanied by systemic as well as local effects. The body responds to kinetic energy transfer to it by local and systemic inflammation. The inflammation is triggered by mechanosensitive ion channel proteins PIEZO1 and PIEZO2 receptors on the cell surface, which detect pressure changes and open ion channels. Cells can actively release danger signals (e.g., molecules which are normally not extracellular, like mitochondrial components) or can release their components due to necrosis. The innate immune system differentiates the 'injured self' from the 'intact self' and initiates an inflammatory response via cellular and humoral mechanisms. This metabolic response to trauma traditionally was divided into an *ebb phase* and a *flow phase* by Cuthbertson in 1932:[1]

> *The ebb phase is relatively short lived and corresponds to the period of severe shock characterized by depression of enzymatic activity and oxygen consumption. After effective resuscitation has been accomplished with restoration of adequate oxygen transport, the flow phase comes into play.*

The flow phase can be divided into:

- A catabolic phase with fat and protein mobilization associated with increased urinary nitrogen excretion and weight loss.
- An anabolic phase with restoration of fat and protein stores, and weight gain.

The appropriate protective flow phase is characterized by:

- A normal or slightly elevated blood glucose level
- Increased glucose production
- Normal or slightly elevated free fatty acid levels, with increased flux
- A normal or elevated insulin concentration
- High-normal or elevated levels of catecholamine and glucagon
- A normal blood lactate level
- Elevated oxygen consumption
- Increased cardiac output
- Elevated core temperature

These responses are marked by hyperdynamic circulatory changes, signs of inflammation, glucose intolerance, and muscle wasting.

3.1.2 Initiating Factors

The magnitude of the metabolic response depends on the degree of trauma and concomitant contributory factors such as hypovolaemia (blood loss), infection, tissue necrosis, and pre-existing systemic disease. The response will also depend on the age and sex of the patient, the genetic composition, the underlying nutritional state, and the timing of treatment and its effectiveness. In general, the more severe the injury (i.e., the greater the degree of tissue damage), the greater the metabolic response.

The metabolic response alterations seem to be less aggressive in children and the elderly and in the premenopausal female. Starvation and nutritional depletion also modify the response. Patients with poor nutritional or immunological status have a reduced metabolic response to trauma compared to healthy well-nourished patients,

DOI: 10.1201/9781003258124-5

whilst burns and severe traumatic brain injury (TBI) cause a relatively greater response than other mechanical injuries.

Wherever possible, efforts should be made to reduce the magnitude and duration of the initial insult, since by doing so it may be possible to reduce the extent of the metabolic changes. Thus, aggressive resuscitation, control of pain and temperature, limiting acidosis, adequate debridement of devitalized tissue, avoidance of unnecessary blood component administration with coagulopathy, and nutritional (preferably enteral) support are critical.

3.1.2.1 HYPOVOLAEMIA

Hypovolaemia, specifically tissue hypoperfusion, is the most potent precipitator of the metabolic response. This is due primarily to decreased circulating blood volume from trauma, and capillary leak, the latter occurring mostly from disruption of the endothelial glycocalyx due to activation of the inflammatory process. (See Section 3.2.) Simultaneously, there is activation of systemic responses with activation of the coagulation cascade and contraction of bleeding vessels and platelet activation (both by thromboxane A2).

The damaged vessel exposes collagen and, with the endothelial release of tissue factor, results in fibrin deposition and, ultimately, mature clot formation approximately 24 hours later. The initial response of the cardiovascular system is to increase cardiac output (CO) by increasing stroke volume (SV, or myocardial contractility), heart rate, and vasoconstriction of peripheral blood vessels, all due to catecholamine release.[2]

Renin secretion from the juxtaglomerular apparatus is increased with conversion of angiotensinogen to angiotensin I and angiotensin II by the lungs and liver. The latter causes vasoconstriction and stimulates aldosterone secretion by the adrenal cortex with sodium and water reabsorption. Simultaneously, due to the hypotension, antidiuretic hormone (ADH) is secreted from the hypothalamus and pituitary, also with reabsorption of water.

3.1.2.2 INFLAMMATION

The *innate* immune response is initiated by tissue injury which activates a diverse response via release of damage-associated molecular patterns (DAMPs) and pathogen-associated molecular patterns (PAMPs) which bind to pattern recognition receptors (PRRs) of four main classes: Toll-like receptors (TLRs), NOD-like receptors

(NLRs), RIG-I-like receptors (RLRs), and C-type lectin receptors (CLRs).[3]

DAMPs include formyl peptides, cytochrome C, cardiolipin, heat shock protein 70 (HSP70), high-mobility group box 1 (HMGB1), and cell-free DNA (cfDNA). PAMPs may be involved through translocation from gut ischaemia, although there is evidence that this is not an important acute cause of inflammation in humans with traumatic injury.[3]

PRRs, through activation of intracellular kinases, activate nuclear factor kappa B (NFκB) with transcription of proinflammatory cytokines and interferons via interferon release factor (IRF). Uncontrolled activation of endogenous inflammatory mediators and cells manifests as the systemic inflammatory response syndrome (SIRS) which is accompanied by activation of the neuro-endocrine system with mobilization of peripheral white blood cells, resulting in leucocytosis. As such, SIRS is characterized by elevated interleukin-1 (IL-1), IL-2, IL-6, IL-12, tumour necrosis factor (TNF), interferon (IFN), and the complement components C3a and C5a.[3]

These cytokines – in particular, TNF and IL-18 – stimulate NK cells, macrophages, and T cells and increase the production of inducible nitric oxide synthase (iNOS) from the endothelium with production of nitric oxide (NO) and cyclo-oxygenase (both causing vasodilatation), and activation of coagulation by release of tissue factor.

The cellular *adaptive* immune response follows the acute activation of the innate immune response. This is initiated by activation of the antigen-presenting cell (APC) by the PRR–DAMP/PAMP complex which presents antigens via the major histocompatibility complex class II to undifferentiated T lymphocytes. This, along with cytokines from the APC and cluster of differentiation 80 (CD80) or CD86, activates and results in differentiation of T cells. B cells are simultaneously activated, differentiate into memory B cells and plasma cells, and are responsible for the production of immunoglobulins (see **Figure 3.1**).

After tissue injury, DAMPs and/or PAMPs bind to PRRs on APCs. This results in the release of proinflammatory cytokines via NFkB, NETosis (NETs are neutrophil extracellular traps) via TLR4, and, via the oligomerization of NLRs, inflammasomes are formed and activate Pro-IL-1B and Pro-IL-18. Activated APCs activate T cells and B cells. T cells differentiate into effector T cells: T helper cells (Th1 and Th2) and T regulatory cells (T-regs).

Simultaneously, there is initiation of an anti-inflammatory response. Myeloid cells (macrophages and

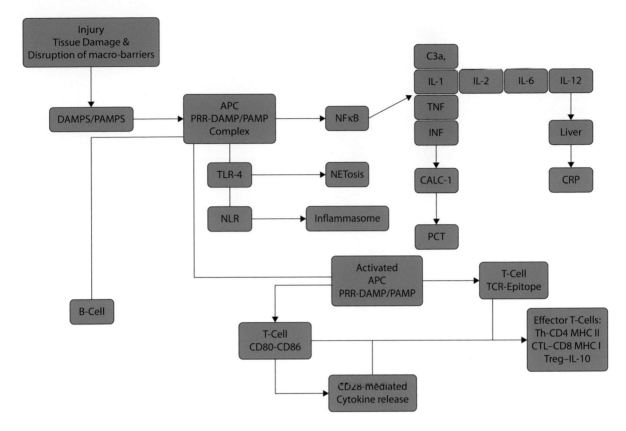

Figure 3.1 Injury-induced immune activation.[3]

neutrophils) are consumed along with the release of growth factors and cytokines. These, in concert with activation of the sympathetic nervous system with release of catecholamines, stimulate production and release of myeloid cells from the bone marrow and lymphoid tissue which results in a relative lymphopenia.

Trauma-induced inflammation can lead to aberrant myeloid differentiation with production of myeloid-derived suppressor cells (MDSCs) which, through stimulation of CD40 cells, upregulate the programmed death ligand 1 (PD-L1), suppressing T-cell proliferation and upregulating T-regulatory cells (T-regs. These latter regulate the inflammatory response through stimulation of IL-0 which inhibits the effects of IL-1, IL-6, and IL-8 and TNFα. MDSCs also directly increase secretion of IL-10 Hand TGFß which further stimulate T-regs and favour a type II macrophage response responsible for tissue repair. MDSCs deplete L-arginine, a substrate for NO production in macrophages, to improve bactericidal activity, and they moderate T-cell function, proliferation, and

maturation.[4] MDSCs also increase reactive oxygen species (ROS) production which induces T-cell apoptosis and, through formation of peroxynitrites, reduces T-cell responsiveness (see **Figure 3.2**).

Following injury consumption of myeloid cells, cytokine release and adrenergic activation stimulate the bone marrow and lymphoid tissue to increase the differentiation and release of myeloid cells (emergency myelopoiesis) at the expense of lympho- and haematopoiesis. This results in the activation of an aberrant differentiation pathway and the release of MDSCs. MDSCs have pleiotropic immunosuppressive consequences via the stimulation of CD40 and upregulation of T-cell protein death 1 (PD1) receptors, inducing T-cell suppression and apoptosis. MDSCs also secrete anti-inflammatory cytokines, and they depress the T-cell intracellular signalling by the increased metabolism of L-arginine. Finally, MDSCs increase T-cell apoptosis and responsiveness via the release of ROS.

Endothelial dysfunction is a critical component of the inflammatory response. The endothelial glycocalyx (EG)

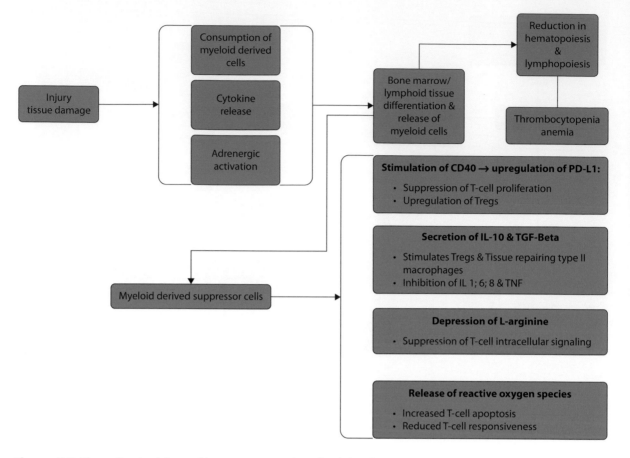

Figure 3.2 The pathophysiology of immunosuppression after injury.[3]

is a non-circulating 1 mm thick fluid layer on the endothelial surface, within which are membrane-bound glycoproteins and glycosaminoglycans.[5] The EG functions to separate cellular blood components from the endothelium and maintains osmotic tension of the intravascular compartment.[6] The inflammatory response, specifically TNFα and oxidative stress, causes disruption of the EG, exposing the endothelium and allowing adhesion, clumping, and activation of platelets with degranulation and release of vasoactive substances. This, along with tissue factor release, promotes coagulation and capillary leak.[7]

3.1.2.3 THE CONSEQUENCES OF THE PRO- AND ANTI-INFLAMMATORY RESPONSES

SIRS can lead ultimately to multiple organ dysfunction syndrome (MODS) and multiple organ failure (MOF), which are associated with a mortality rate of up to 50%. Early after severe injury or sepsis, the pro-inflammatory response predominates, and SIRS and shock also predominate. Thereafter, recovery may occur; however, if the suppressive response is excessive, it leads to immunosuppression and greatly increased susceptibility to nosocomial infections, which are frequently seen in severely injured and critically ill patients.

3.1.2.4 COAGULATION AND INFLAMMATION

Coagulation and inflammation are closely interlinked processes, as depicted in **Figure 3.3**.

Pro-inflammatory mediators have a role in triggering the clotting cascade by stimulating the release of tissue factor from monocytes and the vascular endothelium, leading to thrombin formation and a fibrin clot. At the same time, thrombin stimulates the inflammatory response by activating NFκB and suppresses natural anticoagulant responses by activating thrombin-activatable fibrinolysis inhibitor (TAFI). This overall

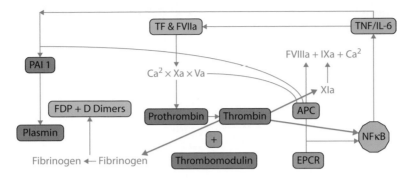

Figure 3.3 The relationship between coagulation and inflammation. *Abbreviations*: APC, activated protein C; EPCR, endothelial protein C receptor; FDPs, fibrin degradation products; IL-6, interleukin-6; NfκB, nuclear factor kappa B; PAI1, plasmin activator inhibitor-1; TF, tissue factor; TNF, tumour necrosis factor.

procoagulant response leads to microvascular thrombosis and is implicated in MOF associated with sepsis. On the other hand, thrombin binding to endothelial thrombomodulin generates activated protein C (APC), which is an endogenous anticoagulant, inhibiting factors 5 and 8. It also binds to an endothelial protein C receptor which has an inhibitory effect on transcription via NFκB. Plasminogen activator inhibitor-1 (PAI1) is a procoagulant molecule that inhibits tissue plasminogen activation, thrombomodulin, and APC. PAI1 is released by platelets as well as endothelium in response to inflammation, damage, or ischaemia. This adds to the perturbation of the coagulation process and contributes to bleeding as clotting factors are consumed.

3.2 HORMONAL MEDIATORS

In response to trauma, many circulatory hormones are altered. Adrenaline (epinephrine), noradrenaline (norepinephrine), cortisol, and glucagon are increased, whilst certain others are decreased. The sympathetic–adrenal axis is a major system by which the body's response to injury is activated.

3.2.1 Hypothalamus–Pituitary Axis[8]

The hypothalamus is the highest level of integration of the stress response. The major efferent pathways of the hypothalamus are endocrine via the pituitary, and the efferent sympathetic and parasympathetic systems. In contrast, the cholinergic system is now recognized to have a variety of anti-inflammatory effects. The pituitary gland responds to trauma with increased levels of adrenocorticotrophic hormone (ACTH), prolactin, and growth hormone, whilst the remaining hormones are relatively unchanged.

Pain receptors, osmoreceptors, baroreceptors, and chemoreceptors stimulate or inhibit ganglia in the hypothalamus to induce sympathetic nerve activity. The neural endplates and adrenal medulla secrete catecholamines. Pain stimuli via the pain receptors also stimulate secretion of endogenous opiates, β-endorphin, and pro-opiomelanocorticotrophin (precursor of the adrenocorticotrophin [ACTH]), which modifies the response to pain and reinforces the catecholamine effects. The β-endorphin has little effect but serves as a marker for anterior pituitary secretion.

Hypotension, hypovolaemia in the form of a decrease in left ventricular (LV) pressure, and hyponatraemia stimulate secretion of vasopressin, ADH from the supra-optic nuclei in the anterior hypothalamus, aldosterone from the adrenal cortex, and renin from the juxtaglomerular apparatus of the kidney. The increase in aldosterone secretion results in conservation of sodium and, thereby, water. As osmolality increases, the secretion of ADH increases, and more water is reabsorbed, thereby decreasing the serum osmolality (negative feedback control system).

Hypovolaemia stimulates receptors in the right atrium (RA), and hypotension stimulates receptors in the carotid artery. This results in activation of paraventricular hypothalamic nuclei, which secrete pituitary-releasing hormone from the median eminence into capillary blood, which stimulates the anterior pituitary to secrete ACTH. ACTH stimulates the adrenal cortex to secrete cortisol and aldosterone. Changes in glucose concentration influence the release of insulin from the β cells of the pancreas, and high amino acid levels affect the release of glucagon from the α cells.

3.2.2 Adrenal Hormones

Plasma cortisol and glucagon levels rise following trauma. The degree is related to the severity of injury. The function of glucocorticoid secretion in the initial metabolic response is uncertain, since the hormones have little direct action, and primarily they seem to augment the effects of other hormones such as the catecholamines.

3.2.3 Pancreatic Hormones

There is a rise in the blood sugar following trauma related to insulin resistance which occurs due to increases in adrenaline, growth hormone, and glucagon.[9]

3.2.4 Renal Hormones

Aldosterone secretion is increased by several mechanisms. The renin–angiotensin mechanism is the most important. When the glomerular arteriolar inflow pressure falls, the juxtaglomerular apparatus of the kidney secretes renin, which acts with angiotensinogen to form angiotensin I. This is converted to angiotensin II, a substance that stimulates production of aldosterone by the adrenal cortex. Reduction in sodium concentration stimulates the macula densa, a specialized area in the tubular epithelium adjacent to the juxtaglomerular apparatus, to activate renin release. An increase in plasma potassium concentration also stimulates aldosterone release. Volume losses and a fall in arterial pressure stimulate release of ACTH via receptors in the RA and the carotid artery.

3.2.5 Other Hormones

Atrial natriuretic factor (ANF) or peptide (ANP) is a hormone produced by the atria, along with brain or B-type natriuretic peptide (BNP) produced by the ventricular muscle cells, in response to an increase in vascular volume and thus distension and pressure.[10] ANF and BNP produce similar increases in glomerular filtration and pronounced natriuresis and diuresis to decrease intravascular volume by inhibition of aldosterone which also minimizes kaliuresis. In addition, ANP causes disruption of the EG, as described above, which acutely decreases intravascular volume.

3.3 EFFECTS OF THE VARIOUS MEDIATORS

3.3.1 Hyperdynamic State

Following illness or injury, the systemic inflammatory response occurs, which manifests with tachycardia, widened pulse pressure (PP), and a greater CO. There is an increase in the metabolic rate, with an increase in oxygen consumption, increased protein catabolism, and hyperglycaemia.

There is no 'normal' cardiac index. It could be normally abnormal, in that the cardiac index may exceed a theoretical normal of 4.5 L/min/m² after severe trauma in those patients able to respond. This is usually accompanied by a decrease in systemic vascular resistance (SVR) due to endothelial NO release with an increase in microcirculatory oxygen delivery. This hyperdynamic state elevates the resting energy expenditure significantly above normal, total body oxygen consumption (VO_2) is increased, and, due to the metabolic response and increased metabolic rate, core temperature may be increased. The response of the heart may also be abnormally normal, where the CO fails to rise appropriately or may even be depressed. In this case, oxygen delivery and therefore consumption may fall to values of less than 100 mL/min/m² (theoretical normal = 120–160 mL/min/m²). Mitochondrial dysfunction due to reactive oxidant production may limit utilization of oxygen for oxidative phosphorylation.

The amount of adenosine triphosphate (ATP) synthesized by an adult is considerable. However, there is no reservoir of ATP or creatinine phosphate; therefore, mitochondrial injury and a decrease in oxygen delivery result in rapid deterioration of ATP production (via glycolysis), and lactate is produced. Because of anaerobic glycolysis, only two ATP equivalents instead of 34 are produced from 1 mol of glucose in the Krebs cycle. Lactate is formed from pyruvate, which is the end product of glycolysis. It is normally reconverted to glucose in the Cori cycle in the liver. However, in shock, the oxidative reduction (redox) potential declines, and conversion of pyruvate to acetyl coenzyme A (acetyl-CoA) for entry into the Krebs cycle is inhibited. Lactate therefore accumulates because of impaired hepatic gluconeogenesis due to hepatic hypoperfusion, causing metabolic acidosis.

Lactic acidosis after injury equals mitochondrial dysfunction. Mitochondria drive cellular energy transformation from food to ATP, and control cell death and cell reproduction, that is, 'power, sex, suicide'.[11] This correlates with the Injury Severity Score (ISS) and is an early and important clinical sign of acute blood loss, reflecting tissue hypoperfusion. Persistent lactic acidosis can be indicative of inadequate resuscitation and predictive of the development of MOF and acute respiratory distress syndrome (ARDS). Lactate can, however, also be elevated by liver injury, alcohol, and various drugs.

3.3.2 Water and Salt Retention

Secretion of ADH from the supra-optic nuclei in the anterior hypothalamus is stimulated by volume reduction and increased osmolality of the plasma. The latter is due mainly to increased sodium content of the extracellular fluid. Volume receptors are in the atria and pulmonary arteries, and osmoreceptors are located near ADH neurones in the hypothalamus. ADH acts mainly on the connecting tubules of the kidney but also on the distal tubules to promote reabsorption of water. This adds to the potential for fluid overload and, along with excessive crystalloid administration and capillary leak, can lead to the development of oedema.

Aldosterone acts mainly on the distal renal tubules to promote reabsorption of sodium and bicarbonate and increased excretion of potassium. According to Stewart's principles, the increase in sodium increases the strong ion gap which causes the bicarbonate to rise to maintain electrical neutrality.[12] This metabolic alkalosis may impair release of oxygen from haemoglobin; however, this is generally more than balanced by the lactic acidosis described above. After injury, urinary sodium excretion may fall to 10–25 mmol/24 hours and potassium excretion may rise to 100–200 mmol/24 hours.

Aldosterone also modifies the effects of catecholamines on cells, thus affecting the exchange of sodium and potassium across all cell membranes. The release of large quantities of intracellular potassium into the extracellular fluid may cause a significant rise in serum potassium, especially if renal function is impaired.

3.3.3 Effects on Substrate Metabolism

3.3.3.1 CARBOHYDRATES

Critically ill patients develop a glucose intolerance which resembles that found in diabetic patients. This is a result of both increased mobilization and decreased uptake of glucose by the tissues. The turnover of glucose is increased, and the serum glucose is higher than normal.

As blood glucose rises during the phase of hepatic gluconeogenesis, blood insulin concentration rises, sometimes to very high levels. Provided that the liver circulation is maintained, gluconeogenesis will not be suppressed by hyperinsulinaemia or hyperglycaemia, because an accelerated rate of glucose production in the liver is required for clearance of lactate and amino acids, which are not able to be used for protein synthesis. This period of breakdown of muscle protein for gluconeogenesis, and the resultant hyperglycaemia, characterize the catabolic phase of the metabolic response to trauma.

The glucose level following trauma should be monitored carefully in the intensive care unit. The optimum blood glucose level remains controversial; excessive levels of glucose correlate directly with infectious complications, particularly in surgical or injury wounds. However, in the patient with major traumatic injury, especially with TBI, a higher minimum threshold level with a maximum level of 10 mmol/L[13] should be maintained. Control of the blood glucose is best achieved by titration with intravenous (IV) insulin, based on a protocol which stringently avoids hypoglycaemia. Measurements should initially be performed hourly, and when stable the interval can be increased. However, because of the degree of insulin resistance associated with trauma, the quantities required may be considerably higher than normal. However, overaggressive control of blood glucose increases the risk of hypoglycaemia and must be avoided.

Enteral nutrition is preferred but parenteral nutrition may be required, and this will exacerbate the difficulty of glucose control. Glucose remains the safest energy substrate following major trauma: 60%–75% of the caloric requirements should be supplied by glucose, with the remainder being supplied as a fat emulsion.

3.3.3.2 FAT

A major source of energy following trauma is adipose tissue. Lipids stored as triglycerides in adipose tissue are mobilized when insulin falls below 25 units/mL. Initially, because of the suppression of insulin release by the catecholamine spike after trauma, as much as 200–500 g of fat may be broken down early after severe trauma.[14] Catecholamines and glucagon activate adenyl cyclase in the fat cells to produce cyclic adenosine monophosphate (cAMP). This activates lipase, which promptly hydrolyses triglycerides to release glycerol and fatty acids. Growth hormone and cortisol play minor roles in this process as well. Glycerol provides substrate for gluconeogenesis in the liver, which derives energy by β-oxidation of fatty acids, a process inhibited by hyperinsulinaemia.

The free fatty acids provide energy for all tissues and for hepatic gluconeogenesis.

3.3.3.3 AMINO ACIDS

The intake of protein by a healthy adult is between 80 and 120 g of protein – 1 to 2 g protein/kg/day. This is equivalent to 13–20 g of nitrogen per day. In the absence of an exogenous source of protein, amino acids are principally derived from the breakdown of skeletal muscle protein. Following trauma or sepsis, the release rate of amino acids increases by three to four times. This manifests as marked muscle wasting, in other words, loss of lean body mass.

Cortisol, glucagon, and catecholamines play roles in this reaction. The mobilized amino acids are utilized for gluconeogenesis or oxidation in the liver and other tissues, but also for synthesis of acute-phase proteins required for immunocompetence, clotting, wound healing, and maintenance of cellular function.

After severe trauma or sepsis, as much as 20 g/day of urea nitrogen is excreted in the urine. Since 1 g urea nitrogen is derived from 6.25 g degraded amino acids, this protein wastage is up to 125 g/day. One gram of muscle protein represents 5 g wet muscle mass. The patient in this example would be losing 625 g of muscle mass per day. A loss of 40% of body protein is usually fatal, because failing immunity leads to overwhelming infection. Nitrogen excretion usually peaks several days after injury, returning to normal after several weeks. This is a characteristic feature of the metabolic response to illness.

The most profound alterations in metabolic rate and nitrogen loss occur after burns and may persist for months.

3.3.3.4 THE GUT

The intestinal mucosa requires rapid synthesis of amino acids. Depletion of amino acids results in atrophy of the mucosa, causing failure of the mucosal barrier. This may lead to bacterial translocation from the gut to the portal system. The extent of bacterial translocation in trauma has not been defined. In fact, the evidence for the relationship between gut barrier dysfunction and translocation is circumstantial.[15]

The presence of food in the gut lumen is a major stimulus for mucosal cell growth and the intestinal mucosa.

Food intake is invariably interrupted after major trauma, and the supply of glutamine may be insufficient for mucosal cell growth. Early nutrition (within 24–48 hours), and early enteral rather than parenteral feeding, may prevent or reduce these events.

3.4 THE ANABOLIC PHASE

During this phase, the patient is in a positive nitrogen balance, regains weight, and restores fat deposits. The hormones which contribute to anabolism are growth hormones, androgens, and 17 beta-ketosteroids. However, reversal of catabolism following injury is critically dependent on resolution of the inflammatory response, adequate protein and energy intake, and early mobilization.[16,17]

3.5 CLINICAL AND THERAPEUTIC RELEVANCE

Survival after injury depends on a balance between the extent of cellular damage, the efficacy of the metabolic response, and the effectiveness of treatment.

The degree to which the body can compensate for injury is astonishing, although sometimes the compensatory mechanisms may work to the patient's disadvantage. Adequate resuscitation is critical; however, over-resuscitation has emerged as an important factor contributing to a worse outcome, leading to the concept of de-resuscitation (see Chapter 17). After blood losses have been replaced, in the absence of invasive monitoring, it is difficult to determine when adequate additional crystalloid has been administered; however, the presence of oedema indicates fluid overload, and if hypotension persists, vasopressors are necessary.

Rapid resuscitation, control of haemorrhage, maintenance of oxygen delivery to the tissues, removal of devitalized tissue or pus, and control of infection are the cornerstones. The best metabolic therapy is excellent surgical care.

3.6 SHOCK

3.6.1 Definition of Shock

Shock is defined as inadequate delivery of oxygenated blood to the tissues, which is termed tissue hypoxia.

Shock, at first, leads to reversible ischaemia-induced cellular injury. If the process is sufficiently severe or protracted, it ultimately results in irreversible cellular and organ injury and dysfunction. The precise mechanisms responsible for the transition from reversible to irreversible injury and death of cells are not clearly understood, although the biochemical/morphological sequence in the progression of ischaemic cellular injury has been well elucidated.[18]

By understanding the events leading to cell injury and death, we may be able to intervene therapeutically in shock by protecting sub-lethally injured cells from irreversible injury and death.

3.6.2 Classification of Shock[19]

The classification of shock is of practical importance if the pathophysiology is understood in terms that make an impact on therapy. Although the basic definition of shock – decreased delivery of oxygen (and nutrients) to the tissues – remains inviolate, five types of shock, based on a distinction not only in the pathophysiology but also in the management of the patients, are recognized.

- Hypovolaemic (usually secondary to trauma)
- Cardiogenic:
  - Cardiac compressive (e.g., cardiac tamponade)
  - Obstructive (e.g., mediastinal compression)
- Distributive (inflammatory, e.g., septic shock or trauma)
- Neurogenic

3.6.2.1 HYPOVOLAEMIC SHOCK

Hypovolaemic shock is caused by a decrease in the intravascular volume. If reduced significantly, both pressure and flow decrease. With a significant decrease in filling pressure, there is a consequent decrease in SV. CO may be temporarily maintained by a compensatory tachycardia, and with continuing hypovolaemia, blood pressure (BP) is maintained by reflex increases in peripheral and, importantly, splanchnic vascular resistance and myocardial contractility mediated by neurohumoral mechanisms.

Preload influences cavity size and increases muscle shortening, as do exogenous or intrinsic inotropes. Cavity size and muscle shortening determine SV, and heart rate and SV determine CO. CO and SVR determine the BP. According to La Place's law, cavity size increases myocardial wall tension (tension ∞ radius), and as afterload is effectively the transmural tension developed by the myocardium, the cavity size, BP, and intrathoracic pressure determine afterload which negatively impacts muscle shortening.

- BP is determined by CO × SVR.
- SV is determined by the preload, by the contractility of the myocardium, and by the afterload.

Cardiac Output (CO) = Stroke Volume (SV) × Heart Rate (HR)

Contractility of the heart is improved by inotropic agents. The product of the SV and the heart rate determines the CO (**Figure 3.4**). CO and the SVR generate the BP. Diminished CO in patients with pump failure may be associated with a fall in BP; however, compensatory vasoconstriction can maintain the BP for prolonged periods. An exaggerated rise in SVR can lead to further depression of cardiac function by increasing ventricular afterload which is determined by the systolic pressure and the radius of the left ventricle (La Place). The LV radius

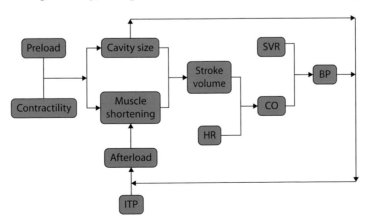

Figure 3.4 Haemodynamic response.

is related to end-diastolic volume (preload) and systolic pressure to the impedance to blood flow in the aorta, and the SVR (**Figure 3.4**).

BP is a poor surrogate for CO.

Inotropes can hide poor cardiac function.

Hypovolaemic shock is divided into four classes (see **Table 3.1**).

Class I and Class II shock represent compensated shock. When blood volume loss exceeds 30% (Class III and Class IV shock), the compensatory mechanisms are no longer effective and the decrease in CO causes tissue hypoxia. Tissues attempt to maintain oxygen consumption and viability by increasing oxygen extraction. Eventually, however, even this compensatory mechanism fails, and tissue hypoxia leads to lactic acidosis, hyperglycaemia, and failure of the sodium pump with swelling of the cells from water influx.

3.6.2.1.1 Clinical Presentation

The classic features of hypovolaemic shock are hypotension, tachycardia, pallor secondary to vasoconstriction, sweating, cyanosis, hyperventilation, confusion, and oliguria. Cardiac function can be depressed without gross clinical haemodynamic manifestations, as the heart shares in the ischaemic insult. Systemic arterial hypotension increases coronary ischaemia, causing rhythm disturbances and decreased myocardial performance. If heart failure occurs, as in a patient with myocardial ischaemia, LV end-diastolic pressure may rise, causing pulmonary oedema. In the setting of hypovolaemia, however, this is less common.

Hyperventilation secondary to lactic acidosis may maintain arterial oxygen pressure (PaO_2) at near-normal levels, but there is a compensatory fall in arterial blood CO_2 pressure ($PaCO_2$). Later, pulmonary insufficiency may supervene from contusion, fluid overload, and/or ARDS and, if myocardial dysfunction occurs, pulmonary oedema.

Renal function is also critically dependent on renal perfusion, with oliguria an inevitable feature of prolonged hypovolaemia. This may be exacerbated by raised intra-abdominal pressure (intra-abdominal hypertension) which can occur due to fluid overload and following abdominal surgery. During volume loss, renal blood flow falls correspondingly with the BP. Anuria occurs when the systolic BP falls to around 50 mmHg as a function of hypoxia of the renal medulla, and the oliguria is a protective measure. Thus, urine output is a good indicator of peripheral perfusion.

Pitfall

On admission, after catheterization, **discard the urine drained** (which was passed before the injury occurred – *check for haematuria first!*), then monitor urine output.

3.6.2.2 CARDIOGENIC SHOCK[20]

When the heart fails to produce an adequate CO, even though the end-diastolic volume is normal, cardiogenic shock is said to be present. Intravascular obstructive shock results when intravascular obstruction occurs, on either the right or the left side of the heart. On the right side, causes include pulmonary embolism and ARDS with hypoxaemia, where both cause pulmonary hypertension; on the left, aortic stenosis; and on both, tamponade.

Cardiac function is often impaired in shocked patients, even if myocardial damage is not the primary cause. Reduced myocardial function in shock can result from arrhythmias secondary to ischaemia or contusion, myocardial ischaemia from systemic hypotension and variations in blood flow, myocardial lesions from high circulatory levels of catecholamines (takotsubo), and,

Table 3.1 Classes of Hypovolaemic Shock

Class	Blood Loss (%)	Volume	Pulse Rate	Blood Pressure	Pulse Pressure	Resp. Rate
Class I	15	< 750 mL	< 100	Normal	Normal	14–20
Class II	30	750–1500 mL	> 100	Normal	Decreased	20–30
Class III	40	1500–2000 mL	> 120	Decreased	Decreased	30–40
Class IV	> 40	> 2000 mL	> 140	Decreased	Decreased	> 35

with severe inflammation, peroxynitrite-mediated damage to the myocardium.[21,22]

Other forms of cardiogenic shock include those conditions in which the patient may have a nearly normal resting CO but cannot increase this appropriately. CO is therefore reduced because of a reduced SV in the setting of impaired contractility due to ischaemia, infarction, cardiomyopathy, or direct trauma with mechanical complications or those that may occur with an acute myocardial infarction, such as acute mitral valvular regurgitation or ventricular septal rupture.

3.6.2.2.1 Cardiac Compressive Shock

The pathophysiology of cardiac compressive shock is very different from that of cardiogenic shock. External forces compress the thin-walled chambers of the heart (the atria and the right ventricle), the great veins (systemic or pulmonary), or any combination of these. Impaired diastolic filling will result. Clinical conditions capable of causing compressive shock include pericardial tamponade, tension pneumothorax, positive-pressure ventilation with large tidal volumes or high airway pressures (especially in a hypovolaemic patient), an elevated diaphragm (as in pregnancy), displacement of abdominal viscera through a ruptured diaphragm, and the abdominal compartment syndrome (e.g., from ascites, abdominal distension, abdominal or retroperitoneal bleeding, or a stiff abdominal wall, as in a patient with deep burns to the torso).

The consequence of this compression is an increase in right atrial pressure (RAP) without an increase in volume, impeding venous return and reducing end-diastolic volumes and provoking hypotension.

3.6.2.2.1.1 *Cardiac Tamponade*

This follows blunt or penetrating trauma and is a classic example of compressive cardiac shock. As a result of the presence of blood in the pericardial sac, the atria are compressed and cannot fill adequately. The systolic BP falls below 90 mmHg; there is a narrowed PP and a pulsus paradoxus exceeding 10 mmHg. Distended neck veins may be present, with cyanosis visible over the head and supraclavicular area unless the patient is hypovolaemic as well. Heart sounds are muffled. The limited compliance of the pericardial sac means that a very small amount (< 25 mL blood) may be enough to cause decompensation.

Similarly, tension pneumothorax can also produce compressive heart failure. In the patient with chest trauma and hypotension, the problem usually can be identified immediately, from decreased breath sounds, hyperresonance of the affected side, and displacement of the trachea to the opposite side. Neck veins also may be distended.

Pitfall

Immediate release of the tension, prior to waiting for an X-ray, is required to prevent cardiac arrest, reduction in myocardial reserve, or an inability to mobilize myocardial reserves due to pharmacologic beta-adrenergic blockade or underlying clinically silent ischaemia.

3.6.2.3 DECREASED LV FILLING PRESSURES

Tamponade will decrease venous return to the RA, as will elevated intrathoracic pressure as occurs in tension pneumothorax and positive-pressure ventilation with large tidal volumes or high airway pressures (especially in the hypovolaemic patient). Diaphragmatic rupture with displacement of the liver into the chest may also increase intrathoracic pressure.

In pregnancy, particularly in the supine position, compression of the inferior vena cava (IVC) will decrease venous return, as will elevated intra-abdominal pressure (e.g., from ascites, abdominal distension, abdominal or retroperitoneal bleeding, or a stiff abdominal wall, as in a patient with deep burns to the torso).

3.6.2.3.1 Clinical Presentation

The clinical picture will depend on the underlying cause. Clinical signs of peripheral vasoconstriction may be prominent but may be less so with a marked inflammatory response in which vasodilatation occurs. With LV dysfunction, pulmonary congestion is frequent, and oliguria is almost always present. Pulmonary oedema causes severe dyspnoea and possibly central cyanosis, and clinically there would be an S3 gallop and inspiratory crackles, with bats-wing pulmonary infiltrates, upper lobe blood diversion, and Kerley B lines visible on X-ray. A systolic murmur appearing after myocardial infarction suggests mitral regurgitation or septal perforation.

Haemodynamic findings consist of a systolic arterial pressure less than 90 mmHg; decreased CO, usually less than 1.8 L/min/m²; and a pulmonary arterial wedge pressure (PAWP) greater than 20 mmHg. However, cardiogenic shock can occur without the PAWP being elevated. This may be a result of excess diuretic therapy acutely, capillary leak, plasma blood loss, or RV compromise (e.g., right-sided infarct, pulmonary embolus, or tamponade). These latter patients will have a reduced SV but normal LV function. They will only respond to fluids if hypovolaemia is present.

3.6.3 Distributive (Inflammatory) Shock[23]

Dilatation of the capacitance reservoirs in the body occurs with release of DAMPs and PAMPs because of cytokine-mediated upregulation of inducible NO synthase with endothelial production of NO. Prolonged hypovolaemia may cause cellular death also, with release of DAMPs such as cfDNA. In these settings, vasodilatation with an inadequate myocardial response will cause hypotension.

Decreased oxygen delivery or reactive oxidant-mediated mitochondrial injury decreases the ability to produce ATP, and anaerobic metabolism ensues. This occurs both with major trauma and with sepsis, frequently in the setting of low vascular resistance. The ultimate cause of death in shock is failure of cellular energy production, reflected by a decline in oxygen consumption. There is a narrowing of arterial–mixed venous oxygen difference as an indication of reduced oxygen extraction, which often precedes the fall of CO. Inadequate oxidative phosphorylation leads to anaerobic metabolism and a severe metabolic acidosis due to lactate formation.

The clinical features include altered mental status, tachycardia, tachypnoea, hypotension, warm extremities with bounding pulses in early shock, hypo- or hyperthermia, and decreased urine output.

3.6.4 Neurogenic Shock

Neurogenic shock is a hypotensive syndrome in which there is loss of adrenergic tone and dilatation of the arterial and venous vasculature. The CO is normal, or may even be elevated, but because the total peripheral resistance is reduced, the patient is hypotensive with a reduced perfusion pressure. In trauma, it often occurs due to spinal cord injury. A simple example of this type of shock is syncope (*vasovagal syncope*). It is caused by a strong vagal discharge resulting in a bradycardia associated with dilatation of the small vessels of the splanchnic bed, decreasing the CO.

3.6.4.1 CLINICAL PRESENTATION

Commonly seen with high spinal cord injury, the patient usually has weakly palpable peripheral pulses, warm extremities, and brisk capillary filling, and may be anxious. The PP is wide, with both systolic and diastolic BP being low. Heart rate is below 100 beats per minute, and there may even be a bradycardia. However, the diagnosis of neurogenic shock should only be made once other causes of shock have been excluded, since the common cause is injury, and there may be other injuries present causing a hypovolaemic shock in parallel.

3.6.5 Measurements in Shock

In physics, flow is directly related to pressure and inversely related to resistance. This universal flow formula is not dependent on the type of fluid and is also applied to the flow of electrons. In electricity, it is expressed as Ohm's law. This law applies just as appropriately to blood flow.

$$Flow = \frac{\text{Pressure}}{\text{Peripheral resistance}}$$

From this law, it can be deduced that shock is just as much a state of elevated resistance as it is a state of low BP. However, the focus should remain on flow rather than simply on pressure, since most drugs that result in a rise in pressure do so by raising the resistance, which in turn decreases flow, whilst simultaneously increasing work and oxygen consumption by the myocardium.

3.6.5.1 CARDIAC OUTPUT

Blood flow is dependent on CO, which is determined by three factors (**Figure 3.4**):

- Preload, or the volume entering the heart.
- Contractility of the heart.
- Afterload, or the resistance against which the heart must function to deliver the SV. This can be expressed as the tension developed in the LV wall.

These three factors are interrelated to produce the systolic ejection from the heart. Up to a point, the greater the preload, the greater the CO. As myocardial fibres are stretched by the preload, the tension developed increases according to the Frank–Starling principle. However, an excessive increase in preload leads to pulmonary/systemic venous congestion without further improvement in cardiac performance. The preload is a positive factor in cardiac performance up the slope of the Frank–Starling curve but not beyond the point of cardiac decompensation.

3.6.5.2 **INDIRECT MEASUREMENT OF FLOW**

In many patients in shock, simply laying a hand upon their extremities will help to determine flow by the cold clammy feeling of hypoperfusion, which may be due to increased vascular resistance in hypovolaemic shock or due to an inadequate myocardial response to systemic vasodilation. Probably the most important clinical observation to determine adequate oxygen delivery to a visceral organ indirectly will be the urine output. The kidney responds to decreased oxygen delivery with several compensatory changes to protect its own perfusion. Over a range of BP, the kidneys maintain a nearly constant blood flow. If the BP decreases, the kidney's autoregulation of resistance results in dilatation of the vascular bed. It keeps flow constant by lowering the resistance, even though the pressure has decreased. This allows selective shunting of blood to the renal bed.

For practical purposes, if a patient is producing a normal quantity of normal-quality urine, then they are not in shock. In addition, a normal Glasgow Coma Scale (GCS) can also be used to evaluate the adequacy of oxygen delivery in the patient with shock.

3.6.5.3 **DIRECT MEASUREMENTS**

3.6.5.3.1 Central Venous Pressure (CVP) (See also Chapter 17)

Markers of inadequate perfusion and therefore oxygen delivery are an elevated lactate, a decreased central venous oxygen saturation ($ScvO_2$), and a > 6 mmHg difference between the partial pressure of central venous carbon dioxide (CO_2) and that of the arterial blood. A central venous catheter allows venous access and can be used to evaluate CO with invasive cardiac monitoring. Unfortunately, it is not of value in determining fluid status either as a single measurement or in the change following fluid bolus.[24]

The RAP determines venous return, as the RA filling pressure is a function of the pressure in the peripheral venous system, which is in the region of 7 mmHg, and the pressure in the RAP which must be lower than 7 mmHg. In normal circumstances, it is usually in the region of 0 to 2.[25]

The CVP therefore reflects the RV filling pressure, and an elevation indicates RV dysfunction or increased intrathoracic pressure. If it is elevated, a cardiac echo should be performed to confirm the cause, such as cardiac tamponade, pulmonary embolism, RV ischaemia, or contusion, and a clinical examination to exclude tension pneumothorax should also be performed.

3.6.5.3.2 Routes of Cannulation

Cannulation of the central venous system is generally achieved using the subclavian, jugular, or femoral route. The site used is determined to an extent by the type of injury, the body habitus of the patient, and the expertise of the operator. A set protocol should be employed which involves handwashing, bare below elbows, gown, gloves, mask, skin cleansing with 2% chlorhexidine solution, draping as per a surgical procedure, and then using a tightly fitting securement device with a chlorhexidine-impregnated pledget covering the insertion site.

The subclavian route is often preferred in the trauma patient, particularly when the status of the cervical spine is unclear.

Ultrasonic guidance is recommended to reduce the incidence of complications, such as arterial cannulation, pneumothorax, or tracheal or thoracic duct perforation. The internal jugular route or, occasionally, the external jugular route is commonly utilized as well under ultrasonic guidance. It provides ease of access, especially under operative conditions.

The femoral route is often easier to access; however, the infection rate is higher, particularly in the obese patient.

Pitfall

Avoid femoral lines if major abdominal injury is present. Placing the cannula inside the abdominal cavity can be particularly misleading if blood is present inside the abdominal cavity, since aspiration of the cannula will yield blood and thus a false sense of security. In addition, if there is iliac or caval injury, the fluids instilled will fill the abdominal cavity rather than the circulation! Again, the use of ultrasound can reduce catheter insertion complications.

3.6.5.3.3 Systemic Arterial Pressure

Systemic arterial pressure reflects the product of the peripheral resistance and the cardiac output. Measurement can be indirect or direct. Indirect measurement involves the use of a BP cuff with auscultation of the artery to determine systolic and diastolic BP. Direct measurement involves placement of a catheter into the lumen of the artery, with direct measurement of the pressure.

In patients with hypovolaemic shock who have an elevated SVR, there is often a significant difference obtained between the two measurements. In patients with increased vascular resistance, low cuff pressure does not necessarily indicate hypotension. Failure to recognize this may lead to dangerous errors in therapy.

Conversely, in vasodilatory shock, diastolic arterial pressure (DAP) is mainly determined by vascular tone and is constant from ascending aorta to peripheral vessels. If the diastolic pressure is low, this indicates vasodilation and could indicate a need for early use of vasopressors. Low DAP (<50 mmHg) may also impair LV perfusion, especially with tachycardia, as coronary perfusion occurs mainly during diastole.[26]

Cannulation of the brachial artery is not recommended because of the potential for thrombosis and for ischaemia of the lower arm and hand.

3.6.5.4 NON-INVASIVE CARDIAC MONITORING

Cardiac echocardiography is useful to assess RV and LV function and to exclude tamponade. It is also useful to help diagnose pneumothorax and pulmonary oedema.

A collapsed IVC has been assumed to indicate fluid depletion, but the mean end-diastolic dimension correlates with mean RA pressure, so IVC diameter is an indirect indicator of CVP and has the same limitations. A lack of respiratory variation indicates a lower likelihood of fluid responsiveness, but respiratory variation may merely indicate large variations in intrathoracic pressure. There are numerous situations where it would be inaccurate, and it cannot be relied upon to give accurate information.[27]

3.6.5.5 INVASIVE HAEMODYNAMIC MONITORING

3.6.5.5.1 Uncalibrated Systems

Various devices utilize PP analysis, with an algorithm that compensates for age- and gender-related changes in vascular tone, to estimate CO. The main determinants of PP are SV and aortic impedance, and many studies have shown that PP can accurately follow changes in SV.[28]

A PP <40 mmHg is clearly low and reflects a decreased SV, which could be due to a decreased preload or severe systolic dysfunction. These devices can calculate SV, SV variation (SVV), and SVR in addition; however, both SVV and PP variation are reliable predictors of fluid responsiveness only when Tidal Volume (TV) ≥ 8 mL/kg and the patient is fully mechanically ventilated. They can be used to distinguish trends in response to resuscitation but are also of no value with atrial fibrillation, pulmonary embolism, tamponade, aortic stenosis, RV infarct, and raised intra-abdominal pressure, and they cannot distinguish between an elevation in CO due to fluid bolus and administration of an inotrope.

3.6.5.5.2 Calibrated Systems

These utilize the thermodilution technique, whereby cold saline is injected into the central line, and the time taken for a decrease in temperature is recorded in a femoral arterial line. These systems then relate the measured CO to the recorded PP, such that the SV so derived is more accurate. These devices measure additional parameters, such as extravascular lung water and global end-diastolic volume index, which estimate fluid status even with the presence of the confounders described above for uncalibrated systems. They are seldom used, however, in the acute resuscitation phase.

3.7 ENDPOINTS IN SHOCK RESUSCITATION

The ultimate measurement of the impact of shock must be at the cellular level. The most convenient measurement is a determination of the blood gases. Measurement of PaO_2, $PaCO_2$, pH, base deficit (BD), and arterial lactate will supply information on oxygen delivery and utilization of energy substrates.

When there is inadequate delivery of nutrients and oxygen to the tissues, as occurs in shock, the cells shift to anaerobic metabolism within 3–5 minutes. In the absence of aerobic metabolism, lactate and pyruvate accumulate, which have toxic effects on normal physiology. These products of anaerobic metabolism can be seen because of the 'oxygen debt'. There is some buffer capacity in the body that allows this debt to accumulate within limits, but it must ultimately be shut off by adequate oxygen and nutrient delivery.

Acidosis has significant consequences in compensatory physiology. Oxyhaemoglobin dissociates more readily as acidosis worsens. Despite the salutary effect on oxyhaemoglobin dissociation, acidosis may have a negative effect on oxygen delivery, as endogenous (and exogenous) catecholamines are physiologically less effective in an acid environment.

The adequacy of resuscitation is best assessed by declining lactate levels, the trend of the ScvO$_2$, and the central venous/arterial CO$_2$ difference where one aims for a value of ≤ 6 mmHg.

3.7.1 Post-Shock and Multiple Organ Failure Syndromes

Although the primary consequence of sepsis following trauma and shock is the development of MOF, the ultimate cause of death in shock is failure of energy production, as reflected by a decline in oxygen consumption (VO$_2$) to less than 100 mL/min/m^2. Circulatory insufficiency is responsible for this fall in energy, compounded by impairment of cellular oxidative phosphorylation by DAMPs such as cfDNA and PAMPs such as endotoxin and endogenously produced substances, such as toxic reactive oxidant species.

In shock, whether hypovolaemic or septic, energy production is insufficient to satisfy cellular requirements. In the presence of oxygen deprivation and cellular injury, the conversion of pyruvate to acetyl-CoA for entry into the Krebs cycle is inhibited. Lactic acid accumulates, and the oxidation reduction potential falls. Although lactate is normally used by the liver via the Cori cycle to synthesize glucose, hepatic gluconeogenesis may fail in hypovolaemic or septic shock because of hepatocyte injury and inadequate circulation. Terminally, the lactic acidosis cannot necessarily be corrected by improvement of circulation and oxygen delivery once the cells are irreparably damaged.

In the low-output shock state, plasma concentrations of free fatty acids and triglycerides rise to high levels because ketone production by beta-oxidation of fatty acids in the liver is reduced, suppressing the acetoacetate–beta-hydroxybutarate ratio in the plasma.

The post-shock sequel of inadequate nutrient flow, therefore, is progressive loss of function. The rate at which this loss occurs depends on the cell's ability to switch metabolism, to convert alternate fuels to energy, and to increase extraction of oxygen from haemoglobin, and on the compensatory collaboration of failing cells and organs whereby nutrients may be shunted selectively to more critical systems. Not all cells are equally sensitive to shock nor similarly refractory to restoration of

function when adequate oxygen delivery is achieved. As cells lose function, the reserves of the organ composed of those cells are depleted until impaired function of the organ results. These organs function in systems, and a 'system failure' results. Multiple system failures occurring in sequence lead to the collapse of the organism.

3.7.2 Management of the Shocked Patient

The primary goal of shock resuscitation is the early establishment of adequate oxygen delivery (DO$_2$). The calculated variable of DO$_2$ is the product of CO and arterial oxygen content (CaO$_2$). By convention, CO is indexed to body surface area and expressed as cardiac index (CI), and when multiplied by CaO$_2$, yields an oxygen delivery index (DO$_2$I). Normal DO$_2$I is roughly 450 mL/min/m^2.

CaO$_2$ and DO$_2$I are calculated as follows:

$$CaO_2 \, (mL.O_2 / dL = [Hb](g/dL.) \times 1.36 mL.O_2 / gHb \\ \times SaO_2 (\%) + [PaO_2 (mmHg) \\ \times 0.003 mL.O_2 / mmHg]$$

$$DO_2I (mL / min / m^2) = CI (L / min / m^2) \\ \times CaO_2 (mL / dL) \times 10 dL / L$$

where *Hb* is haemoglobin concentration, *SaO$_2$* is haemoglobin oxygen saturation, *PaO$_2$* is arterial oxygen tension, and there is a 0.003 solubility of O$_2$ in blood.

Early work demonstrated that the initial 'survivor' response to traumatic stress is to become hyperdynamic. Supranormal resuscitation based on the DO$_2$I was therefore proposed. Subsequent randomized controlled trials have failed to demonstrate improved outcomes with goal-directed supranormal therapy, and, in fact, this strategy increased acute coronary syndromes, MOF, and death.

CI may be normally abnormal, as in the hyperdynamic state, or abnormally normal where it does not increase appropriately according to demand. It has been suggested that, if monitoring cardiac index, one should initially aim at a value > 3.8 L/min/m^2 as a resuscitation goal.[29]

The purpose of distinguishing the different pathophysiologic mechanisms of shock becomes important when treatment must be initiated. The final aim of treatment is to restore aerobic cellular metabolism. This requires restoration of adequate flow of oxygenated blood (which is dependent on optimal oxygenation of sufficient red blood cells, i.e., haematocrit, and adequate CO). The initial focus is securing a patent airway and controlling ventilation to prevent inadequate alveolar ventilation and oxygenation.

Restoration of optimal circulating blood volume, enhancing CO using inotropic agents and/or mean arterial pressure (MAP) through vasopressors, the correction of acid–base disturbances and metabolic deficits, and the combating of sepsis are all vital in the management of the shocked patient.

3.7.2.1 OXYGENATION

The severely traumatized, hypovolaemic, or septic patient has an oxygen demand that may exceed twice the normal. However, the traumatized shocked patient usually cannot generate the additional respiratory effort required, and therefore often develops respiratory failure followed by a lactic acidosis due to tissue hypoxaemia.

In some patients, an oxygen mask may be enough to maintain oxygen delivery to the lungs. In more severe cases, endotracheal intubation and ventilatory assistance may be necessary. It is important to distinguish between the need for *intubation* and the need for *ventilation*.

Early intubation is preferable to cardiac collapse.

3.7.2.2 AIRWAY INDICATIONS FOR INTUBATION

- Obstructed airway
- Inadequate gag reflex

3.7.2.3 BREATHING INDICATIONS FOR INTUBATION

- Inability to breathe (e.g., paralysis, either spinal or drug induced)
- Tidal volume less than 5 mL/kg

3.7.2.4 BREATHING INDICATIONS FOR VENTILATION[30]

- Inability to oxygenate adequately. PaO_2 less than 60 mmHg (7.9 kPa) on 40% O_2 or SpO_2 of less than 90% on oxygen.
- A respiratory rate of 30 breaths or more per minute and excessive ventilatory effort.
- A $PaCO_2$ of greater than 45 (6 kPa) mmHg with metabolic acidosis, or greater than 50 mmHg (6.6 kPa) with normal bicarbonate levels.

3.7.2.5 CIRCULATORY INDICATION FOR INTUBATION

- Systolic BP less than 75 mmHg despite resuscitation

3.7.2.6 DISABILITY INDICATIONS FOR INTUBATION

- High spinal injury with inability to breathe.
- Coma (GCS < 9/15)

3.7.2.7 ENVIRONMENTAL INDICATION FOR INTUBATION

- Core temperature of < 32° C

If ventilatory support is instituted, the goals are relatively specific. The respiratory rate should be adjusted to ensure a $PaCO_2$ of between 35 and 40 mmHg (4.6–5.3 kPa). This will avoid a respiratory alkalosis and a shift of the oxyhaemoglobin dissociation curve to the left, which results in an increased affinity of haemoglobin for oxygen, and significantly decreases oxygen availability to tissues. A respiratory alkalosis also causes vasoconstriction of cerebral vessels and further decreases oxygen delivery to the brain. For this reason, hyperventilation and hypocapnoea are no longer seen as appropriate for the management of brain injury.

The arterial PaO_2 should be maintained at 80–100 mmHg (10.6–13.2 kPa) with the lowest possible inspired oxygen concentration, and values >120 mmHg should be avoided.[31]

It has also been shown that increased respiratory effort requires a disproportionate share of the total CO for the respiratory muscles and, therefore, other organs are deprived of necessary blood flow and lactic acidosis is potentiated. Mechanical ventilation may help to reverse this lactic acidosis, particularly if neuromuscular blockade is used. This latter intervention may be of value for 48 hours, as it decreases respiratory work and improves ventilator/patient synchrony.[32]

3.7.3 Fluid Therapy for Volume Expansion

The preferred in-hospital strategy is balanced blood component therapy. In the pre-hospital setting, this strategy is also implemented in some countries (primarily Helicopter Emergency Medical Services [HEMS] operations). Crystalloid (i.e., Ringer's lactate) should be discouraged in the initial treatment of trauma patients, if balanced blood component therapy is available.

3.7.3.1 HYPOTENSIVE RESUSCITATION

In 1994, Bickell et al. concluded that patients with penetrating torso trauma in hypovolaemic shock who were not given IV fluids during transport and emergency department evaluation had a better chance of survival than those who received conventional volume resuscitation.[33]

However, the only difference in survival was in the subgroup with pericardial tamponade. In animal studies, IV fluids have been shown to inhibit platelet aggregation, dilute clotting factors, modulate the physical properties of thrombus, and cause increases in BP that can mechanically disrupt clot. Thus, the benefit of restricted resuscitation volumes was possibly because the reduced BP limited the amount of blood loss. In the typical civilian trauma centre, blunt trauma is the most common form of injury, and inadequate resuscitation leads to further organ injury due to inadequate oxygen delivery, particularly with TBI. Thus, whilst the ideal approach is not known, the optimum systolic BP for a patient with uncontrolled haemorrhage appears to be approximately 90 mmHg. MAP should be approximately 70 mmHg, for both the military environment and, likely, the civilian setting also. However, a pre-hospital study by Schreiber et al. suggested benefit of an even lower systolic BP of 70 mmHg.[34] However, care must be exercised in cardiac patients and the elderly.

A meta-analysis of 30 studies evaluated hypotensive resuscitation, defined as limiting fluid resuscitation to maintain adequate organ perfusion, with a systolic BP of approximately 70–80 mmHg or a MAP of approximately 50 mmHg. This showed a statistically significant decrease in mortality (risk ratio [RR]: 0.50; 95% confidence interval [CI]: 0.40–0.61). There was no difference between groups observed for AKI, but there was a protective effect regarding multiple organ dysfunction and ARDS.[35]

3.7.4 **Route of Administration**

3.7.4.1 **INTRAVENOUS DEVICES**

As with all IV lines, the shorter the line and the wider the diameter, the faster the flow. For the same bore of line, but with variable lengths, flow rates vary.

14G via peripheral cannula	Full flow
14G via 20 cm central line	33% reduction in flow
14G via 70 cm central line	50% reduction in flow

A minimum of two lines is required in the severely injured or hypotensive patient. In all cases of hypovolaemic shock, two large-bore peripheral lines are essential. A central line is most useful for monitoring but can be used for transfusion as well. The monitoring line should be a central venous line. The subclavian route is preferable since this approach avoids any movement of the head in a patient whose neck has not yet been cleared. The jugular and femoral routes are less preferable because of issues with securing the lines and with earlier sepsis at the insertion site due to movement.

3.7.4.2 **INTRAOSSEOUS DEVICES**

Intraosseous infusion is the process of injecting directly into the marrow of a bone to provide a non-collapsible entry point into the venous system. This technique is used in emergency and military situations to provide fluids and medication when IV access is not feasible. A comparison of IV, intramuscular, and intraosseous routes of administration concluded that in children, the intraosseous route is demonstrably superior to the intramuscular route, and comparable to the IV route.[36] Insertion in adults requires less than a minute, and flow rates of up to 125 mL/min have been achieved.

Pitfall

Note that these only work with pressure bag systems.
The devices are for emergency resuscitation and should be removed within 24 hours.

3.7.5 **Pharmacologic Support of Blood Pressure**

SV is controlled by ventricular preload, afterload, and contractility. Ventricular preload is influenced primarily by the volume of circulating blood, but afterload and contractility can be enhanced by pharmacological agents. Reducing the SVR with vasodilators can be a very effective means of improving CO when systemic pressures or cardiac-filling pressures are normal or elevated, but it is not currently recommended for acute trauma.

Pitfall

The catecholamines shift the metabolism to anaerobic in nature and will worsen or sustain the metabolic acidosis. They also contribute to coagulopathy (due to endotheliopathy, shredding glycocalyx) and increase the risk of sepsis, as they formulate complexes with iron, which is essential for, and therefore potentiates, bacterial growth.

3.7.5.1 NOREPINEPHRINE (NORADRENALINE)

The preferred inotropic agent for acute trauma is noradrenaline (norepinephrine). It is a sympathetic neurotransmitter with potent inotropic effects. It activates myocardial β-adrenergic receptors and vascular α-adrenergic receptors. It is used in the treatment of shock and hypotension characterized by low SVR and unresponsiveness to fluid resuscitation.

3.7.5.2 EPINEPHRINE (ADRENALINE)

Adrenaline is a natural catecholamine with both α- and β-adrenergic agonist activity. The pharmacological actions are complex. The primary difference between noradrenaline and adrenaline is that the latter has more B1 effects, and it is more likely to cause a tachycardia. It also causes a transient increase in lactate in the first 24 hours which is not related to worsening oxygen delivery.

Both agents increase the SVR, systolic and diastolic BP, coronary and cerebral blood flow, inotropism, and myocardial oxygen requirement.[37] The initial dose is 0.03 μg/kg/min, titrated upwards until the desired effect is achieved.

3.7.5.3 DOPAMINE

Dopamine hydrochloride is a chemical precursor of noradrenaline which stimulates dopaminergic, β_1-adrenergic, and α-adrenergic receptors in a dose-dependent fashion. Low doses of dopamine (<3 μg/kg/min) produce cerebral, renal, and mesenteric vasodilatation, and venous tone is increased. Urine output is increased, but there is no evidence to show that this is in any way protective to the kidneys. At doses greater than 10 μg/kg/min, however, the α-adrenergic effects predominate. This results in marked increases in SVR, pulmonary resistance, and increases in preload due to marked arterial, splanchnic, and venous constriction. It increases systolic BP without increasing diastolic BP or heart rate. Dopamine is seldom used anymore, as it is uncertain as to what dose would cause specific effects and it has been associated with an increased number of adverse events.[38]

3.7.5.4 DOBUTAMINE

Dobutamine is a synthetic sympathomimetic amine that has potent inotropic effects by stimulating β_1- and α_1-adrenergic receptors in the myocardium. Dobutamine has a 'balanced' effect on the peripheral α receptors and as such does not have a pressor effect. For this reason, it is seldom used in sepsis or trauma. Its primary use is in cases of myocardial dysfunction, where inotropism without an increase in afterload is desired.

In hypovolemic traumatic shock, the therapy should consist of fluid replacement, preferably with blood products. If there is major trauma, however, as discussed above, DAMPs may increase production of NO via inducible NO synthase, and a pressor would decrease the volume of fluid required to ensure adequate resuscitation. This also decreases the need for 'de-resuscitation' (i.e., the removal of fluid overload which is associated with a worse outcome).[39]

3.7.6 Prognosis in Shock

The prognosis of the shocked patient depends on the duration of the shock, the underlying cause, and the pre-existing vital organ function. The prognosis is best when the duration is kept short by early recognition and aggressive correction of the circulatory disturbance and when the underlying cause is known and corrected.

Occasionally, shock does not respond to standard therapeutic measures. Unresponsive shock requires an understanding of the potential occult causes of persistent physiologic disturbances. These correctable causes include:

- Underappreciated volume losses with inadequate fluid resuscitation and a failure to assess the response to a fluid challenge.
- Overcautious resuscitation in the presence of cardiac disease.
- Hypoxaemia caused by inadequate ventilation, barotrauma to the lung, pneumothorax, or cardiac tamponade.
- Undiagnosed or inadequately treated sepsis.
- Uncorrected acid–base or electrolyte abnormalities.
- Unrecognized adrenal insufficiency or hypothyroidism.
- Drug/alcohol toxicity.

3.7.6.1 RECOMMENDED PROTOCOL FOR SHOCK

3.7.6.1.1 Military Experience

Recent military experience from the Iraq war has shown the value of *damage control resuscitation*.[40,41] (See Section 6.2, 'Damage Control Resuscitation [DCR]'.) This implies that damage control techniques are used from the time of injury, minimizing the time between injury and care, and controlling the bleeding and contamination through use of minimal clear fluids, early fresh whole blood, early resuscitation, and early damage control surgery. The military use of whole blood has minimized some of the risks of component therapy and has also shown that survival is improved. From this philosophy has developed a change in protocol in civilian practice towards minimizing crystalloid resuscitation (restrictive or limited resuscitation; not hypotensive) and early use of whole blood and mixed products to maintain the coagulation profile as normal as possible.

3.7.6.1.2 Initial Resuscitation

A. Major trauma patients arriving in shock (SBP <90 mmHg and/or HR >130 bpm) are initially considered to be in haemorrhagic shock. Correction should be aimed at damage control through surgical control of bleeding, and damage control resuscitation (see Chapter 6).

B. Patients with major torso trauma requiring ongoing resuscitation should have a central venous line placed in the emergency department when time allows for it.

C. Early CVP >8 mmHg (before extensive volume loading) suggests cardiogenic or cardiac compressive shock.

D. Low CVP despite volume loading suggests ongoing bleeding. Endpoints are currently vague. At present, the rational compromise is volume-limited resuscitation (SBP = 90 mmHg, and HR <130 bpm) with moderate volume loading until haemorrhage is controlled.

E. Patients at risk for trauma-induced coagulopathy (TIC) should have a massive transfusion protocol initiated (see Chapter 4: "Transfusion in Trauma").

ANAESTHESIOLOGICAL CONSIDERATIONS

- Consider succinctly letting the surgeon know at an appropriate time:
  - Ongoing blood loss
  - Metabolic state (e.g., base deficit or lactate)
  - Vasopressor requirements
  - Overview of coagulation
- Consider asking the surgeon at an appropriate time:
  - Is the patient clotting clinically?
  - How does the perfusion of vital organs look clinically (e.g., bowel)?
  - What are the available treatment options?

REFERENCES

1. Cuthbertson D. Observations on disturbance of metabolism produced by injury of the limbs. *Q J Med.* 1932;**25**:233–6.
2. Kolecki P. Hypovolemic Shock Clinical Presentation. 2022; https://emedicine.medscape.com/article/760145-clinical (accessed online August 2023).
3. De Jager PP, Smith O, Pool R, Bolon S, Richards GA. Review of the pathophysiology and prognostic biomarkers of immune dysregulation after severe injury. *J Trauma Acute Care Surg.* 2021 Feb 1;**90(2)**:e21–e30. doi: 10.1097/TA.0000000000002996.
4. Rosenthal MD, Rosenthal C, Patel J, Jordan J, Go K, Moore FA. Arginine in the critically Ill: can we finally push past the controversy? *Int J Crit Care Emerg Med.* 2016;**2**. doi: 10.23937/2474-3674/1510017.
5. Yilmaz O, Afsar B, Ortiz A, Kanbay M. The role of endothelial glycocalyx in health and disease. *Clin Kid J.* 2019 Apr 23;**12(5)**:611–19. doi: 10.1093/ckj/sfz042. eCollection 2019 Oct.
6. Woodcock TE, Woodcock TM. Revised Starling equation and the glycocalyx model of transvascular fluid exchange: an improved paradigm for prescribing intravenous fluid therapy. *Br J Anaesth.* 2012;**108**:384–94. doi: 10.1093/bja/aer515.
7. Iba T, Levy JH. Derangement of the endothelial glycocalyx in sepsis. *J Thromb Haemost.* 2019;**17**:283–94. doi: 10.1111/jth.14371.
8. Lilly MP, Gann DS. The hypothalamic-pituitary-adrenal immune axis. *Arch Surg.* 1992;**127(12)**:1463–74. doi: 10.1001/archsurg.1992.01420120097017.
9. Porte D, Robertson RP. Control of insulin by catecholamines, stress, and the sympathetic nervous system. *Federal Proceedings.* 1973;**32**:1792–96.

10. Rao S, Pena C, Shurmur S, Nugent K. Atrial natriuretic peptide: structure, function, and physiological effects: a narrative review. *Curr Cardiol Rev.* 2021;**17(6)**:e051121191003. doi: 10.2174/1573403X17666210202102210.

11. Lane N. *Power, Sex, Suicide: Mitochondria and the Meaning of Life (Oxford Landmark Science)*, 2nd Edn. Oxford University Press. 2005.

12. Kishen R, Honoré PM, Jacobs R, Joannes-Boyau O, De Waele E, De Regt J, et al. Facing acid–base disorders in the third millennium – the Stewart approach revisited. *Int J Nephrol Renov Dis.* 2014;**7**:209–17. doi: 10.2147/IJNRD.S62126.

13. Alhatemi G, Aldiwani H, Alhatemi R, Hussein M, Mahdai S, Seyoum B. Glycemic control in the critically ill: less is more. *Cleveland Clinic J Med.* 2022;**89**:191–199. doi: 10.3949/ccjm.89a.20171.

14. Ram AD, Davenport M. Metabolic Response to Injury and Sepsis. In: Sinha CK, Davenport, M. eds. *Handbook of Pediatric Surgery*. Springer Cham. ISBN: 978-3-030-84466-0. 2022. doi: 10.1007/978-3-030-84467-7_4.

15. Li S, Liu P, Liu Y, Huang J, Wu X, Ren J. Intestinal rehabilitation in critical illness. *World J Surg Infect.* 2022;**1**:30–7. https://www.worldsurginfect.com/text.asp?2022/1/1/30/347770

16. Hickmann CE, Castanares-Zapatero D, Deldicque L, Van den Berghe P, Caty G, Robert A, et al. Impact of very early physical therapy during septic shock on skeletal muscle: a randomized controlled trial. *CCM.* 2018;**46(9)**:1436–43. doi: 10.1097/CCM.0000000000003263.

17. Bear DE, Wandrag L, Merriweather JL, Connolly B, Hart N, Grocott MPW, et al. The role of nutrition support in the physical and functional recovery of critically ill patients: a narrative review. *Crit Care.* 2017;**21**:226 doi: 10.1186/s13054-017-1810-2.

18. Wu M.-Y, Yiang G.-T, Liao W.-T, Tsai AP.-Y, Cheng Y.-L, Cheng P.-W, Li C.-Y, Li C.-J: Current mechanistic concepts in ischemia and reperfusion injury. *Cell Physiol Biochem.* 2018;**46**:1650–67. doi: 10.1159/000489241.

19. Hendy A, Bubenek-Turconi ŞI. The diagnosis and hemodynamic monitoring of circulatory shock: current and future trends. *J Crit Care Med* (Targu Mures). 2016 Aug 10;**2(3)**:115–23. doi: 10.1515/jccm-2016-0018.

20. Brener MI, Rosenblum HR, Burkhoff D. Pathophysiology and advanced hemodynamic assessment of cardiogenic shock. *Methodist Debakey Cardiovasc J.* 2020 Jan-Mar;**16(1)**:7–15. doi: 10.14797/mdcj-16-1-7.

21. Komamura K, Fukui M, Iwasaku T, Hirotani S, Masuyama T. Takotsubo cardiomyopathy: pathophysiology, diagnosis, and treatment. World J *Cardiol.* 2014;**6(7)**:602–9. Published online 2014 Jul 26. doi: 10.4330/wjc.v6.i7.602.

22. Ferdinandy P, Danial H, Ambrus I, Rothery RA, Schulz R. Peroxynitrite is a major contributor to cytokine-induced myocardial contractile failure. *Circ Res.* 2000;**87**:241–7. doi: 10.1161/01.RES.87.3.241.

23. Lessnau K-D. Distributive Shock. Medscape 2022; https://emedicine.medscape.com/article/168689-print.

24. Marik PE, Baram M, Vahid B. Does central venous pressure predict fluid responsiveness? A systematic review of the literature and the tale of seven mares. *Chest.* 2008;**134(1)**:172–8. doi: 10.1378/chest.07-2331.

25. *Cardiovascular Physiology*. In: Mohrman DE, Heller L. (eds), 9e. McGraw Hill, 2018. https://accesscardiology.mhmedical.com/content.aspx?bookid=2432&sectionid=190800303 (accessed November 28, 2022).

26. Hernandez G, Messina A, Kattan E. Invasive arterial pressure monitoring: much more than mean arterial pressure! *Intensive Care Med.* 2022;**48**:1495–97. doi: 10.1007/s00134-022-06798-8.

27. Via G, Tavazzi G, Price S. Ten situations where inferior vena cava ultrasound may fail to accurately predict fluid responsiveness: a physiologically based point of view. *Intensive Care Med.* 2016 Jul;**42(7)**:1164–7. doi: 10.1007/s00134-016-4357-9. Epub 2016 Apr 23.

28. Kobe J, Mishra N, Arya VK, Al-Moustadi W, Nates W, Kumar B. Cardiac output monitoring: technology and choice. A*nn Card Anaesth.* 2019 Jan-Mar;**22(1)**:6–17. doi: 10.4103/aca.ACA_41_18.

29. Russell A, Rivers EP, Giri PC, Jaehne AK, Nguyen HB. A physiologic approach to hemodynamic monitoring and optimizing oxygen delivery in shock resuscitation. *J Clin Med.* 2020 Jun 30;**9(7)**:2052. doi: 10.3390/jcm9072052.

30. Richards GA, Hardcastle TC, Hodgson RE. Ventilation in the Trauma Patient: A Practical Approach. In: Velmahos G, Degiannis E, Doll D. eds. *Penetrating Trauma*. Springer, Berlin, Heidelberg. 2017. doi: 10.1007/978-3-662-49859-0_13.

31. Asehnoune K, Taccone FS, Singer M. High oxygen level in traumatic brain injury patients. Never ending story? *Intensive Care Med.* 2022;**48**:1772–74. doi: 10.1007/s00134-022-06903-x.

32. Papazian L, Forel J-M, Gacouin A, Penot-Ragon C, Perrin G, Loundou A, et al. Neuromuscular blockers in early acute respiratory distress syndrome. *N Engl J Med.* 2010;**363**:1107–116. doi: 10.1056/NEJMoa1005372.

33. Bickell WH, Wall MJ, Pepe PE. Immediate versus delayed resuscitation for hypotensive patients with penetrating torso injuries. *N Engl J Med.* 1994 Oct 27;**331(17)**:1105–9. doi: 10.1056/NEJM199410273311701.

34. Schreiber MA, Meier EN, Tisherman SA, Kerby JD, Newgard CD, Brasel K, et al ROC Investigators. A controlled resuscitation strategy is feasible and safe in hypotensive trauma

patients: results of a prospective randomized pilot trial. *J Trauma Acute Care Surg.* 2015 Apr;**78(4)**:687–95; discussion 695–7. doi: 10.1097/TA.0000000000000600.

35. Owattanapanich, N., Chittawatanarat, K., Benyakorn, T, Sirikun J. Risks, and benefits of hypotensive resuscitation in patients with traumatic hemorrhagic shock: a meta-analysis. *Scand J Trauma Resusc Emerg Med.* 2018 Dec;**26(1)**:107: doi.org/10.1186/s13049-018-0572-4.

36. Moore GP, Pace SA, Busby W. Comparison of intraosseus, intramuscular, and intravenous administration of succinyl choline. *Pediatric Emergency Care.* 1989 Dec;**5(4)**:209–10. doi: 10.1097/00006565-198912000-00001.

37. Myburgh JA, Higgins A, Jovanovska A, Lipman J, Ramakrishnan N, Santamaria J; CAT Study investigators. A comparison of epinephrine and norepinephrine in critically ill patients. *Intensive Care Med.* 2008 Dec;**34(12)**:2226–34. doi: 10.1007/s00134-008-1219-0. Epub 2008 Jul 25. PMID: 18654759.

38. De Backer D, Biston P, Devriendt J, Madl C, Chochrad D, Aldecoa C, et al: SOAP II Investigators. Comparison of dopamine and norepinephrine in the treatment of shock. *N Engl J Med.* 2010 Mar 4;**362(9)**:779–89. doi: 10.1056/NEJMoa0907118. PMID: 20200382

39. Malbrain MLNG, Martin G, Ostermann M. Everything you need to know about deresuscitation. *Intensive Care Med.* 2022;**48**:1781–86. doi: 10.1007/s00134-022-06761-7.

40. Cap AP, Pidcoke HF, Spinella P, Strandenes G, Borgman MA, Schreiber M, et al. Damage control resuscitation. *Mil Med.* 2018 Sep 1;**183(suppl_2)**:36–43. doi: 10.1093/milmed/usy112.

41. Leibner E, Andreae M, Galvagno SM, Scalea T. Damage control resuscitation. *Clin Exp Emerg Med.* 2020 Mar;**7(1)**:5–13. doi: 10.15441/ceem.19.089. Epub 2020 Mar 31.

Recommended Reading

Advanced Cardiovascular Life Support Provider Manual. American Heart Association, Dallas, Texas. 2020. ISBN 978-1616697723.

Evans L, Rhodes A, Alhazzani W, Antonelli M, Coopersmith CM, French C, et al. Surviving sepsis campaign: international guidelines for management of sepsis and septic shock. *Crit Care Med.* 2021 Nov 1;**49(11)**:e1063–e143. doi: 10.1097/CCM.0000000000005337.

Lane N. *Power, Sex, Suicide: Mitochondria and the Meaning of Life (Oxford Landmark Science)*, 2nd Edn. Oxford University Press. 2005.

Marino PL. ed. *The ICU Book*, 4th Edn. Wolters Kluver Health/Lippincott Williams and Wilkins, Philadelphia PA, USA. 2014.

Transfusion in Trauma **4**

Transfusion of blood and blood components is a fundamental part of trauma management, and approximately 40% of the 13 million units of blood transfused in the United States each year are used in emergency resuscitation. The principles of resuscitating a patient in haemorrhagic shock are governed by damage control resuscitation principles which were first described in 2007.[1] Damage control resuscitation is designed to normalize physiology by restoring intravascular volume and oxygen-carrying capacity whilst normalizing coagulation with the components that have been lost. This is best done with fresh whole blood (FWB) or the closest equivalent, including either liquid cold-stored whole blood or red blood cells (RBCs), plasma, and platelets given in a 1:1:1 ratio.[2,3]

4.1 INDICATIONS FOR TRANSFUSION

4.1.1 Oxygen-Carrying Capacity

Anaemia is a decrease in the O_2-carrying capacity of blood, defined by a decrease in circulating red cell mass (to below 24 mL/kg in females and 26 mL/kg in males). Anaemia will result in an increase in cardiac output at a haemoglobin (Hb) level of < 7 g/dL (4.0 mmol/L). Oxygen extraction increases as O_2 delivery falls, ensuring a constant O_2 uptake by the tissues. Normal humans can survive an 80% loss of red cell mass if they are normovolaemic and normothermic. The threshold for O_2 delivery to maintain adequate tissue oxygenation is at a haematocrit of 10% and a Hb level of 3 g/dL (1.8 mmol/L) when breathing 100% O_2 with a normal metabolic rate.

Volume-dependent markers (such as haematocrit and Hb) are poor indicators of anaemia because they are concentrations which are affected by the relative volume of the RBC mass and plasma volume. Even after haemorrhage control is achieved, the Hb will continue to drop, as the increase in intravascular volume is usually dominated by an increase in plasma volume from equilibration and crystalloid resuscitation.

Pitfall

Early in haemorrhagic shock, whole blood is being lost. The whole blood left behind will have the same haematocrit and Hb, and so **it is not possible to assess the patient using these parameters**, which will only alter after refilling of the circulation and, with transfusion, will be reflected by a relatively small reduction in haematocrit and Hb.

4.2 TRANSFUSION FLUIDS

4.2.1 Colloids

4.2.1.1 STARCHES

The use of starches is contraindicated in the actively bleeding patient, since starches deplete the factor VIII–von Willebrand factor complex, and may make the actively bleeding patient more coagulopathic from both factor depletion and dilution coagulopathy. Hydroxyethyl starch is an independent risk factor for acute kidney injury and death after blunt trauma.[4]

4.2.1.2 ALBUMIN

Human albumin has not been evaluated for acute resuscitation, although animal experimentation suggests it may be appropriate. The Saline versus Albumin Fluid Evaluation (SAFE) study in 2007 tested saline versus albumin in the intensive care unit (ICU) and suggested an increased mortality in trauma patients, particularly in patients with traumatic brain injury (TBI).

DOI: 10.1201/9781003258124-6

Pitfall

Neither starches nor albumin should be used in trauma resuscitation.

4.2.2 **Blood**

4.2.2.1 FRESH WHOLE BLOOD

Humans are O_2-dependent organisms, and O_2 depletion causes major damage within minutes. Thus, in the exsanguinating patient, RBCs are transfused in order to improve O_2 transport, although older blood does not carry oxygen well. Evidence from military studies has suggested the advantage of FWB in the resuscitation and survival of the exsanguinating patient.[5] The rationale is that FWB has more functions than merely being an O_2 transport medium and provides:

- Oncotic pressure and protection from endothelial and glycocalyx damage (from plasma).
- Near 100% clotting factor and platelet function.
- Temperature homeostasis (from warm circulating fluid).
- FWB offers blood at close to 37 °C, RBCs, plasma, and platelets in natural proportions, to address the need of the exsanguinating patient for O_2 and oncotic pressure. A 500 mL unit of FWB has:
  - A haematocrit of 38%–50%.
  - 50,000–400,000/mm^3 fully functional platelets.
  - 100% activity of clotting factors diluted only by the anticoagulant.
  - Excellent oxygen-carrying ability.

In addition, the viability and flow characteristics of fresh RBCs are better than those of their stored counterparts, which have metabolic depletion and membrane dysfunction. The safe use of FWB requires the availability of healthy, pre-screened donors and is generally not available in civilian settings. Even with the use of rapid tests for transfusion-transmitted diseases (TTDs) which are approximately 85% sensitive, the safety of FWB cannot be guaranteed, and for this reason it is not US Food and Drug Administration (FDA)-approved for use in the United States.

FWB can be stored warm for 8 hours. After 8 hours, it is still considered fresh when stored at 4 °C for 48 hours. After 48 hours, it is considered cold-stored whole blood which can be stored for 21 days in citrate–phosphate–dextrose (CPD) solution and 35 days in CPA–adenine (CPDA-1) solution. Platelet count diminishes substantially after approximately 5 days, and whilst the labile clotting factors V and VIII decline within 24 hours, clotting as measured by thromboelastography (TEG) is only impaired to a clinically significant degree after 21 days.[6] Some blood suppliers leukoreduce whole blood which results in decreased platelet count and function.[7] Liquid cold-stored whole blood can be fully tested for TTDs and is FDA-approved, but it does not have equivalent positive effects on coagulation due to gradual depletion of coagulation factors, platelets, and platelet function.

4.2.2.2 STORED WHOLE BLOOD

Some of the benefits of whole blood – including an inherently balanced resuscitation, relatively less anticoagulant when compared to equivalent volumes of blood components, and the logistic ease of administration – can be realized with stored whole blood. Stored whole blood with a 14–21-day shelf life is substantially easier to provide than FWB in many circumstances. In recent years, several civilian centres have evaluated the use of cold-stored low-titre type O whole blood for the resuscitation of acutely injured patients. Initial observational results appear promising with an associated survival benefit and very few adverse events, including haemolysis. Clinical results have not been compared in any large clinical study and as such, despite some theoretical differences, should be considered effectively equivalent by clinicians in the context of trauma. Increased volumes of cold-stored whole blood for use in initial massive transfusion are now the subject of a randomized controlled trial (Trauma Resuscitation with Low-Titre Group O Whole Blood or Products [TROOP]). The goal of this clinical trial is to compare the effectiveness of unseparated whole blood (referred to as *low-titre group O whole blood*) and the separate components of whole blood (including red cells, plasma, platelets, and cryoprecipitate) in critically injured patients who require large-volume blood transfusions.[8] The US military's Tactical Combat Casualty Care guidelines prefer stored over FWB, essentially for reasons of supply.

4.2.2.3 PACKED RED BLOOD CELLS

Previous haemorrhage management involved resuscitation with excessive amounts of crystalloids and transfusion of RBCs in high ratios compared to other components which diluted native clotting factors, causing hypocoagulation.[9] This additional fluid aggravated the coagulopathy initiated from the moment of injury due to:

- Loss of warm blood and replacement with cooler fluid, resulting in decreased body temperature
- Resuscitation with acidic solutions that are high-chloride-containing products, resulting in acidosis
- Dilution of coagulation factors
- Raising blood pressure in the absence of improved coagulation capacity, resulting in displacing established clots

4.2.2.4 SYNTHETIC BLOOD AND BLOOD PRODUCTS[10]

Synthetic biology adopts an engineering design approach to create innovative treatments that are dependable, scalable, and customizable to individual patients. Interest in substitutes for allogenic blood components, primarily RBCs and platelets, increased in the 1980s because of concerns over infectious disease transmission. However, only now, with emerging synthetic approaches, are such substitutes showing genuine promise. Affordable alternatives to donated blood would be of enormous benefit worldwide. Several approaches to replacing the oxygen-carrying function of red cells are under advanced investigation. Haemoglobin-based oxygen carriers incorporate modifications to reduce the renal toxicity and nitric oxide scavenging of free haemoglobin. Whilst use of earlier-generation haemoglobin-based oxygen carriers may be limited to circumstances in which blood transfusion is not an option, recent advances in chemical modification of haemoglobin may eventually overcome such problems. Another approach encases haemoglobin molecules in biocompatible synthetic nanoparticles. An alternative is the *ex vivo* production of red cells in bioreactors, with or without genetic manipulation, which offers the potential of a universal donor product. Various strategies to manufacture synthetic platelets are also underway, ranging from simple phospholipid liposomes encapsulating adenosine diphosphate (ADP) and decorated with fibrinogen fragments, to more complex capsules with multiple receptor peptide sequences. *Ex vivo* production of platelets in bioreactors is also possible including, for example, platelets derived from induced pluripotent stem cells that are differentiated into a megakaryocytic lineage.

4.2.3 Component Therapy (Platelets, Fresh Frozen Plasma [FFP], and Cryoprecipitate)

4.2.3.1 PLATELETS[11]

The body has large reserves of platelets, sequestrated in the spleen, liver, and endothelium, that are mobilized when there is a need. A fall in platelet count occurs somewhat later than the loss of clotting factors. Trauma patients rarely develop thrombocytopenia (platelet count <100,000/mm[3]), although platelet dysfunction due to hypothermia and other factors is common. Spontaneous bleeding rarely occurs if the platelet count is greater than 30,000/mm[3].

Hypothermia affects platelet adhesion more than enzymes at temperatures above 34 °C, whilst it affects all aspects of coagulation below 34 °C. There is general agreement that the indications for platelet transfusion are:

- *Prophylaxis*: If the platelet count <15,000/mm.
- *Pre-surgery*: Platelet count <50,000/mm[3].
- *Active bleeding*: Platelet count <100,000/mm[3].
- One unit increases the platelet count by 10,000/mm[3] platelets.
- One mega-unit (5 units) of apheresis platelets increases the platelet count by 50,000/mm[3].

Platelets are the most problematic component of damage control resuscitation. Platelets are typically stored at room temperature for up to 5 days and agitated. The short half-life is due to the risk of bacterial contamination. There is evidence that cold-stored platelets have greater haemostatic efficacy, and they can be stored up to 21 days.[12] Cold platelets are approved for use in the United States for up to 3 days. A special exception can be obtained from the FDA to store platelets up to 21 days when standard platelets are not available. Cold platelets are used by the US military and stored up to 21 days in battlefield settings.

The short life span of platelets and the need for constant stirring have led to research into deep-frozen platelets (−80 °C). Evidence suggests that platelets at that temperature retain function for 4 years. The need for stirring is eliminated, as well as the dependence on the 'walking blood bank' which is utilized in the military situation. The Massive Transfusion of Frozen Blood (MAFOd) study protocol initiated from the Dutch Army is currently evaluating the non-inferiority of deep-frozen platelets versus room-temperature-stored platelets.[13]

Platelets can be distributed as single-donor platelets equivalent to the number of platelets present in a single unit of whole blood or as apheresis platelets (megaunits), a unit of which is equivalent to the number of platelets in 4–6 units of whole blood (different country dependent). Using damage control principles, a unit of apheresis platelets is transfused with equivalent units of RBCs and plasma. Platelets are typically suspended in plasma.

4.2.3.2 PLASMA: FFP OR FREEZE-DRIED PLASMA (FDP)

Plasma utilized in damage control resuscitation may come in the form of liquid plasma, thawed plasma, FDP, or FFP. Liquid plasma has never been frozen and has superior factor function due to the absence of loss of function due to freezing and thawing. Liquid plasma can be stored for up to 26 days with minimal factor degradation, and it is immediately available for high ratio transfusion.

FFP is much less logistically feasible in damage control resuscitation due to the need to thaw units which may take up to 30 minutes. This problem can be partially mitigated by thawing units for future use. Thawed FFP can be stored for up to 5 days with minimal factor degradation, but this practice results in increased waste. Type AB plasma is the universal donor, but type A plasma is also frequently used for this purpose.

Current evidence suggests that most patients will require 1 unit of plasma for every unit of blood transfused. A unit of plasma also contains most of the citrate anticoagulant from the unit of blood from which it was originally derived. It contains about 0.5 g fibrinogen, and normal levels of pro- and anticoagulants. Solvent-detergent-related/lyophilized/freeze-dried plasma was previously thought to hold about 20% less of the above per unit given; however, more recent research shows that FFP is equivalent to FDP.

Potential advantages of plasma are:

- It contains all coagulation factors, although not all in equal concentration.
- It is preferred to cryoprecipitate, which contains 50% content of most normal coagulation factors, apart from fibrinogen, factor VIII, and von Willebrand factor.

4.2.3.3 CRYOPRECIPITATE

Cryoprecipitate contains fibrinogen, the factor VIII–von Willebrand factor complex, and fibrin-stabilizing factor XIII. Cryoprecipitate may not be required in all cases of trauma. One unit (250 mL) of FFP contains 0.5 g fibrinogen; one unit of cryoprecipitate contains 0.25 g fibrinogen, but in 10 mL (rather than 250 mL). Therefore, in most cases, FFP will meet the needs required. However, if a rapid increase in fibrinogen is needed, early cryoprecipitate is a useful adjunct.[14]

The CRYOSTAT trials are currently in progress: CRYOSTAT-1 was a feasibility study which suggested that early cryoprecipitate therapy maintained acceptable blood fibrinogen levels during active bleeding, with a signal for reduced mortality in the treatment arm of the study.[15] CRYOSTAT-2 will test the effect of early cryoprecipitate (within 90 minutes of admission) compared to standard blood transfusion therapy and is due for completion in 2023. A 2-year retrospective trauma quality improvement project review of trauma patients receiving 4 or more units of RBCs showed an association between cryoprecipitate use and improved survival.[16]

4.2.3.4 FIBRINOGEN CONCENTRATE

The use of fibrinogen concentrate has been reported in trauma patients. The RETIC (Reversal of Trauma Induced Coagulopathy Using Coagulation Factor Concentrates or Fresh Frozen Plasma) trial was a single-centre, open-label, randomized trial comparing initial treatment with 15 mL/kg FFP or 50 mg/kg fibrinogen concentrate based on rotary thromboelastomerography (RoTEM) parameters. The trial showed that a single dose of fibrinogen concentrate was more likely to restore normal coagulation in severely injured trauma patients based on RoTEM and resulted in a lower bleeding score.[17]

4.3 EFFECTS OF TRANSFUSING BLOOD AND BLOOD PRODUCTS

Stored packed red blood cells (pRBCs) (stored for a maximum of 42 days with current FDA-approved storage solutions) develop defects proportionate to the duration of storage that assume greater clinical significance when transfused rapidly or in large quantities, such as in critically ill patients.

4.3.1 Metabolic Effects

- There is storage-related decreased adenosine triphosphate (ATP) which precedes RBC membrane deformability and its survival during storage.

- Degradation of 2,3-diphosphoglycerate (2,3-DPG) occurs after 7–10 days in storage. 2,3-DPG is an enzyme affecting the affinity of Hb for O_2. After 7 days of storage, the O_2-transporting ability of Hb drops by two-thirds. Adenine added to pRBCs may restore levels of 2,3-DPG *in vivo* after transfusion.
- Increased ammonia release occurs due to the release of intracellular protein after disruption of the red cell membrane during storage.
- Blood products are stored in citrate which chelates calcium, a critical component of nearly every reaction of coagulation.

> *Early replacement of calcium in the form of calcium gluconate or calcium chloride is critical for normal coagulation function. (See Coagulation triad vs. the Deadly Diamond – hypocalcaemia.)*

4.3.2 **Hyperkalaemia**

Serum potassium levels rise in stored blood as the efficiency of the Na+/K+ pump decreases. Transfused blood may have a potassium concentration of > 40 mmol/L. Transient hyperkalaemia may occur as a result, but often does not need correction.

4.3.3 **Coagulopathy of Trauma[9]**

Biochemical reactions within the body require a specific and narrow temperature and pH range to go ahead. The coagulation cascade is inhibited, even in the presence of all the clotting factors, when the tissue pH is below 7.2 and the temperature is below 34 °C. This progression of events is known as *trauma-induced coagulopathy* (TIC). TIC differs from acute traumatic coagulopathy that occurs as a result of massive tissue trauma and acidosis and occurs endogenously within moments of injury mediated through the protein C pathway. Endothelial damage resulting in third spacing and glycocalyx damage is directly proportional to the volume of crystalloid infused, and these processes are mitigated by transfusion of plasma. Fibrinolysis, fibrinogen dysfunction, platelet dysfunction, and endotheliopathy are all worsened by crystalloid resuscitation, and this dysfunction is mitigated by FWB transfusion. It is important to detect the acute coagulopathy of trauma (ACT) and TIC as early as possible (see **Figure 4.1**).

Coagulation tests, such as prothrombin time/international ratio (PT/INR), activated partial thromboplastin time (APTT), fibrinogen concentration, and platelet counts, have traditionally been used. Conventional coagulation assays either focus on one artificial aspect of clotting (PT/APTT) or report concentrations as in the case of fibrinogen or platelets which may not correlate with

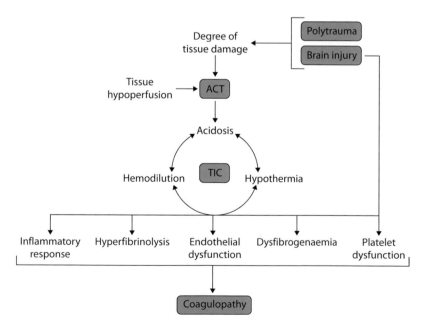

Figure 4.1 Pathophysiology of ACT and TIC. *Abbreviations*: ACT, acute traumatic coagulopathy; TIC, trauma-induced coagulopathy (TIC).

function. Increasingly, the transfusion of blood components is guided by viscoelastic haemostatic assays (VHAs) such as TEG or RoTEM. (See Section 4.5.2.) These assays focus on whole blood clotting and are functional in nature. However, in the face of continued bleeding, despite surgical control, blood products may need to be given empirically. VHAs may be performed at point of care and provide results within minutes, guiding adjunctive therapies given in addition to empiric damage control resuscitation.

4.3.4 **Other Risks of Transfusion**

4.3.4.1 TRANSFUSION-TRANSMITTED INFECTIONS

- Hepatitis A, B, C, and D
- Human immunodeficiency virus (HIV) 'window period'
- Cytomegalovirus
- Atypical mononucleosis and a swinging temperature that can be present for 7–10 days post transfusion
- Malaria
- Brucellosis
- Yersinia
- Syphilis

4.3.4.2 HAEMOLYTIC TRANSFUSION REACTIONS

- *Incompatibility*: ABO, rhesus (type the blood), and 26 other surface antigens (screen for these)
- To very cold blood, overheated blood, or pressurized blood
- Immediate generalized reaction (plasma)

4.3.4.3 IMMUNOLOGICAL COMPLICATIONS

- *Major incompatibility reaction*: Usually caused by 'wrong blood' due to administrative errors.
- *Graft-versus-host disease*: This is rare but often fatal.
- *Transfusion-related acute lung injury (TRALI)*.
- *Immunomodulation*: Reports on transplant and oncology patients have supplied evidence that transfusion induces a regulatory immune response in the recipient that increases the ratio of suppressor to helper T cells. These changes may make the trauma patient more susceptible to infection.

4.3.4.4 FACTORS IMPLICATED IN HAEMOSTATIC FAILURE

- *Hypothermia*: Blood is stored at 4 °C, but body temperature is 37 °C, so the body needs to provide 1255 kJ of energy to heat each unit of blood to body temperature.

- *Acidosis*: From citrate and lactate.
- Dilution, depletion, and decreased production of red cells and platelets.
- *Diffuse intravascular coagulation*: There is a consumption of clotting factors and platelets within the circulation, which are trapped in the microvascular thrombi created due to fibrin disposition.
- *Extrinsic*: Tissue thromboplastins, for example blunt trauma and surgery, and burns.
- *Intrinsic*: Endothelial injury, endotoxin, hypothermia, hypoxia, acidosis, and platelet activation.
- Fibrinolysis.
- Consumption of red cells and platelets.
- Protein C activation.
- Hypocalcaemia.

Despite the extensive list quoted above, there is limited evidence about the risks of pRBC transfusion, although pRBC transfusion is an independent risk factor for:

- Increased nosocomial infections (wound infection, pneumonia, sepsis).
- Multiple organ failure and systemic inflammatory response syndrome.
- Longer ICU and hospital lengths of stay, increased complications, and increased mortality.
- Pre-storage leukocyte depletion of RBC transfusion reduces complication rates, with some studies showing a reduction in infectious complications.
- There is a relationship between receiving a transfusion and contracting TRALI and acute respiratory distress syndrome (ARDS).
- Transfusion, pRBCs, and FFP increase the risk for deep vein thrombosis (DVT) in trauma patients.

4.4 **ADJUNCTS TO ENHANCE CLOTTING**

There has been extensive interest in the provision of adjuncts to enhance clotting as part of the resuscitation of the trauma patient. These include the following.

4.4.1 **Prothrombin Complex Concentrate (PCC)**

Prothrombin complex concentrate is produced by combining plasma from thousands of patients and then isolating the complex which contains the vitamin

K–dependent factors as well as anticoagulants including proteins C and S, anti-thrombin III, and heparin.[18] Overall, it is procoagulant, but it is balanced by anticoagulant factors. PCC undergoes multiple viral inactivation steps, and anti-HLA (human leukocyte antigen) antibodies are reduced. PCC can be rapidly reconstituted with a small volume, and 3000 IUs increase coagulation factors by 40%–80%. Newer plasma-factor concentrates and prothrombin concentrates (e.g., Octaplex® [Octapharma, Vienna, Austria] and Haemosolvex® [NBI, Pinetown, South Africa]) have produced evidence that these may be a better option than FFP and FDP in trauma with smaller volumes and similar clotting enhancements, although these are currently primarily approved for warfarin reversal and acute haemophilia crises. PCC rapidly reverses the anticoagulation effects of coumadin much faster than plasma and is approved for use by the FDA for this purpose in patients requiring life-saving procedures or with life-threatening bleeds. In a retrospective, propensity-matched TQIP study, the use of PCC in combination with plasma for non-anticoagulated trauma patients was associated with improved survival and decreased rates of acute kidney injury and ARDS.[19,20] Due to its relatively short half-life, PCC is given with vitamin K.

4.4.2 Tranexamic Acid (TXA)

Tranexamic acid may be indicated in patients in haemorrhagic shock and patients in whom a massive transfusion protocol has been activated. The effect of TXA is to 'stabilize' a *formed* blood clot and prevent its breakdown. It does not alter the formation, only the stability, and is primarily reflected in the Ly30 seen in VHA studies (see Section 4.5.2).

The CRASH-2 trial showed a significant reduction in mortality with the use of TXA;[21] however, although the trial involved 20,000 subjects, fewer than half of the patients required red cell transfusion, and in those who were transfused, the two arms utilized the same amount of blood, and the mortality rates in both arms did not correlate with those in other studies. In addition, no injury severity comparisons were included. Study of the use of TXA in the military context showed improved coagulation and survival, especially in those patients requiring massive transfusion (the MATTERs Study).[22]

The STAAMP trial was a prospective randomized trial inclusive of over 900 patients comparing the use of TXA to placebo in trauma patients with either hypotension or tachycardia.[23] Overall, there was no survival benefit in

the group that received TXA. Subgroup analysis revealed that patients who received TXA within 1 hour of injury, and patients with an initial systolic blood pressure (SBP) < 70 mmHg, had improved survival.

The TXA in TBI trial (CRASH-3 trial), which was another large randomized trial, concluded that patients with reactive pupils and/or a mild to moderate Glasgow Coma Scale (GCS) score may have benefited from TXA in the trial because they had less intracranial bleeding at baseline. However, because bleeding occurs soon after injury, treatment delay reduces the benefit of TXA.[24] Patients with moderate to severe TBI who received a 2 g bolus of TXA in the field had increased survival and improved disability rating scores compared to patients who received placebo or 1 g in the field and a 1 g infusion in the hospital.[25] Some regions are now giving a 2 g bolus of TXA in the field for both haemorrhagic shock and TBI.

Current European guidelines (sixth edition)[26] recommend administration of TXA:

- For patients who are bleeding or at risk of significant haemorrhage as soon as possible and within 3 hours after injury at a loading dose of 1 g infused over 10 minutes, followed by an intravenous (IV) infusion of 1 g over 8 hours.
- En route to the hospital.
- Not waiting for the results from a viscoelastic assessment.
- Not waiting for a viscoelastic assessment.
- At a dose of 1 g intravenously administered over 10 minutes, then 1 g intravenously administered over 8 hours, although newer studies suggest a single dose of 2 g may be more effective.
- In adult trauma patients with severe haemorrhagic shock (SBP < 75 mmHg), with known predictors of fibrinolysis, or verified fibrinolysis by TEG (LY30).

Whilst TXA's use pre-hospital and in-hospital in Europe is ubiquitous, in many other countries, including the United States,[27] its use is not routine, or is reserved only for rural environments with long transport times and for patients with uncontrollable bleeding.

4.4.3 Desmopressin (DDAVP)

Desmopressin potentiates the function of platelets and is indicated only for functional platelet disorders, secondary to platelet inhibitors such as aspirin, clopidogrel, ticagrelor, prasugrel, and so on; renal or hepatic failure; haemophilia A; and von Willebrand disease.

4.4.4 **Recombinant Activated Factor VIIA**

Interest has focussed on recombinant activated factor VIIa (rFVIIa, or NovoSeven). This was initially developed as an adjunct for the treatment of haemophilia. However, following its successful use in controlling the bleeding in a trauma patient, there was considerable interest in its use. A large multicentre trial in 2005[28] showed a reduction in red cell transfusion requirements in blunt trauma patients, and the drug has been used extensively 'off-label'. A further large trial in 2008 showed a reduction in blood product usage of 3.6 units in blunt injury, but the study sample was too small to show significance on mortality or for penetrating injury.[29]

Consequently, rFVIIa is not widely considered, but it is still utilized in certain countries and in some military situations. A suitable protocol appears in **Table 4.1**.

4.5 **MONITORING THE COAGULATION STATUS**

Ideally, the use of blood components should be guided by laboratory tests of clotting function. This is part of the concept of personalized medicine, or, in trauma, part of the concept of goal-directed therapy, giving the patient only what is needed and avoiding transfusions not needed. Haemostasis according to the cell-based model is described in the phases of initiation, amplification, and propagation, from clot formation to clot lysis, with participation of all circulating plasma and cellular components. Thrombin generation is central for clot development and strength. It primarily occurs on the surface of activated platelets, and, hence, platelets and thrombin generation are closely related to the development of coagulopathy.

4.5.1 **Traditional Assays**

- *International normalized ratio* (*INR*): Extrinsic
- *Partial thromboplastin time* (*PTT*): Intrinsic
- *D-dimer values* (*fibrinolysis*)

All of the above assays are cost-effective if frequently done, but all take time to return results which are likely to be misleading to clinical decision-making in the context of rapidly evolving trauma coagulopathy.

Table 4.1 Guidelines for the Use of rFVIIA

Definition
This guideline describes the use of rFVIIa as an *adjunct* in the management of coagulopathy following trauma with massive bleeding or the need to enter the massive transfusion protocol.

Issue
The blood bank will issue the required rFVIIa for administration immediately **after completion** of the 6th and 12th units of transfused blood.

Limitation
rFVIIa should **only** be used:
- **If all** surgical **bleeding has been controlled.**
- **In the presence of active bleeding.**
- **Where possible, its use should be backed up with a thromboelastogram**.
  - Increased R (reaction time) despite fresh frozen plasma.
- After transfusion of > 6 units of red cells or whole blood.
- If the platelet count is > 50,000/mm³.
- If the pH is > 7.2.
- If the temperature is > 34 °C.

Blood specimens
Disseminated intravascular coagulopathy screen:
- Full blood count and platelets
- Fibrinogen
- TEG or RoTEM, or, if not available: prothrombin time, activated partial thromboplastin time, thrombin time, International Normalized Ratio, D-dimer

Dose
The dose of rFVIIa should be 90 µg/kg, but may be as high as 120 µg/kg
- Round UP to the nearest 1.2 mg
  (*Example*: A 75 kg male receives 75 × 90 µg/kg = 6.75 mg rFVIIa. Round UP to 7.2 mg.)
If the patient continues to bleed:
- Repeat the dose after 1 hour and after 3 hours from first dose.
- Repeat the dose after completion of the **12th** unit of transfused blood.

End points of administration
The first of:
- Cessation of bleeding
  or
- Three doses

4.5.2 **Viscoelastic Haemostatic Assays (VHAs):[30,31] Thromboelastography (TEG) and Rotary Thromboelastomerography (RoTEM)**

The VHA technology results in a visual profile, or trace, and variables with a reference value (see **Figure 4.2a** and **4.2b**). Briefly, the collected whole-blood sample is placed in a specially designed small cup (< 1 cc). A pin that is connected to a detector system (a torsion wire in TEG, and an optical detector in RoTEM) is suspended in the blood, and the cup and pin are oscillated relative to each other, with movement initiated from either the cup (TEG) or the pin (RoTEM). As fibrin strings form between the cup and pin, the transmitted rotation from the cup to pin (TEG) or the impedance of the rotation of the pin (RoTEM) is detected at the pin and a trace is generated, as seen in **Figure 4.2a** (TEG) and **4.2b** (RoTEM). The standard assays can be accelerated with kaolin activation and tissue factor in TEG (RapidTEG),

and tissue factor or kaolin activation, respectively, in the ExTEM and InTEM assays in RoTEM. Several other dedicated assays are available from both technologies. The contribution of fibrinogen to clot strength can be evaluated in the functional fibrinogen assay in TEG and the FibTEM assay in RoTEM. New VHAs are the portable cartridge-driven bedside devices TEG 6® (Haemonetics, Signy-Centre, Switzerland) and RoTEM Sigma® (Werfen, Bedford, MA, USA). Many results are available within 10 minutes in the form of a curve (**Figure 4.1a** or **4.1b**), although completion of the test out to LY30 can take close to an hour. Measured parameters include (see **Table 4.3**):

- *R time (reaction time)/Clotting time*: The latency from the time at which the blood is placed in the cup until the clot begins to form.
- *The α (alpha) angle*: The progressive increase in clot strength which is primarily determined by the rate of fibrin crosslinking.

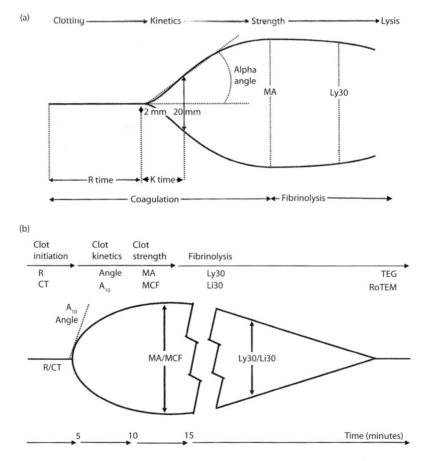

Figure 4.2 (a) Thromboelastogram (TEG), and (b) rotary thromboelastogram (RoTEM). *Abbreviations*: α (Alpha) angle, clot strength; A_{10}, amplitude after 10 minutes; CT, clotting time; K time, kinetic time; Ly30 and Ly30/Li30, fibrinolysis after 30 minutes; MA, maximum amplitude – maximum clot strength; MCF, maximum clot firmness; R time, reaction time.

Table 4.2 Interpretation of the Parameters of the TEG and RoTEM

Measurement	TEG Parameter (Normal Range)	RoTEM Parameter (Normal Range)
Clotting factor activity	R time (3–8 minutes)	CT_{ExTEM} (38–79 second) CT_{InTEM} (100–240 second)
Kinetics to maximum clot strength	K time (1–3 min)	
Rate of increase in clot strength	α (alpha) angle (55°–69°)	$A10_{ExTEM}$ (43–65 mm)
Maximum strength of the clot	MA (51–69 mm)	MCF_{ExTEM} (50–72 mm)
Fibrinolysis at 30 minutes	LY30 (< 4%)	LI30 (94%–100%)
Fibrinogen activity (level)	FF_{MA} (14–24 mm)	FibTEM MCF (9–16 mm)
Thrombelastography (TEG®): R, reaction time CT, clottng MCF time K time, kinetic time α, Alpha angle MA, maximum amplitude FFMA, functional fibrinogen Ly30, fibrinolysis after 30 minutes	Rotational thromboelastometry (RoTEM®): ExTEM, Extrinsically activated RoTEM InTEM, Intrinsically activated RoTEM FibTEM, Fibrin based extrinsically activated RoTEM A10, Amplitude after 10 min MCF, maximum clot firmness LI30, fibrinolysis after 30 minutes Fib, fibrinogen	

- *K time (kinetic time)*: The K time starts where the R time ends, and it ends when the curve is at 20 mm amplitude.
- *MA (maximum amplitude)*: The maximal clot strength.
- *LY30*: Amount of thrombolysis after 30 minutes, expressed as a percentage of the MA.

VHAs allow for goal-directed haemostatic therapy, thereby only treating with what is needed. They offer substantial support to decision-making during the resuscitation, as they give real-time accurate information on the coagulation status of the trauma patient, and facilitate the differentiation between pathological abnormality and surgically correctable bleeding.

See **Table 4.2** for interpretation of the curves and their management. Furthermore, it is possible to decide whether the bleeding is surgical or coagulopathic/pathological, which clotting factors are missing, the function of platelets, and whether fibrinolysis is evolving normally. Transfusion of blood components, coagulation factors, and additional medication can be administered rationally, based on the results. See **Table 4.3** for goal-directed management. This can also be presented as a pictogram graphically interpreting the VHAs for staff. See **Figure 4.3**, and a cartoon interpreting the graphics for staff **Figure 4.4**.

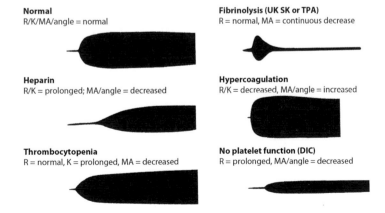

Normal
R/K/MA/angle = normal

Fibrinolysis (UK SK or TPA)
R = normal, MA = continuous decrease

Heparin
R/K = prolonged; MA/angle = decreased

Hypercoagulation
R/K = decreased, MA/angle = increased

Thrombocytopenia
R = normal, K = prolonged, MA = decreased

No platelet function (DIC)
R = prolonged, MA/angle = decreased

Figure 4.3 Abnormal appearance of the thromboelastogram. *Abbreviations*: DIC, disseminated intravascular coagulopathy; K, kinetic time; MA, maximum amplitude; R, reaction time; SK, streptokinase; TPA, tissue plasminogen activator; UK, urokinase.

Table 4.3 Goal-Directed Administration of Haemostatic Products and Medication, Based on TEG and RoTEM

TEG	RoTEM	Coagulopathy	Treatment options
R 10–14 min	ExTEM CT 80–100 second	Coagulation factors ↓	FFP 20 mL/kg
	InTEM CT 200–240 second		
R >14 min	ExTEM CT > 100 second	Coagulation factors ↓↓	FFP 30 mL/kg rFVIIA (see **Table 3.5**)
	InTEM CT > 240 second		
FF$_{MA}$ 7–14 mm	FibTEM MCF 6–9 mm	Fibrinogen ↓	FFP 20 mL/kg or cryoprecipitate 3 mL/kg or fibrinogen concentrate 20 mg/kg
FF$_{MA}$ 0–7 mm	FibTEM MCF 0–6 mm	Fibrinogen ↓↓	FFP 30 mL/kg or cryoprecipitate 5 mL/kg or fibrinogen concentrate 30 g/kg
K (kinetic) time	> 4 minutes		Cryoprecipitate 5 mL/kg or fibrinogen concentrate 30 mg/kg or rFVIIA (see **Table 4.5**)
α angle	<65°		Cryoprecipitate 5 mL/kg or fibrinogen concentrate 30 mg/kg or DDAVP
MA 45–49 mm and FF$_{MA}$ > 14 mm	ExTEM A$_{10}$ 35–42 mm and FibTEM ≥ 10 mm	Platelets ↓	Platelets 5 mL/kg
	ExTEM MCF <50 mm and FibTEM ≥10 mm		
MA < 45 mm and FF$_{MA}$ > 14 mm	ExTEM A$_{10}$ < 35 mm and FibTEM ≥ 10 mm	Platelets ↓↓	Platelets 10 mL/kg
Ly30 > 3 (–8)%	ExTEM LI30 < 94%	Hyperfibrinolysis	TXA 10 g or 10–20 mg/kg
Difference in R Hep TEG versus standard TEG R > 2 min	InTEM CT / HEPTEM CT > 1.25	Heparinization	Protamine 50–100 mg or FFP 10–20 mL/kg

TXA – Tranexamic acid
FFP – Fresh frozen plasma
rFVIIA – Recombinant Factor VIIa
Sec – Seconds
ExTEM – Extrinsically activated RoTEM

InTEM – Intrinsically activated ROTEM
FibTEM – Fibrin based extrinsically activated ROTEM
HepTEM – Addition of heparinase, allowing analysis of heparinised samples

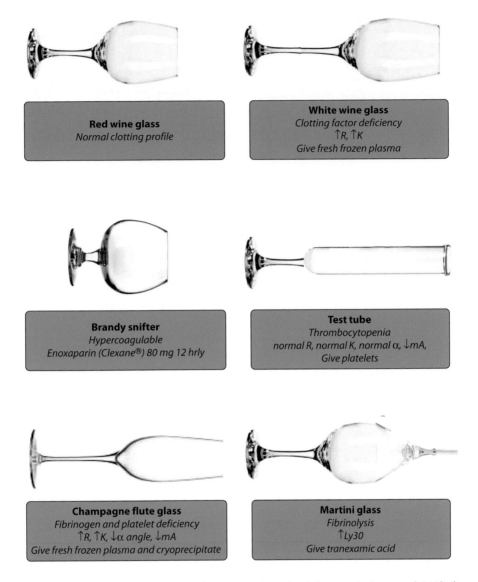

Figure 4.4 Graphics interpreting management of common viscoelastic haemostatic assay (VHA) abnormalities.

During a massive transfusion when coagulation status is rapidly changing, VHAs can be used in addition to damage control resuscitation to decide adjunctive therapies.[32]

4.6 **AUTOTRANSFUSION**

Intraoperative and postoperative blood salvage and alternative methods for decreasing transfusion may lead to a significant reduction in allogenic blood usage.

Autotransfusion eliminates the risk of incompatibility and the need for crossmatching; the risk of transmission of disease from the donor is also eliminated. Autotransfusion is a safe and cost-effective method of sustaining RBC mass whilst decreasing demands on the blood bank. However, cell salvage in trauma patients is logistically challenging, as, in the trauma patient, autotransfusion typically involves the collection of blood shed from wounds and into body cavities – especially the chest, abdomen, and drains.

Modern autotransfusion devices are basically of two types:

- Collection of blood that is anticoagulated with heparin or citrate, and then run through a system in which it is washed and centrifuged, before being re-transfused.

  Reinfusion after filtration is less labour intensive and provides blood for transfusion quickly. Whole blood is returned to the patient with platelets and proteins intact, but free Hb and procoagulants are also reinfused. A high proportion of the salvaged blood is returned to the patient, and the most recent devices do not require mixing of the blood with an anticoagulant solution. In-line filters are essential when autotransfusion devices are used. These filters remove gross particles and macroaggregates during collection and reinfusion, thus minimizing microembolization.[33]

- Cell-washing and centrifugation techniques require a machine and (usually) a technician to be the sole operator. This latter requirement can limit the utility of the devices in everyday practice. The cell-washing cycle produces red cells suspended in saline with a haematocrit of 55%–60%. This solution has minimal free Hb, procoagulants, and bacteria. However, bacteria have been shown to adhere to the iron in the Hb molecule; and washing, therefore, does not eliminate the risk of infection.

In practical terms, bleeding from the chest seems ideal for immediate autotransfusion, as the contents of the thoracic cavity are sterile, in contrast with abdominal bleeding, where visceral injury and contamination may coexist. The simplest effective method is to use the sterile chest drain container. Saline is used to create the fluid valve at the end of a chest drainage tube, to which is added 1000 IU fractionated heparin. The contents of the bottle may be hung and (using a microfilter to collect microaggregates) immediately reintroduced intravenously.

Autotransfusion is generally contraindicated in the presence of bacterial or malignant cell contamination (e.g., and open bowel, infected vascular prostheses, etc.), unless no other RBC source is available and the patient is in a life-threatening situation. However, there are several studies showing the practice may not be as unreasonable as previously thought.[34,35]

Cell salvage techniques have been shown to be cost-effective and useful in some trauma patients (e.g., in splenic trauma with significant blood loss), but further studies are indicated to clarify the indications.

4.7 MASSIVE HAEMORRHAGE AND MASSIVE TRANSFUSION PROTOCOLS (MHPs/MTPs)

4.7.1 Definition

Blood volume is approximately 70 mL/kg.

Massive transfusion has traditionally been defined as:

- Replacement of 100% of the patient's blood volume in less than 6 hours
- Transfusion of 10 units of RBCs in 24 hours
- Administration of 50% of the patient's blood volume in 1 hour

This definition is problematic from the standpoint that patients who die early with high-intensity transfusion may not survive long enough to receive 10 units and patients with low-intensity bleeding may reach 10 units over 24 hours whilst never being in haemorrhagic shock. The critical administration threshold (CAT) was described to address both of these issues and is defined as greater than or equal to 3 units of RBCs transfused in the first hour.[36]

There is a danger of death when blood loss is more than 150 mL per minute or 50% of blood volume in 20 minutes. Each trauma unit should have a policy for massive transfusion, which should be activated as soon as a potential candidate is admitted.

Pitfall

The MHP/MTP protocol should be activated **early** if there is *ongoing* active bleeding necessitating more than 2 units of blood transfused, since at that point there will already be depletion of all the components, which need replacement.

Also germane to the initial period of massive blood transfusion are the potential complications of acidosis, hypothermia, and hypocalcaemia. Hypothermia (<34 °C) causes platelet sequestration and inhibits the release of platelet factors that are important in the intrinsic clotting pathway. Hypothermia has consistently been associated with a poor outcome in trauma patients. Core temperature often falls insidiously because of exposure at the scene and in the emergency department, and because of the administration of resuscitation fluids stored at ambient temperature.

The use of bicarbonate in the treatment of systemic acidosis remains controversial. Administration of sodium bicarbonate may cause a leftward shift of the oxyhaemoglobin dissociation curve, reducing tissue O_2 extraction, and may worsen intracellular acidosis caused by carbon dioxide production.

Pitfall

Use of sodium bicarbonate in the acidotic trauma patient is associated with an increase in mortality.[37]

The acidosis is usually due to raised sodium lactate – a reflection of tissue hypoxia, and best dealt with by improving the oxygen delivery to tissues, not treating numbers!

Hypocalcaemia caused by citrate binding of ionized calcium does not occur until the blood transfusion rate exceeds 100 mL per minute (equivalent to 1 unit every 5 minutes). Decreased serum levels of ionized calcium depress myocardial function before impairing coagulation. Calcium gluconate or calcium chloride should be reserved for cases in which there is electrocardiogram (ECG) evidence of QT interval prolongation or, in rare instances, for cases of unexplained hypotension during massive transfusion, or where the active (ionized) fraction is >1 mmol/l on a blood-gas result.

Pitfall

Waiting for ECG evidence of QT interval prolongation or unexplained hypotension during massive transfusion is unwise.

4.7.2 Massive Transfusion Protocol

An algorithm of coordinated action incorporating many hospital departments (surgery, blood bank, ICU, anaesthesiology) is activated upon the arrival of a trauma patient with massive haemorrhage. The protocol provides roles for the personnel, actions to be taken, medications, and blood products to be transfused. The target is increased survival of these patients. MTPs should include delivery of boxes of blood either as low-titre type O whole blood (LTOWB) or balanced ratios of RBCs, plasma, and platelets until bleeding is stopped. Early on, calcium should be empirically given, and calcium levels should be followed throughout the MTP. TXA should be considered early.

Viscoelastic testing should be performed often to guide adjunctive therapies. Ideally, an individual is assigned these tasks, allowing other members of the team to focus on the patient. Massive transfusions tend to be chaotic, and assigning a member of the team to organize the MTP can result in a much better organized resuscitation (see **Table 4.4** and **Figure 4.5**).

4.8 LOCAL HAEMOSTATIC ADJUNCTS

4.8.1 Overview[38]

Haemostatic substances can be used after surgical haemostasis in trauma surgery to secure the surface of the wound. Tissue adhesives are used alone or in combination with other haemostatic measures.

The main indications for using adhesives are:

- To arrest non-surgical haemorrhage
- To secure the wound area to prevent subsequent bleeding

Various forms of fibrin sealants are available and are suitable for treating solid-organ injuries. The different presentations make some suitable for superficial bleeding surfaces, and others easier to apply in deep lacerations. Some are readily available, whilst preparation is time-consuming in others. It is important that the surgeon knows what haemostatic agents are available and how and where they can be used.

4.8.2 Tissue Adhesives

4.8.2.1 FIBRIN

Of the adhesives currently available, fibrin glue is the most suitable for treating injuries to the solid organs and retroperitoneum. It is also possible to make autologous fibrin from the patient's own blood (with the Vivostat system; Vivolution, Birkerød, Denmark); the fibrin is

Table 4.4 Example of a Massive Transfusion or Haemorrhage Protocol (MTP or MHP)

Definition

- The replacement of 100% of the patient's blood volume in less than 6 hours
- The administration of 50% of the patient's blood volume in 1 hour

Activation

- The protocol will be activated **automatically by the blood bank** after 2 units of packed red blood cells (pRBCs) have been issued to a patient, *and* a request for a further 4 units of blood or more is subsequently requested within any 24-hour period. A prospective tool utilizing PR > 120 bpm and BP <90 *and* free blood in the abdomen can be used.[19]
- Activation can also be done at the discretion of the treating physician.
- It is essential that the protocol activation is based on criteria available on admission and not on parameters calculated after hours (e.g., blood loss), since by that time the salvation potential is zeroed.

Blood specimens

Group and crossmatch:

- Leukodepleted blood should be used wherever it is available.
- Crossmatched blood if available.
- Uncrossmatched group O blood.

The following **baseline blood specimens** are required:

- Full blood count, including platelets
- Prothrombin time (PT), activated partial thromboplastin time (aPTT), thrombin time, International Normalized Ratio (INR), fibrinogen, D-dimer, thromboelastogram (TEG), or RoTEM

The following are required **after every 6 units of transfused blood**:

- Repeat baseline blood samples
- Full TEG or RoTEM

Avoid hypothermia (patient and transfused fluid)

- Use an appropriate blood warmer.
- Keep the patient warm using an appropriate patient-warming device.
- Maintain a warm environment.

Blood and blood products

The blood bank will issue the following products (as part of a 2- or 6-unit 'massive transfusion pack'):
Note: Multiple **2-unit packs** are preferable, as they can be returned if the 'cold chain' is intact.

- Two units or 6 units of pRBCs using the *freshest blood available*
- Two units or 6 units of **thawed** fresh frozen plasma (FFP)
- Two units or 5–6 units of platelets (apheresis unit – individual laboratory dependent)
  or
  For every 5–6 units of blood issued:

- One apheresis unit of platelets ('platelet megaunit'). *Note*: May be 5 or 6 units of pooled platelets.

(Continued)

Table 4.4 (*Continued*) Example of a Massive Transfusion or Haemorrhage Protocol (MTP or MHP)

Administration

Microaggregate filters are **not** advised.

Once administration of the 'massive transfusion pack' blood is begun, administer all the above in a
1:1:1 ratio (blood:FFP:platelets) or **6:6:1/5:5:1/4:4:1** (blood:FFP:apheresis unit of platelets – depends on local interpretation of a platelet megaunit). After every 6 units of red cells, if ongoing bleeding or need for transfusion is present:

- Give a further 4 units of FFP if PT or aPTT is > 1.5 times mid-normal or according to TEG/RoTEM.
- Give 10 units of cryoprecipitate if fibrinogen < 1 g/L or according to TEG/RoTEM.
- Give 10 mL 10% calcium chloride only if the above additional doses are given.
- Give at least 1 megaunit of pooled platelets if the platelet count is <75,000/mm^3.
  Return all unused 'massive transfusion packs' to the blood bank as soon as possible.

End points of transfusion

- Any active surgical bleeding has been controlled.
- No further need for red cells.
- Temperature > 35 °C.
- pH > 7.3.
- Fibrinogen > 1.5 g/L.
- INR better than 1.5, PT less than 16 seconds, and aPTT less than 42 seconds.
- Haemoglobin 8–10 g/dL (4–6 mmol/L).

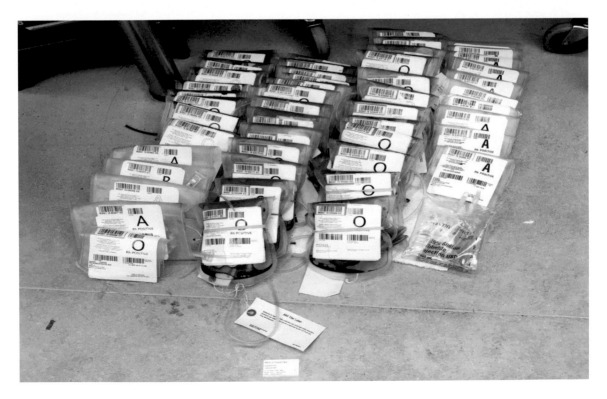

Figure 4.5 Example of a well-organized massive transfusion protocol (MTP).

applied with a sprayer. The necessary volume of blood (125 mL) can be drawn in the emergency room, and the autologous adhesive is ready within 30 minutes.

Fibrin sealant function is based on the transformation of fibrinogen to fibrin. Fibrin promotes clotting and tissue adhesion through accelerated clotting function. The reaction is the same as in the last phase of blood clotting. One such heterologous fibrin is Tisseel®/Tissucol® (Baxter Hyland Immuno, Vienna, Austria). Heterologous fibrin is a biological two-component adhesive that has high concentrations of fibrinogen and factor XIII, which, together with thrombin and calcium, result in clotting. Resorption time and resistance to tearing depend on the size and thickness of the glue layer, and on the proportion by volume of the two components. The fibrin sealant is best applied with a sprayer or syringe injection system such as the Tissomat® sprayer (Baxter Hyland Immuno).

4.8.2.2 **PATCHES**

4.8.2.2.1 TachoSil®

TachoSil (Baxter Hyland Immuno) is a fixed, ready-to-use combination of a collagen sponge coated with a dry layer of the human coagulation factors fibrinogen and thrombin, making it easy to employ. It is most suitable for oozing from the raw surfaces of solid organs or to seal air leaks from lung injuries. It is available in most countries in Europe and Australasia.

4.8.2.2.2 HemoPatch®

Similarly, HemoPatch (Baxter Hyland Immuno) has recently become available.

HemoPatch is a soft, thin, and flexible patch consisting of a porous collagen matrix, which facilitates clotting, coated on one side with a thin protein-binding layer (pentaerythritol polyethylene glycol ether tetra-succinimidyl glutarate [NHS-PEG]) which allows rapid adhesion (within 2 minutes) via electrophilic crosslinking. The patch consequently has a dual-method mechanism of action, in which the two components interact to achieve hemostasis by sealing off the bleeding surface and initiating the body's own clotting mechanisms. The patch is resorbed within 6–8 weeks.

4.8.2.2.3 Collagen Fleece

Even after surgical haemostasis, deep parenchymal injuries can require a resorbable tamponade; here, collagen fleece (e.g., TissoFleece, Baxter Hyland Immuno) is suitable. Collagen fleece is composed of heterologous collagen fibrils obtained from devitalized connective tissue and is fully resorbable. Collagen fleece promotes the aggregation of thrombocytes when in contact with blood. The platelets degenerate and liberate clotting factors, which in turn activate haemostasis. The spongy structure of the collagen stabilizes and strengthens the coagulate. Another alternative for deep parenchymal injuries is FloSeal® (Baxter, Deerfield, IL, USA).

Fibrin glue and collagen fleece are used preferentially to treat mild bleeding. Before application, the bleeding surface should be tamponaded and compressed with a warm pad for a few minutes. Immediately after removal of the pad, air is first sprayed alone, followed by short bursts of fibrin. This creates a surface that is free from blood and nearly dry when the fibrin glue is sprayed onto it. A dry field is essential for most fibrin sprays in order to secure adequate haemostasis.

If collagen fleece is to be applied, a thin layer of fibrin is sprayed onto the fleece, which, in turn, is pressed onto the wound. After a few moments' compression, the fleece is sprayed with fibrin glue. The thickness of the fibrin layer will depend on the size and depth of the injury.

4.8.3 **Local Haemostatic Adjuncts**

4.8.3.1 **CHITOSAN (CELOX [MEDITRADE, CREWE, UK]) AND HEMCON (HEMCON MEDICAL TECHNOLOGIES, PORTLAND, OR, USA)**

Celox gauze is composed of chitosan which is a granular product made from a natural polysaccharide derived from chitin found in shellfish. Chitosan is the deacetylated form of chitin. In the form of an acid salt, chitosan demonstrates mucoadhesive activity. Chitosan stops bleeding by bonding with RBCs and gelling with fluids to produce a sticky pseudoclot. This reaction is not exothermic and has been used successfully within body cavities. Theoretically, chitosan will function in a coagulopathic environment since it is not dependent on endogenous coagulation. Chitosan is broken down by enzymatic action within the body to produce glucosamine. The dressing is sold as pads or bandages and has been shown to have bacteriostatic properties. This product is largely used by the British military.

4.8.3.2 MINERAL ZEOLYTE (QUIKCLOT® [Z-MEDICAL, WALLINGFORD, CT, USA])

QuikClot Combat Gauze is imbedded with kaolin. Kaolin is an inorganic mineral that functions by potently activating factor XII, producing accelerated clotting through the extrinsic clotting cascade. This reaction is exothermic. This is the same product that is used to accelerate clot formation in thrombelastography. QuikClot Combat Gauze does not produce an exothermic reaction, and it is carried by the US military and is present in standardized Stop the Bleed kits sold commercially in the United States.

Both QuikClot and Celox come in the format of packable gauzes that are ideal for bleeding wounds. They are approved for external use only.

REFERENCES AND RECOMMENDED READING

References

1. Holcomb JB, Jenkins D, Rhee P, Johanniqman J, Mahoney P, Mehta S, et al. Damage control resuscitation: directly addressing early coagulopathy of trauma. *J Trauma*. 2007;**62**:307–10. doi: 10.1097/TA.0b013e3180324124.

2. Holcomb JB, Tilley BC, Baraniuk S, Fox EE, Wade CE, Podbielski JM, et al. Transfusion of plasma, platelets, and red blood cells in a 1:1:1 vs a 1:1:2 ratio and mortality in patients with severe trauma: the PROPPR randomized clinical trial. *JAMA*. 2015 Feb 3;**313(5)**:471–82. doi: 10.1001/jama.2015.12.

3. Holcomb JB, del Junco DJ, Fox EE, Wade CE, Cohen MJ, Schreiber MA, et al. The Prospective, observational, multicenter, major trauma transfusion (PROMMTT) study. *J Trauma Acute Care Surg*. 2013 Jul;**75(1 Suppl 1)**:S1–2. doi: 10.1097/TA.0b013e3182983876.

4. Allen CJ, Valle EJ, Jouria JM, Schulman CI, Namias N, Livingstone AS, et al. Differences between blunt and penetrating trauma after resuscitation with hydroxyethyl starch. *J Trauma*. 2014 Dec;**77(6)**:859–64; discussion 864. doi: 10.1097/TA.0000000000000422.

5. Nessen SC, Eastridge BJ, Cronk D, Craig RM, Berséus O, Ellison R, et al. Fresh whole blood use by forward surgical teams in Afghanistan is associated with is associated in improved survival compared to component therapy without platelets. *Transfusion*. 2013;**53(Suppl 1)**:107S–13S. doi: 10.1111/trf.12044.

6. Jobes D, Wolfe Y, O'Neill D, Calder J, Jones L, Sesok-Puzzini D, et al. Toward a definition of "fresh" whole blood: an in vitro characterization of coagulation properties in refrigerated whole blood for transfusion. *Transfusion*. 2011 Jan;**51(1)**:43–51. doi: 10.1111/j.1537-2995.2010.02772.x.

7. Remy KE, Yazer MH, Saini A, Mehanovic-Varmaz A, Rogers SR, et al. Effects of platelet-sparing leukocyte reduction and agitation methods on in vitro measures of hemostatic function in cold-stored whole blood. *JTACS*. 2018;**84**:S104–S14. doi: 10.1097/TA.0000000000001870.

8. Jansen J. Principal Investigator. Trauma Resuscitation With Low-Titer Group O Whole Blood or Products (TROOP) Study. Personal Communication. July 2023. https://clinicaltrials.gov/study/NCT05638581 (accessed July 2023).

9. Hess JR, Brohi K, Dutton RP, Hauser CJ, Holcomb JB, Kluger Y, et al. The coagulopathy of trauma: a review of mechanisms. *J Trauma*. 2008 Oct;**65(4)**:748–54. doi: 10.1097/TA.0b013e3181877a9c. Review.

10. Cap AP, Cannon JW, Reade MC. Synthetic blood and blood products for combat casualty care and beyond. *J Trauma Acute Care Surg*. 2021 Aug 1;**91(2S Suppl 2)**:S26–S32. doi: 10.1097/TA.0000000000003248. PMID: 34324470.

11. Ishikura H, Kitamura T: Trauma-induced coagulopathy and critical bleeding: the role of plasma and platelet transfusion. *J Intensive Care*. 2017 Jan 20;**5(1)**:2. doi: 10.1186/s40560-016-0203-y.

12. Reddoch-Cardenas KM, Bynum JA, Meledeo MA, Nair PM, Wu X, Darlington DN, et al. Cold-stored platelets: a product with function optimized for haemorrhage control. *Transfus Apher Sci*. 2019 Feb;**58(1)**:16–22. doi: 10.1016/j.transci.2018.12.012. Epub 2018 Dec 30.

13. Rijnhout TWH, Noorman F, Van der Horst RA, Tan ECTH, Viersen VVA, van Waes OJF, et al. The haemostatic effect of deep-frozen platelets versus room temperature-stored platelets in the treatment of surgical bleeding: MAFOD – study protocol for a randomized controlled non-inferiority trial. *Trials*. 2022 Sep 24;**23(1)**:803. doi: 10.1186/s13063-022-06739-2.

14. Endo A, Senda A, Otomo Y, Firek M, Kojima M, Coimbra R. Clinical benefits of early concurrent use of cryoprecipitate and plasma compared with plasma only in bleeding trauma patients. *Crit Care Med*. 2022 Oct 1;**50(10)**:1477–85. doi: 10.1097/CCM.0000000000005596. Epub 2022 Jul 17.

15. Davenport R, Curry N, Fox E, Thomas H, Lucas J, Evans A, et al. Early and Empirical High-Dose Cryoprecipitate for Hemorrhage After Traumatic Injury: The CRYOSTAT-2 Randomized Clinical Trial. *JAMA*. 2023 Nov 21;**330(19)**:1882–1891. doi: 10.1001/jama.2023.21019.

16. Ditillo M, Hanna K, Castanon L, Zeeshan M, Kulvatunyou N, Tang A, et al. The role of cryoprecipitate in massively transfused patients: results from the Trauma Quality Improvement Program database may change your mind. *J Trauma Acute Care Surg*. 2020 Aug;**89(2)**:336–43. doi: 10.1097/TA.0000000000002764.

17. Innerhofer P, Fries D, Mittermayr M, Innerhofer N, von Langen D, Hell T, et al. Reversal of trauma-induced coagulopathy using first-line coagulation factor concentrates or fresh frozen plasma (RETIC): a single-centre, parallel-group, open-label, randomised trial. *Lancet Haematol.* 2017 Jun;**4(6)**:e258–e71. doi: 10.1016/S2352-3026(17)30077-7. Epub 2017 Apr 28.

18. Tanaka, K.A, Mazzei M, Durila, M. Role of prothrombin complex concentrate in perioperative coagulation therapy. *J Intensive Care.* 2014 Oct 29;**2(1)**:60. doi: 10.1186/s40560-014-0060-5. collection 2014.

19. Sarode R, Milling TJ, Rafai MA, Mangione A, Schneider A, Durn BL, et al. Efficacy and safety of a 4-factor prothrombin complex concentrate in patients on vitamin K antagonists presenting with major bleeding: a randomized, plasma-controlled study, phase IIIb study. *Circulation.* 2013 Sep 10;**128(11)**:1234–43. doi: 10.1161/CIRCULATIONAHA.113.002283. Epub 2013 Aug 9.

20. Zeeshan M, Hamidi M, Feinstein AJ, Gries L, Jehan F, Sakran J, et al. Four-factor prothrombin complex concentrate is associated with improved survival in trauma-related haemorrhage: a nationwide propensity-matched analysis. *J Trauma Acute Care Surg.* 2019 Aug;**87(2)**:274–81. doi: 10.1097/TA.0000000000002262.

21. CRASH-2 Trial Collaborators. Effects of tranexamic acid on death, vascular occlusive events, and blood transfusion in trauma patients with significant haemorrhage (CRASH-2): a randomised, placebo-controlled trial. *Lancet.* 2010 Jul 3;**376(9734)**:23–32. doi: 10.1016/S0140-6736(10)60835-5. Epub 2010 Jun 14.

22. Morrison JJ, Dubose JJ, Rasmussen TE, Midwinter MJ. Military application of tranexamic acid in trauma emergency resuscitation (MATTERs) study. *Arch Surg.* 2012 Feb;**147(2)**:113–9. doi: 10.1001/archsurg.2011.287. Epub 2011 Oct 17.

23. Guyette FX, Brown JB, Zenati MS, Early-Young BJ, Adams PW, Eastridge BJ, et al. Tranexamic acid during prehospital transport in patients at risk for haemorrhage after injury: a double-blind, placebo-controlled, randomized clinical trial. (STAAMP Trial). *JAMA Surg.* 2020 Oct 5;**156(1)**:11–20. doi: 10.1001/jamasurg.2020.4350.

24. CRASH-3 Intracranial Bleeding Mechanistic Study Collaborators. Tranexamic acid in traumatic brain injury: an explanatory study nested within the CRASH-3 trial. *Eur J Trauma Emerg Surg.* 2021 Feb;**47(1)**:261–8. doi: 10.1007/s00068-020-01316-1. Epub 2020 Feb 19.

25. Rowell SE, Meier EN, McKnight B, Kannas D, May S, Sheehan K, et al. Effect of out-of-hospital tranexamic acid vs placebo on 6-month functional neurologic outcomes in patients with moderate or severe traumatic brain injury. *JAMA.* 2020 Sep 8;**324(10)**:961–74. doi: 10.1001/jama.2020.8958.

26. Rossaint R, Afshari A, Bouillon B, Cerny V, Cimpoesu D, Curry N, et al. The European guideline on management of major bleeding and coagulopathy following trauma: sixth edition. *Crit Care.* 2023 Mar 1;**27(1)**:80. doi: 10.1186/s13054-023-04327-7.

27. Napolitano LM. Prehospital tranexamic acid: what is the current evidence? Trauma *Surg Acute Care Open.* 2017; Jan 13;**2(1)**:e000056. doi: 10.1136/tsaco-2016-000056. eCollection 2017.

28. Boffard KD, Riou B, Warren B, Choong PI, Rizoli S, Rossaint R, et al. NovoSeven Trauma Study Group. Recombinant factor VIIa as adjunctive therapy for bleeding control in severely injured trauma patients: two parallel randomized, placebo-controlled, double-blind clinical trials. *J Trauma.* 2005;**59(1)**:8–15; discussion 15–18.

29. Hauser CJ, Boffard K, Dutton R, Bernard GR, Croce MA, Holcomb JB, et al., for the CONTROL Study Group. Results of the CONTROL Trial: efficacy and safety of recombinant activated factor VII in the management of refractory traumatic hemorrhage. *J Trauma.* 2010;**69**:489–500. doi: 10.1097/TA.0b013e3181edf36e.

30. Stensballe J, Ostrowski SR, Johansson PI. Viscoelastic guidance of resuscitation. *Curr Opin Anaesthesiol.* 2014 Apr;**27(2)**:212–8. doi: 10.1097/ACO.0000000000000051.

31. TEG/ROTEM. Available from www.surgicalcriticalcare.net/Guidelines (accessed online August 2023).

32. Hartmann J, Walsh M, Grisoli A, Thomas AV, Shariff F, McCauley R, et al. Diagnosis and treatment of trauma-induced coagulopathy by viscoelastography. *Semin Thromb Hemost.* 2020;**46(2)**:134–46. doi: 10.1055/s-0040-1702171.

33. Hughes LG, Thomas DW, Wareham K, Jones JE, John A, Rees M. Intra-operative blood salvage in abdominal trauma: a review of 5 years' experience. *Anaesthesia.* 2001 Mar;**56(3)**:217–20. doi: 10.1046/j.1365-2044.2001.01832.x.

34. Bowley DM, Barker P, Boffard KD. Intraoperative blood salvage in penetrating abdominal trauma: a randomised controlled trial. *World J Surg.* 2006 Jun;**30(6)**:1074–80. doi: 10.1007/s00268-005-0466-2.

35. Hardcastle TC. We ask the experts: autotransfusion for the provision of blood in lower-and-middle-income countries. *World J Surg.* 2021;**45(7)**:1979–81. doi: 10.1007/s00268-021-06089-1.

36. Savage SA, Sumislawski JJ, Zarzaur BL, Dutton WP, Croce MA, Fabian TC. The new metric to define large-volume hemorrhage: results of a prospective study of the critical administration threshold. *J Trauma Acute Care Surg.* 2015 Feb;**78(2)**:224–9; discussion 229-30. doi: 10.1097/TA.0000000000000502.

37. Wilson RF, Spencer AR, Tyburski JG, Dolman H, Zimmerman LH. Bicarbonate therapy in severely acidotic trauma patients increases mortality. *J Trauma Acute Care Surg.* 2013 Jan;**74(1)**:45–50; discussion 50. doi: 10.1097/TA.0b013e3182788fc4.

38. Tompeck AJ, Reham Gajdhar A, Dowling M, Johnson SB, Barie PS, Winchell RJ, et al. A comprehensive review of topical hemostatic agents: the good, the bad, and the novel. *J Trauma and Acute Care Surg.* 2020 Jan;**88(1)**:e1–e21. doi:10.1097/TA.0000000000002508.

Recommended Reading

Hess JR, Holcomb JB, Hoyt DB. Damage control resuscitation: the need for specific blood products to treat the coagulopathy of trauma. *Transfusion.* 2006;**46(5)**:685–6. doi: 10.1111/j.1537-2995.2006.00816.x.

Johansson PI, Ostrowsky SR, Secher NH. Management of major blood loss: an update. *Acta Anaesthesiol Scand.* 2010;**54**:1039–49. doi: 10.1111/j.1399-6576.2010.02265.x. Epub 2010 Jul 6.

Marino PL. Blood Components. In: *The ICU Book*, 4th Edn. Wolters Kluwer Health/Lippincott Williams & Wilkins, Philadelphia PA., USA. 2014.

Moore EE, Moore HB, Chapman MP, Gonzalez E, Sauia A. Goal-directed hemostatic resuscitation for trauma induced coagulopathy: maintaining homeostasis. *J Trauma Acute Care Surg.* 2018 Jun;**84(6 Suppl 1)**:S35–S40. doi: 10.1097/TA.0000000000001797.

Pre-Hospital and Emergency **5**
Trauma Care

5.1 **RESUSCITATION IN THE PRE-HOSPITAL SETTING AND EMERGENCY DEPARTMENT**

A trauma system is an integrated collaboration of healthcare providers, agencies, and institutions dedicated to the control of the entire spectrum of injury from effective prevention to efficient societal reintegration of injury survivors. At the system's core is coordinated and comprehensive care of acutely injured patients within a defined geographic area. Its services are multidisciplinary and comprehensive and encompass a continuum that includes all phases of patient need.

> *The major goal of an inclusive trauma system is complete control of all aspects of injury, from effective prevention to successful societal reintegration of injury victims.*

Patients with life-threatening injuries represent approximately 10%–15% of all patients hospitalized for injuries.[1] Overtriage of minimally injured patients will impair trauma centre efficiency, whereas undertriage of severely injured patients will increase the risk of preventable death and disability.

For triage purposes, to ensure the patient will go to the closest and most appropriate facility, the scene Injury Severity Score (ISS) is used. Some authors have defined severe trauma as a patient who has an ISS greater than 15, and these patients should go to a level 1 trauma centre.[2-4] Information available in the pre-hospital phase and primary survey should be used and communicated to the receiving facility to help them to prepare for the patient's arrival. Pre-hospital time to definitive care must be minimized.[5]

A standardized handover approach, utilizing the MIST (also known as [AT]MIST, for age/name/sex, time, mechanism, injuries, signs, and treatment) handover, should be used (**Table 5.1**). During this patient handover, there should be a pause in activity (a moment of silence) to allow the pre-hospital staff to give all the necessary information to the receiving healthcare providers. This 'listening' pause is critical for accurate handover of information.

5.2 **MANAGEMENT OF MAJOR TRAUMA**

The principles of management for patients suffering major trauma are:

- Preparation of the trauma room, trauma team, and resources before arrival of the patient.
- Rapid simultaneous assessment and resuscitation where all life-threatening injuries are addressed according to Advanced Trauma Life Support Course® (ATLS) principles.
- A complete physical examination.
- Life-saving intervention to stop bleeding.
- Serial monitoring of the patient's response to resuscitation.
- Diagnostic adjunctive studies *matched to haemodynamic stability*.
- A tertiary survey once the patient is stable and mobile.

Effective civilian trauma systems should include easy notification and arrival of a pre-hospital team to the injured patient. The composition and skill level of this

DOI: 10.1201/9781003258124-7

Table 5.1 The (AT)MIST Handover

		Trauma / Medical Handover
(A)	**Age**	• Name, age, and sex
(T)	**Time**	• Time of incident and expected time of arrival
M	**Mechanism of injury** **Medical complaint**	• Speed, mass, height, restraints, number and type of collisions, helmet use and damage, and weapon type • Medical onset, duration, and history
I	**Injuries sustained** **Illness**	• Pain, deformity, injuries, and injury patterns • STEMI/stroke/previous conditions/previous medications
S	**Signs and symptoms**	• *Vitals*: Initial/Current/Worst • RR, SPO_2, $ETCO_2$, and blood gases • HR and BP • *GCS*: Eyes ____ Motor ____ Verbal ____ Total ____ / 15

T	**Treatment**	• Use the ABCDE approach to systematize management:
		  ○ Tubes, lines (location and size), and fluids
		  ○ Medications and response
		  ○ Immobilization and dressings

team are highly variable within different countries and regions. Nonetheless, life-saving manoeuvres, notification of the nearest and most suitable hospital, preferably a trauma centre, and swift transport are paramount in reducing trauma-related mortality.

Notification of the hospital emergency department (ED), although often not possible, is highly desirable as it allows preparation of human, technical, and logistic resources, such as an operating theatre, massive transfusion protocol (MTP), and imaging, to manage the patient in a timely fashion.

The trauma team should be alerted in time and provided with available pre-hospital information. On arrival of the patient in the ED, the trauma team should start the resuscitation immediately and collect as much information as possible. In addition to patient symptoms, necessary information includes mechanism of injury and the presence of pre-existing medical conditions and medications that may influence the critical decisions to be made. Time to achieve haemorrhage control and necessary interventions is critical: 62% of all trauma patients who die in hospital die within the first 4 hours of hospitalization.[6] The majority either bleed to death or die from primary or secondary injuries to the central nervous system. To reduce this mortality, prompt restoration of adequate tissue oxygenation and perfusion

as well as control of haemorrhage are critical. As such, the initial diagnostic workup must be both expeditious and focussed on potentially life-threatening injuries. To maximize resuscitative efforts and to avoid missing life-threatening injuries, various protocols for resuscitation have been developed, of which ATLS[7] is a model and is considered the 'gold standard'.

The ATLS protocol provides a standardized physiologic-based method to resuscitation aiming at maintaining oxygen supply to the cells: airway, breathing, circulation, disability, and exposure (ABCDE). This sequential, longitudinal approach is helpful, as it treats first what kills first. But with a larger trauma team, a horizontal approach, as is proposed by the European Trauma Course, is also feasible, with team members dedicated to airway, ventilatory, and circulation management. Simultaneous assessment and resuscitation can take place under the guidance of a designated team leader, who should be qualified in trauma resuscitation and proficient in non-technical skills. The surgeon can usually fill this role, as the patient may require a surgical decision early on. Other specialities can integrate the team, such as emergency medicine, critical care, and anaesthesiology. The latter is particularly relevant as a team member, not only for the expert airway skills but also because it ensures a continuum of care from the ED to the operating room (OR), should the patient require operative intervention.

Guideline times for the length of stay in the ED are prompted by physiology as follows:

- **For the unstable patient, time in the ED should be no longer than 30 minutes (unless surgery is performed in the ED), and the unstable patient should be in either the OR, an interventional suite, or the intensive care unit (ICU) within 30 minutes.**
- **For the stable patient, time in the ED should be no longer than 30–60 minutes before computed tomography (CT) imaging or admission to the ICU.**

5.2.1 Resuscitation

Resuscitation is traditionally performed in the <C>ABCDE format, where <C> involves controlling exsanguinating bleeding, intravenous (IV) placement, and resuscitation with blood (preferred) or crystalloid solutions. Bleeding control in the pre-hospital or ED settings may include direct pressure, haemostatic dressings, pelvic binder, and tourniquet application. Resuscitative endovascular balloon occlusion of the aorta (REBOA; see Chapter 15) is still finding a role.

5.2.1.1 CIVILIAN PRE-HOSPITAL TOURNIQUET USE

Simple yet underused, civilian pre-hospital tourniquet application was independently associated with a sixfold mortality reduction in patients with peripheral vascular injuries. More aggressive pre-hospital application of extremity tourniquets in civilian trauma patients with extremity haemorrhage and traumatic amputation is warranted,[8] *provided that they are applied correctly.*

Pitfall

- The tourniquet must be placed proximal to the injury and secured 'tightly' enough to stop arterial inflow.
- It is essential to document the time of application of the tourniquet (there is usually a white tag on the tourniquet itself to write this down). It is very easy to miss this, which may result in tissue ischaemia and extremity compartment syndrome!
- Always try to limit the time of application and put it as close to the injury as possible.

- Venous tourniquets (tourniquets placed tightly enough to stop venous flow but not higher-pressure arterial flow) can often exacerbate rather than stop bleeding.

Resuscitation itself is divided into two components:

- The primary survey and initial resuscitation
- The secondary survey and continuing resuscitation

All patients undergo the primary survey of airway, breathing, circulation, disability, and exposure (<C>ABCDE). Only those patients who become haemodynamically stable will progress to the secondary survey, which focusses on a complete head-to-toe physical examination that directs further diagnostic studies. The great majority of patients who remain haemodynamically unstable require immediate intervention even before the secondary survey.

5.2.1.2 PRIMARY SURVEY

The priorities of the primary ABCDE survey are:

- Establishing a patent airway whilst maintaining cervical spine immobilization.
- Adequate ventilation.
- Maintaining circulation (including intravascular volume and cardiac function).
- Assessing the global neurological status.
- Complete exposure of the patient whilst maintaining normothermia.

5.2.1.2.1 Airway

Patients with extensive trauma who are unconscious, have severe facial trauma or inhalation burns, and are not protecting their airway, or who are in shock, may benefit from immediate endotracheal intubation,[9,10] which may often happen at the pre-hospital level. Airway priorities are to clear the upper airway, to establish high-flow oxygen initially with a bag mask, and to proceed immediately to a definitive airway (cuffed tube in the trachea). The cervical spine must be protected during intubation. Intubation via the oral route is successful in most injured patients, and the GlideScope® (Verathon, Bothell, WA, USA) may be a helpful adjunct if available. On rare occasions, a surgical airway might be indicated as an emergency.

Patients who may require a surgical airway include those with a laryngeal fracture, severe facial fractures, inhalation burns, or a penetrating injury of the neck or throat.

ANAESTHETIC PITFALL

- Always identify potentially difficult airways and be prepared with rescue devices that would include a bougie, video laryngoscope, combination endotracheal tube (ETT), laryngeal mask, and surgical airway.
- The decision to intubate should not be delayed. However, in patients with indication for intubation who need emergency surgery, for instance for severe intra-abdominal bleeding, intubation may be considered in the OR, provided that the patient can be swiftly transferred to the OR, oxygenation is guaranteed, and the airway is not in immediate danger. Intubation in the OR can be accomplished with more resources (human and technical). Moreover, drug-assisted intubation can precipitate cardiovascular collapse, which the surgical team can readily manage with a laparotomy if the patient is already in the OR and the surgical field prepped and draped.
- The decision of where to intubate is an individual, case-by-case decision, varies with local conditions, and requires good communication within the team (ED doctors, surgeon, and anaesthesiologist).
- Ensure tracheal placement of both with confirmation of end-tidal CO_2 on multiple breaths.

5.2.1.2.2 Breathing

Patients with respiratory compromise are not always easy to detect. Simple parameters such as the respiratory rate (RR), adequacy of breathing, and, if possible, a measuring of the saturation (pulse oximeter) should be assessed within the first minute after arrival. One of the most important things is to detect a tension pneumothorax, necessitating immediate decompression by finger thoracostomy followed by the insertion of a chest tube. Previously placed in the mid-clavicular line, the 10th edition of ATLS now suggests needle thoracostomy in the pleural cavity within the 'triangle of safety' in the standard tube thoracostomy position (5th intercostal space, mid to anterior axillary line).[11] However, the use of the finger thoracostomy may be preferable, as the needle may lacerate the lung – especially in blunt injury patients with decreased air entry due to pulmonary contusion. Intubated patients are usually on positive-pressure ventilation, and in time-critical conditions such as in the pre-hospital setting, a thoracostomy incision alone with an occlusive dressing sealed in three of the four sides can often be enough. The chest tube could be inserted upon arrival at the hospital. Other immediate threats to life, for example massive haemothorax, flail chest and pulmonary contusion, and tracheal–bronchial injury, must be identified, and treatment instituted urgently.

5.2.1.2.3 Circulation

Simultaneous with airway and ventilatory management, a quick assessment of the patient will determine the degree of shock present. Shock is a clinical diagnosis but may be subtle in the early stages, often only manifesting in a decreased pulse pressure. A quick first step is to feel an extremity. As it progresses, the extremities will be cool and pale, lack venous filling, and have poor capillary refill; the pulse will be thready; and consciousness will be diminished. Extended focussed assessment with sonography for trauma (eFAST) is the gold standard screening tool.

In trauma, hypotension is haemorrhagic shock until proven otherwise, but there are other causes of shock in trauma that should be kept in mind. The status of the neck veins must be noted. A patient who is in shock with flat neck veins is assumed to have hypovolaemic or neurogenic shock until proven otherwise. If the neck veins are distended, the most likely possibilities are:

- Tension pneumothorax
- Pericardial tamponade
- Myocardial contusion (cardiogenic shock)
- Myocardial infarction (cardiogenic shock)
- Air embolism

Pitfall

Note that the absence of distended neck veins does not exclude these diagnoses because the circulating volume may be so depleted that the circulation is empty.

Tension pneumothorax should always be the number one diagnosis in the physician's differential diagnosis of shock, since it is the life-threatening injury that is easiest to treat in the ED. A simple tube thoracostomy is the definitive management.

Pericardial tamponade is most encountered in patients with penetrating injuries to the torso but can also be seen in blunt trauma. Approximately 25% of all patients with such cardiac injuries will reach the ED alive. The diagnosis can often be made clinically by high index of suspicion with penetrating injuries in the pericardial box with distended neck veins and poor peripheral perfusion, and a few will have pulsus paradoxus. Ultrasound is a reliable diagnostic modality, and eFAST should be performed immediately.

Pitfall

- Needle aspiration may cause bleeding or be blocked by a clot and is unreliable.
- Subxiphoid window is neither an adequate diagnostic procedure nor a good treatment option in traumatic haemopericardium.
- If the patient is *in extremis*, proceed immediately to an emergency room thoracotomy.
- If the patient is more stable, proceed to a planned resuscitative thoracotomy in the OR.
- In stable patients, a sternotomy is the access incision of choice.

Myocardial contusion is a rare cause of cardiac failure in the trauma patient. However, myocardial infarction from coronary occlusion is not uncommon in the elderly. It may be the cause of the initial crash.

Air embolism[12] represents air in the systemic circulation caused by a bronchopulmonary venous fistula. Air embolism occurs in 4% of all major thoracic injuries. Thirty-five per cent of the time it is due to blunt trauma, usually a laceration of the pulmonary parenchyma by a fractured rib. In 65% of patients, it is due to gunshot wounds or stab wounds. The surgeon must be vigilant when pulmonary injury has occurred. Any patient who has no obvious head injury but has focal or lateralizing neurological signs may have air bubbles occluding the cerebral circulation. Any intubated patient on positive-pressure ventilation who has a sudden cardiovascular collapse is presumed to have either tension pneumothorax or air embolism to the coronary circulation.

Definitive treatment of massive air embolism requires immediate thoracotomy followed by clamping of the hilum of the injured lung to prevent further embolism, followed by expansion of the intravascular volume. Open cardiac massage, IV adrenaline (epinephrine), and venting the left heart and aorta with a needle to remove residual air may be required. The pulmonary injury is treated definitively by oversewing the laceration or resecting a lobe.

If the patient's primary problem in shock is blood loss, the intention is to stop the bleeding. If this is not possible, the priorities are:

- To gain venous access to the circulation.
- To obtain a blood sample from the patient.
- To determine where the volume loss is occurring.
- To give appropriate resuscitation fluids – whole blood or blood products.
- To prevent and treat coagulopathy.
- To prevent hypothermia.

Access can be a large-bore (14G) peripheral IV in one of the non-injured extremities or intraosseous access in the humeral head or tibia, until large-calibre access is achieved. These may be placed pre-hospital. Large-bore peripheral IVs are preferred, but intraosseous lines are often quicker and more successful.[13]

Alternatively, a central line may be inserted, **preferably by the subclavian route**, using an 8.5 French gauge (FG) introducer assisted by sonography if necessary. Ultrasonographic placement via the jugular route is an option, but these are easy to dislodge.

Pitfall

- With insertion of the IV line, any access distal to the possible source of bleeding should be avoided.
- A femoral line is contraindicated if there is the possibility of major iliac, or inferior caval, injury. Two large-bore peripheral lines are also adequate.

As soon as the first IV line has been established, baseline blood work is obtained that includes haematocrit, toxicology, blood type, and crossmatching, and a screening battery of laboratory tests if the patient is older and has premorbid conditions. Blood-gas determinations should be obtained early during resuscitation.

The third priority is to determine where the patient may have blood loss.

As a guideline, major clinical shock results from bleeding into only five sites (see **Table 5.2**). There are two sources providing visible bleeding: external and long bone fractures of the extremities; and three sources for occult blood loss: the thorax, the abdomen inclusive of the retroperitoneum, and the pelvis.

'One on the floor, and four more'.

Table 5.2 'Blood on the Floor and Four More': Five Sites for Major Blood Loss	
Visible Bleeding	
External bleeding	• Blood on the floor • Remember that much of this may be pre-hospital
Extremities	• Fractures and soft tissue injuries of the limbs • Exclude by clinical examination and long bone X-ray
Occult Bleeding	
Chest	• Internal bleeding into the chest • Exclude by chest X-ray or eFAST
Abdomen	• Internal bleeding into the abdomen • Exclude by eFAST
Pelvis	• Bleeding from pelvic fractures (usually retroperitoneal) • Exclude radiologically

Fifty per cent of patients with significant haemoperitoneum have no clinical signs. Thus, if the patient's chest and pelvis X-rays are normal, the femur is not fractured, and there is no external bleeding, the patient who remains in shock must be suspected of having ongoing haemorrhage in the abdomen and may require immediate laparotomy to avoid death from haemorrhage.

By doing the eFAST immediately, one can exclude the abdomen as a potential source of bleeding, but retroperitoneal haemorrhage can still be missed. Unstable patients with a positive focussed assessment with sonography in trauma (FAST) must go immediately to the OR,

and all further investigations should be done postoperatively once the patients are stable.

> *In the haemodynamically unstable patient, do not delay mandated therapeutic interventions whilst waiting to obtain non-critical diagnostic tests (e.g., CT scan).*

The fourth priority for the resuscitating physician is recognition of the need for activation of a MTP in a patient with ongoing bleeding. Although whole blood is preferred, especially in the military situation, it is commonly difficult to obtain whole blood from modern blood banks, forcing the use of blood components. Loss of more than 2 units of blood and ongoing bleeding which requires blood transfusion should invoke a predefined massive bleeding protocol (most current massive haemorrhage protocols [MHPs] and MTPs aim at predefined ratios of packed red blood cells:fresh frozen plasma:platelets, mimicking whole blood) monitored by frequent coagulation tests, conventional laboratory tests–clotting studies, and more functional goal-directed haemostasis using viscoelastic measures such as thromboelastography (TEG) or rotary thromboelastometry (RoTEM) when available. Use pharmacological haemostatic adjuncts (topical and systemic) such as tranexamic acid (TXA), when indicated (see Chapter 4: 'Transfusion'). Blood components such as red blood cells, liquid plasma, fibrinogen, and cryoprecipitate are now used in several systems, including Helicopter Emergency Medical Systems (HEMS).

The use of crystalloids should be restricted due to the complications associated with clear fluids, and permissive hypotension is preferable in unstable bleeding patients in both pre-hospital and ED settings until haemorrhage control is achieved (Chapter 6: 'Damage Control Resuscitation').

The criteria for adequate resuscitation are simple and straightforward:

• Keep atrial filling pressure at normal levels.
• Give enough fluid to achieve adequate urinary output (0.5 mL/kg per hour in the adult, 1.0 mL/kg per hour in the child).
• Maintain peripheral perfusion.

In elderly patients with extensive traumatic injuries, utilizing an invasive haemodynamic monitor may be prudent because it will be used to direct a sophisticated multifactorial resuscitation in the OR or ICU.

Resuscitation should be directed to achieve adequate oxygen delivery and oxygen consumption.

5.2.1.2.4 Neurological Status (Disability)

The next priority during the primary survey is to quickly assess neurological status and to initiate diagnostic and treatment priorities. The key components of a rapid neurological evaluation are:

- Determine the level of consciousness.
- Observe the size and reactivity of the pupils.
- Check eye movements and oculovestibular responses.
- Document skeletal muscle motor responses and spontaneous movement of extremities.
- Determine the pattern of breathing.
- Perform a peripheral sensory examination.

Neurological status is often described using the Glasgow Coma Scale (GCS, 3/15–15/15).

Note: In the intubated patient (unable to verbalize), GCS may be expressed either out of 10 (/10) or as intubated with no score for 'Verbal' (/15T).

In patients who present with a significantly altered level of consciousness (GCS ≤11/15) because of either head trauma or medications administered prior to arrival in the ED, the 'D' component of resuscitation can be abbreviated to an assessment of the GCS, the pupils, the presence of lateralizing signs, and the presence of a Cushing's reflex (hypertension and bradycardia). If in addition to a GCS ≤11, there are any of the above additional findings, this indicates that the patient likely has critically raised intracranial pressure. In consultation with senior staff, consideration should be given to osmotherapy (hypertonic saline or mannitol) and hyperventilation whilst prioritizing the CT scan (see Section 5.3.1: Head Trauma; and Chapter 12).

A decreasing level of consciousness is the single most reliable indication that the patient may have a serious head injury or secondary insult (usually hypoxic, hypoglycaemic, or hypotensive) to the brain. Consciousness has two components: awareness and arousal. Awareness is manifested by goal-directed or purposeful behaviour. The use of language is an indication of functioning cerebral hemispheres. If the patient attempts to protect himself from a painful insult, this also implies cortical function. Arousal is a crude function that is simple wakefulness. Eye-opening, either spontaneous or in response to stimuli, is indicative of arousal and is a brainstem function. Coma is a pathological state in which both awareness and arousal are absent, eye-opening does not occur, there is no comprehensible speech detected, and the extremities move neither to command nor appropriately to noxious stimuli. By assessing all components and making sure the primary reflexes (pupillary, ankle, knee, biceps, and triceps) are assessed, and repeating this examination at frequent intervals, it is possible to both diagnose and monitor the neurological status in the ED. An improving neurological status reassures the physician that resuscitation is improving cerebral blood flow. Neurological deterioration is strong presumptive evidence of either a mass lesion or significant neurological injury. A CT scan (including the cervical spine) should be done as soon as possible.

> *We recommend cervical vessel CT angiography to exclude injury in **all** patients with significant blunt cerebral injury. Urgent neurosurgical/vascular involvement is recommended.*

Pitfall

Patients with high cervical or upper thoracic spinal cord injuries can suffer from neurogenic shock that will often present with hypotension and bradycardia. The diagnosis of neurogenic shock can only be made when haemorrhagic shock has been excluded, as such patients can have asymptomatic abdominal trauma due to the sensory level of spinal cord injury. The treatment of neurogenic shock is to restrict fluids and use inotropes.

5.2.1.2.5 Environment

The clothes are to be removed to examine the whole patient. A logroll must be performed, especially after penetrating injuries, to identify all wounds, but it may be delayed in patients with significant pelvic or spinal trauma until they are in a more stable condition. In penetrating wounds, markers should be put on the wounds for the radiological examination.[14] Always correlate if there is an equal amount of bullet wounds, and, if not, try to find a bullet that is lodged inside of the patient. The patient is at risk of hypothermia, and warming measures should be promptly instituted.

The body temperature of trauma patients decreases rapidly, and if the 'on-scene time' has been prolonged, for example by entrapment, patients arrive in the resuscitation room hypothermic. This is aggravated by the administration of cold fluids, the presence of abdominal or chest wounds, and the removal of clothing.

> *Patients can be expected to drop their core temperature by 1–2 °C per hour.*

All fluids need to be at body temperature or above, and there are rapid infusor devices available that will warm fluids at high flow rates prior to infusion. Patients can be placed on warming mattresses, and their environment kept warm using warm air blankets. Early measurement of the core temperature is important to prevent heat loss that will predispose to problems with coagulation. Hypothermia will shift the oxygen dissociation curve to the left, reduce oxygen delivery, reduce the liver's ability to metabolize citrate and lactic acid, and aggravate coagulopathy, and it may produce arrhythmias.

> *A 'cold' patient with a core temperature below 34 °C will have significantly impaired oxygen transport, and coagulation.*

5.2.1.2.6 Resuscitation Adjuncts

The minimum diagnostic studies that should be considered in the haemodynamically unstable patient as part of the primary survey include:

- FAST ultrasound
- Chest X-ray
- Plain film of the pelvis
- Blood-gas analysis

A FAST examination may be helpful:

- To assess whether there is blood in the abdomen or chest (eFAST).
- To exclude cardiac tamponade.
- eFAST will assess for pneumothorax as well.

It must be emphasized that resuscitation should not cease during these films, and the resuscitating team must wear protective lead aprons. Optimally, the X-ray facilities and especially the CT scanner are juxtaposed to the ED, but the essential X-rays can all be obtained with a portable machine.

> *Only stable patients can go to the CT scanner – the 'Doughnut of Death'.*

Pitfall

On completion of the primary survey, it is often useful to pause briefly, to allow the person leading the resuscitation team to ensure all team members are aware of what has been found, and the likely clinical trajectory. This allows team members to properly share the mental model of what the patient's problems are and what will be done next. It also allows team members to raise any concerns they might have about ongoing patient management.

5.2.1.3 SECONDARY SURVEY

Finally, if the patient stabilizes, a secondary survey and diagnostic studies are carried out. However, if the patient remains unstable, he or she should be taken immediately to the OR to achieve surgical haemostasis, or to the surgical ICU.

The patient must have a full 'top-to-toe' and 'front-to-back' examination.

5.2.1.3.1 The Haemodynamically Normal Patient

There is ample time for a full evaluation of the patient, and a decision can be made regarding surgery or non-operative management. CT scanning is currently the modality of choice.

5.2.1.3.2 The Haemodynamically Stable Patient

The stable patient, who is not haemodynamically normal but who is maintaining blood pressure and other parameters with resuscitation, will benefit from investigations aimed at establishing:

- Whether the patient has bled into the abdomen.
- Whether the bleeding has stopped.

Thus, serial investigations of a quantitative nature will allow the best assessment of these patients. CT scan is the modality of choice, provided awareness of the fact that the patient may decompensate.

5.2.1.3.3 The Haemodynamically Unstable Patient

Efforts must be made to try to define the cavity where bleeding is taking place (e.g., the chest, pelvis, or abdominal cavity). Negative chest and pelvic X-rays leave the abdomen as the most likely source. Diagnostic modalities are of necessity limited. FAST is effective for detecting free fluid in the abdomen and pericardium but is operator-dependent – haemodynamic instability caused by intraperitoneal haemorrhage is likely to be readily found, but a negative FAST does not exclude intra-abdominal bleeding. FAST can be performed without moving the patient from the resuscitation area, since an unstable patient should not have a CT scan, even if it were to be readily available next to the resuscitation room. Diagnostic peritoneal lavage (DPL) can also be considered in mass casualty incidents when there is a lack of CT scanners due to a larger number of patients, or in low-resource environments.

5.2.2 **Management of Penetrating Trauma**

Many forces can act on the torso to cause injury to the outer protective layers or the contained viscera. Penetrating trauma is most often due to knives, missiles, and impalement. Knife wounds and impalement usually involve low-velocity penetration, and mortality is directly related to the organ injured. Secondary effects such as infection are due to the nature of the weapon and the material (i.e. clothing and other foreign material) that the missile carries into the body tissue. Infection is also influenced by spillage of contents from an injury to a hollow viscus organ, time since injury, and control of contamination.

An important component of the physical examination is to describe the penetrating wound. It is imperative that surgeons do not label the entrance or exit wounds unless common sense dictates it – an example is a patient with a single penetrating missile injury with no exit. However, in general, it is best to describe whether the wound is circular or ovoid and whether there is surrounding stippling (powder burn) or bruising from the muzzle of a weapon. Similarly, stab wounds should be described as longitudinal, triangular-shaped (hunting knives), or circular depending on the instrument used.

> *Experience has shown that surgeons who describe wounds as entrance or exit may be wrong as often as 50% of the time. Forensic pathology experience is required!*

> *Surgeons should be focussed on treating the injuries caused rather than forensics.*

It is good practice to place radio-opaque markers, such as paper clips or vitamin E tablets (which are radio-opaque), on the skin pointing to the various wounds on the chest wall, which aid in determining the missile track. It is recommended that an 'unfolded' paper clip be placed on any anterior penetrating injury, and a 'folded' one on any posterior injury (**Figure 5.1**).[14] This also can be useful for stab wounds. Tracking the missile helps to determine which visceral organs may be injured and whether there is potential transgression of the diaphragm and/or mediastinum.

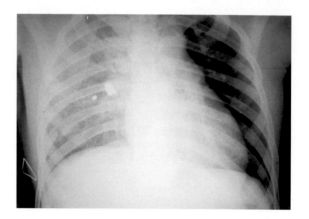

Figure 5.1 Chest X-ray in penetrating injury showing the use of skin markers.

In the pre-hospital setting, patients with penetrating torso trauma should be treated with a 'scoop and run' modality, where on-scene time is minimized. Procedures should rather be performed *en route* to the hospital instead of at the scene of the incident.

5.3 **EMERGENCY DEPARTMENT SURGERY**

The emergency management of a critically injured trauma patient continues to be a substantial challenge. It is essential to have a very simple, effective plan that can be put into place to meset the challenges presented by resuscitating the moribund patient. ATLS principles apply throughout.

As a basic consideration, for all major trauma victims with a systolic blood pressure of less than 90 mmHg, there is a 50% likelihood of death, which, in one-third of cases, will occur within the next 30 minutes if the bleeding has not been controlled. If death is likely to occur in the next 5 minutes, it is essential to determine in which body cavity the lethal event will occur, as the only chance of survival will be the immediate control of haemorrhage.

If death is likely to occur in the next hour, there is time to proceed with an orderly series of investigations and, time permitting, radiographic or other diagnostic aids to determine precisely what is injured, and to effect an operative plan for the management of this life-threatening event.

5.3.1 Head Trauma

In the event of severe facial (and often associated severe neck) injuries, surgical control of the airway may be necessary, using ATLS described techniques.

It is unusual but possible to exsanguinate from a massive scalp laceration ('Blood on the floor...'). For this reason, it is essential to control the vascular scalp laceration with rapidly placed surgical clips or primary pressure and immediate suturing, using deep sutures, rather than staples, and a pressure dressing which often simply covers ongoing bleeding.

A more common cause of death is from intracranial mass lesions. Extradural haematomas and subdural haematomas can be rapidly lethal. A rapid diagnosis of an ipsilateral dilated pupil with contralateral hemiplegia is diagnostic of mass lesion with significant enough intracranial pressure to induce herniation. This requires immediate decompression. Head elevation, loosening a cervical collar, chemical sedation, and paralysis may all decrease intracranial pressure. The use of mannitol or hypertonic saline is useful as a temporizing adjunct only.

Moderate hyperventilation produces mild hypocapnia, and vasoconstriction is only used immediately prior to neurosurgical intervention.

Attention should be paid to monitoring the end-tidal carbon dioxide, as a proxy for $PaCO_2$, which should not be allowed to fall below 35 mmHg (4 kPa). This should decrease intracranial volume and therefore intracranial pressure. There should be an immediate positive effect that usually lasts long enough to obtain a 3D CT scan to determine a specific site of the mass lesion and the type of haematoma. This will direct the surgeon specifically to the location of the craniotomy for removal of the haematoma.

IV mannitol should be administered as a bolus injection in a dose of 0.5–1.0 g/kg or as hypertonic (7.5%) saline in a dosage of 1 mmol/kg. This should not delay any other diagnostic or therapeutic procedures.

5.3.2 Chest Trauma

Lethal injuries to the chest include tension pneumothorax, massive haemothorax, cardiac tamponade, and transected aorta.

Tension pneumothorax is diagnosed clinically with deviation of the trachea away from the lesion (a late sign), hypertympany on the side of the lesion, and decreased breath sounds on the affected side. There may be elevated jugular venous pressure in the neck veins unless the patient is hypovolaemic, which is very common in critically injured patients. This is a clinical diagnosis, and once made, an immediate needle or finger thoracostomy and tube thoracostomy should be performed to relieve the tension pneumothorax. The tube should then be placed to underwater seal on suction. Massive haemothorax is also treated with tube thoracostomy in the ED; 1500 cc of initial blood output or ongoing shock without other potential sources should prompt an exploratory thoracotomy.

It is far better to perform a thoracotomy in the OR, through either an anterolateral approach or a median sternotomy, with good light and assistance and the potential for autotransfusion and potential bypass, than it is to attempt heroic emergency surgery in the resuscitation suite. However, if the patient is pulseless or agonal, or has a systolic blood pressure in the 40 mmHg or lower range despite volume resuscitation, there is no choice but to proceed immediately with a left anterior thoracotomy to relieve the tamponade and control the penetrating injury to the heart. This procedure allows the surgeon to relieve cardiac tamponade, temporize any cardiac or great vessel injuries, perform open cardiac massage, and place a descending thoracic aortic cross clamp to limit infradiaphragmatic exsanguination whilst maintaining perfusion to the coronary and cerebral vasculature.

Once return of spontaneous circulation (ROSC) is achieved and injuries are temporized, the patient is immediately transported to the OR for definitive repair. If there is an obvious penetrating injury to either the left or the right ventricle, the injury should initially be controlled with digital pressure.

Make sure the entire heart is delivered from the pericardium and inspected for wounds. Temporize cardiac wounds with a finger, skin staples, or a vascular clamp before attempting suture repair in the ED.

The options for repair include suture repair, use of staples, or a Foley catheter can be introduced into the hole and the balloon distended with traction to create tamponade. The open end of the Foley should be clamped to prevent blood egress through the catheter lumen. Once the bleeding is controlled, the wound can be easily sutured. The chance of survival after emergency thoracotomy is better after a penetrating than blunt trauma mechanism.

Pitfall

Great care should be taken to apply minimal traction on the Foley – just enough to allow sealing. Excessive traction will pull the catheter out and extend the wound by tearing the muscle.

Massive haemorrhage from intercostal vessels secondary to multiple rib fractures will frequently stop without operative intervention. This is also true for most bleeding from the lung. It is helpful to collect the shed blood from the hemithorax into an autotransfusion collecting device and return it to the patient. If required, a non-anatomic pulmonary resection or tractotomy is often effective to control parenchymal haemorrhage.

Blunt aortic injury is usually diagnosed with a widened mediastinum and confirmed with a CT scan (see Chapter 8 on chest injuries). Once the diagnosis has been made, it is useful to maintain control of hypotension in the less than 100 mmHg range,[15] so as not to precipitate free rupture from the transection, until stenting or operative repair can take place.

Note: Abdominal injury generally takes priority over thoracic aortic injury.

5.3.3 Abdominal Trauma

Significant intra-abdominal or retroperitoneal haemorrhage can be a reason to go rapidly to the OR. The abdomen may be distended and dull to percussion and may be diffusely tender. Ultrasound (FAST) is a useful tool, as it is specific for blood in the peritoneum, but it is operator-dependent. A positive FAST result in an unstable patient is an indication for immediate laparotomy. Conversely, a negative FAST result does not exclude intra-abdominal bleeding, and repeat FAST or other investigations need to be considered. In the presence of shock, a positive FAST exam or positive diagnostic peritoneal aspiration (DPA) or DPL should prompt immediate exploratory laparotomy.

The decision to operate for bleeding should be based on the haemodynamic status.

Non-operative management, including the use of angiography with embolization in selected cases with abdominal bleed, has become the treatment of choice in haemodynamically stable patients with liver and spleen injuries regardless of injury grade (see Chapter 9 on the individual organ systems).

The CT scanner is highly sensitive and very specific for the type, character, and severity of injury to a specific organ. However, patients whose condition is unstable should **not** be considered for CT.

5.3.4 Pelvic Trauma

Pelvic fractures can be a significant cause of haemorrhage and death. It is essential to return the pelvis to its original configuration as swiftly as possible. As an emergency procedure, a compressing sheet, or commercially available pelvic binders, can be used. There are also external fixation devices, such as the external fixator or C-clamp, which can be placed in the resuscitation suite and return the pelvis to its normal anatomy. However, their fixation may be time-consuming, requires skill, and may not present advantages over the non-invasive binders for initial management. It decreases the volume of the pelvis and helps to compress the haematoma in the pelvis. Since approximately 85% of pelvic bleeding is venous, compressing the haematoma usually stops most pelvic bleeding.

Pitfall

For this reason, the use of REBOA may not always achieve the desired result.

If the patient continues to be hypotensive, resuscitation should continue, and, depending on the resources available, a CT angiogram or operative intervention should be considered. Angiography will identify the presence of significant arterial bleeding in the pelvis, which then can be embolized immediately. If the patient is exsanguinating from the pelvic injury or is haemodynamically unstable, and you don't have angiography immediately available, extraperitoneal packing of the pelvis should be performed, and if an intra-abdominal cause is suspected, the packing should be combined with a damage control laparotomy. Proximal aortic control may, on occasion, be required. The REBOA technique (see Section 15.3) has recently been introduced as an alternative to surgery in several EDs (and even a few pre-hospital settings), but the benefit over surgery remains largely unproven.

5.3.5 **Long Bone Fractures**

Lone bone fractures, particularly of the femur, can bleed significantly. The damage control approach to fractures is external fixation. The immediate treatment for a patient who is hypotensive from haemorrhage from a femoral fracture is to put traction on the distal limb, pulling the femur into alignment. This not only realigns the bones but also reconfigures the cylindrical nature of the thigh. This has an immediate tamponading effect on the bleeding in the muscles of the thigh. It is frequently necessary to maintain traction with a commercially available traction splint. Attention should be paid to the distal pulses to be sure that there is continued arterial inflow. If the pulses are absent, an arteriogram should be performed to determine whether there are any injuries to major vascular structures. This can be done in the ED if necessary.[16] A determination is then made as to the timing of arterial repair and bony fixation.

Re-establishing perfusion to the limb takes priority over fracture treatment.

Pitfall

Ensure there are no tibial or fibular fractures prior to placing a patient into any traction splint. This 'floating knee' scenario can lead to a stretch injury to the popliteal artery when traction is applied.

5.3.6 **Peripheral Vascular Injuries**

Peripheral vascular injuries are not in themselves life-threatening, providing that the bleeding is controlled. However, it is critical to assess whether ischaemia and vascular continuity are present, since this will influence the overall planning.

Every ED should have access to a simple flow Doppler monitor to assess pressures and flow. If there is any doubt over whether the vessel is patent, the ankle–brachial index should be measured, and if it is less than 0.9, an arteriogram is mandatory. In any patient with hard signs – that is, active bleeding, pulselessness, bruit, or pulsatile hematoma – the patient must go to theatre. In patients with pulses but soft signs like proximity or more than 10% in differential pressure, a CT angiogram should be done to identify vascular injuries. If there is any doubt, consideration should be given to the use of CT angiography if immediately available, or alternatively the ED angiogram.[16]

5.4 **SUMMARY**

The decision of whether to operate in the ED or in the OR should be made based on an overview of the urgency and the predicted outcome.

It is useful to have a well-thought-out plan for dealing with the critically injured trauma patient so that both clinical diagnosis and relevant investigations can be performed immediately, and an operative or non-operative therapeutic approach implemented.

There is no future in altering only the geographical site of death.

5.5 ANAESTHESIOLOGICAL CONSIDERATIONS

Table 5.3 Anaesthesiological Considerations

- Penetrating torso trauma in the pre-hospital setting should be transported as quickly as possible to a trauma centre ('scoop and run'). Lifesaving interventions should be performed *en route* to the hospital ('scoop and play'). Minimize time on-scene.
- Prepare the trauma centre for the patient, activate a massive transfusion protocol, call relevant personnel for immediate surgery etc.
- Preventable pre-hospital deaths are often due to haemorrhage, so it is important to prioritize haemorrhage control (C-ABC). Use early TXA if bleeding is suspected.
- **STOP** (minimize) the bleeding with e.g., direct pressure, a tourniquet, or pelvic binders.
- Use plasma for haemorrhagic shock, unless there is obvious red blood cell loss.
- Restrictive use of crystalloids, but only in patients with active bleeding if blood components are not available.
- *Suspected pneumothorax*: Use open thoracostomy (size of a finger) instead of needle decompression in intubated patients, and include a chest drain (with valve) in spontaneously breathing patients.
- Chest compressions should take lower priority (but not abandoned) than treating reversible causes of traumatic cardiac arrest.
- For tracheal intubation in comatose trauma patients (GCS <9) due to traumatic brain injury, use relaxants and hypertonic saline.
- Be careful if inducing patients in haemorrhagic shock; consider a delay of intubation until damage control surgery in-hospital. Always reduce anaesthesia dosage considerably for induction.
- Consider succinctly letting the surgeon know at an appropriate time:
- Ongoing blood loss
- Metabolic state (e.g., base deficit or lactate)
- Vasopressor requirements
- Overview of coagulation
- Consider asking the surgeon at an appropriate time:
- Is the patient clotting clinically?
- How does the perfusion of vital organs look clinically (e.g., bowel)?
- What are the available treatment options?

REFERENCES AND RECOMMENDED READING

References

1. Committee on Trauma. Resources for Optimal Care of the Injured Patient (2022 Standards). Chicago, IL, USA, American College of Surgeons, 2014. Available from www.facs.org (accessed online July 2023).
2. Ciesla DJ, Kerwin AJ, Tepas III, J. Trauma systems, Triage, and Transport. In: Moore EE, Feliciano DV, Mattox KL. eds. *Trauma*, 9th edn. New York, NY, USA, McGraw-Hill Education 2017: 54–76. https://accesssurgery.mhmedical.com/content.aspx?bookid=2952&sectionid=249116391 (accessed online August 2023)
3. Baker SP, O'Neill B, Haddon W, Long WB. The Injury Severity Score: a method for describing patients with multiple injuries and evaluating emergency care. *J Trauma* 1974 Mar;**14**:187–96.
4. American Association for the Advancement of Automotive Medicine. *The Abbreviated Injury Scale: 2015 Revision.* Barrington, IL, American Association for the Advancement of Automotive Medicine, 2015. Available from: https://www.aaam.org/abbreviated-injury-scale-ais/ (accessed July 2023).

5. Seamon MJ, Fisher CA, Gaughan J, Lloyd M, Bradley KM, Santora TA, et al. Prehospital procedures before emergency department thoracotomy: "scoop and run" saves lives. *J Trauma*. 2007 Jul;**63(1)**:113–20. doi: 10.1097/TA.0b013e31806842a1.

6. Trunkey DD. Trauma. Accidental and intentional injuries account for more years of life lost in the U.S. than cancer and heart disease. *Sci Am* 1983;**249**:28–35. doi: 10.1038/scientificamerican0883-28

7. American College of Surgeons. *Advanced Trauma Life Support®: Student Course Manual*, 10th edn. Chicago IL, USA, American College of Surgeons, 2018.

8. Teixera GR, Brown CVR, Emigh B, Long M, Foreman M, Eastridge B, Gale S, et al. Civilian prehospital tourniquet use is associated with improved survival in patients with peripheral vascular injury. *J Am Coll Surg*. 2018 May;**226(5)**:769–76.e1. doi: 10.1016/j.jamcollsurg.2018.01.047.

9. Jacobs LM, Berrizbeitia LD, Bennett B, Madigan C. Endotracheal intubation in the prehospital phase of emergency medical care. *JAMA*. 1983;**250(16)**:2175–7.

10. Taryle DA, Chandler JE, Good JT, Potts DE, Sahn SA. Emergency room intubations – complications and survival. *Chest*. 1979 May;**75**:541–3. doi: 10.1378/chest.75.5.541

11. Inaba K, Branco BC, Eckstein M, Shatz DV, Martin MJ, Green DJ, et al. Optimal positioning for emergent needle thoracostomy: a cadaver-based study. *J Trauma*. 2011 Nov;**71(5)**:1099–103; discussion 1103.). doi: 10.1097/TA.0b013e31822d9618

12. Yee ES, Verrier ED, Thomas AN. Management of air embolism in blunt and penetrating trauma. *J Thor Cardiovasc Surg*. 1983 May;**85(5)**:661–8.

13. Chreiman KM, Dumas RP, Seamon MJ, Kim PK, Reilly PM, Kaplan LJ, et al. The intraosseous have it: A prospective observational study of vascular access success rates in patients in extremis using video review. *J Trauma Acute Care Surg*. 2018 Apr;**84(4)**:558–63. doi: 10.1097/TA.0000000000001795.

14. Brooks A, Bowley DMG, Boffard KD. Bullet markers – a simple technique to assist in the evaluation of penetrating trauma. *J R Army Med Corps*. 2002 Sep;**148(3)**:259–61. doi: 10.1136/jramc-148-03-07.

15. Mosquera VX, Marini M, Lopez-Perez JM, Muñiz-Garcia J, Herrera IM, Cao I, et al. Role of conservative management in traumatic aortic injury: comparison of long term results of conservative, surgical and endovascular treatment. *J Thorac Cardiovasc Surg*. 2011 Sep;**142(3)**:614–21. doi: 10.1016/j.jtcvs.2010.10.044. Epub 2011 Jan 26.

16. MacFarlane C, Saadia R, Boffard KD. Emergency room arteriography: a useful technique in the assessment of peripheral vascular injuries. *J Roy Coll Surg Edin*. 1989 Dec;**34(6)**:310–13.

Recommended Reading

American College of Surgeons. *Advanced Trauma Life Support Course for Doctors: Student Course Manual*, 10th edn. Chicago, American College of Surgeons, 2018.

Jacobs LM, ed. *Advanced Trauma Operative Management*. Chicago/Woodbury, CT, American College of Surgeons/Ciné-Med Publishing, 2010.

Committee on Trauma. *Resources for Optimal Care of the Injured Patient (2022 Standards)*. Chicago, IL, USA, American College of Surgeons, 2014. Available from www.facs.org (accessed online 27 July 2023)

Damage Control 6

6.1 INTRODUCTION

The term *damage control* originated in the US Navy to describe the protocol used to save a ship which has suffered catastrophic structural damage from sinking, placing a heavy emphasis on the limitation and containment of fires and flooding.[1]

The concept of damage control in surgery was introduced over a century ago. The Australian-Scottish surgeon James Hogarth Pringle first described compression with packing and clamping as a method of controlling bleeding in severe liver trauma in 1908.[2] However, with the failure to understand the underlying physiological rationale, the results were disastrous.

It was not until 1976 that temporary perihepatic packing as an alternative to hepatectomy for high-grade liver injuries was first reported by Lucas and Ledgerwood.[3] The true survival benefit of this technique was undeniable by 1981, when Feliciano reported a 90% survival rate in 10 patients who were temporarily packed with severe liver injuries.[4] In 1986, Stone et al. introduced the initial abortion laparotomy, often referred to as the 'bail out laparotomy'. This included repair of major vessels, resected bowel left in discontinuity, holes closed with purse-string sutures, injured ureters ligated, and the use of intra-abdominal packs placed for tamponade which was implemented in the face of ongoing coagulopathy.[5] Eleven of 17 patients deemed with a lethal coagulopathy survived, as compared with 1 of 14 patients treated using traditional strategies of definitive repair regardless of the physiologic condition of the patient. This concept and its application to trauma of 'damage control surgery' were first coined and popularized by Rotondo and Schwab in 1993 to describe the damage control objective: to delay the imposition of additional surgical stress at a moment of physiological frailty.[6]

Damage control concepts are not restricted to the abdomen and extend to every cavity in the body as well as vascular damage control. The need for damage control in children is much less common; however, they are much more prone to hypothermia given their large surface area and small body volume – although the physiological parameters are very different, the principles are the same. At the other end of the spectrum, the application of damage control to the elderly, who have decreased physiological reserve and high morbidity and mortality, has also been successful, with survival of greater than 50% when damage control is applied to this group.[7] Damage control surgery (DCS) may be performed in smaller hospitals before transfer to a larger centre. DCS procedures, on properly selected patients, can be life-saving, and may have to be performed in any hospital admitting trauma cases.[8]

> *Damage control has been proven to save life, but it does come with a higher morbidity and longer ICU/hospital stay.*

The application of damage control principles has influenced military care and disaster planning. The need to triage mass casualty scenarios makes an abbreviated surgical and damage control approach advantageous in maximizing the use of limited resources to many patients in a restricted time span or space. A recent prospective observational military study reported that damage control was utilized in 77% of abdominal operations performed in Afghanistan and was safe.[9] The study concluded that damage control resuscitation (DCR)/DCS was the optimal approach to abdominal war injury and should be considered in logistical planning for future military operations. Events such as the Boston Marathon bombing showed that the critical patient surge placed on hospitals within minutes of an incident was well handled with good outcomes when the abbreviated DCS strategy was used to manage all patients.[9]

DOI: 10.1201/9781003258124-8

DCS is now defined as rapid termination of an operation after control of life-threatening bleeding and contamination, followed by correction of physiologic abnormalities and definitive management. This modern strategy involves a staged approach to multiply injured patients designed to avoid or correct the 'lethal triad' of hypothermia, acidosis, and coagulopathy before definitive management of injuries.[10] The goal is to focus on the body physiology and align the objectives of the surgical and anaesthetic intervention with the resuscitation objectives as an overarching damage control principle.

Damage control is divided into:

- **Identification of the patient for damage control**
- **Damage control resuscitation**
  - **Hypotensive resuscitation**
  - **Haemorrhagic resuscitation**
- **Damage control surgery**
  - **Stop the bleeding and contamination.**
- **ICU for restoration of physiology**
- **Definitive surgery**
- **Abdominal closure**

The primary goal is to temporize management of major injuries with directed resuscitation and staged surgery, to allow for resuscitation and restoration of normal physiology.

6.2 DAMAGE CONTROL RESUSCITATION

6.2.1 Overview

The optimal strategy for the management of the haemorrhaging patient is now termed *damage control resuscitation* and is a critical adjunct to the application of DCS, with which it occurs in parallel. Major principles of DCR include stopping the bleeding, permissive hypotension, minimization of crystalloid, transfusion of a balanced ratio of blood products, and goal-directed correction of coagulopathy.

6.2.2 Goals

DCR is the proactive, anticipatory treatment that presents with critical injury and shock. DCR priorities include urgent control of visible bleeding, and the following.[11,12]

6.2.2.1 PERMISSIVE HYPOTENSION

Permissive hypotension is resuscitation only to a pressure which allows organ *perfusion* ('hypotensive resuscitation'), rather than achieving *normotension*. Permissive hypotension is a strategy to reduce blood loss by limiting systolic blood pressure (SBP) to the minimum necessary to maintain perfusion of vital organs.[13]

In massively bleeding patients, raising blood pressure to normal levels before achieving surgical haemostasis has been shown to worsen bleeding by displacing clot formed during the body's attempt at primary haemostasis ('popping the clot'). The strategy is not new, and was reported during the First World War, when Cannon stated that 'if the pressure is raised before the surgeon is ready to check any bleeding that may take place, blood that is sorely needed may be lost'. The goals of fluid resuscitation include controlling bleeding, restoring lost blood volume, and regaining tissue perfusion and organ function. Different target SBP values may be considered for different traumas: 60–70 mmHg for penetrating trauma, 80–90 mmHg for blunt trauma without traumatic brain injury (TBI), and 100–110 mmHg for blunt trauma with TBI. Whilst each clinical scenario is complex and variable, regardless of the blood pressure goals, the aim should attempt for the shortest possible time in order to limit vital organ ischaemia. The importance of early surgical haemostasis and the need for the DCR concept to be applied must be emphasized.[14]

6.2.2.2 MINIMIZE THE USE OF CRYSTALLOID AND NON-BLOOD PRODUCTS

Minimize the use of crystalloid, and early use of blood products and during resuscitation. Before the advent of DCR, isotonic crystalloids were a major component of fluid therapy for patients presenting with traumatic haemorrhagic shock. In the 1980s era of 'supranormal' resuscitation, crystalloid was utilized to drive cardiac output and oxygen delivery to above normal levels. This resulted in the inability to close abdominal walls due to massive intestinal and retroperitoneal oedema, abdominal compartment syndrome (ACS), multiple organ failure (MOF), and death. Additional observational studies demonstrated increased incidence of dilutional coagulopathy, acute respiratory distress syndrome (ARDS), multiple organ dysfunction syndrome (MODS), and mortality in severely injured trauma patients.[15] Closer examination of aggressive fluid therapy in surgical patients demonstrated intracellular oedema that disrupted many vital biochemical processes, including pancreatic insulin synthesis and secretion, hepatocyte glucose metabolism, and cardiac myocyte excitability.[16]

Minimizing the volume of pre-hospital infusion of crystalloids in hypotensive trauma patients has shown a survival benefit. In a retrospective study from Brown, over 1,200 blunt trauma patients were dichotomized into high (>500 mL) and low (≤500 mL) groups based on infusion of pre-hospital crystalloid, and they were stratified by the presence of pre-hospital hypotension.[17] The investigators reported that there was no difference in mortality in patients with pre-hospital hypotension, but >500 mL pre-hospital crystalloid was associated with increased mortality (hazard ratio [HR] = 2.5, 95% confidence interval [CI] = 1.3–4.9) and increased coagulopathy by admission international normalized ratio (INR) (odds ratio [OR] = 2.2, 95% CI = 1.0–4.9) in patients without pre-hospital hypotension. In a retrospective study by Ley, investigators found that infusion of ≥1.5 L of crystalloid in the emergency department was independently associated with increased mortality.[18] Although the safe volume of crystalloid is yet to be determined, it is clear that large infusions of crystalloid are dangerous and even relatively small volumes may be harmful.

6.2.2.3 BLOOD PRODUCT ADMINISTRATION WITH A BALANCED RATIO OF PACKED RED BLOOD CELLS (PRBCS), FRESH FROZEN PLASMA (FFP), AND PLATELETS

A ratio of 1:1:1 has been suggested and proven safe by a large, randomized controlled trial (PROPPR). This has been shown to reduce exsanguination, which is an early cause of death in these patients (9.2% vs. 14.6% in a 1:1:2 group; difference = −5.4% [95% CI = −10.4% to −0.5%, P = .03]), and is at least as safe as a less balanced approach, with no differences in complication rates such as ARDS, MOF, venous thromboembolism, and sepsis.[19] Early and aggressive administration of blood and blood products has been shown to improve survival after trauma-related haemorrhagic shock. Lost blood volume should be replaced by blood products aiming at near equal ratios of PRBCs:FFP:platelets.[20,21] Such regimens have demonstrated improved outcomes. Data suggest that plasma-based resuscitation when compared to crystalloids is better at preserving endothelial integrity. FFP administration after haemorrhagic shock has anti-inflammatory properties and a potential glycocalyx-restoring capacity.[22]

Ultimately, a 1:1:1 ratio is an attempt to re-create what is actively being lost in the bleeding patient, and

in certain environments properly crossmatched whole blood (WB) may also be used. WB in a military setting can take the form of a walking blood bank, which allows immediate access to warm and fresh WB, and where the blood type of the available population is already known. In a civilian setting, WB is often cold-stored, and this has been proven to be a safe transfusion option.[23]

WB has been shown to be significantly more effective than a standard balanced resuscitation. WB patients had a 9% reduction in bleeding complications and a surprising 48% mortality benefit. Hazelton et al. showed improved survival at 24 hours with a 37% mortality reduction (HR = 0.63, 95% CI = 0.41–0.96, P = 0.03), as well as at 30 days (HR = 0.53, 95% CI = 0.31–0.93, P = .02).[24] Whilst it is a safe and potentially improved resuscitative option, not all areas have access to WB, and it requires collaboration between emergency medicine systems, trauma surgeons, traumatologists, and blood bankers.[25]

6.2.2.4 TRANEXAMIC ACID (TXA)

The addition of TXA (1 g bolus up to 3 hours after injury, followed by a 1 g perfusion for 8 hours) has shown a reduction in mortality after severe injury in certain situations. (See Chapter 4: 'Transfusion in Trauma'.)

6.2.2.5 GOAL-DIRECTED HAEMOSTASIS

Targeting coagulopathy with goal-directed haemostasis, using viscoelastic assays such as thromboelastography (TEG) or rotary thromboelastometry (RoTEM), if available, may be used to guide product therapy.[26]

6.2.2.6 AVOID HYPOTHERMIA

Hypothermia below 35 °C has a profound impact on oxygen delivery, as well as on surgical site infection rates after trauma laparotomy. Hypothermia also adversely affects coagulation as well as cardiac output and function in most bodily organs.[27]

6.2.2.7 RESTORATION OF NORMOCALCAEMIA

Recent research has alluded that an early supplement of calcium will reduce morbidity and mortality in the massively hypovolaemic trauma patient.[28]

The Eastern Association for the Surgery of Trauma (EAST) guidelines on DCR[29] addressed its requirements (see **Table 6.1**).

Table 6.1 Pitfalls: Do's and Don'ts

DO

- Cover only one side of the swab. Covering both sides impedes drainage by preventing capillary wicking through the weave of the swab.
- Insert the sandwich with the plastic side against the bowel.
- Insert the sandwich as a 'diamond', with the points tucked in at top and bottom of the incision, and laterally.

DO NOT

- Make any holes (slits) in the membrane. Holes would allow the suction to be transmitted directly to the serosa of the bowel, with possible risk of fistula formation.
- Have a vacuum above a maximum of 25 mmHg. Higher suction pressures, especially in a cold hypotensive patient, transmitted directly on to the bowel may exceed capillary pressure.
- Preferably avoid the commercial equivalents (e.g., VAC®, Kinetic Concepts Incorporated [KCI], San Antonio, TX, USA; or Renasys®, Smith and Nephew, London, UK) currently. These should be reserved for the definitive closure of a wound, both for cost reasons and due to the higher vacuum suction pressure often present.

6.2.3 **Massive Transfusion/Haemorrhage Protocol (MTP/MHP)**

The implementation of a massive transfusion protocol (MTP, also called massive haemorrhage protocol [MHP]) is recommended, which will allow the ready availability of blood products. Availability of a MTP has been shown to be associated with a reduction in organ failure and improved 30-day survival after severe trauma.[30] (See Chapter 4: 'Transfusion in Trauma'.)

6.3 **DAMAGE CONTROL SURGERY**

6.3.1 **Overview**

DCS is a technique whereby the surgeon minimizes operative time and surgical intervention in the grossly unstable patient. The primary reason for this is to minimize hypothermia, metabolic acidosis, and coagulopathy (the

lethal triad), and, more recently highlighted, hypocalcaemia (the 'deadly diamond').

The focus is exclusively on life-saving surgical procedures (bleeding and contamination control), thus permitting earlier and more successful resuscitation and normalization of the physiology. After a postoperative intensive care resuscitation and stabilization period, the patient is returned to the operating room as soon as physiologically possible for definitive surgical care (e.g., restoration of bowel continuity). Although the principles are sound, extreme care needs to be exercised to avoid overutilization of the concept, causing secondary insults to viscera. Furthermore, surgery must be appropriate to minimize activation of the inflammatory cascade and the consequences of systemic inflammatory response syndrome (SIRS) and organ dysfunction.

6.3.2 **Lethal Triad and Deadly Diamond**

6.3.2.1 **HYPOTHERMIA**

Hypothermia is defined as a core temperature below 35° C and has a profound impact on outcome in trauma patients. The stages of hypothermia are defined as:

- *Mild hypothermia*: Core temperature 32–35 °C (90–95 °F)
- *Moderate hypothermia*: Core temperature 28–32 °C (82–90 °F)
- *Severe hypothermia*: Core temperature < 28 °C (<82 °F)

Hypothermia has notable effects on platelets, platelet function, fibrinogen, and coagulation factors. Jurkovich et al. found that mortality increased significantly in trauma patients with a core temperature less than 34 °C and approached 100% in trauma patients with a core temperature less than 32 °C.[31] Physiologic effects included decreased heart rate and cardiac output, increased systemic vascular resistance, arrhythmias, decreased glomerular filtration rate, impaired sodium absorption, and central nervous system depression.

Common laboratory techniques cannot identify those effects because blood samples are usually warmed to 37 °C before analysis and do not fully reflect the *in vivo* situation. Temperatures below 35 °C have been shown to have prolonged prothrombin time (PT) and partial thromboplastin time (PTT).

Rewarming should be initiated as soon as possible. Rewarming techniques can be categorized as passive external rewarming, active external rewarming, and active internal core rewarming. Passive external rewarming is used for mild hypothermia where the patient is covered with blankets or other types of insulation. Generally, it is recommended to rewarm at a rate between 0.5 and 2 °C per hour. For patients who are in need of additional rewarming, active external rewarming is indicated for moderate to severe hypothermia (<32 °C) which involves a combination of warm blankets, heating pads, radiant heat, warm baths, and forced warm air applied directly to the patient's skin. Active internal rewarming is the most aggressive strategy in patients with severe hypothermia (<28 °C).

Endovascular rewarming is the method of choice for patients not requiring extracorporeal life support (ECLS). Endovascular temperature-control catheters are a less invasive alternative to extracorporeal blood rewarming in patients who are not in cardiocirculatory arrest. These devices utilize a femoral catheter that circulates temperature-controlled water inside a closed catheter tip in the femoral vein, warming or cooling blood as it flows past the tip. Several ECLS techniques can be used to treat hypothermic patients by rewarming blood outside the body: veno-venous rewarming, haemodialysis, continuous arteriovenous rewarming (CAVR), cardiopulmonary bypass (CPB), and extracorporeal membrane oxygenation (ECMO).

Active core rewarming also can be accomplished by warm lavage of several body cavities. Gastric, colonic, and bladder lavage have slower rates of increasing temperature (1.0–1.5 °C per hour) secondary to a limited area for heat exchange. Peritoneal dialysis with normal saline, Ringer's lactate, or a dialysate solution heated to 40–45 °C at a rate of 6–10 L per hour has been shown to increase body temperature by 1–3 °C per hour when combined with heated oxygen. It should be emphasized that all of these methods are slow and are to be used in the patient with moderate to severe hypothermia only if extracorporeal blood warming is unavailable.[24]

6.3.2.2 ACIDOSIS

Acidosis is defined as an arterial pH < 7.35, and in trauma patients it is the result of poor perfusion to the tissues from haemorrhage. This results in a tissue oxygen demand that far exceeds oxygen delivery and overall decreased cardiac output severely impairing oxygen delivery to the tissues. The body's cells are forced to utilize anaerobic metabolism instead of the normal aerobic metabolism, resulting in the production of lactic acid. The detrimental effects of acidosis include depressed myocardial contractility, diminished inotropic response to catecholamines, ventricular arrhythmias, increased intracranial pressure, and worsened coagulopathy. An additional cause of acidosis in the trauma patient is excessive resuscitation using unbalanced crystalloid solutions such as normal saline. With a pH of around 5.5, normal saline can result in a hyperchloraemic metabolic acidosis which only compounds the existing lactic acidosis and increases systemic tissue inflammation and coagulopathy. Although Ringer's lactate has a pH of 6.5, it is an imperfect substitute that contains lactate and is incompatible with many medications and blood products. The degree of acidosis upon arrival to the ICU after a damage control procedure directly correlates with mortality. In a study by Aoki et al., all patients who returned to the ICU after damage control laparotomy (DCL) with a pH less than or equal to 7.2 died, whereas 88% of patients who returned with a pH greater than 7.33 lived. All patients whose pH was between 7.2 and 7.33 and whose PTT was less than or equal to 78.7 seconds died. Eighty-two percent of patients survived if their pH was between 7.2 and 7.33 and their PTT was greater than 78.7 seconds.[32]

6.3.2.3 COAGULOPATHY

After initiating MTP with either balanced resuscitation or WB, targeting trauma-induced coagulopathy with goal-directed haemostatic resuscitation, and using viscoelastic assays such as TEG, RoTEM with platelet mapping, if available, may be used to guide product therapy.[26] These viscoelastic studies allow for point-of-care and real-time testing of the patient's WB. Viscoelastic studies have been shown to improve upon clinical judgement and need for MTP as well as guide resuscitation efforts. As these tests can be repeated throughout the process of a prolonged resuscitation effort, they allow for a more customizable resuscitation based on the patient's physiologic derangements rather than a fixed ratio of product.

6.3.2.4 HYPOCALCAEMIA

Calcium plays several important physiologic roles in multiple organ systems; the negative haemodynamic effects of hypocalcaemia are crucial to address in trauma patients. The negative ramifications of hypocalcaemia are intrinsically linked to components of the lethal triad of acidosis, coagulopathy, and hypothermia. Hypocalcaemia has direct and indirect effects on each portion of the lethal triad, supporting calcium's potential position as a fourth component in this proposed lethal diamond. Trauma patients often present with hypocalcaemia in the setting of severe haemorrhage secondary to trauma, which can be worsened by necessary transfusion and resuscitation. The critical consequences of hypocalcaemia in the trauma patient have been repeatedly demonstrated with the associated morbidity and mortality.[33] It remains poorly defined when to administer calcium, though current data suggest that earlier administration may be advantageous.

6.3.3 Damage Control in the Thorax

DCS principles are applicable to thoracic trauma, although there is a dearth of data. In the largest series, mortality was 23%. Predictors included a higher Injury Severity Score (ISS), renal failure, continuous renal replacement therapy, and ECMO. All survivors were neurologically intact and dialysis free.

Patients with severe chest trauma and marked physiologic derangement can benefit from damage control thoracic surgery. Thoracic packing and temporary vacuum closure avoid thoracic compartment syndrome. Timing of thoracic closure is based on physiology. Whilst complications were common, mortality was acceptable in this group of severely injured, metabolically depleted, challenging patients.[34]

6.3.4 Damage Control in the Abdomen

There are five critical decision-making stages of DCS: Stage I, patient selection, and decision to perform damage control; Stage II, operation, and intraoperative assessment of laparotomy; Stage III, resuscitation in the ICU; Stage IV, definitive procedures after returning to the operating room; and Stage V, abdominal wall reconstruction.

6.3.4.1 STAGE 1: PATIENT SELECTION

Proper patient selection is crucial to optimize outcomes following DCS. All patients should undergo a very rapid trauma evaluation, and appropriate DCR. The duration of this stage is dictated by the patient's physiologic stability as well as the underlying pathology. Delays to the operating room must be avoided, and this is particularly relevant in patients with intracavitary bleeding after gunshot wounds, where any delay in excess of 10 minutes is associated with a three times higher risk of mortality. Rapid manoeuvres to control external bleeding (tourniquets, digital control of bleeding, etc.) are indicated as transition to the operating room occurs.

The treatment of bleeding is to stop the bleeding.

In any hospital managing trauma or a high number of emergency surgical cases, protocols for massive transfusion supporting haemostatic resuscitation should be in place and supported by anaesthesia, blood bank, and intensive care staff. The inclusion of the anaesthesiologist in the emergency room resuscitation team is essential. The surgeon is well advised to call for an additional surgeon to assist, if available.

The indications to consider in selecting a patient for damage control are:

- Haemodynamic instability
  - SBP < 90 mmHg and not responding to resuscitation
- Temperature < 35° C
- Metabolic instability
  - Temperature < 35° C
  - pH < 7.2
  - Base excess ≥ –5 and worsening
  - Serum lactate > 5 mmol/L
- Coagulopathy
  - Abnormal viscoelastic haemostatic assays (VHAs): TEG or RoTEM
  - PT > 16 seconds
  - PTT > 60 seconds
- Surgical anatomy
  - Complex life-threatening injuries (e.g., major vascular injury or moderate vascular injury with complex hollow viscus injuries, complex liver injury, exsanguinating retroperitoneal pelvis, multi-cavitary exsanguination, etc.)
  - Anticipated need for a time-consuming surgical procedure in a patient with a suboptimal response to resuscitation
  - Inability to perform the definitive repair in a timely fashion
  - Demand for non-operative control of other injuries, for example a fractured pelvis
  - Inability to approximate the abdominal incision
  - Association with severe injuries in other organs or regions, such as severe head trauma requiring craniotomy in a patient whose abdominal injuries would require a lengthy procedure
- Environment and/or resource demands
  - Blood requirement requiring a MTP
  - Operating time greater than 60 minutes

- Logistics
  - Multiple patients/mass casualty situation
- Minimal resources
  - For example, personnel, medical equipment, and safety concerns

It is critical to identify these potential scenarios before the patient becomes metabolically unsalvageable. The decision to deploy a damage control physiologic-based approach should be done to prevent this metabolic deterioration from occurring in the first place. It can often be a decision that is made at the very beginning of the surgical intervention.

If resources allow, the use of a hybrid operating room expedites definitive haemorrhage control and can complement damage control therapy in the exsanguinating patient.

> *Irrespective of the setting, a coagulopathy is the single most common reason for abortion of a planned procedure or curtailment of definitive surgery. It is important to abort the surgery before the coagulopathy becomes obvious.*

The technical aspects of the surgery are dictated by the injury pattern.

6.3.4.2 STAGE 2: OPERATIVE HAEMORRHAGE AND CONTAMINATION CONTROL

The primary objectives are as follows.

6.3.4.2.1 Initial Incision

A generous midline laparotomy incision is necessary to allow for wide retraction of the abdominal wall and rapid visualization of the liver, abdominal great vessels, and all other retroperitoneal structures. Rapid control of the largest source of blood loss is critical, and in those cases with several sources of bleeding and manual pressure, packing and temporary ligation may be necessary. Each case is unique in presentation; however, the principle is to control active large blood loss first.

6.3.4.2.2 Haemorrhage Control

The operative process works through the following:

- Arrest arterial and major venous bleeding. Failure to control ongoing bleeding will lead to the patient's demise:
  - Major arterial bleeding must be controlled at the index procedure. A temporary intravascular shunt is preferred for named vessels; however, ligation may be required to save an exsanguinating patient.
- Temporary intravascular shunting (see **Figure 6.1**):
  - Use tubing approximately 50% of the diameter of the vessel being shunted.
  - Allow 3–4 cm of the tube in each end of the vessel.
  - The shunt can be either a straight (linear) shunt (**Figure 6.1a**, e.g., for iliac vessels, portal vein, etc.) or a 'pig-tail' shunt (**Figure 6.1b**) where access is difficult.

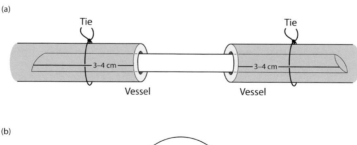

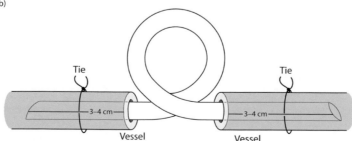

Figure 6.1 Diagram of an intravascular shunt: (a) Straight shunt, and (b) 'pig-tail' shunt.

- Tamponade using wraps or packs.
- Occlusion of inflow into the bleeding organ (e.g., Pringle's manoeuvre for bleeding liver).
- Repair or ligation of accessible blood vessels.
- Intraoperative or postoperative catheter-directed embolization.

6.3.4.2.3 Control of Contamination (Hollow Viscus Organs)

- Defects in the bowel or hollow viscus organs can be controlled with simple suturing or stapler applications.
- Damaged segments can be resected with clamps or staples.
- Biliary and genitourinary injuries can be temporized with external drainage (T-tube, ureterostomy, etc.).
- Pancreatic injuries should be widely drained and packed.

Avoid definitive repair, restoration of intestinal continuity, stoma formation, and creation of feeding access at this stage.

Pitfall

Avoid definitive repair, restoration of intestinal continuity, stoma formation, and creation of feeding access at this stage. However, ensure there is no potential for gross contamination; otherwise, the patient's status may quickly deteriorate due to overwhelming immune-inflammatory activation, potentiated by the initial tissue destruction, operative trauma, and shock.

6.3.4.2.3.1 *Copious Wash-Out*

At the end of the procedure, before temporary closure, the abdominal cavity must be washed out with copious (several litres of) warmed normal saline, especially if there has been gross contamination. After washing out, attempt to suction all fluid and leave the cavity as dry as possible.

6.3.4.2.3.2 *Temporary Abdominal Closure (TAC)*

The abdominal cavity should be temporized to prevent heat and moisture loss, and to protect the viscera.

Temporary abdominal closure is required when any combination of the factors listed above under damage control, or re-look surgery, exists. Patients with multiple injuries who have undergone protracted surgery with massive volume resuscitation to maintain haemodynamic stability will often develop tissue interstitial oedema. This may predispose them to the development of ACS or may simply make primary closure impractical. In addition, significant enteric or other contamination will raise the risk of intra-abdominal sepsis, or the extent of tissue damage may raise doubt over the viability of any repair; these conditions usually mandate planned re-laparotomy and thus a temporary closure.

In these circumstances, a temporary abdominal closure is required. The needs of such a closure can be summarized as:

- Fast
- Inexpensive
- Keeps the abdominal contents inside the abdominal cavity
- Allows drainage of fluid
- Minimizes sepsis
- Facilitates delayed primary fascial closure

Vacuum-based closure is recommended for the management of the open abdomen. A review of the literature available suggests that negative-pressure wound vacuum therapy may have improved fascial closure rates and may be associated with improved outcomes over alternative abdominal closure techniques (e.g., mesh, Velcro, and bag-type dressings).

Many temporary closure systems are available, of which the most cost-effective is the 'sandwich technique' first described by Schein in 1986.[35]

A sheet of self-adhesive incise drape (Opsite®, Smith and Nephew, London, UK; or Steri-Drape® or Ioban®, 3M, St. Paul, MN, USA) is placed flat and sticky side up, and an abdominal swab is placed upon it. The objective is to create a non-stick membrane on one side of the abdominal swab to place against the visceral organs. The size should be large enough that, when inserted, the sheet will extend laterally to the paracolic gutters, and 10 cm cranial and caudal to the incision. This technique results in a composite sheet with a membrane (i.e. the drape) on one side, and an abdominal swab on the other. The membrane is utilized as a lay-on over the bowel and abdominal organs, with the margins 'tucked in' under the edges of the open sheath as far as the paracolic gutters, with only the membrane in contact with the bowel. The abdominal swab is on the external surface.

Pitfalls: Do's and Don'ts

DO

- Cover only one side of the swab. Covering both sides impedes drainage by preventing capillary wicking through the weave of the swab.
- Insert the sandwich with the plastic side against the bowel.
- Insert the sandwich as a 'diamond', with the points tucked in at the top and bottom of the incision, and laterally.

DO NOT

- Use commercial equivalents (e.g., VAC®, Kinetic Concepts Incorporated [KCI], San Antonio, TX, USA; or Renasys®, Smith and Nephew) in the immediate care of the wound. These should be reserved for the definitive closure of a wound, for both cost reasons and the higher vacuum suction pressure often present.
- Make any holes (slits) in the membrane. Holes would allow the suction to be transmitted directly to the serosa of the bowel, with possible risk of fistula formation.
- Have a vacuum above a maximum of 25 mmHg. Higher suction pressures, especially in a cold hypotensive patient, transmitted directly on to the bowel may exceed capillary pressure.

The drainage of serosanguinous fluid that occurs is best dealt with by placing a pair of drainage tubes (e.g., sump-type nasogastric tubes or closed-system suction drains) with the tips placed in the caudal end of the incision, brought out through *separate* cranial end stab incisions. The tubes are placed to lie on either side of the incision, *under* the edge of the anterior abdominal peritoneum, utilizing continuous low-vacuum suction.

A self-adhesive sheet is placed to cover the placed drainage tubes and incision, with a margin of 20 cm around the incision, to avoid air leakage, thus providing a closed system (the 'sandwich'; **Figures 6.2 and 6.3**).

Pitfall

The 'Bogota bag' and towel clips, etc., **should no longer be used**, and for temporary abdominal closure, no sutures should be placed in the sheath, nor skin, although recent evidence suggests there may be a role for whipstitch to the skin as a skin-only closure.[36]

The timing of transfer of the patient from the operating room to the ICU is critical. Control of bleeding and contamination must be achieved. On the other hand,

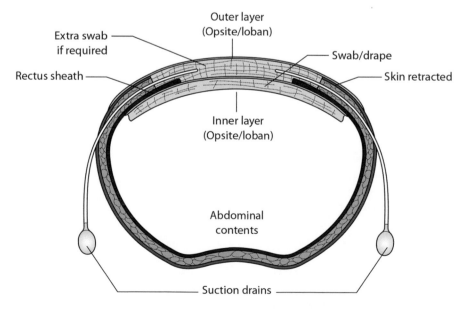

Outer layer
(Opsite/Ioban)

Extra swab
if required

Rectus sheath

Swab/drape

Skin retracted

Inner layer
(Opsite/Ioban)

Abdominal
contents

Suction drains

Figure 6.2 Diagrammatic representation of the sandwich technique for temporary abdominal closure.

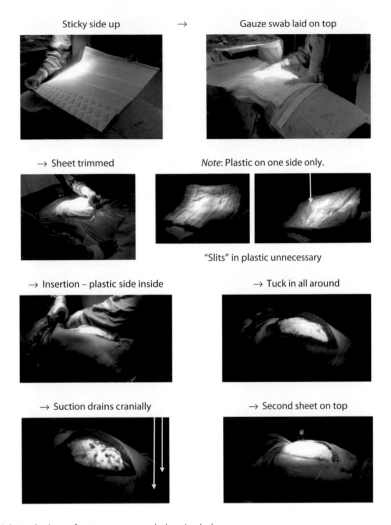

Figure 6.3 Sandwich technique for temporary abdominal closure.

once haemostasis has been properly achieved, it may not be necessary to abort the procedure in the same fashion.[37]

- **Prompt transfer to the ICU is cost-effective; premature transfer is counterproductive.**
- **Patient transfer to the ICU after DCS is a key moment and should entail proper operative notes (including the number of swabs left in the abdomen, the number and location of shunts) and predicted timing of the planned second-look. Excellent communication between the surgeon, anaesthesiologist, and intensive care specialist is key to a successful outcome, and this handover should not be neglected. Also, this is the opportunity to debrief the OR team.**

- **If the physiological condition allows and there is suspicion of other severe injuries (e.g., head trauma), a patient who did not undergo full-body CT may have one at this stage. Otherwise, severely ill patients are better transported to the ICU for ongoing resuscitation.**

6.3.4.3 STAGE 3: PHYSIOLOGICAL RESTORATION IN THE ICU

Priorities in the ICU are as follows:

Restoration of body temperature

- Passive rewarming using warming blankets, convection blankets, warmed fluids, heat lamps, elevation of the ambient room temperature, etc.

- Active rewarming with either external or internal methods as appropriate
- Extracorporeal blood warming if indicated and/or available.

Optimization of oxygen delivery

- Volume loading to restore circulating blood volume
- Haemoglobin optimization to a haemoglobin level of 8–10 g/dL (80–100 g/L, 4–6 mmol/L)
- Monitoring of cardiac output
  - Correction of acidosis to a pH > 7.3
  - Ultrasonic cardiac output devices
  - Cardiac output monitors if appropriate
- Measurement and correction of lactic acidosis to less than 2.5 mmol/L
- Inotropic support as required, but not prioritized over *adequate* blood product resuscitation

Correction of clotting profiles

- Blood component repletion
- Assessment and normalization of any coagulopathy
  - Coagulation studies
- TEG or RoTEM

Improvement of physiological endpoints, as evidenced by

- Lactate clearance
- Mixed venous oxygen saturation (SvO$_2$)
- Urine output
- Haemodynamics
- Resolution of acidaemia
- Inotropic support decreased once intravascular volume has been repleted.

Monitoring for and minimizing the incidence of intra-abdominal hypertension (IAH) and ACS

- Measurement of intra-abdominal pressure (IAP)
  - Foley (bladder) catheter
  - Intragastric catheter

Recognition of additional injuries

- Review of injury mechanism, presentation, and those steps in standard trauma resuscitation, along with diagnostics and therapies that were not completed, to facilitate damage control.
- Tertiary survey
- Additional imaging as needed.
- Review of history, comorbid conditions, and medications.

6.3.4.4 STAGE 4: DEFINITIVE SURGERY

The patient is returned to the operating room as soon as physiological stability has been achieved. Ideally this would be within 24–48 hours, as delaying beyond 48 hours can be detrimental; however, the timing for this is determined by:

- The indication for damage control in the first place
- The pattern of injury
- The physiological response to resuscitation, warming, and evaluation as above.

Patients with ongoing bleeding despite correction of the other parameters require immediate return to the operating room or angiography suite.

Patients who develop major ACS must undergo re-look surgery early, and any further underlying causes must be corrected. This can and does occur even in the patient with a temporary abdominal closure.

Every effort must be made to return *all* patients to the operating room within 24–36 hours of their initial surgery. By leaving matters longer, other problems such as ARDS, SIRS, and sepsis may intervene (cause or effect) and may preclude further surgery.

6.3.4.4.1 The 'Re-Look Laparotomy'

The re-look laparotomy may be:

- *Planned*: That is decided upon at the time of the initial procedure and usually for reasons of contamination or questionable tissue viability, for retrieval of intra-abdominal packs, or for further definitive surgery after damage control.
- *On demand*: That occurs when evidence of intra-abdominal complication develops. In these cases, the principle applies of re-operation 'when the patient fails to progress according to expectation'. Failure to act in these circumstances may have dire consequences in terms of morbidity and mortality.

Re-exploration should be thorough, with careful evaluation for previously undiagnosed injuries. If the patient's physiological parameters deteriorate again, then the damage control philosophy should be reapplied with aggressive resuscitation, abbreviated laparotomy, and possible adjunctive procedures such as angiography, pelvic stabilization, and evaluation of extraabdominal injury. In many cases, repacking combined with aggressive correction of physiologic endpoints including coagulopathy, along with further warming and coagulopathy, are necessary.

If a stoma (colostomy or ileostomy) is needed, the stoma is positioned more laterally, between the musculature of the anterior and mid-axillary lines. The rectus fascia and musculature are thereby spared for future reconstruction, and the stoma is positioned well away from the midline wound, thus minimizing contamination. As the abdominal wall is reapproximated, the stoma will move toward the anterior midline.

6.3.4.5 STAGE 5: ABDOMINAL WALL CLOSURE

Once the patient has completed definitive surgery and no further operations are contemplated, the abdominal wall can be closed. In most series, most patients had the fascia closed after the first re-look, or within 7 to 8 days from injury. This varies greatly depending on patient size and body habitus, time to achieve physiologic stabilization, volume of fluid used to resuscitate, and injuries sustained.

6.3.4.5.1 Delayed Primary Abdominal Closure

Delayed closure will be required once the reasons for the temporary surgery have been removed or treated. This is usually possible after an interval of 24–48 hours (or longer). Usually, the abdominal wall can be closed in layers using normal closure techniques. However, this should only be performed when no further surgery is contemplated and should be accomplished without any fascial tension.

If the abdominal viscera are protruding above the fascia in the supine anesthetized patient, further management with temporary closure (vacuum assisted) is recommended. Return to the operating room after another 24–48 hours of intensive care, and fluid mobilization in most cases will then allow primary fascial closure. Both the surgeon and anaesthetist must be aware of the danger of causing ACS as a result of the closure, and intra-abdominal or respiratory pressures must be closely monitored.

6.3.4.5.2 Secondary Abdominal Closure

If, for various reasons, a delayed primary closure is not possible, then it will be necessary to accept (but minimize) the defect that results. The skin of the abdominal wall and the underlying fascia retract, and thus prevent a primary closure from being achieved. During the period of the open abdomen, in this situation, several techniques are usually combined to get to a point where the fascia can be closed without tension and safely. The goal is to achieve fascial closure, and subsequent skin closure.

Methods involved which will minimize or reduce the eventual defect include:

- Closure of skin only, allowing the formation of a hernia.
- Biologic material such as human (AlloDerm) or porcine (Permacol) dermal matrix used as mesh early to prevent hernia formation, providing skin coverage.
- Continued vacuum-assisted temporary abdominal closure such as VAC (KCI) and Renasys (Smith and Nephew) until granulation over bowel occurs, for subsequent split-thickness skin grafting.
- If a synthetic mesh is left *in situ*, skin coverage of the resulting defect by split-grafting or flap transfer; *never use a polypropylene-only mesh.*
- Grafts using Vicryl® mesh (Johnson and Johnson. New Brunswick, NJ, USA) or Gore-Tex® sheets (W L Gore and associates Inc. Flagstaff AZ USA) or other synthetic sheets
- Biologic meshes – human dermal matrix (AlloDerm® - LifeCell, Bridgewater NJ, USA) or porcine dermal matrix (Permacol – Covidien, Mansfield MA, USA)
- Split-thickness skin grafts directly on granulated bowel or mesh.
- For large hernias, often the need for later reconstruction using different techniques such as component separation and flap construction.
- A Wittmann patch.
- A multitude of tension-assist devices are now available.

An absorbable mesh of polyglycolic acid such as Vicryl (Johnson & Johnson) elicits minimal tissue reaction and ingrowth. Thus, it has a low risk of infection or fistula formation.

Membranes such as polytetrafluoroethylene (PTFE, or Gore-Tex, WL Gore and Associates), which elicit minimal tissue reaction and ingrowth, and thus minimize risk of infection or fistula formation, can be used, but this is considerably costlier. Recently, composite meshes have shown promise. The mesh can then have a skin graft placed upon it (or even directly on bowel), and definitive abdominal wall reconstruction can take place at a later stage.

Should any mesh be used and left *in situ*, however, the resulting defect will require skin coverage by split-grafting or flap transfer.

6.3.5 PLANNED HERNIA

A planned hernia approach aims at skin coverage with subsequent delayed abdominal wall reconstruction. Conditions favouring a planned hernia strategy include the inability to reapproximate the retracted abdominal wall edges, sizeable tissue deficit, risk of tertiary ACS, inadequate infection source control, anterior enteric fistula, and poor nutritional status of the patient. Various techniques have been applied. Autologous split-thickness skin grafting over the visceral content of the abdomen allows coverage of the exposed bowel. Maturation of the skin graft requires about 6–12 months, after which the grafted skin can be easily removed from the bowel surface for reconstruction.

Bridging mesh is often employed, and absorbable mesh is preferred. Non-absorbable mesh (polypropylene mesh, etc.) has been abandoned because of infection and high rates of fistula formation.

More commonly, a component separation is performed. A large relaxing incision is placed in the exterior oblique muscle component of the anterior rectus muscle bilaterally. This can be combined with mobilization of the rectus muscle from the posterior fascial sheath to provide local advancement across the hernia defect. Modification of this technique has been described with division of the internal oblique to the arcuate line. Large abdominal wall defects can be reconstructed with pedicular or microvascular flaps. The most commonly used is the tensor fascia lata (TFL) flap.

6.3.6 OUTCOMES

Although DCS is widely assumed to reduce mortality in critically injured patients, survivors often suffer substantial morbidity. Patients who undergo damage control procedures are at high risk of ARDS, MOF, and death. DCL has also been associated with increased rates of fascial dehiscence, infection, incisional hernia, and enteric suture line failure.[39] A cautionary tale of potential overuse of DCL was reported by Higa et al., where a practice paradigm shift was implemented to decease the utilization of DCL over a 3-year period. This resulted in a decreased mortality rate for patients requiring open laparotomy from 21.9% in 2006 to 12.9% in 2008 (p = 0.05). The decreases in average costs and charges are projected to result in savings of $2.2 million and $5.8 million, respectively.[38] The potential overuse of DCL is being reported in the literature by the trauma community, recognizing complications of patients who underwent DCL but may have safely been closed at the first operation.[40] As the pendulum of the use of DCL swings, there is little debate that, if applied appropriately, the development of DCL has revolutionized the care of severely injured trauma patients.

Inappropriate Damage Control is just as much of an error as no Damage Control.

6.4 DAMAGE CONTROL ORTHOPAEDICS (DCO)[41]

Early definitive internal fixation of long bones and the axial skeleton is preferable in most haemodynamically normal or polytrauma patients or for those who respond to the initiated haemostatic resuscitation. Patients *in extremis*, not responding to resuscitation, with high intracranial pressures as well as difficulties in ventilation and coagulopathy, would benefit from temporary external fixation followed by staged definitive internal fixation. The concept is called *damage control orthopaedics* (DCO) due to the abbreviated surgery to allow physiological recovery and planned definitive care at a later stage.

DCO involves, but is not limited to, haemorrhage control, revascularization (via shunts), contamination control (debridement and irrigation), temporary skeletal stabilization (external fixation, percutaneous screws, traction, plasters, fasciotomies, guillotine amputations, and any combinations of these). DCO as a default term means lifesaving procedures on a critically injured patient with seriously compromised physiology (patient mode).

When it is specified, it can mean 'limb mode', ranging from isolated limb salvage without systemic physiological compromise to temporary spanning eternal fixation of grossly swollen limbs with major articular fractures.

The DCO 'resource mode' refers to a situation where local personal or material resources are not available or are overwhelmed by the complexity of the injury and/or the number of injured patients.

The goals of DCO are to limit ongoing haemorrhage and soft tissue injury through efficient fracture stabilization, whilst minimizing additional physiological insult. Normal damage control principles are followed, such as avoiding the deadly diamond of hypothermia, coagulopathy, hypocalcaemia, and acidosis, and minimizing secondary injury to organ systems (kidney, brain, etc.). External fixation is employed for long bone fractures and pelvic injuries. Surgical wound toilet and fasciotomies may be required.[42]

REFERENCES AND RECOMMENDED READING

References

1. U.S. Navy. *Surface Ship Survivability*. United States, Naval War Publications, 19962.

2. Pringle JH. V. Notes on the arrest of hepatic hemorrhage due to trauma. *Ann Surg*. 1908;**48(4)**:541–9.

3. Lucas CE, Ledgerwood AM. Prospective evaluation of hemostatic techniques for liver injuries. *J Trauma*. 1976 Jun;**16(6)**:442–51. doi: 10.1097/00005373-197606000-00003

4. Feliciano DV, Mattox KL, Jordan Jr GL. Intra-abdominal packing for control of hepatic hemorrhage: a reappraisal. *J Trauma*. 1981 Apr;**21(4)**:285–90. doi: 10.1097/00005373-198104000-00005

5. Stone HH, Strom PR, Mullins RJ. Management of the major coagulopathy with onset during laparotomy. *Ann Surg*. 1983 May;**197(5)**:532–5. doi: 10.1097/00000658-198305000-00005

6. Rotondo MF, Schwab CW, McGonigal MD, Phillips GR, Fruchterman TM, Kauder DR, et al. Damage control: an approach for improved survival in exsanguinating penetrating abdominal injury. *J Trauma*. 1993 Sep;**35(3)**:375–82; discussion 382–3.

7. Newell MA, Schlitzkus LL, Waibel BH, White MA, Schenarts PJ, Rotondo MF. "Damage control" in the elderly: futile endeavour or fruitful enterprise? *J Trauma*. 2010. Nov;**69(5)**:1049–53. doi: 10.1097/TA.0b013e3181ed4e7a

8. Gastes J, Arabian S, Biddinger P, Blansfield J, Burke P, Chung S, et al. The initial response to the Boston Marathon Bombing: Lessons to prepare for the next disaster. *Ann Surg*. 2014 Dec;**260(6)**:960–6. doi: 10.1097/SLA.0000000000000914

9. Smith IM, Beech ZKM, Lundy JB, Bowley DM. A prospective observational study of abdominal injury management in the contemporary military operations: Damage control laparotomy is associated with high survivability and low rates of fecal diversion. *Ann Surg*. 2015 Apr;**261(4)**:765–73. doi: 10.1097/SLA.0000000000000657

10. Schrieber M. Damage control surgery *Crit Care Clin*. 2004 Jan;**20(1)**:101–18. doi: 10.1016/s0749-0704(03)00095-2

11. Holcomb JB, Jenkins D, Rhee P, Johannigman J, Mahoney P, Mehta S, et al. Damage control resuscitation: directly addressing the early coagulopathy of trauma. *J Trauma*. 2007 Feb;**62(2)**:307–10. doi: 10.1097/TA.0b013e3180324124

12. Hess JR, Holcomb JB, Hoyt DB. Damage control resuscitation: the need for specific blood products to treat the coagulopathy of trauma. *Transfusion*. 2006 May;**46(5)**:685–6. doi: 10.1111/j.1537-2995.2006.00816.x

13. Lamb CM, MacGoey P, Navarro AP, Brooks AJ. Damage control surgery in the era of damage control resuscitation. *Br J Anaes*. 2014 Aug;**113(2)**:242–9. doi: 10.1093/bja/aeu233

14. Schreiber MA, Meier EN, Tisherman SA, Kerby JD, Newgard CD, Brasel K, et al. ROC Investigators. A controlled resuscitation strategy is feasible and safe in hypotensive trauma patients: results of a prospective randomized pilot trial. *J Trauma Acute Care Surg*. 2015 Apr;**78(4)**:687–95; discussion 695–7. doi: 10.1097/TA.0000000000000600

15. Shah SK, Uray KS, Stewart RH, Laine GA, Cox CS. Resuscitation-induced intestinal edema, and related dysfunction: state of the science. *J Surg Res*. 2011;**166(1)**:120–30. doi: 10.1016/j.jss.2009.09.010. Epub 2009 Sep 29.

16. Chang R, Holcomb J. Optimal fluid therapy for traumatic hemorrhagic shock. *Crit Care Clin*. 2017 Jan;**33(1)**:15–36. doi: 10.1016/j.ccc.2016.08.007

17. Brown JB, Cohen MJ, Minei JP, Maier RV, West MA, Billiar TR, et al. Goal-directed resuscitation in the prehospital setting: a propensity-adjusted analysis. *J Trauma Acute Care Surg*. 2013;**74(5)**:1207–12. doi: 10.1097/TA.0b013e31828c44fd

18. Ley EJ, Clond MA, Srour MK, Barnajian M, Mirocha J, Margulies DR, et al. Emergency department crystalloid resuscitation of 1. 5 L or more is associated with increased mortality in elderly and nonelderly trauma patients. *J Trauma*. 2011;**70(2)**:398–400. doi: 10.1097/TA.0b013e318208f99b

19. Holcomb JB, Tilley BC, Baraniuk S, Fox EE, Wade CE, Podbielski JM, et al. Transfusion of plasma, platelets, and red blood cells in a 1: 1: 1 vs a 1: 1: 2 ratio and mortality in patients with severe trauma: the PROPPR randomized clinical trial. *Jama*. 2015 Feb 3;**313(5)**:471–82. doi: 10.1001/jama.2015.12

20. Gunter OL, Jr. Au BK, Isbell JM, Mowery NT, Young PP, Cotton BA. Optimising outcomes in damage control resuscitation: identifying blood product ratios associated with improved survival. *J Trauma*. 2008 Sep;**65(3)**:527–34. doi: 10.1097/TA.0b013e3181826ddf

21. Holcomb JB, Wade CE, Michalek JE, Chisholm GB, Zarzabal LA, Schreiber MA, et al. Increased plasma and platelet to red blood cell ratios improves outcome in 466 massively transfused civilian trauma patients. *Ann Surg*. 2008 Sep;**248(3)**:447–58. doi: 10.1097/SLA.0b013e318185a9ad

22. Kozar RA, Peng Z, Zhang R, Holcomb JB, Pati S, Park P, et al. Plasma restoration of endothelial glycocalyx in a rodent model of hemorrhagic shock. *Anesthesia & Analgesia*. 2011 Jun;**112(6)**:1289–95.

23. Gallaher JR, Dixon A, Cockcroft A, Grey M, Dewey E, Goodman A, et al. Large volume transfusion with whole blood is safe compared with component therapy. *Journal of Trauma and Acute Care Surgery*. 2020 Jul 1;**89(1)**:238–45. doi: 10.1097/TA.0000000000002687

24. Hazelton JP, Ssentongo AE, Oh JS, Ssentongo P, Seamon MJ, Byrne JP, et al. Use of cold-stored whole blood is associated with improved mortality in hemostatic resuscitation of major bleeding: a multicenter study. *Annals of Surgery*. 2022 Oct 1;**276(4)**:579–88. doi: 10.1097/SLA.0000000000005603. Epub 2022 Jul 18.

25. Torres CM, Kent A, Scantling D, Joseph B, Haut ER, Sakran JV. Association of whole blood with survival among patients presenting with severe hemorrhage in US and Canadian adult civilian trauma centers. *JAMA Surg*. 2023 May 1;**158(5)**:532–40. doi: 10.1001/jamasurg.2022.6978

26. Brill JB, Brenner M, Duchesne J, Roberts D, Ferrada P, Horer T, et al. The role of TEG and RoTEM in damage control resuscitation. *Shock (Augusta, Ga.)*. 2021 Dec 1;**56(1S)**:52–61. doi: 10.1097/SHK.0000000000001686.

27. Patt A, McCroskey BL, Moore EE. Hypothermia-induced coagulopathies in trauma. *Surg Clin North Am*. 1988 Aug;**68(4)**:775–85. doi: 10.1016/s0039-6109(16)44585-8.

28. Ditzel RM, Anderson JL, Eisenhart WJ, Rankin CJ, DeFeo DR, Oak S, et al. A review of transfusion- And trauma-induced hypocalcemia: Is it time to change the lethal triad to the lethal diamond? *J Trauma Acute Care Surg*. 2020 Mar;88(3):434–439. doi: 10.1097/TA.0000000000002570

29. Cannon JW, Khan MA, Raja AS, Cohen MJ, Como JJ, Cotton BA, et al. Damage control resuscitation in patients with severe traumatic hemorrhage: A practice management guideline from the Eastern Association for the Surgery of Trauma. *J Trauma Acute Care Surg*. 2017 Mar;**82(3)**:605–17. doi: 10.1097/TA.0000000000001333

30. Cotton BA, Au BK, Nunez TC, Gunter OL, Robertson AM, Young PP. Predefined massive transfusion protocols are associated with a reduction in organ failure and postinjury complications. *J Trauma*. 2009 Jan;**66(1)**:41–8; discussion 48–9. doi: 10.1097/TA.0b013e31819313bb.

31. Jurkovich GJ, Greiser WB, Luterman A, Curreri PW. Hypothermia in trauma victims: an ominous predictor of survival. *J Trauma*. 1987 Sep;**27(9)**:1019–24.

32. Aoki N, Wall MJ, Demsar J, Zupan B, Granchi T, Schreiber MA, et al. Predictive model for survival at the conclusion of a damage control laparotomy. *Am J Surg*. 2000 Dec;**180(6)**:540–4; discussion 544–5.

33. Kronstedt S, Roberts N, Ditzel R, Elder J, Steen A, Thompson K, et al. Hypocalcemia as a predictor of mortality and transfusion. A scoping review of hypocalcemia in trauma and hemostatic resuscitation. *Transfusion*. 2022 Aug;**62(Suppl 1)**:S158–66. doi: 10.1111/trf.16965. Epub 2022 Jun 24.

34. O'Connor JV, DuBose JJ, Scalea TM. Damage control thoracic surgery: management and outcomes. *J Trauma Acute Care Surg*. 2014 Nov; **77(5)**: 660–65. doi: 10.1097/TA.0000000000000451.

35. Schein M, Saadia R. Jamieson JR, Decker GA. The 'sandwich technique' in the management of the open abdomen. *Br J Surg*. 1986;73:369–70. doi: 10.1002/bjs.1800730514

36. Collins R, Dhanasekara CS, Morris E, Marschke B, Dissanaike S. Simple suture whipstitch closure is a reasonable option for many patients requiring temporary abdominal closure for blunt or penetrating trauma. *Trauma Surg Acute Care Open*. 2022 Oct 21;**7(1)**:e000980. doi: 10.1136/tsaco-2022-000980

37. Matsuda M, Sawano M. Single-staged laparotomy versus multiple-staged laparotomy for traumatic massive hemoperitoneum with hemodynamic instability: a single-center, propensity score-matched analysis. *BMC Surg [Internet]*. 2022;22(1):1–7. doi: 10.1186/s12893-022-01660-6

38. Rasilainen SK, Mentula PJ, Leppäniemi AK. Vacuum and mesh-mediated fascial traction for primary closure of the open abdomen in critically ill surgical patients. *Br J Surg*. 2012 Dec;**99(12)**:1725–32. doi: 10.1002/bjs.8914

39. George MJ, Adams SD, Harvin J, McNutt MK, Love JD, Albarado R, Moore LJ, et al. The effect of damage control laparotomy on major abdominal complications: A matched analysis. *Am J Surg*. 2018 Jul;**216(1)**:56–59. doi: 10.1016/j.amjsurg.2017.10.044. Epub 2017 Nov 11.

40. Guillermo H, Friese R, O'Keeffe T, Wynne J, Bowlby P, Ziemba M, et al. Damage Control Laparotomy: a vital tool once overused. *J Trauma*. 2010 Jul;**69(1)**:53–9. doi: 10.1097/TA.0b013e3181e293b4

41. Edgington J, Szatkowski J. Evaluation, Resuscitation and Damage Control Orthopaedics. https://www.orthobullets.com/trauma/1005/evaluation-resuscitation-and-dco (accessed online September 2023).

42. Guerado E, Bertrand ML, Cano JR, Cerván AM, Galán A. Damage control orthopaedics: state of the art. *World J Orthop.* 2019 Jan 18;**10(1)**:1–13. doi: 10.5312/wjo.v10.i1.1

Recommended Reading

Chovanes J, Cannon JW, Nunez TC. The evolution of damage control surgery. *Surg Clin North Am.* 2012 Aug; **92(4)**:859–75, vii–viii. doi: 10.1016/j.suc.2012.04.002

Cirocchi R, Abraha I, Montedori A, Farinella E, Bonacini I, Tagliabue L, et al. Damage control surgery for abdominal trauma. *Cochrane Database Syst Rev.* 2010;(1):CD007438.

Godat L, Kobayashi L, Costantini T, Coimbra R. Abdominal damage control surgery and reconstruction: World Society of Emergency Surgery position paper. *World J Emerg Surg.* 2013 Dec;**17(8)**:53. doi: 10.1186/1749-7922-8-53.

Acknowledgements

Additional material provided by Nick Bedrin MD, Martin Schreiber MD, and Albert Chi MD.

Part 3

Anatomical and organ system injury

The Neck 7

7.1 OVERVIEW

The high density of critical vascular, aerodigestive, and neurological structures within the neck makes the management of penetrating injuries difficult and contributes to the morbidity and mortality seen in these patients. Before World War II, non-operative management of penetrating neck trauma resulted in mortality rates of up to 15%. Therefore, the exploration of all neck wounds penetrating the platysma muscle became mandatory. However, due to the high rate of negative and non-therapeutic interventions seen with this policy (up to 50%), selective non-operative management (SNOM) has become the 'gold standard' for the management of penetrating neck injuries (PNIs). The current iteration of the policy relies on the liberal use of computed tomography (CT) angiography in patients who are haemodynamically and physiologically stable or normal and without any hard signs of vascular or aerodigestive injuries. Immediate surgical exploration is indicated for those who arrive in shock or with obvious signs of vascular or aerodigestive injury irrespective of zone of penetration ('no-zone approach').

7.2 MANAGEMENT PRINCIPLES: PENETRATING CERVICAL INJURY

7.2.1 Initial Assessment and Definitive Airway

Patients with signs of significant neck injury, with active bleeding or an expanding haematoma, will require prompt exploration. However, the initial assessment and management of the patient should be conducted according to Advanced Trauma Life Support® (ATLS) principles.[1]

The major initial concern in any patient with a penetrating neck wound is securing the airway and initial control of active haemorrhage. Supplemental oxygen is critical. Oxygenate the patient with simple measures first (i.e. basic airway-opening techniques).

Intubation in these patients is complicated by the possibility of associated cervical spine injury, laryngeal trauma, and large haematomas in the neck. Appropriate protective measures for possible cervical spine injury must be implemented. A rapid risk–benefit assessment must be done in the presence of a deteriorating airway. Cervical spine immobilization techniques make endotracheal intubation more difficult and, in the updated Eastern Association for the Surgery of Trauma (EAST) guidelines, are not recommended[2].

The route of intubation must be carefully considered in these patients, since it may be complicated by distortion of anatomy, haematoma, dislodging of clots, laryngeal trauma, and cervical spinal injury. It may be possible to place an endotracheal tube over a bronchoscope, enter the trachea under direct vision, and then slide the endotracheal tube into place. Use of the fibre-optic portable video laryngoscope (Glidescope Go®, Verathon, Bothell, WA, USA) or a bougie may prove useful, but always be prepared for a surgical airway.

UK military experience in Afghanistan is that most patients can be managed with a rapid sequence induction (RSI) of anaesthesia, followed by endotracheal intubation with a relatively small tube (e.g., size 6.5 mm or 7.0 mm inner diameter [ID] in an adult male) aided by a gum-elastic bougie or stylet.

Patients have also been managed by a vapour induction of anaesthesia (supplemented with small boluses of ketamine – 10 mg intravenous [IV]), laryngoscopy whilst still breathing, and then endotracheal intubation. Once the cords are seen, a bougie can be introduced and the paralytic agent given, thereby avoiding the patient coughing and dislodging a clot on intubation.

DOI: 10.1201/9781003258124-10

Ketamine-based delayed sequence intubation (DSI) or ketamine-only breathing intubation (KOBI) using video-laryngoscopy can also be used in certain circumstances.

Pitfalls

- If it becomes immediately evident that the trachea cannot be intubated following RSI, a surgeon **must** be scrubbed and ready to perform a cricothyroidotomy (or tracheostomy, if the larynx is involved),
- The treating doctor should choose the technique he/she is most familiar with and have an alternative escape plan in place.

Patients with hard signs of significant neck injury, and those whose condition is unstable, should be explored urgently in the operating room with good light, good instruments, and good assistance, once rapid initial assessment has been completed and the airway has been secured.

Hard signs are regarded as:

- Airway compromise
- Massive subcutaneous emphysema/air bubbling through the wound
- Expending or pulsatile haematoma
- Active bleeding
- Shock
- Neurological deficit
- Haematemesis

Tracheostomy has no routine place in the emergency department. Cricothyroidotomies should be converted to formal tracheostomies within about 48 hours.

ANAESTHETIC PITFALLS

- Be aware that bleeding into the airway will rapidly obscure the view of the cords.
- Laryngeal mask airways (LMAs) do **not** provide a definitive airway in the presence of complex neck injuries but can be used to attempt oxygenation prior to endotracheal tube intubation or surgical airway.
- Endotracheal intubation should be considered at a very early stage in the presence of a large or expanding haematoma, before the anatomy is lost. Subsequent cricothyroidotomy or emergency percutaneous tracheostomy (only to be considered if the enabling environment, with extensive experience in the technique, is available) can be technically difficult, as by entering the haematoma planes, torrential bleeding via the skin incision may result.
- Immediate ventilation assessment should be performed after any surgical airway procedure, given the high incidence of pneumothoraces resulting from either PNI or surgical incisions.

Note: The use of paralysing agents in these patients should be used as a last resort and with extreme caution, since the airway may be held open only by the patient's own use of muscles. Abolishing the use of muscles in such patients may result in the immediate and total obstruction of the airway and, with no visibility due to the presence of blood, may result in catastrophe. Ideally, local anaesthetic spray should be used with sedation, and a cricothyroidotomy (below the injury) should be considered when necessary.

Managing complicated airway injuries should be rehearsed along with backup plans for alternate techniques to secure the airway if the initial plan fails. The decision as to what technique is the most appropriate should be made rapidly and jointly by the surgeon, anaesthesiologist, and trauma team leader.

There should be no hesitation in performing an emergency cricothyroidotomy should circumstances warrant it.

7.2.2 Control of Haemorrhage

Control of haemorrhage should be done by direct pressure where possible. If the neck wound is *not* bleeding, do not probe or finger the wound, as the clot may be dislodged. If the wound is actively bleeding, the bleeding should be controlled by digital pressure or, if this is ineffective, a Foley catheter may be inserted into the wound and the balloon inflated. This is often useful for stopping haemorrhage deep in the neck. Always clamp the Foley catheter after insertion. Occasionally, the wound may need to be sutured around the catheter to produce the required tamponade.

With larger wounds, haemostatic gauze could be packed tightly into the neck wound and hand pressure applied. The remainder of the gauze can then be used over the wound. The gauze should not be removed until the patient is in a safe place.

Pitfall

This may result in converting external haemorrhage into concealed bleeding deep within the neck if tamponade is not achieved, which will further compromise an already compressed airway. Hence, it is important to secure an early definitive airway. More than one Foley catheter is sometimes needed.

7.2.3 **Injury Location**

Traditionally, division of the neck into anatomical zones (**Figure 7.1**) helped the categorization and management of neck wounds:

- *Zone I* extends from the level of the sternal notch to the lower border of the cricoid cartilage. Within Zone I lie the great vessels, the trachea, the oesophagus, the thoracic duct, and the upper mediastinum and lung apices.
- *Zone II* includes the area between the cricoid cartilage and the angle of the mandible. Enclosed within its region are the carotid and vertebral arteries, jugular veins, pharynx, larynx, oesophagus, and trachea.
- *Zone III* includes the area above the angle of the mandible to the base of the skull, the pharynx, and the distal extracranial carotid and vertebral arteries, as well as segments of the jugular veins.

Injuries in Zone II are readily evaluated and exposed operatively. In trauma centres with a high volume of penetrating trauma, a decision on immediate surgery can be reached on clinical grounds without any preoperative investigations. Zones I and III are difficult to assess clinically and to access operatively. Therefore, in those two zones, it is important in the physiologically stable patient to proceed with diagnostic workup so that the presence or absence of injury is established, and the possibility of dealing with it without an operative procedure is decided (e.g., embolization of a bleeding artery), as, should an operation be necessary, this will be facilitated by knowing the type of injury and its topography. As mentioned before, the clinical findings of the patient are the determinants to select the use of surgery or CT angiography irrespective of which zone is injured.

The no-zone approach for haemodynamically stable patients who can undergo investigation (CT angiography and contrast swallow, if indicated) has become favoured for this patient subgroup and is the currently accepted management strategy in penetrating neck trauma.[3,6]

When possible, all penetrating injuries of the neck, irrespective of zone, should be investigated using CT angiography.

NEVER blind-probe a wound of the neck or perform a mini-exploration in the emergency department.

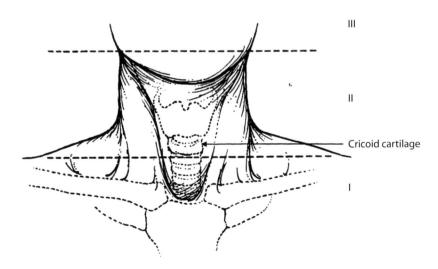

III

II

Cricoid cartilage

I

Figure 7.1 Anterior view showing zones of the neck.

Pitfall

Don't assume that a wound in one zone means an injury in that zone. Not infrequently, a wound in one zone is associated with an injury in quite another area. For example, a long knife may penetrate the skin in Zone I or II, but the injury may lie in the superior mediastinum. Similarly, bullets and missile fragments often transgress zone boundaries. Either may cross the midline, giving rise to contralateral injured structures.

7.2.4 Mechanism

Gunshot wounds carry a higher risk of major injury than stab wounds because of their tendency to penetrate deeper and their ability to damage tissue outside the tract of the missile due to cavitation or a percussion wave injury.

7.2.5 Frequency of Injury

The carotid artery and internal jugular vein are the most frequently injured vessels. Due to its relatively protected position, the vertebral artery is involved less frequently. The larynx and trachea, and pharynx and oesophagus, are frequently injured. The spinal cord is damaged less often, but injury should not be ruled out until examination has confirmed its integrity, particularly in patients with gunshot wounds.

7.2.6 Use of Diagnostic Studies

In the stable patient without indications for immediate neck exploration, additional studies are often obtained, including mandatory angiography, endoscopy, contrast radiography, and bronchoscopy.

7.2.6.1 COMPUTED TOMOGRAPHY SCANNING WITH CONTRAST: CT ANGIOGRAPHY[7]

Modern CT scanners have provided a means of creating a three-dimensional (3D) image of high quality. Not only is CT angiography diagnostic, but access may allow it to be therapeutic as well, as open angiography allows arterial embolization as well as the stenting of a particular vessel. CT angiography should include both internal and external carotid arteries on both sides (four-vessel CT angiography) as well as the vertebral arteries, preferably with 3D reconstruction. This imaging modality has been recognized to be both highly sensitive and specific in detecting vascular, laryngotracheal, and many pharyngo-oesophageal injuries. It can also provide information on the trajectory of the wound track and include the thorax as a high-risk area for injury. All patients with Zone I and III neck injuries should undergo CT angiography when vital signs are stable. The ability to evaluate other neck structures during the same procedure is an advantage. Slightly delayed repeat images can provide information about the venous systems as well. Have a low threshold to do CT angiograms for stable Zone II cases as well, the so-called no-zone approach.[6,8]

7.2.6.2 ANGIOGRAPHY

This modality is rarely used for screening in these days of CT angiography; it is only used if the CT angiogram is not conclusive, or the images are obscured by foreign materials like metal fragments. Digital subtraction angiogram may also reduce the amount of contrast required, especially in Zone I or Zone III injuries, where surgical exposure can be difficult. Angiography is useful in excluding injury following damage with shotgun pellets, and in cases of possible embolization.

7.2.6.3 OTHER DIAGNOSTIC STUDIES

The selective management of penetrating neck wounds involves evaluation of the oesophagus, larynx, and trachea. In awake patients, a contrast swallow is usually performed first,[9] followed by a flexible oesophagoscopy in the event of non-diagnosis. Flexible oesophagoscopy has sensitivity close to 100%. Laryngoscopy and bronchoscopy are useful adjuncts in localizing or excluding injury to the hypopharynx or trachea. A recent development is 3D CT reconstruction of the trachea and bronchi which can replace endoscopy in suspected injuries of these anatomical structures.

7.3 MANAGEMENT

The Western Trauma Algorithm (**Figure 7.2**) is used as a guideline for the management of major trauma to the neck.[10]

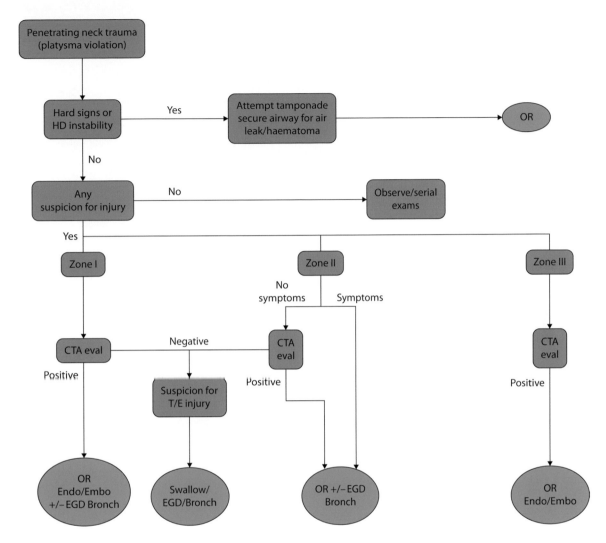

Figure 7.2 Western Trauma Algorithm for the management of penetrating neck trauma. *Abbreviations*: CTA, computed tomography angiogram; EGD, oesophago-gastric digestive tract; HD, haemodynamic instability; T/E, transoesophageal.

The huge developments in endovascular surgery over the past two decades have massively impacted the management of penetrating neck trauma. There are now several endovascular approaches available which offer elegant alternatives to open surgery of the major vessels in the neck and root of the neck. Surgical access to the subclavian vessels is challenging and requires extensive dissection. Endovascular stenting greatly simplifies the management of subclavian artery injuries. Injury to the vertebral artery is also simplified by means of endovascular approaches. As experience with these techniques increases, we are more likely to develop more evidence-based algorithms for the management of these injuries.

Minimal arterial injuries involving tears to the intimal of the artery are increasingly recognized due to the efficacy and ready availability of modern imaging techniques. There is controversy around the management of these injuries. The torn intimal presents a thrombogenic surface to the blood flow and may result in a thrombus being formed which can either embolism or occlude. This may result in a cerebrovascular accident if the flap is in the cerebral circulation, or distal ischaemia if the flap is in the vasculature to the upper limbs. The advent of highly efficacious anti-platelet agents has allowed for many of these injuries to be treated non-operatively. These injuries are relatively infrequent, and there are insufficient data to make firm recommendations. It does appear that the role for non-operative management of these so-called minimal vascular injuries will expand.

The management of carotid artery injury is controversial. The approach depends very much on the neurological status of the patient on presentation. Most authors agree that in the absence of profound neurological deficit, most injuries to the common or internal carotid artery should be explored and repaired either with a primary repair or with the use of an interposition graft. In cases of profound neurological deficit, then revascularization may only make the situation worse.

7.3.1 Mandatory versus Selective Neck Exploration

Recommendations for the management of patients with penetrating cervical trauma depend on the zone of injury and the patient's haemodynamic status. If the platysma is not penetrated, the patient may be observed. Mandatory exploration for PNI in patients with hard signs of vascular or aerodigestive tract injury is still appropriate.

Missed injuries are associated with high morbidity and mortality due to missed visceral injuries, and the negligible morbidity caused by negative exploration is important; however, exploration of all stab wounds of the neck may yield a high rate of non-therapeutic procedures. Thus, the selective management of penetrating neck wounds based on CT evaluation has been recommended.

7.3.2 Management Based on Anatomical Zones

- Zone I injuries require CT angiogram and, if any doubt, a formal angiogram because of the increased association of vascular injuries with penetrating trauma to the thoracic outlet. Angiography helps the surgeon plan the surgical approach.
- For Zone II injuries, without any hard signs and with a haemodynamically stable patient, a CT angiogram is indicated. Unstable patients must go to theatre.
- Zone III injuries require a CT angiogram because of the relationship of the blood vessels to the base of

the skull. Often these injuries can be best managed by either non-operative techniques or manoeuvres remote from the injury site, such as balloon tamponade or embolization.

Pitfalls

- Early CT angiography may *not* rule out significant injury to the trachea or oesophagus.
- CT angiogram is a better screening tool, as it can diagnose tracheal injuries or identify surgical emphysema that might be suggestive of an aerodigestive injury that requires further investigations.
- Injuries to the oesophagus require a high index of suspicion when interpreting CT scans.
- Isolated venous injuries do not mandate surgical exploration. Only repair when there is ongoing bleeding, worsening neck haematoma, or failure to respond despite the use of adjuncts like a Foley balloon tamponade.

7.4 ACCESS TO THE NECK

The operative approach selected to explore neck injuries is determined by the structures known or suspected to be injured. Surgical exploration should be done formally and systematically in a fully equipped operating room under general anaesthesia with endotracheal intubation.

Blind probing of wounds or mini-explorations in the emergency department should **never** be attempted.

Certainly, patients who present in shock with Zone II injuries are best treated with diagnostic exploration. Even stable patients in Zone II can be treated with operative exploration, although imaging is preferred. Unstable patients with Zone I injuries also undergo operative exploration. The thoracic incision is determined by surgical experience to gain proximal control. Stable patients with Zone I injuries are best assessed by CT angiography. Given the same issues of difficult vascular control in Zone III, stable patients should undergo diagnostic testing.

Whilst surgical dogma advocates operative exploration for Zone III injuries with hypotension, operative exploration can be quite complicated. If an endovascular option is immediately available, that may be wiser in most cases.

(a)

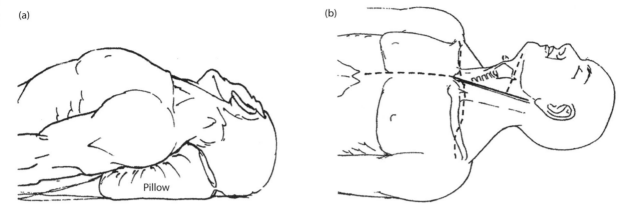

Pillow

(b)

Figure 7.3 Approach to the left side of the neck: (a) Positioning and (b) incisions.

7.4.1 **Position**

Active bleeding from a penetrating wound should be controlled digitally, or with one or multiple Foley catheters inserted, inflated, and clamped. Penetrating wounds to the neck should not be probed, cannulated, or locally explored, because these procedures may dislodge a clot and cause uncontrollable bleeding or air embolism. Skin preparation should include the entire chest and shoulder, extending above the angle of the mandible. The face, neck, and anterior chest should be prepped and widely draped. The patient is placed in the supine position on the operating table with the arms tucked at the sides. If possible, the head should be extended and rotated to the contralateral side. A sandbag may be placed between the shoulder blades, and the neck extended and rotated away from the side of injury – provided that the cervical spine has been cleared preoperatively (**Figure 7.3**(a)).

7.4.2 **Incision**

Always expect the worst! Plan the incision to provide optimal access for early vascular source control or immediate access to the airway. The most universal approach is via an incision along the anterior border of the sternomastoid, which can be lengthened proximally and distally, extended to a median sternotomy, or augmented with lateral extensions (**Figure 7.3(b)**).

A collar incision gives the best exposure for the anterior trachea

Having made the sternocleidomastoid muscle incision, the platysma is divided, and the sternomastoid is retracted laterally to expose the fascial sheath covering the internal jugular vein. The vein cannot be mobilized until the common facial vein is divided. Omohyoid muscle is the only strap muscle that crosses the carotid sheath obliquely and acts as a landmark for the common carotid artery. Lateral retraction of the jugular vein and underlying carotid artery allows access to the trachea, oesophagus, and thyroid, and medial retraction of the carotid sheath and its contents will allow the dissection to proceed posteriorly to the prevertebral fascia and vertebral arteries. Posterior to the carotid sheath, the sympathetic chain lies on the longus colli, which separates it from the transverse processes of the cervical vertebrae (**Figures 7.4** and **7.5**).

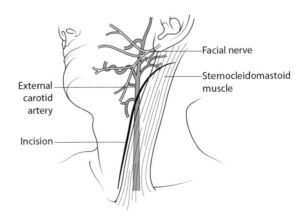

Facial nerve

Sternocleidomastoid muscle

External carotid artery

Incision

Figure 7.4 Approach to the left side of the neck: Initial incision.

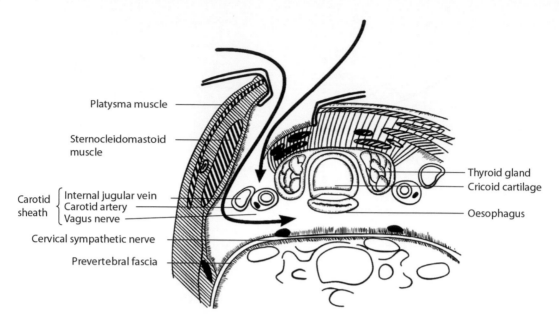

Figure 7.5 Approach to the left side of the neck showing retraction of the platysma and sternomastoid muscles.

7.4.3 **Surgical Access**

7.4.3.1 **ACCESS TO THE GREAT VESSELS (SEE FIGURE 7.6)**

Surgical access to the subclavian artery is influenced by the site of the injury. Injuries to the proximal or first part of the artery generally require a median sternotomy to access the origins of the subclavian artery to ensure proximal control. This is different on the right and left.

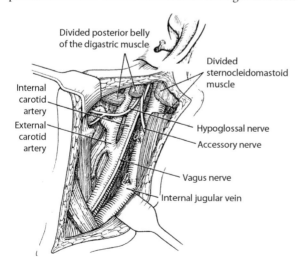

Figure 7.6 Approach to the left side of the neck with divided sternomastoid and digastric muscles.

On the right side, the subclavian is usually the point at which the innominate artery divides into the right common carotid and right subclavian artery. On the left, the subclavian comes directly off the arch of the aorta. Proximal control is then followed by distal control. This usually requires supraclavicular dissection through the sternocleidomastoid muscle onto the scalene fat pad. The scalene fat pad is then dissected off the anterior scalene muscle, taking care to preserve the phrenic nerve. The phrenic nerve is the only nerve in the body to run from lateral to medial. The subclavian artery will be found behind the anterior scalene muscle. The section of the artery behind the clavicle can be difficult to access. Division of the clavicle should be avoided, as it generally results in a non-union of the clavicle and presents long-term morbidity for the patient.

Access to the carotid artery is generally much easier, and the dissection is along the anterior border of the sternocleidomastoid muscle. The muscle is retracted laterally, and the carotid sheath is opened. This will be facilitated by dividing the facial vein which drains directly into the internal jugular vein and crosses anteriorly to the artery. The sheath contains the common carotid artery, the internal jugular vein, and the vagus nerve. Dissection must be performed onto the carotid artery, which should be gently slung and controlled above and below the injury. Repair should involve either a primary repair or the use of autologous interposition graft.

Access to the internal carotid artery is more difficult, and the bifurcation must be identified. Care must be taken not to damage the accessory nerve as it enters the sternocleidomastoid muscle and the glossopharyngeal nerve as it crosses in front of the internal carotid artery. Liberal division of the digastric muscle belly will enhance access. The difficulty with this artery is in obtaining distal control, as the internal carotid enters through the carotid canal into the base of the skull. Dividing the styloid process may provide extra exposure to the internal carotid artery before it enters the base of the skull. Dislocating the mandible is often described but rarely performed. Modern endovascular approaches provide elegant solutions to injuries to the internal carotid artery.

7.4.3.2 ZONE I[11]

Zone I vascular injuries at the base of the neck require aggressive management. Frequently, uncontrollable haemorrhage will require immediate thoracotomy for initial proximal control. In an unstable patient, quick exposure often may be achieved via a median sternotomy and a supraclavicular extension.

The location of the vascular injury will dictate the definitive exposure. For right-sided great vessel injuries, a median sternotomy with a supraclavicular extension allows optimal access. On the left side, a high (3rd or 4th interspace) left anterolateral thoracotomy may provide initial proximal control. Further operation for definitive repair may require a sternotomy, or extension into the right side of the chest or up into the neck. 'Trapdoor' or 'clamshell' incisions are **not** recommended. They are often difficult to perform, do not significantly improve the exposure, but significantly increase the morbidity postoperative disability. Avoid injury to the phrenic and vagus nerves as they enter the thorax. In the stable patient in whom the vascular injury has been confirmed by CT, the right subclavian artery or the distal two-thirds of the left subclavian artery can be exposed through an incision immediately superior to the medial third of the clavicle. Injuries to the vessels behind the clavicle can be controlled by combining supra- and infraclavicular incisions. The clavicle does *not* need to be divided or resected. Grafts can easily be tunnelled underneath the bone, avoiding risk to the subclavian vein.

- Injuries to the internal jugular vein should be repaired if possible. In severe injuries that require extensive debridement, ligation is preferred. Venous interposition grafts should not be performed.

- Vertebral artery injuries are generally found to have been injured only on angiographic study. These rarely require surgical repair, as they are best dealt with by angioembolization. Operative exposure may be difficult, and it may be easier to ligate it at its origin off the subclavian artery, or pass a size 3 or 4 Fogarty catheter into the lumen and inflation of the balloon to provide tamponade. This may be left permanently if required, with small incidence of neurological damage. Venous bleeding can be stopped by packing around the area of injury.

- The area of bleeding can also be controlled by Ligaclips® (Johnson & Johnson, Brunswick, NJ, USA) and packing the area with bone wax.

Many carotid artery injuries can be managed with intraluminal stenting. This approach is now used most frequently in situations where arterial lesions are not surgically accessible or when anticoagulation is contraindicated.

7.4.3.3 ZONE II

Zone II injuries are explored by an incision made along the anterior border of the sternocleidomastoid muscle, as for carotid endarterectomy. An extended collar incision or bilateral incisions along the anterior edge of the sternocleidomastoid muscles may be used for wounds that traverse both sides of the neck. Proximal and distal control of the blood vessel is obtained. If the vessel is actively bleeding, direct pressure is applied to the bleeding site whilst control is obtained. Use of anticoagulation is optional. If there are no injuries that preclude its use, heparin may be given in the management of carotid injuries. Vascular shunts are rarely needed in patients with carotid injuries, especially if the distal clamp is applied proximal to the bifurcation of the internal and external carotid arteries. Repair techniques for cervical trauma do not differ significantly from those used for other vascular injuries.

The oesophagus is a left-sided structure in Zone II, so it is best approached from the left side. The trachea and thyroid should be mobilized medially to expose the upper oesophagus.

7.4.3.4 ZONE III

Zone III injuries, at the very base of the skull, are complex and should be explored with great care. Access is often extremely difficult, and on rare occasions, it may not be possible to control the distal stump of a high internal carotid artery injury. Bleeding from this injury can be controlled either temporarily or permanently by inserting a Fogarty catheter into the distal segment and inflating the balloon. The catheter is secured, transected, and left in place. It may be necessary to control the internal carotid artery from within the cranial cavity (usually the realm of the neurosurgeon).

7.4.3.5 ACCESS TO THE AERODIGESTIVE TRACT

The aerodigestive tract structures are central and can be accessed via an anterior sternocleidomastoid incision or via a collar incision. Mobilizing the thyroid gland will expose the trachea and the oesophagus. Passing a rigid nasogastric tube will help to digitally identify the oesophagus. Care must be taken to not damage the recurrent laryngeal nerves.

7.4.4 Priorities

- The first concern in the patient with a penetrating injury of the neck is early control of the airway.
- The next concern is to stop bleeding, by either digital pressure or using a Foley catheter.
- The stability of the patient determines the appropriate diagnostic and treatment priorities. Never make the operation more difficult than necessary by inadequate exposure. Adequate exposure of the area involved is critical.
- The intraoperative decisions are influenced by the patient's preoperative neurological status. If the patient has no neurological deficit preoperatively, the injured vessel should be repaired. (The one exception may be if a complete obstruction of blood flow is found at the time of surgery, because restoration of flow may cause distal remobilization or haemorrhagic infarction.)
- Operative management of the patient with a carotid injury and a preoperative neurological deficit is controversial. Vascular reconstruction should be performed in patients with mild-to-moderate deficits in whom retrograde flow is present. Ligation is rarely recommended for patients with severe preoperative neurological deficits greater than 48 hours old, and without evidence of retrograde flow at the time of operation.

If associated injuries allow, 5,000–10,000 units of heparin as a bolus should be given before any of the arteries in the neck are occluded.

Because they have no branches, the common and internal carotid arteries can be safely mobilized for some distance from the injury to ensure a tension-free repair. Complex venous injuries can be ligated if not amenable to repair.

7.4.4.1 CAROTID ARTERY[12]

For exposure of the proximal carotid artery in Zone I, the artery is exposed by division of the omohyoid muscle between the superior and inferior bellies. More proximal control may require a midline sternotomy.

Exposure of the carotid artery in Zone III is obtained by ligating the middle thyroid and common facial veins and retracting the internal jugular laterally together with the sternocleidomastoid. The vagus nerve, lying posteriorly within the carotid sheath, must be preserved. The occipital artery and inferior branches of the *ansa cervicalis* may be divided. To expose the carotid bifurcation, the dissection is carried upwards to the posterior belly of the digastric muscle, which is divided behind the angle of the jaw. Care must be taken to find and preserve the hypoglossal nerve, which runs forward across both the internal and external carotid artery to enter the floor of the mouth. It usually is found either at the lower border of the posterior belly of the digastric, or just deep to that muscle (**Figure 7.6**).

All significant penetrating carotid artery lesions should be repaired when technically feasible, either primarily or with patch angioplasty. If a segment of artery is lost, interposition graft or internal-to-external carotid artery transposition may be performed.

For distal Zone III carotid injuries, consider angiographic stenting. However, if surgical intervention is required:

- Use nasotracheal intubation, not orotracheal. The tube between the teeth opens the mouth and reduces the space behind the ramus.
- Access to the internal carotid can be improved by dividing the sternocleidomastoid muscle near its origin at the mastoid. Care must be taken not to injure the accessory nerve where it enters the sternomastoid muscle 3 cm below the mastoid, or the glossopharyngeal nerve crossing anteriorly over the internal carotid artery.
- More distal exploration of the internal carotid artery may require unilateral mandibular subluxation, division of the ascending ramus.

- A Langenbeck retractor can be used to pull the upper pole of the mandibular ramus forward, increasing access to the internal carotid artery in Zone III.
- The styloid process may be excised after division of the stylohyoid ligament and styloglossus and stylopharyngeus muscles. The facial nerve lies superficial to these muscles and must be preserved.
- To reach the internal carotid artery where it enters the carotid canal, part of the mastoid bone can be removed. Fortunately, this is rarely required.

7.4.4.2 TRACHEAL INJURIES

The trachea is best accessed via a collar incision. The incision is placed 1–2 cm above the sternal notch and extends laterally to the medial border of the sternocleidomastoid. Take care to ligate the anterior jugular veins. The thyroid isthmus is clamped and divided. This will expose the larynx and cervical trachea. Access to the lower trachea may require partial sternotomy. Circumferential mobilization of the trachea will result in devascularization and should not be performed.

Injuries to the trachea should be closed in a single layer with absorbable sutures. Larger defects may require a fascia flap. One can resect up to two tracheal rings and still manage to do anastomosis. For exceptionally large defects, the endotracheal tube gets placed through the defect whilst the posterior wall gets repaired, and then replace it with an oral endotracheal tube passed through the defect when the anterior wall gets repaired. *These injuries should be drained, preferably with a suction drain.*

7.4.4.3 PHARYNGEAL AND OESOPHAGEAL INJURIES

Oesophageal injuries are often missed at neck exploration. Injuries to the hypopharynx and cervical oesophagus may also be difficult to diagnose preoperatively. Perforations of the hypopharynx or oesophagus should be closed in two layers if possible, although the mucosal layer is the key to leakproof repair. The site should be widely drained. Identification may be aided by the passage of a nasogastric tube. For devastating oesophageal injuries requiring extensive resection and debridement, a cutaneous oesophagostomy for feeding, and pharyngostomy for diversion, may be necessary.

7.4.5 **Midline Visceral Structures**

The trachea, oesophagus, and thyroid are approached by retracting the carotid sheath laterally. The inferior thyroid artery should be divided laterally near the carotid artery, and the thyroid lobe is lifted anteriorly to expose the trachea and oesophagus posteriorly. Oesophageal identification is aided by passing a large dilator or nasogastric tube. The recurrent laryngeal nerves should be carefully preserved: the left nerve runs vertically in the tracheo-oesophageal groove, but the right nerve runs obliquely across the oesophagus and trachea from inferolateral to superomedial. Both nerves are at risk of injury with circumferential mobilization of the oesophagus. Bilateral exposure of the midline structures may require transverse extension of the standard incision.

7.4.6 **Root of the Neck**

The structures at the root of the neck can be approached by extending the incision laterally above the clavicle. The clavicular head of the sternocleidomastoid is divided, and the supraclavicular fat pad is cleared by blunt dissection. This fat pad is a constant feature, even in the thinnest of individuals. It is complicated in its removal because it contains many small blood vessels, lymph nodes, and the thoracic duct. Removal reveals the scalenus anterior muscle, with the phrenic nerve crossing it from the lateral side. Division of the scalenus anterior, with preservation of the phrenic nerve, allows access to the second part of the subclavian artery. The distal subclavian artery can be exposed by a further infraclavicular incision and obtaining control of the proximal axillary artery, or dividing the clavicle at its mid-point, and dissecting away the subclavius muscle and fascia.

The clavicle should **not** be resected, as this leads to considerable morbidity. However, if required to fix the divided bone, the periosteum should be approximated with strong polyfilament absorbable sutures, or a miniplate can be inserted.

7.4.7 **Collar Incisions**

These are rarely used unless there is absolute certainty that the injury is limited to the area about to be exposed. In trauma in general, it is wiser to make incisions that can be extended both proximally and distally. It may be preferable to use bilateral sternomastoid incisions that can be joined for bilateral injuries in the form of a 'U'.

Some surgeons adopt the collar incisions. Horizontal or 'collar' incisions placed either over the thyroid or higher up over the thyroid cartilage can sometimes be useful to expose bilateral injuries or injuries limited to the larynx or trachea. The transverse incision is carried through the platysma, and subplatysmal flaps are then developed: superiorly up to the thyroid cartilage notch, and inferiorly to the sternal notch. The strap muscles are divided vertically in the midline and retracted laterally to expose the fascia covering the thyroid. The thyroid isthmus can be divided to expose the trachea. A high collar incision, placed over the larynx, is useful for repairing isolated laryngeal injuries.

7.4.8 Vertebral Arteries

The proximal part of the vertebral artery is approached via the anterior sternomastoid incision, with division of the clavicular head of the sternomastoid. The internal jugular vein and common carotid artery are mobilized, the vein is retracted medially, and the artery and nerve are retracted laterally. The proximal vertebral artery lies deeply between these structures. The vertebral artery is crossed by branches of the cervical sympathetic chain and on the left side by the thoracic duct. The inferior thyroid artery crosses in a more superficial plane, just before the vertebral artery enters its bony canal.

Access to the distal vertebral artery is challenging and rarely needed. The contents of the carotid sheath are retracted anteromedially, and the prevertebral muscles are longitudinally split over a transverse process above the level of the injury. The anterior surface of the transverse process can be removed with a small rongeur, or a J-shaped needle may be used to snare the artery in the space between the transverse processes.

The most distal portion of the vertebral artery can be approached between the atlas and the axis after division of the sternocleidomastoid near its origin at the mastoid process. The prevertebral fascia is divided over the transverse process of the atlas. With preservation of the C2 nerve root, the levator scapulae and splenius cervicus muscles are divided close to the transverse process of the atlas. The vertebral artery can now be visualized between the two vertebrae and may be ligated with a J-shaped needle. This area of dissection is more commonly the province of a neurosurgeon, if available.

Neck exploration wounds are closed in layers after acquiring homeostasis. Drainage is usually indicated, mainly to prevent haematomas and sepsis.

ANAESTHESIOLOGICAL CONSIDERATIONS

- Plan with your team!
- Continue 'damage control resuscitation.'
- Time is of the essence; only strictly needed procedures are allowed to delay CT scan for diagnosis and potential neurosurgical treatment.
- Rapid sequence intubation with care of cervical spine, avoidance of increased intracranial pressure (ICP) (coughing/straining), maintenance of mean arterial pressure (MAP) (hence, cerebral perfusion pressure), and avoidance of obstruction of cerebral venous drainage (tube ties, neck position, etc.).
- Monitor end-tidal CO_2 and ventilate to normocapnia (confirm with blood gas when possible).
- Take care of the neck during intubation and surgery. Consider manual inline stabilization of the cervical spine.
- Insert an arterial line, but if this is proving difficult, avoid delay, defer the arterial line, and allow the surgeons to commence the surgery.
- Prevention of secondary brain injury is the aim.
- Maintain MAP, normocapnia, and normoglycaemia; avoid hypothermia.
- Be aware of fluid balance and blood loss, and replace as required; replace clotting factors and platelets as indicated.
- Elevate the head end of the operating table 10° if blood pressure is maintained.
- Oxygen delivery to the brain cells is improved by securing the airway; assuring proper ventilation and oxygenation; restoring adequate circulation, oxygen-carrying capacity, and perfusion pressure; and aiming for reducing cerebral oedema by facilitating venous drainage (head up) and adequate serum sodium levels.

- Oxygen demand is reduced by adequate sedation using anaesthetics that can reduce the $CMRO_2$ (cerebral metabolic rate of oxygen).
- In combined injuries (not single traumatic brain injury [TBI]), compromises of the above-mentioned aims often must be done.
- Ketamine is safe in TBI patients and can be used in the acute setting until haemodynamics is under control. Thereafter, propofol is mostly used for short-term anaesthesia/sedation maintenance.
- Insert a nasogastric tube if the anterior skull base has been cleared of fractures (otherwise, insert an orogastric tube).
- Consider succinctly letting the surgeon know at an appropriate time:
  - Ongoing blood loss
  - Metabolic state (e.g., base deficit or lactate)
  - Vasopressor requirements
  - Overview of coagulation
- Consider asking the surgeon at an appropriate time:
  - Is the patient clotting clinically?
  - How does the perfusion of vital organs look clinically (e.g., bowel)?
  - What are the available treatment options?
- Patients with trauma above the diaphragm → venous access below the diaphragm
  - Femoral central line or a tibial intraosseous line
- Penetrating neck injuries
  - Risk of distortion of anatomy, making intubation impossible: early intubation
  - Bag-mask ventilation: risk of the positive pressure displacing air into violated soft tissue spaces → distorting the airway anatomy

SPECIFIC GUIDELINES

- Major trauma to face and neck:
  - In some patients, a surgical airway may be the first option.
  - If RSI is an option, consider a double setup.
    - *Double setup* refers to simultaneous preparation for orotracheal intubation and surgical airway.
    - Enables shift instantly from an attempt at orotracheal to surgical airway.
- Surgical exploration of distal carotid – Zone III – requires a nasotracheal tube because an orotracheal tube reduces the space behind the mandibular ramus.
- Plan the extubation in neck trauma.
  - Airway may be lost due to rebleeding, or because of the risk of bilateral laryngeal nerve palsy.

TRAUMATIZED AIRWAY

- *If the airway appears stable*: Assessment, planning, and intervention in optimal conditions.
- *Identify crash airway (no time available)*: Exposed trachea/lacerated trachea; airway obstruction; SpO_2 <90%.
- *Operating room*: More space, better lighting, and staff more familiar with the tracheostomy.
- Always consider maintaining spontaneous ventilation.
- Laryngoscopy and mask ventilation impossible in some scenarios.
- Don't perform induction of anaesthesia if you are not able to oxygenate the patient with face mask or laryngeal mask and a bag.
- Consider awake cricothyrotomy or tracheotomy as the first approach in some scenarios, or as the rescue plan.
- *In a patient with a bleeding airway, positioning is paramount*: upright, or lateral decubitus position to allow gravity to assist moving blood out of the airway; don't force patient positioning.
- Grasp exposed trachea from a stab wound by applying towel clip or clamp at the inferior tracheal portion to prevent its retraction into the chest.

CLOTHESLINE INJURY

- *High-level suspicion*: hoarseness, emphysema, crepitation, stridor.
- Clear view of the cords does not guarantee successful endotracheal intubation.
- Avoid blind placement of a tracheal tube into a lacerated tracheal segment because it can create a false lumen outside the trachea or convert a partial tracheal laceration into a complete transection.
- Even the gentle placement 'gum-elastic bougie' may create an airway obstruction.
- Positive-pressure ventilation above the lesion should be avoided, if possible.
- Maintaining spontaneous ventilation is generally a safer approach.
- Endotracheal tube placement should ideally be performed with visualization of the airway using a flexible intubating endoscope (FIE).
  - If RSI is chosen:
    - *Modified rapid sequence induction*: No cricoid pressure, no positive-pressure ventilation.
    - Tracheal tube placed at introitus of cords and only advanced under direct vision via fiberscope.
    - Surgeons scrubbed and equipment prepared for immediately surgical airway if failed intubation.
    - Accessing the trachea based on the level of the airway breach.
- Video laryngoscope with a channelled blade requires less pharyngeal retraction.

LEFORT III FRACTURES

- Have available at least two suction devices.
- Mid-face fractures associated with:
  - Head and cervical spine injuries.
  - Fractured skull base – leakage cerebrospinal fluid.
- Bilateral mandibular fractures.
  - Risk of airway obstruction.
    - Reduced by upright positioning – dangerous if spinal cord injury present.
  - Allow patient to assume the most comfortable position.
- Mandibular condylar fracture
  - Fragment might prevent mouth opening.

REFERENCES AND RECOMMENDED READING

References

1. American College of Surgeons. *Advanced Trauma Life Support®: Student Course Manual*, 10th edn. American College of Surgeons, Chicago IL, USA. 2018.
2. Velopulos CG, Shihab HM, Lottenberg L, Feinman M, Raja A, Salomone J, Haut ER. Prehospital spine immobilization/spinal motion restriction in penetrating trauma: A practice management guideline from the Eastern Association for the Surgery of Trauma (EAST). *J Trauma Acute Care Surg.* 2018 May;**84(5)**:736–44. doi: 10.1097/TA.0000000000001764
3. Amico F, Bendinelli C, Balogh ZJ. Penetrating neck trauma: No zone no problem? *ANZ J Surg.* 2021 Jun;**91(6)**:1051–2. doi: 10.1111/ans.16930
4. Ibraheem K, Khan M, Rhee P, Azim A, O'Keeffe T, Tang A, et al. "No zone" approach in penetrating neck trauma reduces unnecessary computed tomography angiography and negative explorations. *J Surg Res.* 2018 Jan;**221**:113–20. doi: 10.1016/j.jss.2017.08.033
5. Shiroff AM, Gale SC, Martin ND, Marchalik D, Petrov D, Ahmed HM, et al. Penetrating neck trauma: a review of management strategies and discussion of the 'No Zone' approach. *Am Surg.* 2013 Jan;**79(1)**:23–9. doi: 10.1177/000313481307900113
6. Chandrananth ML, Zhang A, Voutier CR, Skandarajah A, Thomson BNJ, Shakerian R, Read DJ. 'No zone' approach to the management of stable penetrating neck injuries: a systematic review. *ANZ J Surg.* 2021 Jun;**91(6)**:1083–90. doi: 10.1111/ans.16600
7. Osborn TM, Bell RB, Qaisi W, Long WB. Computed angiography as an aid to clinical decision making in the selective management of penetrating injuries of the

neck: a reduction in the need for operative exploration. *J Trauma* 2008 Jun;**64(6)**:1466–71. doi: 10.1097/TA.0b013e3181271b32

8. Nowicki JL, Stew B, Ooi E. Penetrating neck injuries: a guide to evaluation and management. *Ann R Coll Surg Engl.* 2018 Jan;**100(1)**:6–11

9. Nel L, Whitfield Jones L, Hardcastle TC. Imaging the oesophagus after penetrating cervical trauma using water soluble contrast alone: simple, cost effective and accurate. *Emerg Med J.* 2009 Feb;**26(2)**:106–8. doi: 10.1136/emj.2008.063958

10. Sperry JL, Moore EE, Coimbra R, Croce M, Davis JW, Karmy-Jones R, et al. Western Trauma Association critical decisions in trauma: penetrating neck trauma. *J Trauma Acute Care Surg.* 2013;**75(6)**:936–40. doi: 10.1097/TA.0b013e31829e20e3

11. George SM Jr, Croce MA, Fabian TC, Mangiate EC, Kudsk KA, Voeller, Pate JW. Cervicothoracic arterial injuries: recommendations for diagnosis and management. *World J Surg.* 1991 Jan-Feb;**15(1)**:134–9; discussion 139–40. doi: 10.1007/BF01658986

12. Fabian TC, George SM Jr, Croce MA, Mangiante EC, Voeller GR, Kusdk KA. Carotid artery trauma: management based on mechanism of injury. *J Trauma* 1990 Aug;**30(8)**: 953–61;discussion961.doi:10.1097/00005373-199008000-00003

Recommended Reading

Demetriades D, Asensio J, Velmahos G, Thal E. Complex problems in penetrating neck trauma. *Surg Clin North Am.* 1996 Aug;**76(4)**:661–83. doi: 10.1016/s0039-6109(05)70475-8

Feliciano DV. Penetrating cervical trauma. Current concepts in penetrating trauma, IATSIC symposium, international surgical society, Helsinki, Finland, August 25–29, 2013. *World J Surg.* 2015; **39(1)**:1363–72.

Moeng MS, Boffard KD. Penetrating neck injuries. *Review Scand J Surg.* 2002;**91(1)**:34–40. doi: 10.1177/145749690209100106

The Chest 8

8.1 OVERVIEW

Thoracic injury constitutes a significant problem in terms of mortality and morbidity. Somewhat less clearly defined is the extent of appreciable morbidity following chest injury, most usually the long-term consequences of hypoxic brain damage, chronic pain, and opiate dependency that may be present.

A significant proportion of deaths occur virtually immediately (i.e., at the time of injury) from rapid exsanguination, and patients with thoracic injury who reach hospital may die in hospital as the result of mis-assessment or delays in initiation of definitive treatment. These deaths may occur *early*, often due to blood loss, or *late* as the result of respiratory failure, multiple organ failure, and sepsis.

Most life-threatening thoracic injuries can be promptly treated after identification with simple and effective techniques that can be performed by any trained physician (supplemental oxygen, analgesia, and intercostal drainage insertion). Thoracotomy (sternotomy) is required in less than 5% of blunt cases and in about 15%–20% of penetrating cases, although it can be as high as 30% in some areas.

Life-saving procedures like an emergency department thoracotomy (EDT, also called emergency room thoracotomy [ERT]) are usually related to patients *in extremis* with penetrating injury and have specific indications. Indiscriminate use of EDT, however, especially in blunt trauma, will not alter patient outcome, but will increase the risk of communicable disease transmission to health workers and expenses in an otherwise resource-limited environment.

Injuries to the chest wall and thoracic viscera can directly impair oxygen transport mechanisms. Hypoxia and hypovolaemia resulting from thoracic injury may worsen traumatic brain injuries (TBIs) (secondary injury) or may directly cause cerebral oedema due to hypercapnoea.

Conversely, shock and/or brain injury can secondarily aggravate thoracic injuries and hypoxaemia by disrupting normal ventilatory patterns or by causing loss of protective airway reflexes and aspiration.

The lung is a target organ for secondary injury following shock and remote tissue injury. Microemboli formed in the peripheral microcirculation embolize to the lung, causing ventilation–perfusion mismatch and right heart failure.

8.2 THE SPECTRUM OF THORACIC INJURY

Thoracic injuries, whether blunt or penetrating, are grouped into two types.

8.2.1 Immediately Life-Threatening Injuries

Thoracic injuries may result in rapid death (within minutes) by causing either airway obstruction, impaired gas exchange, or shock. Common injuries are:

- Airway obstruction
- Breathing (impaired gas exchange)
- Shock

> *Remember the anagram ATOMC ('atomic'): Airway obstruction, tension pneumothorax, open pneumothorax, massive haemothorax, cardiac tamponade.*

8.2.2 Potentially Life-Threatening Injuries

Injuries resulting in death within hours or days are related to:

- Pneumothorax
- Haemothorax
- Flail chest and multiple fractured ribs
- Pulmonary contusion
- Traumatic diaphragmatic herniation
- Tracheobronchial tree disruption

DOI: 10.1201/9781003258124-11

- Blunt aortic rupture (contained)
- Blunt cardiac injury
- Oesophageal laceration

Penetrating wounds traversing the mediastinum frequently damage several mediastinal structures and are thus more complex in their evaluation and management; the same applies to transitional injuries in the neck or thoraco-abdominal area.

8.3 PATHOPHYSIOLOGY OF THORACIC INJURIES

The well-recognized pathophysiological changes occurring in patients with thoracic injuries are essentially the result of:

- Impaired ventilation (hypercapnoea) due to airway obstruction, restricted chest wall motility, and abnormal diaphragmatic function.
- Impaired gas exchange (hypoxaemia) at the alveolar level (lung contusion and high-volume parenchymal air leaks)
- Impaired cardiac output and poor tissue perfusion (shock) due to haemorrhage, cardiac compression, and air embolus.

An approach to the patient with a thoracic injury must therefore take all these elements into account. Specifically, hypoxia at a cellular or tissue level results from inadequate delivery of oxygen, with development of acidosis and associated hypercapnoea. The late complications resulting from mis-assessment of thoracic injuries are directly attributable to these processes.

Penetrating chest injuries should be obvious. Exceptions include small puncture wounds such as those caused by ice picks or secondary ballistic fragments. Bleeding from the lung is generally minimal due to the low pressure within the pulmonary system. Exceptions include wounds to the great vessels as they exit over the apex of the chest wall to the upper extremities, or injury to any systemic vessel that may be injured in the chest wall, such as the internal mammary or intercostal vessels.

Penetrating thoraco-abdominal injuries generate more controversy. These will require an aggressive approach, particularly with anterior wounds. If the wound is between one posterior axillary line and the other and obviously penetrates the abdomen, laparotomy may be indicated. If peritoneal penetration has occurred or is strongly suspected, a laparotomy is indicated, especially in patients

with abnormal physiology or haemodynamic abnormality. Other options include diagnostic-therapeutic laparoscopy or thoracoscopy to evacuate clots from the chest, to identify and repair a diaphragmatic injury, and occasionally to repair large parenchymal tears (see Section 9.3.1).[1]

In the haemodynamically unstable patient with penetrating injury to the upper torso whose bleeding is occurring into the chest cavity, it is important to insert a chest tube as soon as possible during the initial assessment and resuscitation. In the patient *in extremis* who has chest injuries or in whom there may be suspicion of a transmediastinal injury, bilateral chest tubes are indicated. X-ray is *not* required to insert a chest tube, but it *is* useful after the chest tubes have been inserted to confirm proper placement, and it may help guide your initial surgical decision-making.

In haemodynamically stable patients, the widespread use, free availability, and training in performing extended focussed assessment with sonography in trauma (eFAST) have further reduced the need for plain radiographies in thoracic trauma. However, a chest X-ray performed in the emergency department (ED) remains the gold standard for diagnosis of a pneumothorax or haemothorax. In these patients, it is preferable to have the X-ray completed before placement of a chest tube. The decrease in air entry may not be due to a pneumothorax, and especially following blunt injury may be due to pulmonary contusion (which will be missed on eFAST) or a ruptured diaphragm with bowel or stomach occupying the thoracic cavity. One caveat is that supine chest radiography may miss up to 30% of small haemo- or pneumothoraces seen in the ED.

When it comes to the removal of chest tubes, bedside thoracic ultrasonography on the fourth intercostal space can reliably determine safe removal of tube thoracostomy after traumatic injury, by excluding the presence of an ongoing pneumothorax, and ensuring a new pneumothorax has not redeveloped by repeating the examination in 4 to 6 hours.[2]

8.3.1 Paediatric Considerations

There are several important considerations in the assessment and management of paediatric and adolescent chest trauma.[3] See also Section 14.1.

- In children, the ribs are more flexible, so the presence of rib fractures implies a high-energy injury, as well as a higher incidence of associated head, thoracic, and abdominal solid organ injuries.[4]

- The rare penetrating cardiac wounds in the paediatric age group have a poorer prognosis than in adults and are associated with a low in-hospital survival rate (< 30%).[5]
- In children, the thymus may be very large, and care should be taken to avoid damage to it.
- The sternum is relatively soft and can be divided using a pair of heavy scissors.

Tip

Intercostal drains should be *tunnelled subcutaneously over at least one rib space* to facilitate later removal without air leaks. The child may not cooperate with a Valsalva manoeuvre, and external compression over the tract may prevent recurrent pneumothorax during removal.

Pneumothoraces after blunt torso trauma are uncommon in children, and most are not identified on the ED chest X-ray. Nearly half of pneumothoraces, particularly occult pneumothoraces (not visible on imaging), can be managed without tube thoracostomy.[6] An important issue in dealing with severe paediatric chest trauma is the unavailability and unsuitability of adult-sized aortic stent grafts for the very rare occasions of traumatic aortic injuries in this age group.

8.4 APPLIED SURGICAL ANATOMY OF THE CHEST

It is useful to broadly view the thorax as a container with an inlet, walls, a floor, and contents.

8.4.1 The Chest Wall

This is the bony 'cage' constituted by the ribs, thoracic vertebral column, and sternum with the clavicles anteriorly and the scapula posteriorly. The associated muscle groups and vascular structures (specifically, the intercostal vessels and the internal thoracic vessels) are further components.

Remember the 'triangle of safety' of the chest. This area is the thinnest region of the chest wall in terms of musculature. This is the area of choice for tube thoracostomy insertion. In this area, there are no significant structures within the walls that may be damaged;

however, note that there is a need to avoid the intercostal vascular and nerve bundle on the undersurface of the rib (**Figure 8.1**).

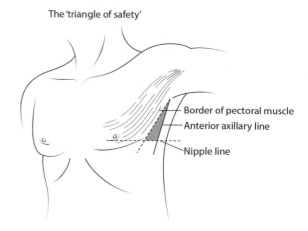

Figure 8.1 Anatomy of the chest wall for placement of a chest drain: The 'triangle of safety'.

8.4.2 The Chest Floor

This is formed by the diaphragm with its various openings. This broad sheet of muscle with its large, trefoil-shaped central tendon has hiatuses through which pass the aorta, the oesophagus, and the inferior vena cava, and it is innervated by the phrenic nerves. The oesophageal hiatus also contains both vagus nerves. The aortic hiatus contains the azygos vein and the thoracic duct.

Pitfall

During normal breathing, the diaphragm moves about 2 cm, but it can move up to 10 cm in deep breathing. During maximum expiration, the diaphragm may rise as high as the fifth intercostal space. Thus, any injury below the fifth intercostal space may involve the abdominal cavity as well.

8.4.3 The Chest Contents

These are:

- The left and right pleural spaces containing the lungs, lined by the parietal and visceral pleurae.

- The mediastinum and its viscera are in the centre of the chest. The mediastinum itself has anterior, middle, posterior, and superior divisions (**Figure 8.2**). The superior mediastinum is contiguous with the thoracic inlet and Zone I of the neck.
- From a functional and practical point of view, it is useful to regard the chest in terms of a 'hemithorax and its contents', both in evaluation of the injury and in choosing the option for access. **Figures 8.3** and **8.4** illustrate the hemithoraces and their respective contents.

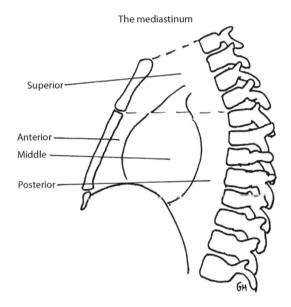

The mediastinum

Figure 8.2 Chest contents.

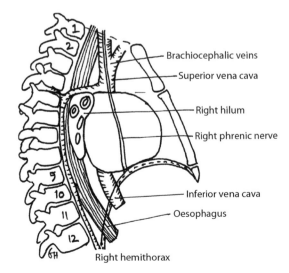

Figure 8.3 Right hemithorax and mediastinum.

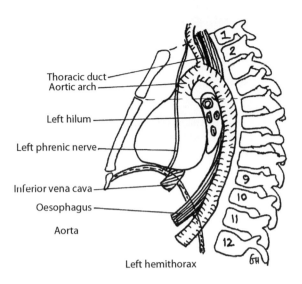

Figure 8.4 Left hemithorax and mediastinum.

8.4.3.1 TRACHEOBRONCHIAL TREE

The trachea extends from the cricoid cartilage at the level of the fifth cervical vertebra, to the carina at the level of the upper border of the sixth thoracic vertebra, where it bifurcates. The right main bronchus is shorter, straighter, and at less of an angle compared with that on the left side. It lies just below the junction between the azygos vein and the superior vena cava, and behind the right pulmonary artery. Due to this anatomic configuration, main stem endotracheal intubations are often right-sided.

8.4.3.2 LUNGS AND PLEURAE

The right lung constitutes about 55% of the total lung mass and has oblique and transverse fissures that divide it into three lobes. The left lung is divided into upper and lower lobes by the oblique fissure. Both lungs are divided into bronchopulmonary segments corresponding to the branches of the lesser bronchi and are supplied by branches of the pulmonary arteries. The right and left pulmonary arteries pass superiorly in the hilum, anterior to each respective bronchus. There are superior and inferior pulmonary veins on each side, the middle lobe usually being drained by the superior vein.

The pleural cavities are lined by parietal and visceral pleurae. The parietal pleura lines the inner wall of the thoracic cage. The visceral pleura is intimately applied to the surface of the lungs and is reflected onto the mediastinum to join the parietal pleura at the hilum.

8.4.3.3 HEART AND PERICARDIUM

The heart lies in the middle mediastinum, extending from the level of the third costal cartilage to the xiphisternal junction. Most of the anterior surface of the heart is represented by the right atrium and its auricular appendage superiorly, and the right ventricle inferiorly. The aorta emerges from the cranial aspect and crosses to the left and posteriorly as the arch. The pulmonary artery extends cranially and bifurcates in the concavity of the aortic arch. The left pulmonary artery is attached to the concavity of the arch of the aorta, just distal to the origin of the left subclavian artery, by the ligamentum arteriosum. The pericardium is a strong fibrous sac that completely invests the heart and is attached to the diaphragm inferiorly.

Pitfalls

- Pericardial tamponade can occur by the sudden accumulation of even a small amount of blood < 200 mL.
- The lateral lying phrenic nerves are in the 3 and 9 o'clock positions on the pericardial sac and should be avoided when performing a pericardiotomy.

8.4.3.4 THE AORTA AND GREAT VESSELS

The thoracic aorta is divided into three parts: the ascending aorta, arch, and descending aorta. The innominate artery (i.e., brachiocephalic artery) is the first branch from the arch, passing upwards and to the right, posterior to the innominate vein. The left common carotid artery and left subclavian artery arise from the left side of the arch.

8.4.3.5 OESOPHAGUS

The oesophagus, approximately 25 cm long, extends from the pharynx to the stomach. It starts at the level of the sixth cervical vertebra and passes through the diaphragm about 2.5 cm to the left of the midline at the level of the 11th thoracic vertebra. The entire intrathoracic oesophagus is surrounded by loose areolar tissue, which allows for rapid spread of infection if the oesophagus is

breached. Another significant anatomical feature is the lack of serosal cover which predisposes to anastomotic failure and poor healing.

8.4.3.6 THORACIC DUCT

The duct arises from the cysterna chyli overlying the first and second lumbar vertebrae. It lies posteriorly and to the right of the aorta. It ascends through the oesophageal hiatus of the diaphragm between the aorta and the azygos vein, anterior to the right intercostal branches from the aorta. It overlies the right side of the vertebral bodies and drains into the venous system at the junction of the left subclavian and internal jugular veins. Injury can result in a left-sided chylothorax.

8.5 DIAGNOSIS

Penetrating injuries to the chest may be clinically obvious. It is, however, important to logroll the patient to make sure that the entire back has been examined. Logrolling is just as important in patients with penetrating trauma as it is in those with blunt trauma, to rule out posterior injuries as well as injuries to the thoracic or lumbar spine.

The surgeon should auscultate each hemithorax, noting whether there are diminished or absent breath sounds.

Ultrasound's primary role is in determining whether a patient has pericardial blood and assessing for the presence of haemopneumothoraces, and it has greater accuracy than a supine plain chest X-ray (eFAST).[7] Ultrasound may also be superior to plain radiography in differentiating between fluid and lung contusion.[8]

Transoesophageal echocardiography (TOE or TEE) is a useful adjunct in determining whether tamponade is present in the haemodynamically stable patient, as well as assessing the heart in patients with blunt cardiac and aortic injuries, but it is rarely used in the acute setting. Trans-thoracic echocardiography (TTO) or TOE should be obtained in all patients with a penetrating cardiac injury immediately after repair to exclude valvular complex and septal abnormalities.

Computed tomography (CT) is **not** routinely used in patients with penetrating chest injury, except in *stable* patients with transmediastinal wounds and those with penetration to the thoraco-abdominal region and suspected diaphragmatic injury and intra-abdominal organ involvement. It may have some utility in determining the extent of pulmonary contusion caused by higher-energy injuries or shotgun blasts but is not generally indicated in the initial resuscitation or treatment of such patients. CT angiography (CTA) can be very useful in the haemo-dynamically stable patient with penetrating injuries to the thoracic outlet or upper chest to delineate potential vascular injuries that may be repaired using stent grafts (arteriovenous fistulas and false aneurysms).

In the patient with penetrating injuries, a chest X-ray remains the 'gold standard' and should be obtained early. It is good practice to place radiopaque objects such as paper clips on the skin over any wounds on the chest wall. X-ray is the key diagnostic study in penetrating injury, since it will not only reveal the presence of a pneumothorax and haemothorax, but also allow projection of a bullet track. Furthermore, missiles often leave metallic fragments outlining the path of the bullet, and areas of pulmonary contusion are additional indicators of the missile track. This is also useful for stab wounds. Tracking the missile helps the surgeon to determine which visceral organs may be injured and whether there is potential transgression of the diaphragm and/or mediastinum. In patients without favourable haemo-dynamics, an additional lateral X-ray view may also help with incision planning.

Ultrasound will not show a bullet track.

In stable blunt trauma patients, CT or CTA is an invaluable screening tool for blunt aortic rupture, to assist with the diagnosis of diaphragmatic injuries and to delineate the anatomy of flail chest and multiple rib fractures to decide if surgical stabilization is indicated.

In victims of blast injury, where there is an associated blast shock wave, the risk of pulmonary contusion is high (see Chapter 20).

Pitfall

Pulmonary contusion following blast only develops significantly 12–24 hours after the injury. It is recommended that a CT of the chest should **not** be done immediately, but rather after 24 hours.

Non-operative management of thoraco-abdominal injuries requires injuries to the diaphragm or abdominal viscera to be excluded. Various modalities have been described to try to identify the trajectory of penetrating injuries in these regions, including triple-contrast CT scan and, recently, CT tractography with radiopaque contrast.[9] Thoracoscopy and laparoscopy have been successful in diagnosing diaphragm penetration. Laparoscopy may have a small advantage in that if the diaphragm has been penetrated, it also allows some assessment of the intraperitoneal viscera; however, in many ways, thoracoscopy is better for assessment of the diaphragm, particularly in the right hemithorax. The disadvantage is that, once an injury has been detected, this does not rule out associated intraperitoneal injuries.

8.6 MANAGEMENT OF SPECIFIC INJURIES

Non-operative management (referring to major surgery) can be used in most penetrating injuries. These patients should be observed in a monitored setting to ensure haemodynamic stability, monitoring of ventilatory status, and output of blood from the pleural cavity.

8.6.1 Damage Control in the Chest

Damage control surgery procedures such as hilar cross-clamping, lung parenchymal tractotomy, packing, and temporary vacuum closure over an intercostal drain can be used.[10] Delayed anatomical closure and reconstruction can be carried out after physiological restoration. Myocutaneous flaps such as latissimus dorsi or pectoralis major may be necessary in patients with significant tissue loss affecting the chest wall secondary to the primary injury or surgical debridement (see Chapter 6: 'Damage Control').

8.6.2 Open Pneumothorax

The incidence of open pneumothorax or significant chest wall injuries following civilian trauma is less than 1% of all major thoracic injuries. Although all penetrating wounds are technically open pneumothoraces, the tissue of the chest wall serves as an effective seal. True open pneumothorax is most often associated with close-range shotgun blasts, high-energy missiles, and slash lacerations caused by long blades (machetes) or boat propellers. There is usually a large gaping wound commonly associated with frothy blood at its entrance. Respiratory sounds can be heard with the to-and-from movement of air. The patient often has air hunger and may be in shock from associated visceral injuries.

The wound should be immediately sealed with an occlusive clean or sterile dressing, such as petroleum jelly–soaked gauze; thin plastic sheets, sealed on three sides to create a valve; or even aluminium foil as a temporary dressing.

Pitfall

Once the chest wound has been sealed, a tube thoracostomy is immediately necessary because of the risk of converting the open pneumothorax into a tension pneumothorax.

Large gaping wounds will invariably require debridement, including resection of devitalized tissue back to bleeding tissue, and removal of all foreign bodies including clothing, wadding from shotgun shells, or debris from the object that penetrated the chest. Most of these patients will require thoracotomy to treat visceral injuries and to control bleeding from the lung or chest wall.

After the wounds have been thoroughly debrided and irrigated, the size of the defect may necessitate reconstruction. The use of synthetic material to repair large defects in the chest wall has mostly been abandoned. Instead, myocutaneous flaps such as latissimus dorsi or pectoralis major have proven efficacy, particularly when cartilage or ribs must be excised. The flap provides prompt healing and minimizes infection to the exposed ribs or costal cartilages. If potential muscle flaps have been destroyed by the injury, a temporary dressing can be placed (damage control), and the patient stabilized in the intensive care unit (ICU) and then returned to the operating room in 24–48 hours for a free myocutaneous graft or alternative reconstruction. Complications include wound infection and respiratory insufficiency, the latter usually due to associated parenchymal injury. Ventilatory embarrassment can persist secondary to the large defect. If the chest wall becomes infected, debridement, wound care, and myocutaneous flaps should be considered.

8.6.3 Tension Pneumothorax (Haemo- or Pneumothorax)

Tension pneumothorax is an immediate threat to life. The importance of making the diagnosis is that it is the most easily treatable life-threatening surgical emergency in the

ED. 'Simple' isolated closed pneumothorax, which is not quite as dramatic, occurs in approximately 20% of all penetrating chest injuries. Haemothorax, in contrast, is present in about 30% of penetrating injuries, and haemopneumothorax is found in 40%–50% of penetrating injuries.

The diagnosis of tension pneumothorax can be difficult in a noisy ED. The classic signs are decreased breath sounds and percussion tympany on the ipsilateral side, and tracheal shift to the contralateral side. The diagnosis is clinical. In the patient who is dying, there should be no hesitation in performing a tube thoracostomy. Massive haemothorax is equally life-threatening.

8.6.4 Massive Haemothorax

Approximately 50% of patients with hilar, great vessel, or cardiac wounds expire immediately after injury. Another 25% live for periods of 5–6 minutes, and, in urban centres, some of these patients may arrive alive in the ED after rapid transport. The remaining 25% live for periods of up to 30 minutes. These two groups of patients require immediate diagnosis and treatment.

The diagnosis of massive haemothorax (like tension pneumothorax) is invariably made by the presence of shock, ventilatory embarrassment, and a shift in the mediastinum *away* from the affected side (as opposed to a shift towards the affected side during plugging or atelectasis).

The classical description of a massive haemothorax, that of 1500 mL of blood, needs to be revised. A massive haemothorax may be present in a patient with blunt or penetrating thoracic injury who has significant physiological derangement but demonstrates moderate output via the chest tube. Therefore, assessing and correctly interpreting the poor physiology and haemodynamic status of the patient as the definition of 'massive', rather than concentrating on obtaining a large blood volume via the chest tube, are the essence of diagnosis.

Chest X-ray or eFAST will confirm the extent of blood loss, but most of the time tube thoracostomy is done immediately to relieve the threat of ventilatory embarrassment. If a gush of blood is obtained when the chest tube is placed, autotransfusion should be considered. There are simple devices that should be available in all major trauma resuscitation centres.

The treatment of massive haemothorax is to control the bleeding source and restore blood volume. In approximately 85% of patients with massive haemothorax, a systemic vessel has been injured such as the intercostal artery or internal mammary artery, and essentially, all such patients will require a thoracotomy. In a few patients, there may be injury to the hilum of the lung or the myocardium. In about 15% of instances, the bleeding is from deep pulmonary lacerations. These injuries are treated by pulmonary tractotomy and oversewing the lesion, making sure that bleeding is controlled to the depth of the lesion, or, in some instances, they are treated by resection of a segment or lobe; pneumonectomy should be avoided in the acute trauma setting due to poor outcome brought about by inability of the remaining lung to acutely compensate and provide appropriate gas exchange.

8.6.5 Retained Haemothorax

Complications of haemothorax or massive haemothorax are almost invariably related to visceral injuries. Failure of non-operative management is considered in patients who continue to bleed from the pleural cavity and those patients who go on to develop a retained haemothorax.

Occasionally, a retained haemothorax may require a cortical peel necessitating thoracoscopy or thoracotomy and removal. The aggressive use of two chest tubes could minimize the incidence of this complication. If there are retained clots, video-assisted thoracoscopy (VATS) is indicated, optimally within 72 hours of the injury, to aid in the removal of these clots and reduce the need for open surgery.[11] Fibrinolytic agents such as streptokinase or activated recombinant tissue plasminogen activator may be instilled into the pleural space in an effort to evacuate the retained blood and avoid surgery; however, these agents may be contraindicated in patients with a high risk of haemorrhage. The Eastern Association for the Surgery of Trauma (EAST) Practice Management Guidelines for the Management of Simple and Retained Haemothorax recommend:[12]

- For stable patients with traumatic haemothorax, we conditionally recommend pig-tail catheters.
- In patients with retained haemothorax, we conditionally recommend VATS rather than thrombolytic therapy.
- In patients with retained haemothorax who need VATS, we recommend that it should be performed early (≤ 4 days).

8.6.6 Tracheobronchial Injuries[13]

Penetrating injuries to the tracheobronchial tree are uncommon and constitute less than 2% of all major thoracic injuries. Disruption of the tracheobronchial tree is suggested by massive haemoptysis, airway obstruction, progressive mediastinal air, subcutaneous emphysema, tension pneumothorax, and significant persistent air leak after placement of a chest tube. Fibre-optic bronchoscopy in the relatively stable patient is a useful adjunct in diagnosis, tracheal tube placement, tracheobronchial removal of inspissated secretions, and postoperative follow-up of tracheobronchial repairs.

Treatment for bronchial injuries is usually straightforward. If it is a minor distal bronchus, there may be persistent air leak for a few days, but it will usually close with chest tube drainage alone with or without negative suction. If, however, there is a significant air leak, or the patient has significant loss of minute volume through the chest tube, usually represented by loss of one-third or more of the inspired tidal volume (200–350 mL) causing significant hypoxia and respiratory acidosis, the chest should be explored, usually through a posterolateral thoracotomy. If possible, the bronchus is repaired with monofilament suture. In some instances, a segmentectomy or lobectomy may be required.

Intrathoracic tracheal injuries secondary to blunt trauma are rare compared to those from penetrating injuries. The presentation is similar in both cases: a tension pneumothorax that fails to re-expand after chest tube insertion with a significant air leak causing severe hypoxia and respiratory acidosis. A thoracotomy for direct repair is the best option to control these injuries, and access is better with an approach from the right side.

8.6.7 Oesophageal Injuries

Penetrating injuries to the thoracic oesophagus are quite uncommon. Injuries to the cervical oesophagus are somewhat more frequent and are usually detected at the time of exploration of Zone I and II injuries of the neck. In those centres where selective management of neck injuries is practised, the symptoms found are usually related to pain on swallowing and dysphagia. Occasionally, patients may present late with signs of posterior mediastinitis – a grave situation with a high mortality rate, even with aggressive and comprehensive treatment. Injuries to the thoracic oesophagus may present with pain, fever, pneumomediastinum, persistent pneumothorax despite tube thoracostomy, purulent pleural effusion, and extravasation of contrast seen on a water-soluble contrast swallow. Flexible oesophagogastroscopy (OGD) is very useful in determining the level and character of the injury, may be used to close minor lacerations with the application of over-the-scope clips, but in untrained hands can easily convert a partial laceration into a complete disruption, worsening the prognosis. The best diagnostic sensitivity is attained with a combination of both contrast-swallow imaging and direct visualization by OGD.

Treatment of cervical oesophageal injuries is relatively straightforward. As noted above, the injury is usually found during routine exploration of penetrating wounds beneath the platysma. Once found, a primary closure is performed. In more devitalizing injuries, it may be necessary to debride and close using drainage to protect the anastomosis. Injuries to the thoracic oesophagus should be repaired if the injury is less than 6 hours old and there are minimal inflammation and devitalized tissue present; however, some centres may perform a primary repair up to 24 hours after injury. A two-layer closure has been used, but a single full-thickness layer of absorbable suture incorporating the mucosa is all that is necessary in most cases with a drainage nearby. Postoperatively, the patient is kept on intravenous support and supplemental nutrition. Antibiotics may be indicated during the 24-hour perioperative period, unless established mediastinal sepsis is present.

A suction drain will prevent pooling of saliva or gastric content.

If the wound is between 6 and 24 hours old, a decision will be necessary to determine whether primary closure can be attempted or whether drainage and nutritional support is the optimal management. Almost all injuries older than 24 hours will not heal primarily when repaired. Open drainage, antibiotics, nutritional support, and consideration of diversion are the optimal management principles. Complications following oesophageal injuries include wound infection, mediastinitis, and empyema.

Non-operative endoscopic self-expanding silicon-coated stent placement in selected cases has been advocated. The main problem with covered stents is the issue of stent migration, as the smooth oesophageal mucosa does not offer a grip surface; this can be overcome by concomitant application of clips to keep the stent in place. Cervical (upper third) and gastro-oesophageal junction injuries are not suitable, due to incomplete sealing by the stent and significant reflux. Some authorities advise a concomitant thoracotomy or thoracoscopy to place mediastinal drains when the stenting method is used. Accurate localization and assessment of the extent of the injury by contrast radiography and endoscopy are mandatory when selecting cases for stenting. As mentioned before, another option of treatment for small

oesophageal lacerations is the application of over-the-scope clips; however, there are limited data to support one technique over the other in the trauma literature.

8.6.8 Diaphragmatic Injuries

See Section 9.3: 'Bowel, Rectum, and Diaphragm'.

8.6.9 Pulmonary Contusion (PC)

Pulmonary contusions represent bruising of the lung and are usually associated with direct chest trauma, high-velocity missiles, and shotgun and other blast injuries. The pathophysiology is the result of ventilation–perfusion mismatch and shunts caused by hypoxic pulmonary vasoconstriction. Its anatomical composition makes the extent of lung damage easily quantifiable on CT scanning. The treatment of significant pulmonary contusion consists primarily of cardiovascular and tailored ventilatory support.

Pitfall

In the past, measures such as systemic steroids to modulate the development of significant systemic inflammatory response syndrome (SIRS), and a policy of fluid restriction with the use of diuretics, were suggested; however, there is no high-level evidence supporting these therapies.

Antibiotics are not generally used, as this will simply select out nosocomial, opportunistic, and resistant organisms. It is preferable to obtain a Gram stain of the sputum and chest X-rays when necessary. If the Gram stain shows the presence of a predominant organism with an associated increase in polymorphonuclear cells, antibiotics are indicated.

8.6.10 Flail Chest (FC)

Traditionally, flail chest, and by extension multiple rib fractures, have been managed by internal splinting ('internal pneumatic stabilization') utilizing positive pressure ventilation, as it treats the associated (often severe) pulmonary contusion whilst it is believed to provide fracture site immobility.

Table 8.1 The PICO Format

P	Patient, Population, or Problem	How would I describe the patient group?
I	Intervention, Prognostic factor, or Exposure	Which main intervention, prognostic factor, or exposure is considered?
C	Comparison or Intervention (if appropriate)	What is the main alternative to compare with the intervention?
O	Outcome you would like to measure or achieve	What can be accomplished, measured, improved, or affected?

Whilst this is undoubtedly the method of choice in most instances, especially in patients who may need ventilatory support for other associated injuries (e.g., TBIs), in general, surgical rib stabilization shortens the recovery time, and facilitates earlier ICU and hospital discharge and earlier return to normal productive activities, when compared with traditional medical therapy.

Several trials and recent meta-analysis have shown considerable benefits with a shortening of ventilation time and in some cases avoidance of invasive ventilation, facilitating the use of non-invasive modalities, reduction of risk for ventilator-associated pneumonia (VAP), improved earlier mobilization, reduced analgesic requirements based on Visual Analogue pain scales application, as well as less incidence of chronic pain and opiate dependence.[14–16]

8.6.11 Fixation of Multiple Fractures of Ribs[17,18]

A flail chest may be stabilized using pins, plates, wires, rods, or, more recently, absorbable plates. Exposure for the insertion of these can be via a conventional posterolateral thoracotomy, via incisions made over the ribs or using VATS.

The EAST guidelines for the open reduction and internal fixation of rib fractures have PICO guidelines.[18] (See **Tables 8.1** and **8.2**.)

The elderly present specific additional problems.[19] See **Table 8.3**.

Table 8.2 Eastern Association for the Surgery of Trauma Practice Management Guideline for Open Reduction and Internal Fixation of Rib Fractures

PICO	Recommendation
PICO Question 1	
In adult patients with flail chest after blunt trauma, should rib ORIF be performed (vs. non-operative management) to decrease mortality; DMV, ICU LOS, and hospital LOS; and incidence of pneumonia and need for tracheostomy; and to improve pain control?	In adult patients with flail chest after blunt trauma, we conditionally recommend rib ORIF to decrease mortality; shorten duration of mechanical ventilation, ICU LOS, and hospital LOS; and decrease incidence of pneumonia and tracheostomy. **We cannot offer a recommendation** for pain control with currently available evidence.
PICO Question 2	
In adult patients with non-flail rib fractures after blunt trauma, should rib ORIF be performed (vs. non-operative management) to decrease mortality and incidence of pneumonia; shorten DMV and hospital LOS; improve pain control; and decrease need for tracheostomy, if applicable?	In adult patients with non-flail rib fractures after blunt trauma, **we cannot offer a recommendation** for any of the outcomes with currently available evidence.

DMV, duration of mechanical ventilation
ICU, intensive care unit
LOS, length of stay
ORIF, operative rib fixation
PICO, patient/population/problem, intervention, comparison, and outcome

Table 8.3 Non-Surgical Management and Analgesia Strategies for Older Adults with Multiple Rib Fractures: A Systematic Review, Meta-Analysis, and Practice Management Guideline

PICO	Recommendation
PICO Question 1	
In adults aged ≥ 65-years-old with ≥ 3 rib fractures (P), should admission to an ICU setting (I) versus admission to a non-ICU setting (C) take place to reduce pneumonia, need for intubation, ventilator days, or mortality (O)?	These studies were retrospective with different definitions. Some studies included older patients [11–13], whilst other studies included all patients. There was little discussion regarding the predetermined critical outcomes. Guidelines for ICU admission were also frequently not followed. Risk of bias was high, and quality of evidence was very low. **This data did not support any quantitative analysis nor any recommendations.**
PICO Question 2	
In adults aged ≥ 65-years-old with rib fractures (P), should routine use of incentive spirometry (I) versus no routine use of incentive spirometry (C), be performed to reduce pneumonia, need for intubation, or mortality (O)?	In assessing the literature, data quality was low with one RCT and three retrospective studies, and no quantitative analysis was possible. However, other factors considered included good therapeutic tolerance, few side effects, and low cost. **Thus, we recommend that incentive spirometry be used to reduce overall pulmonary complications.**
PICO Question 3	
In adults aged ≥ 65-years-old with rib fractures and acute hypoxic respiratory failure refractory to nasal cannula and face mask (P), should non-invasive positive-pressure ventilation (NIPPV: high-flow nasal cannula, bilevel positive airway pressure, or continuous positive airway pressure) (I) versus endotracheal intubation (C) be utilized to reduce pneumonia, need for intubation, days on ventilator, or mortality (O)?	**We recommend that NIPPV be used in carefully selected patients with persistent acute hypoxic respiratory failure as defined as O_2 saturation < 90% on supplemental oxygen ≥ 10 L by face mask after optimizing analgesia and ensuring that patients could protect their airway and avoid complications of airway failure.** Patients whose O_2 saturations do not improve above 90% on NIPPV or who have worsening of their mental status or airway compromise should then proceed to ETT.
PICO Question 4	
In adults aged ≥ 65-years-old with ≥ 3 rib fractures and dyspnoea or refractory pain (P), should ketamine infusion plus structured multimodal pain therapy per institutional protocol (I) versus structured multimodal pain therapy per institutional protocol alone (C) be performed to reduce pain, pneumonia, need for intubation, days on ventilator, or mortality (O)?	Quality of evidence was felt to be low to moderate. **No recommendation for or against the use of ketamine was indicated.**
PICO Question 5	
In adults aged ≥ 65-years-old with ≥ 3 rib fractures and dyspnoea or refractory pain (P), should a thoracic epidural catheter and structured multimodal pain therapy per institutional protocol (I) versus structured multimodal pain therapy per institutional protocol alone (C) be performed to reduce pain, pneumonia, need for intubation, hospital LOS, or mortality (O)?	The group therefore elected to make **no recommendation** for or against epidural analgesia.
PICO Question 6	
In adults aged ≥ 65-years-old with ≥ 3 rib fractures and dyspnoea or refractory pain (P), should nonepidural locoregional anaesthetic (subcutaneous infusion pump or local block) and structured multimodal pain therapy per institutional protocol (I) versus structured multimodal pain therapy per institutional protocol alone (C) be performed to reduce pain, pneumonia, need for intubation, days on ventilator, or mortality (O)?	The final decision was to offer **no recommendation** for or against.

8.6.12 **Pulmonary Laceration**

Lung preservation wherever possible is critically important, with conservative resections if required, using a combination of techniques such as tractotomy, wedge resection, and segmentectomy, reserving lobectomy or pneumonectomy for only the most critical patients. Currently available stapling devices are invaluable. Outcomes following trauma pneumonectomy are poor, with a 50% mortality rate, and should be utilized only when there is no other chance of salvage.

8.6.12.1 **AIR EMBOLISM**[20]

Air embolism is an infrequent event following penetrating trauma. It occurs in 4% of all major thoracic trauma. Sixty-five per cent of the cases are due to penetrating injuries. The key to diagnosis is to be aware of the possibility. The pathophysiology is a fistula between a bronchus and the pulmonary vein. Those patients who are breathing spontaneously will have a pressure differential from the pulmonary vein to the bronchus that will cause approximately 22% of these patients to have haemoptysis on presentation. If, however, the patient has a Valsalva-type respiration or grunts, or is intubated with positive pressure in the bronchus, the pressure differential is from the bronchus to the pulmonary vein, causing systemic air embolism.

These patients present in one of three ways: focal or lateralizing neurological signs, sudden cardiovascular collapse, and froth when the initial arterial blood specimen is obtained. Any patient who has obvious chest injury, does not have obvious head injury, and yet has focal or lateralizing neurological findings should be assumed to have air embolism. Confirmation can occasionally be obtained by fundoscopic examination, which shows air in the retinal vessels. Patients who are intubated and have a sudden unexplained cardiovascular collapse with an absence of vital signs should be immediately assumed to have an air embolism to the coronary vessels. Finally, those patients who have a frothy blood sample drawn for initial blood gas determination will have air embolism.

When a patient comes to the ED *in extremis* and an EDT is carried out, air should always be looked for in the coronary vessels. If air is found, the hilum of the offending lung should be clamped immediately to reduce the ingress of air into the vessels.

The treatment of air embolism is immediate thoracotomy, preferably in the operating room. In most patients, the left or right chest is opened depending on the side of penetration. If a resuscitative thoracotomy has been carried out, it may be necessary to extend this across the sternum into the opposite chest if there is no parenchymal injury to the lung on the left. Definitive treatment is to oversew the lacerations to the lung, in some instances perform a lobectomy, and only rarely a pneumonectomy.

Other resuscitative measures in patients who have asystolic arrest due to air embolism include internal cardiac massage and reaching up and holding the ascending aorta with the thumb and index finger for one or two beats – this will tend to push air out of the coronary vessels and thus establish perfusion. Adrenaline (epinephrine) 1:1000 can be injected intravenously or down the endotracheal tube to provide an alpha effect, driving air out of the systemic microcirculation. It is prudent to vent the left atrium and ventricle as well as the ascending aorta to remove all residual air once the lung hilum has been clamped. This prevents further air embolism when the patient is moved.

Using aggressive diagnosis and treatment, it is possible to achieve up to a 55% salvage rate in patients with air embolism secondary to penetrating trauma.

8.6.13 **Cardiac Injuries**

In urban trauma centres, cardiac injuries are the most common after penetrating trauma, and constitute about 5% of all thoracic injuries. The diagnosis of cardiac injury is usually obvious. The patient presents with exsanguination, cardiac tamponade, and, rarely, acute heart failure. In addition to the well-described globular heart shape on X-rays, a straight left heart border has been associated with the presence of a haemopericardium. Patients with tamponade due to penetrating injuries usually have a wound in proximity, decreased cardiac output, increased central venous pressure manifested as distended jugular veins, decreased blood pressure, decreased heart sounds, narrow pulse pressure, and occasionally paradoxical pulse. A clinician-performed eFAST will demonstrate the presence of pericardial fluid, but in cases where the diagnosis of pericardial tamponade cannot be confirmed on clinical signs and on eFAST ('occult' cardiac injury), several screening and diagnostic modalities are available including measurement of troponins, echocardiogram, and CTA. However, in such cases, if a high index of suspicion remains, a subxiphoid pericardial window will invariably demonstrate blood in the pericardium, thus facilitating the decision to open the chest and examine and repair the heart injury.

The treatment of all cardiac injuries is immediate thoracotomy, ideally in the operating room. In the patient who is *in extremis*, thoracotomy in the ED can be life-saving (see Section 8.9: 'Emergency Department Thoracotomy').

Complications from myocardial injuries include recurrent tamponade, mediastinitis, and post-cardiotomy syndrome. The former can be avoided by placing a mediastinal chest tube or leaving the pericardium open following repair. Most cardiac injuries are treated through a left anterolateral thoracotomy, and only occasionally via a median sternotomy, depending on the patient's haemodynamics and the wound location. If mediastinitis does develop, the wound should be opened (including the sternum), and debridement carried out with secondary closure in 4–5 days.

Another complication is herniation of the heart through the pericardium, which may occlude venous return and cause sudden death. This is avoided by loosely approximating the pericardium after the cardiac injury has been repaired.

8.6.14 **Injuries to the Great Vessels**[21]

Injuries to the great vessels from penetrating forces are infrequently reported. The reason for this is that extensive injury to the great vessels results in immediate exsanguination into the chest, and most of these patients die at the scene of injury.

The diagnosis of penetrating great vessel injury is usually obvious. The patient is in shock, and there is an injury in proximity to the thoracic outlet or posterior mediastinum. If the patient stabilizes with resuscitation, angiography should be performed to localize the injury. Approximately 8% of patients with major vascular injuries do not have clinical signs, stressing the need for angiography when there is a wound in proximity. These patients usually have a false aneurysm or arteriovenous fistula. Treatment of penetrating injuries to the great vessels can almost always be accomplished using lateral repair, since larger injuries that might necessitate grafts are usually incompatible with survival long enough to permit the patient to reach the ED alive.[22] See **Figure 8.5**.

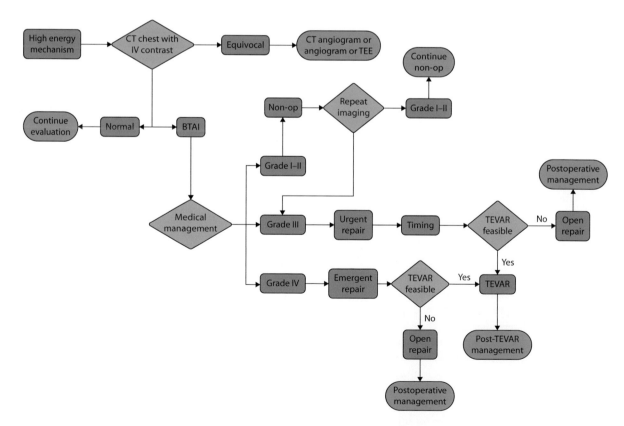

Figure 8.5 Western Trauma Association algorithm for blunt thoracic aortic injury management.

Complications of injuries to the great vessels include rebleeding, false aneurysm formation, and thrombosis. A devastating complication is paraplegia, which usually occurs following blunt injuries but rarely after penetrating injuries, either because of associated injury to the spinal cord, or because at the time of surgery important intercostal arteries are ligated. The spinal cord has a segmental blood supply to the anterior spinal artery (artery of Adamkiewicz), and every effort should be made to preserve the intercostal vessels, particularly those that appear to be larger than normal, as these may constitute an important collateral feeder system.

8.7 **CHEST DRAINAGE**

8.7.1 **Drain Insertion**

Chest tubes are placed according to the technique described in the Advanced Trauma Life Support® (ATLS) programme. The placement is in the triangle between the mid-axillary line, the anterior axillary line, via the fifth intercostal space – the triangle of safety. The optimal site is in the anterior axillary line. Care must be taken to avoid placement of the drain through breast tissue or the pectoralis major muscle.

Pitfall

Drains should **not** be placed through pectoralis major muscle, and **never** through breast tissue.

In the conscious patient, a wheal of 1% lignocaine (Lidocaine) is placed in the skin, followed by a further 20 mL subcutaneously and down to the pleura.

Adequate local anaesthesia is critical. The aim is to block the relevant intercostal nerves. Remember that local anaesthetic may take 5–10 minutes to work adequately.

The chest is prepped and draped in the usual way, and after topical analgesia, an incision is made of about 2–3 cm in length onto the underlying rib (**Figure 8.6**).

Using blunt dissection, the tissue is lifted upwards off the rib, and penetration is made over the top of the rib towards the pleura (**Figure 8.7**). In this manner, damage to the intercostal neurovascular bundle is avoided.

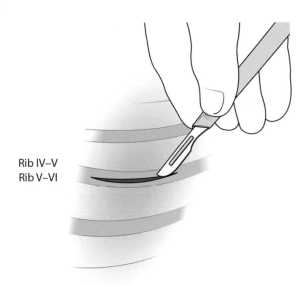

Figure 8.6 Anatomical placement of the incision for a chest drain.

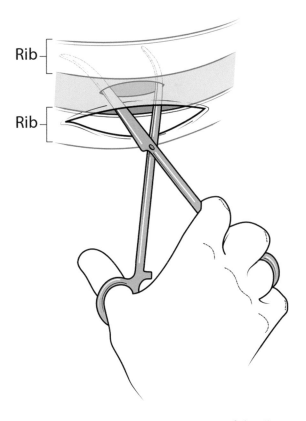

Figure 8.7 Blunt dissection over the top of the rib.

Once the incision has been made, the wound is explored with the index finger for adults and the fifth finger for children. This ensures that the chest cavity has been entered and allows limited exploration of the pleural cavity (**Figure 8.8**). In patients with minor adhesions (e.g., following tuberculosis), it allows the lung tissue to be cleared from the path of the drain.

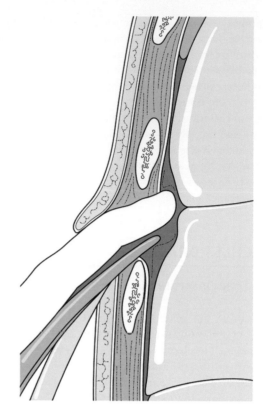

Figure 8.9 Finger and tube (held in forceps) inserted into chest cavity.

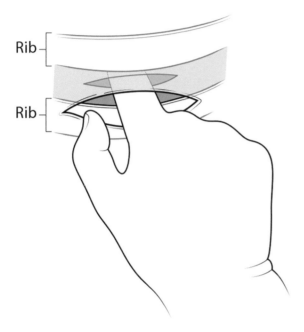

Figure 8.8 Use of a finger to clear adhesions.

Once the tract has been dilatated with the finger, a 28–32G chest tube is inserted. Although data are still accruing, there are reports that small-calibre chest tubes or 'pig-tail' drains may be equally effective in draining pneumo- or haemothoraces, and are perhaps better tolerated by patients.[23,24] The incision should be of sufficient size to allow the introduction of a finger *and* the tube together, allowing the tube to be directed posteriorly and cranially *behind* the lung towards the apex, via the posterior gutter. This provides optimal drainage of both blood and air (**Figure 8.9**).

When the chest tube is in place, it is secured to the chest wall with a size 0 monofilament suture as follows:

- A vertical mattress suture is inserted into the centre of the wound (**Figure 8.10**). A *single* throw is placed in the suture at skin level, and then the suture is knotted halfway up its length.

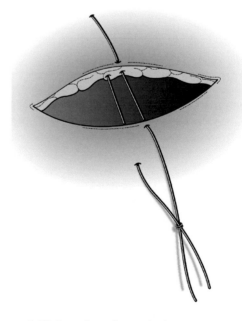

Figure 8.10 Insertion of a vertical mattress suture in the centre of the wound.

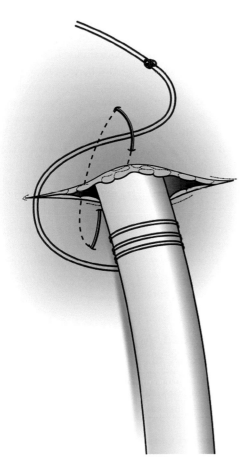

Figure 8.11 Securing the tube: First stage.

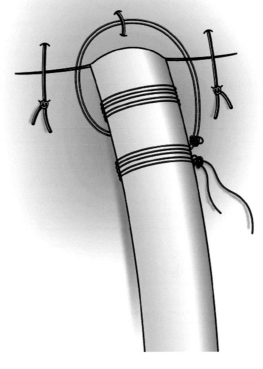

Figure 8.12 Securing the tube: Second stage.

- The suture is then wound around the chest tube until 1 cm before the 'halfway knot' mark is reached. The suture with knot is then threaded *under* the vertical mattress loop (**Figure 8.11**).
- The suture is then tied around the chest tube at the level of the knot, about 1 cm from the skin (**Figure 8.12**).

Additional skin sutures may be needed to close the wound in a linear fashion (**Figure 8.13**).

Pitfalls

- Do not use a 'purse-string' closure, as this is both painful in the long term and less effective. Use a vertical mattress suture.
- Do **not** 'weave' the drain tie (the 'Roman sandal technique') because if it becomes loose, the entire securing suture will be loose. The securing suture should be wound around the drain in one plane, as shown in **Figure 8.12**.

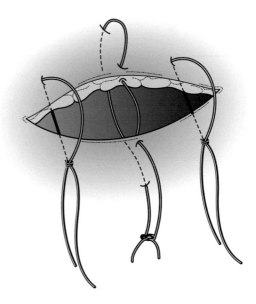

Figure 8.13 Additional simple sutures may be required laterally for full closure.

All connections are taped to prevent inadvertent disconnection or removal of the chest tube.

After the chest tube has been placed, it is prudent to obtain an immediate chest film or further ultrasound, to assess the adequate removal of air and blood, and the position of the tube. If, for any reason, blood accumulates and cannot be removed, another chest tube is inserted. Persistent air leak or bleeding should alert the surgeon that there is significant visceral injury that may require operative intervention.

Pitfall

- The surgeon should be aware that if blood continues to drain, the blood may be entering the chest via a hole in the diaphragm.

8.7.2 Drain Removal

The tube is removed once the lung has expanded. The suture is cut at the 'halfway knot'. The remaining suture is unwound, and the skin can then be pinched, or sealed with petroleum gauze, as the tube is withdrawn (**Figure 8.14**); the preplaced suture, now unwound, is then pulled tight and secured. The wound should thus be closed as a linear incision (**Figure 8.15**).

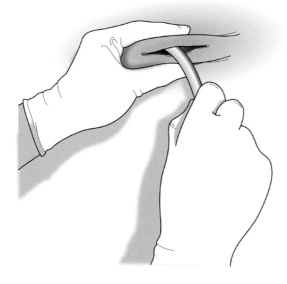

Figure 8.14 Removal of the drain showing pinching of the skin.

Complications of tube thoracostomy include wound tract infection and empyema. With meticulous aseptic techniques, the incidence of both should be well under 1%.

There are enough (class I and II) data to recommend prophylactic antibiotic use in patients receiving tube thoracostomy following chest trauma. The data suggest there may be a reduction in the incidence of pneumonia but **not** empyema in trauma patients receiving prophylactic antibiotics when a tube thoracostomy is placed.[17]

Routine antibiotics are not a substitute for good surgical technique.

On the frequently discussed issue of negative suction, a recent prospective study concluded that routine negative suction confers **no** advantage in patients with uncomplicated traumatic pneumothorax, haemothorax, or haemopneumothorax.[25]

8.8 SURGICAL APPROACHES TO THE THORAX

The choice of approach to the injured thorax should be determined by three factors:

- The hemithorax and its contents
- The stability of the patient
- Whether the indication for surgery is acute or chronic (non-acute)

A useful distinction can be made with respect to indications (**Table 8.4**). It will be noted that the acute indications include all acutely life-threatening situations,

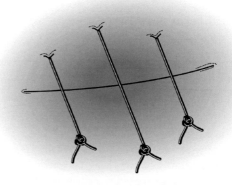

Figure 8.15 End result following drain removal.

Table 8.4 Indications for Surgery in the Thorax

Acute indications	Chronic indications
• Cardiac tamponade	• Unevacuated clotted haemothorax
• Acute deterioration	• Chronic traumatic diaphragmatic hernia
• Vascular injury at the thoracic outlet	• Traumatic atrioventricular fistula
• Loss of chest wall substance	• Traumatic cardiac septal or valvular lesions
• Endoscopic or radiological evidence of tracheal, oesophageal, or great vessel injury	• Missed tracheobronchial injury or tracheooesophageal fistula
• Massive or continuing haemothorax	• Infected intrapulmonary haematoma
• Bullet embolism to the heart or pulmonary artery	
• Penetrating mediastinal injury	

whilst the chronic or non-acute indications are essentially late presentations.

The surgical approaches include:

- Anterolateral thoracotomy
- Median sternotomy
- Bilateral thoracotomy ('clamshell' incision)
- Posterolateral thoracotomy
- (The 'trapdoor' incision) – **Obsolete**

Anterolateral thoracotomy and sternotomy are by far the most utilized incisions. It is **seldom** necessary to resort to the last three mentioned approaches in the acute situation. Of these, the bilateral trans-sternal thoracotomy (the 'clamshell' incision) is complex and somewhat mutilating, with significant postoperative morbidity, but it offers acceptable access in patients *in extremis*, particularly those with gunshot traversing the midline.

In the *unstable* patient, the choice of approach usually will be an anterolateral thoracotomy or median sternotomy, depending upon the suspected injury. In the case of the *stable* patient, the choice of approach must be planned after proper evaluation and workup have clearly identified the nature of the injury.

If time permits, intubation (or reintubation) with a double-lumen endotracheal tube, to allow selective deflation or ventilation of each lung, can be very helpful and occasionally life-saving; however, advice should be sought from an experienced anaesthetist, as this procedure takes time and requires appropriate training.

8.8.1 Anterolateral Thoracotomy

This is the approach of choice in most unstable patients and is utilized for EDT (**Figure 8.16**):

- This approach allows rapid access to the injured hemithorax and its contents.
- It is made with the patient in the supine position with no special positioning requirements or instruments.
- It has the advantages that it:
  - May be extended across the sternum into the contralateral hemithorax (the 'clamshell' incision or bilateral thoracotomy).
  - May be extended downwards to create a thoracoabdominal incision.

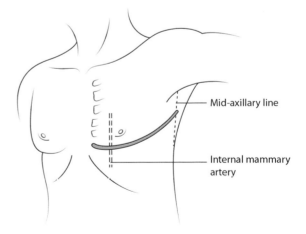

Figure 8.16 Left anterolateral thoracotomy.

This is the approach of choice in injury to any part of the left thorax or an injury above the nipple line in the right thorax. It should be noted that right lower-thoracic injuries (i.e., below the nipple line) usually involve bleeding from the liver. In these cases, the approach should initially be a midline laparotomy, the chest being entered **only** if no source of intra-abdominal bleeding is found.

8.8.1.1 TECHNIQUE

A slight tilt of the patient to the right is advisable; this is achieved by use of either a sandbag or other support, or by tilting the table.

The incision is made through the fourth or fifth intercostal space from the costochondral junction anteriorly to the mid-axillary line posteriorly, following the upper border of the lower rib in order to avoid damage to the intercostal neurovascular bundle.

The muscle groups are divided down to the periosteum of the lower rib. The muscle groups of the serratus anterior posteriorly and the intercostals medially and anteriorly are divided. The trapezius and the pectoralis major are avoided. Care should be taken at the anterior end of the incision, where the internal mammary artery runs and may be transected.

The parietal pleura is then opened, taking care to avoid the internal mammary artery adjacent to the sternal border. These vessels are ligated if necessary.

A Finochietto retractor is placed with the handle away from the sternum (i.e., laterally placed), the ribs are spread, and intrathoracic inspection for identification of injuries is carried out after suctioning. In cases of ongoing bleeding, an autotransfusion suction device is advisable.

Note that it is important to identify the lateral-lying phrenic nerve in its course across the pericardium if this structure is to be opened – the pericardiotomy is made 1 cm anterior and vertical to the nerve trunk in order to avoid damage and subsequent morbidity.

8.8.1.2 CLOSURE

Following definitive manoeuvres, the anterolateral thoracotomy is closed in layers over one or two large-bore intercostal tube drains and after careful haemostasis and copious lavage.

The ribs and intercostal muscles should be closed with synthetic absorbable sutures.

Closure of discrete muscle layers reduces both pain and long-term disability.

The skin is routinely closed.

8.8.2 **Median Sternotomy**

This incision is the approach of choice in patients with a penetrating injury at the base of the neck (Zone I) and the thoracic outlet, as well as to the heart itself. It allows access to the pericardium and heart, the arch of the aorta, and the origins of the great vessels. It has the attraction of allowing upwards extension into the neck (as a Henry's incision), extension downwards into a midline laparotomy, or lateral extension into a supraclavicular approach (**Figure 8.17**). It has the relative disadvantage of requiring a sternal saw or chisel (of the Lebsche type). In addition, the infrequent but significant complication of sternal sepsis may occur postoperatively, especially in the emergency setting. In general, the median sternotomy patient endures less postoperative pain than those who undergo anterolateral thoracotomy.

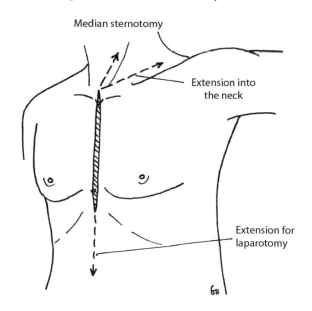

Figure 8.17 Median sternotomy.

8.8.2.1 TECHNIQUE

The incision is made with the patient fully supine, in the midline from the suprasternal notch to below the xiphoid cartilage. A finger-sweep is used to open spaces behind the sternum, above and below. Excision of the xiphoid cartilage may be necessary if this is large and intrusive and can be done with heavy scissors.

Split section (bisection) of the sternum is carried out with a saw (either oscillating or a braided-wire Gigli saw) or a Lebsche knife, commencing from above and moving downwards. This is an important point to avoid inadvertent damage to vascular structures in the mediastinum. In addition, be aware of the possible presence of the large transverse communicating vein, which may be found in the areolar tissue of the suprasternal space of Burns and must be controlled.

8.8.2.2 CLOSURE

- The pericardium is usually left open after trauma to prevent re-accumulation of fluid.
- If closure is considered, use an absorbable suture to avoid adhesion formation.
- Two mediastinal tube drains are brought out through epigastric incisions.
- Closure of the sternotomy is made with horizontal sternal wires or encircling heavy non-absorbable suture (braided, non-absorbable).
- Closure of the linea alba should be by non-absorbable suture.

8.8.3 The 'Clamshell' Thoracotomy

This is the thoracic equivalent of the chevron or 'bucket handle' upper abdominal incision, providing wide exposure to both hemithoraces. It is usually necessary to use this incision only when it becomes necessary to gain access to both hemithoraces.

The clamshell is essentially a bilateral fourth or fifth interspace thoracotomy, linked by division of the sternum, which allows the chest to be opened very widely anteriorly. The sternum is divided using a Gigli saw, chisel, or bone-cutting forceps (**Figure 8.18**).

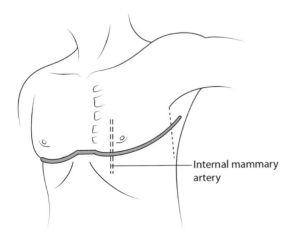

Figure 8.18 Bilateral trans-sternal thoracotomy ('clamshell' thoracotomy).

This rapid incision is particularly effective in those situations where it is important to achieve rapid access to the *opposite* side of the chest, especially posteriorly, such as for:

- Transmediastinal injury
- Lung injury
- Injury on the right, where aortic control may be necessary.

This is the incision which allows access to the most thoracic structures. It has been recently demonstrated through cadaveric studies that the clamshell incision gives access to the most intrathoracic organs, but it is inferior to median sternotomy in accessing upper mediastinal vascular structures.

Pitfall

It is essential to ligate the internal mammary arteries, and to ensure haemostasis prior to closure.

Warning!

The clamshell incision carries a very high morbidity and a high risk of sternal non-union, and it is *very painful*. It should *only* be considered if more limited exposure is impossible. Recovery is slower, with a high postoperative morbidity, and it is mostly permanently incapacitating, due to ongoing movement and non-union of the sternal transection.

8.8.4 Posterolateral Thoracotomy

This approach requires appropriate positioning of the patient and is usually used in the elective setting for definitive lung and oesophageal surgery. It is not usually employed in the acute setting, as access is very limited. It is more time-consuming in approach and closure, since the bulkier muscle groups of the posterolateral thorax are traversed, and scapular retraction is necessary.

8.8.5 'Trapdoor' Thoracotomy

This incision is considered ***obsolete***.

Instead, a combined sternotomy and right clavicular incision may be utilized for distal innominate or proximal right subclavian artery injuries, whilst a combined antero-lateral thoracotomy and separate clavicular incision utilized for left subclavian artery injuries. Resection of the clavicular head may facilitate exposure for each.

8.9 EMERGENCY DEPARTMENT THORACOTOMY

8.9.1 History

Rapid emergency medical response times and advances in pre-hospital care have led to increasing numbers of patients arriving in resuscitation *in extremis*. Salvage of these patients often demands immediate control of haemorrhage and desperate measures to resuscitate them. This has often been attempted in hopeless situations, and a differentiation must be made between the true EDT indications and futile care.

In 1874, Schiff described open cardiac massage, and in 1901, Rehn sutured a right ventricle in a patient presenting with cardiac tamponade. The limited success of EDT in most circumstances, however, prohibited the use of the technique for the next six or seven decades. A revival of interest occurred in the 1970s, when the procedure was initially revived by Ben Taub General Hospital in Houston for the treatment of cardiac injuries. It has subsequently been applied as a means of temporary aortic occlusion in exsanguinating abdominal trauma. More recently, there has been decreased enthusiasm, a more selective approach particularly with respect to blunt trauma, and consideration of other techniques such as resuscitative endovascular balloon occlusion of the aorta (REBOA) (see Section 15.3).

> *There is an extremely high mortality rate associated with all thoracotomies performed anywhere outside the operating theatre, especially when performed by non-surgeons on moribund patients.*

It is important early on to differentiate between the definitions of thoracotomy:

- EDT for patients *in extremis*
  - To control haemorrhage
  - To control the aortic outflow (aortic 'cross-clamping')
  - To perform internal cardiac massage
  - To relieve cardiac tamponade
- *Planned* resuscitative thoracotomy (i.e., in the operating room) in acutely deteriorating patients for control of haemorrhage

With EDT, it is also important to differentiate between:

- Patients with 'no signs of life'
- Patients with 'no vital signs' in whom cardiac electrical activity, pupillary activity, and/or respiratory effort is still evident (This is where cardiac ultrasound can be very helpful.)

Obviously, the results of EDT in these two circumstances will differ.

8.9.2 Objectives

The primary objectives of EDT in this set of circumstances are to:

- Release cardiac tamponade.
- Control intrathoracic bleeding.
- Control air embolism or bronchopleural fistula.
- Permit open cardiac massage.
- Allow for temporary occlusion of the descending aorta to improve coronary and cerebral perfusion and limit subdiaphragmatic haemorrhage.

EDT has been shown to be most productive in life-threatening penetrating cardiac stab wounds, especially when cardiac tamponade is present. Patients requiring EDT for blunt cardiac injury rarely survive, even in established trauma centres. The outcome in the field is even worse. Indications for the procedure in military practice are essentially the same as in civilian practice.

EDT and the necessary rapid use of sharp surgical instruments, as well as exposure to the patient's blood, pose certain risks to the resuscitating surgeon. Contact rates of the patient's blood to the surgeon's skin approximate to 20%. 'Invisible pathogens' such as human immunodeficiency virus (HIV), hepatitis C, and others must be considered. Although the likelihood of a practitioner contracting HIV or hepatitis due to an EDT occupational exposure is exceedingly low, the use of universal precautions minimizes this risk.[26]

8.9.3 Indications and Contraindications

As indicated in EAST's practice management guidelines for adults[27] and children,[28] there are instances where EDT has been shown to have clear benefit (**Table 8.5**).

Table 8.5 An Evidence-Based Approach to Patient Selection for Emergency Department Thoracotomy: A Practice Management Guideline from the Eastern Association for the Surgery of Trauma

PICO	Recommendation
PICO Question 1	
In patients presenting pulseless to the emergency department with signs of life after penetrating thoracic injury (P), does EDT (I) versus resuscitation without EDT (C) improve hospital survival and neurologically intact hospital survival (O)?	**In patients presenting pulseless to the emergency department with signs of life after penetrating thoracic injury, we strongly recommend that patients undergo EDT.** This recommendation is based on moderate quality of evidence and places emphasis on patient preference for improved survival and neurologically intact survival after EDT.
PICO Question 2	
In patients presenting pulseless to the emergency department without signs of life after penetrating thoracic injury (P), does EDT (I) versus resuscitation without EDT (C) improve hospital survival and neurologically intact hospital survival (O)?	**In patients presenting pulseless to the emergency department without signs of life after penetrating thoracic injury, we conditionally recommend that patients undergo EDT.** This recommendation is based on moderate quality of evidence and places emphasis on patient preference for improved survival and neurologically intact survival after EDT, but also acknowledges that elapsed time without signs of life is an important component.
PICO Question 3	
In patients presenting pulseless to the emergency department with signs of life after penetrating extrathoracic injury (P), does EDT versus resuscitation without EDT (C) improve hospital survival and neurologically intact hospital survival (O)?	**In patients presenting pulseless to the emergency department with signs of life after penetrating extrathoracic injury, we conditionally recommend that patients undergo EDT.** This recommendation does not pertain to patients with isolated cranial injuries. This recommendation is based on moderate quality of evidence and places emphasis on patient preference for improved survival and neurologically intact survival after EDT, but also acknowledges that penetrating injuries to all extrathoracic anatomic areas will not have equivalent salvage rates after EDT.
PICO Question 4	
In patients presenting pulseless to the emergency department without signs of life after penetrating extrathoracic injury (P), does EDT versus resuscitation without EDT (C) improve hospital survival and neurologically intact hospital survival (O)?	**In patients presenting pulseless to the emergency department without signs of life after penetrating extrathoracic injury, we conditionally recommend that patients undergo EDT.** This recommendation does not pertain to patients with isolated cranial injuries and is based on low quality of evidence. The majority of subcommittee members believed that most patients would prefer undergoing EDT in hopes of improved survival and neurologically intact survival.
PICO Question 5	
In patients presenting pulseless to the emergency department with signs of life after blunt injury (P), does EDT versus resuscitation without EDT (C) improve hospital survival and neurologically intact hospital survival (O)?	**In patients presenting pulseless to the emergency department with signs of life after blunt injury, we conditionally recommend that patients undergo EDT.** This recommendation is based on moderate quality of evidence and places emphasis on patient preference for improved survival and neurologically intact survival after EDT.
PICO Question 6	
In patients presenting pulseless to the emergency department without signs of life after blunt injury (P), does EDT versus resuscitation without EDT (C) improve hospital survival and neurologically intact hospital survival (O)?	**In patients presenting pulseless to the emergency department without signs of life after blunt injury, we conditionally recommend against the performance of EDT.** This recommendation is based on low quality of evidence and reflects subcommittee group disagreement regarding the strength of the unanimous recommendation against EDT.
Blood-borne pathogen exposure	Regardless, when needlestick or cut exposure transmission rates from known seropositive blood are considered, it is imperative that universal precautions are maintained for all resuscitations.

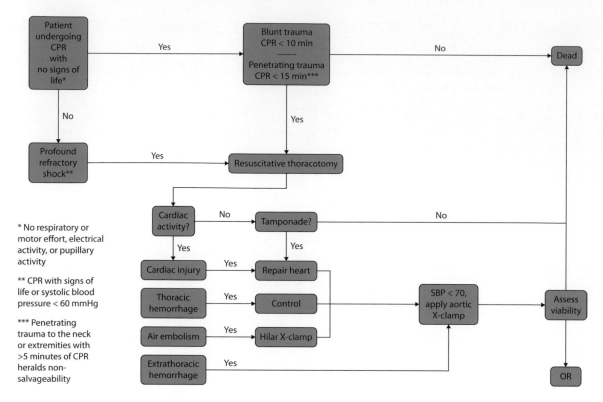

Figure 8.19 Western Trauma Association algorithm for resuscitative thoracotomy.

See also the Western Trauma Association algorithm for resuscitative thoracotomy for adults (**Figure 8.19**)[29] and for paediatric resuscitative thoracotomy (**Figures 14.1** and **14.2**).[30]

Patients who are most likely to benefit are:

- Patients presenting pulseless to the ED with signs of life after penetrating thoracic injury (best survival).
- Patients presenting pulseless to the ED without signs of life after penetrating thoracic injury (assuming reasonable arrest until EDT times, although data are limited, probably < 15 min).
- Patients presenting pulseless to the ED with signs of life after penetrating extrathoracic injury.
- Patients presenting pulseless to the ED without signs of life after penetrating extrathoracic injury. (Assuming reasonable arrest until EDT times, although data are limited, probably < 15 min).
- Patients presenting pulseless to the ED with signs of life after blunt injury.

Less clear benefit occurs for:

- Blunt-injured patients. Not only do blunt-injured patients survive less often after EDT, but also, they more often have severe neurologic impairment after EDT. Whilst exact reasons for this are unknown, this is likely multifactorial, including polytrauma TBI and the absence of a lesion to repair in the ED.
- Patients presenting with moderate post-injury hypotension (blood pressure < 80 mmHg), potentially due to intra-abdominal aortic injury (e.g., an epigastric gunshot wound).
- Major pelvic fractures.
- Active intra-abdominal haemorrhage.

EDT is *contraindicated*:

- In patients presenting pulseless to the ED without signs of life after blunt injury. Consider the use of cardiac ultrasound (perfusing cardiac motion or the presence of hemopericardium) to aid the diagnosis and assess for futility.

8.9.4 **Results**

Outcomes after EDT vary according to injury mechanism, anatomic injury location, and presenting physiology. Pooled data from all prior studies reported in the 2015 EAST Guideline[27] determined that 21% of patients who presented pulseless after penetrating thoracic injury with ED signs of life survived their hospitalization, whilst only 8% of patients who presented pulseless after penetrating thoracic injury without ED signs of life survived. Similarly, 16% of patients who presented pulseless after penetrating extrathoracic injury (e.g., abdomen or extremity) with ED signs of life survived their hospitalization, whilst only 3% of patients who presented pulseless after penetrating extrathoracic injury without ED signs of life survived. When blunt-injured patient EDT survival data were pooled, 5% of patients who presented pulseless after blunt injury mechanisms with ED signs of life survived their hospitalization, whilst < 1% of patients who presented pulseless after blunt injury without ED signs of life survived.

8.9.5 **When to Stop an Emergency Department Thoracotomy**

EDT is a 'team event'. It should not be prolonged unduly but should have specific endpoints. If an injury is repaired and the patient responds, he or she should be moved to the operating room for definitive repair or closure.

EDT should be terminated if:

- Irreparable cardiac or great vessel damage has occurred.
- The patient is identified as having massive head injuries.
- Return of spontaneous circulation (ROSC) is not achieved within 15 minutes.
- A perfusing cardiac rhythm is not maintained to allow transportation to the operating room.

8.9.6 **Technique**

8.9.6.1 **INSTRUMENT REQUIREMENTS**

The numbers of instruments and types of equipment necessary to perform EDT are as follows:

- A scalpel, with a #20 or #21 blade
- Forceps
- A suitable retractor such as a Finochietto chest retractor or a Balfour abdominal retractor
- A Lebsche knife and mallet or Gigli saw for the sternum
- Large vascular clamps, such as Satinsky vascular clamps (large and small)
- Mayo scissors
- Metzenbaum scissors
- Long needle-holders
- Internal defibrillator paddles
- Sutures, swabs, and Teflon pledgets
- Sterile skin preparation and drapes
- Good light

8.9.6.2 **APPROACH**

Two basic incisions are used in EDT: the left anterolateral thoracotomy and the bilateral or clamshell thoracotomy. These are applied based on external wounds or procedural findings.

Routine immediate resuscitation protocols as per ATLS are instituted, and once indications for EDT have been fulfilled, EDT should follow without delay.

Pitfall

If the conditions are not fulfilled, you are embarking upon futile care.

The left anterolateral thoracotomy is the most common site for urgent access. The incision is placed in the fifth intercostal space through muscle, periosteum, and parietal pleura from the sternum anteriorly to the mid-axillary line laterally, following the upper border of rib, and care is taken to avoid the internal mammary artery. This curvilinear incision can be extended as a bilateral incision requiring horizontal division of the sternum and ligation of the internal mammary vessels bilaterally. It affords excellent access to both pleural cavities, the pericardial cavity, and even the abdominal cavity if required.

The median sternotomy affords the best exposure to the anterior and middle mediastinum, including the heart and great vessels, and is typically advocated for penetrating wounds, particularly of the upper chest between the nipples. This can be extended supraclavicularly for access to control subclavian and brachiocephalic vascular injuries.

In general, this incision is not as rapid as the left anterolateral thoracotomy; thus, it is often better utilized for patients in shock in the operating room rather than moribund patients in the ED.

8.10 SURGICAL PROCEDURES

8.10.1 Pericardial Tamponade

- Open the pericardium in a cranial to caudal direction, anterior to the phrenic nerve.
- The pericardial incision is initiated using either a knife or the sharp point of a pair of scissors, and blood and clots are evacuated.
- It is important to examine the whole heart to localize the source of bleeding.
- Temporize the source of bleeding, and transport to the operating room for definitive repair.
- Do not fully close the pericardium after the procedure; drain it.

Pitfall

It is important to identify the phrenic nerve prior to opening the pericardium at least 1 cm anterior to this structure.

8.10.2 Cardiac Injury

Cardiac bleeding points on the ventricle are initially managed with digital pressure, and those on the atria and great vessels by partially occluding vascular clamps (e.g., Satinsky clamps).

If the heart is beating, repair should be delayed until initial resuscitation measures have been completed. If it is not beating, suturing precedes resuscitation.

- Wherever possible, initial control of a myocardial laceration should be digital, whilst the damage is assessed.
- Use 3-0 or 4-0 non-absorbable monofilament sutures tied gently to effect the repair. Pledgets may be helpful.
- Foley catheters may be used to temporarily control haemorrhage prior to definitive repair in the ED or operating theatre. A Foley catheter with a large (30 mL) balloon is preferable.
- Skin staplers may be helpful as a temporizing measure, and will allow control of the bleeding, with minimal manipulation of the heart.

Pitfalls

- There is a real danger of extending the damage if the Foley balloon pulls through the laceration. Use a 30 mL balloon and avoid other than gentle traction.
- Care should be exercised near coronary arteries. Whereas a vertical mattress suture is normally acceptable, it may be necessary to use a horizontal mattress suture under the vessel to avoid occluding it.
- Staples often eventually tear out, so the repair should not be regarded as definitive. Leave the staples in place, and suture around them in a horizontal mattress fashion for definitive repair.

Posterior wounds are more difficult, as they necessitate elevation of the heart before their closure, which can lead to further haemodynamic compromise. Slowly elevating the heart with swabs may be better tolerated, and dosing epinephrine may help. With large wounds of the ventricle or inaccessible posterior wounds, temporary digital inflow occlusion might be necessary to facilitate repair.[31-33]

The great majority of low-pressure venous and atrial wounds can be closed with simple continuous sutures or horizontal mattress sutures of a 3-0 or 4-0 monofilament. Bolstering the suture with Teflon pledgets is **not** essential, but may occasionally be required, particularly if there is surrounding contusion, or there is proximity of the wound to a coronary artery.

If the stab wound or gunshot wound is in proximity to a coronary artery, care must be taken not to suture the vessels. This can be achieved by passing horizontal mattress sutures *underneath* the coronary vessels, avoiding ligation of the vessel.

If the coronary arteries have been transected, two options exist. Closure of proximal coronary vessels can be accomplished in the beating heart using a fine 6-0 or 7-0 polypropylene suture, under magnification if necessary. The second option is to temporarily initiate inflow occlusion and fibrillation. However, both measures have a high risk associated with them. Heparinization is optimally avoided in the trauma patient, and fibrillation in the presence of shock and acidosis may be difficult to reverse. Bypass is usually reserved for patients who have injury to the valves, chordae tendineae, or septum. In most instances, these injuries are not immediately life-threatening, but become evident over a few hours or days following the injury.

Most patients with blunt injuries to the heart who survive the initial resuscitation and require operative intervention can likewise be treated with simple off-pump methods, although more complex injuries may require immediate cardiopulmonary bypass and advanced techniques. Of note, blunt cardiac ruptured tissue is often difficult to suture repair and is easily torn. Pledgets are helpful.

8.10.3 Pulmonary Haemorrhage

- Access is best achieved by anterolateral thoracotomy on the appropriate side.
- With localized bleeding sites, rapid control can be achieved with a vascular clamp placed across the hilum, occluding the pulmonary artery, vein, and main-stem bronchus, or across the affected segment if necessary.
- The affected segment is then dealt with, preferably in controlled circumstances in the operating theatre by local oversewing, segmental resection, or pulmonary tractotomy.

Pulmonary tractotomy is a means of controlling tracts that pass through multiple lung segments where the extent of injury precludes pulmonary resection. It is a means of non-anatomical lung preservation in which one arm of the linear stapler is placed into the lung parenchyma injury tract, and the lung is divided with the stapler to allow blood vessels and airways in the bases to be repaired; the divided edges are then oversewn.

With massive haemorrhage from multiple or indeterminate sites, or widespread destruction of lung parenchyma leaving large areas of non-viable tissue, hilar clamping with a large soft vascular clamp or a large, doubled vessel loop, or a soft catheter across the hilar structures occluding the pulmonary artery, pulmonary vein, and main-stem bronchus, is employed until a definitive surgical procedure can be performed.

Air embolism is controlled by placing a clamp across the hilar structures, and air is evacuated by needle aspiration of the elevated left ventricular apex.

8.10.4 Pulmonary Tractotomy

- This is used where the injury crosses more than one segment, commonly caused by a penetrating injury. Anatomical resection may not be possible.

- Linear staplers can be introduced along both sides of the tract, the tract being divided and then oversewn.
- If staplers are not available, straight soft bowel clamps or long straight haemostatic clamps can be inserted in similar fashion, the parenchyma divided, and haemostatic sutures applied.
- Please note that the apex of the incision (the deep part of the incision) is where blood vessels and bronchi are located; thus, sutures must include this area for the tractotomy to be satisfactory.
- This procedure is part of the 'damage control' techniques for the chest.

8.10.5 Lobectomy or Pneumonectomy[34]

- This is rarely performed, usually done to control massive haemorrhage from the pulmonary hilum.
- Lung preservation should be attempted whenever possible.
- A double-lumen endotracheal tube should be used whenever possible.
- For segmental pneumonectomy, use of the GIA stapler is helpful. The staple line can then be oversewn.
- Medications such as eproprostenol may help reduce pulmonary pressures in these circumstances.

8.10.6 Thoracotomy with Aortic Cross-Clamping

This technique is employed to optimize oxygen transport to vital proximal structures (the heart and brain), maximize coronary perfusion, and possibly limit infradiaphragmatic haemorrhage in both blunt and penetrating trauma.

The thoracic aorta is cross-clamped inferior to the left pulmonary hilum, and the area is exposed by elevating the left lung anteriorly and superiorly. The mediastinal pleura is dissected under direct vision, the aorta being separated by blunt dissection from the oesophagus anteriorly and the prevertebral fascia posteriorly. When properly exposed, the aorta is occluded using a large vascular clamp. It is important that the aortic cross-clamp time be kept to the absolute minimum – that is, that the clamp is removed once effective cardiac function and systemic arterial pressure have been achieved – as the metabolic penalty rapidly becomes exponential once beyond 30 minutes.

Begin unclamping the aortic cross clamp,
one 'click' at a time.

8.10.7 **Aortic Injury**

- Most patients with these injuries do not survive to reach hospital. (Some reported urban penetrating series, report 'no survivors'.)
- Patients who arrive alive usually have contained injuries. It is essential to identify and manage other life-threatening injuries before attempting to characterize and manage the aortic injury.
- Current recommendations support the use of endovascular stenting (endovascular aneurysm repair [EVAR]) for contained aortic injuries, as it carries a lower rate of complications compared to open surgery.
- Open surgery when required must be performed under cardiopulmonary bypass to reduce the risk of paraplegia.

8.10.8 **Tracheobronchial Injury**

- Flexible bronchoscopy is very helpful in assessment.
- Formal repair should be undertaken under ideal conditions, with removal of devitalized tissue.

8.10.9 **Oesophageal Injury**

- Surgical repair is essential; drainage of the mediastinum is mandatory.
- Two-layer repair (mucosal and muscular) has been advocated, but a single full-thickness layer of interrupted sutures incorporating the mucosa seems as effective.
- If possible, the repair should be wrapped in autogenous tissue.
- A feeding jejunostomy may be considered, because the stomach should be preserved in case oesophageal substitution is required later.
- A cervical oesophagostomy is not usually required or recommended; large-bore drains offer similar results to create a controlled fistula.

8.11 **SUMMARY**

Success in the management of thoracic injury in those cases requiring operation lies in the 'team approach', with good anaesthesia and rapid access to the thoracic cavity with good exposure. Thus, good lighting, appropriate instrumentation, functioning suction apparatus, and a 'controlled, aggressive, but calm frame of mind' on the part of the team will result in acceptable, uncomplicated survival figures.

8.12 **ANAESTHESIA FOR THORACIC TRAUMA**

In all chest trauma, decision-making, assistance within the operation, and identifying and treating the injury, anaesthesia plays an important part. There are major differences in the presentation, treatment, and prognosis of a penetrating or blunt thoracic injury. What they have in common is that if they arrive alive in hospital, with vigilant reception on arrival, they stand a fighting chance.

8.12.1 **Penetrating Thoracic Injury**

Depending on the cause of the penetration, the chances of the patient range from excellent (knife, low-energy-dispersing projectile) to very bad with structures (large vessels, heart) damaged beyond repair.

The ATLS 'airway, breathing, circulation' (ABC) principles should focus on signs of tamponade, pneumothorax, and massive air leaks (emphysema), and should not miss hidden injuries such as penetration of the oesophagus in a secondary survey. As a priority, remember to inspect the back of the patient immediately for an exit or entry wound, and mark these with metal markers.

Penetrating thoracic injury is most often treated by chest tube insertion. A massive air leak will alert to large airway penetration, massive blood loss from cardiac and large vessel injury, and food from an oesophageal or stomach injury.

The massive air leak and a substantial airway bleeding should initially be treated by intubation, with either a normal endotracheal tube or a double-lumen tube (DLT). This will allow a flexible bronchoscopy to identify the rupture site and isolate the rupture from the rest of the airway. The single-lumen tube can be positioned past the rupture; the DLT can be used to identify the injured side. The single-lumen tube will allow a type of bronchus blocker in a later stage to assist the operation.

Cardiac tamponade and massive cardiac or large vessel injury will all require an emergency thoracic intervention with anaesthesia prepared for very fast, large blood loss.

8.12.2 **Blunt Thoracic Injury**

Blunt thoracic injury commonly results from motor vehicle crashes, but may also be the result of a fall, being crushed under a large object, a blast injury from an explosion, or a combination of the above. The injury usually works from the outside inwards: via the bony thoracic wall and spine, to the lungs and the mediastinum. The severity of the damage will signify how deep the damage is likely to be. The lungs provide some protection to the mediastinum. Sometimes, however, especially in cases of a blast injury, the force can work from the inside out when the blast wave is swallowed or inhaled, opening the deeper structures, lung, and oesophagus to the blast wave or rapidly expanding shock wave.

Blunt trauma to the heart may lead to a cardiac contusion or chamber rupture. Myocardial contusion should be suspected based on the trauma mechanism and the additional trauma signs: rib fractures, lung contusion, dysrhythmias, sinus tachycardia, or ectopic beats. It can present as a progressive disease where an abnormal 12-lead electrocardiograph (ECG) should lead to a cardiac ultrasound. Signs of left ventricle ischaemia ST-T changes and Q-waves may show. All types of atrioventricular blocks can be a result of the oedema in the cardiac muscle. In TTE or TOE, the valves should be inspected for ruptures, and wall motion abnormalities should be excluded. Intra-aortic balloon counter-pulsation should be considered if there is cardiogenic shock.

Most deaths are from ventricular fibrillation. Management for valve damage may be operative, and for the myocardial contusion just supportive.

For a free wall cardiac rupture, a rapid diagnosis needs to be made using eFAST, CT, TTE, and TOE. A sternotomy will be the most appropriate approach for an isolated cardiac injury. If cardiopulmonary bypass is available, this will facilitate the operation.

8.12.2.1 **CONTAINED LARGE VESSEL RUPTURE OR ANEURYSM**

A contained large vessel rupture can be dealt with by the cardiac surgeon or the interventional radiologist. The thoracic aorta will most often tear at the ligamentum arteriosum where the vessel is restricted in its movement. Support for the intervention will be with a TOE and careful manipulation of the blood pressure to prevent shear stress on the tear. Open repair will follow the same techniques as an elective case, with anaesthetic management consisting of a careful titration of vasodilatation and inotropes on clamping and clamp release. A cardiopulmonary bypass may be necessary.

8.12.2.2 **PULMONARY CONTUSION**

The pulmonary contusion is an entity in development. The initial chest X-ray will not show the complete full-blown contusion, and in the stable patient, CT scan is the modality of choice. The contusion will very often be accompanied by a flail chest. The contusion is a complex of intraparenchymal bleeding, oedema, and alveolar collapse due to reduced surfactant production. This leads to ventilation–perfusion mismatch, shunting, and decreased compliance. Treatment consists of a ventilation strategy where one should realize that the ventilation stressors are primarily exerted on the healthier lung. Low volume, high positive end-expiratory pressure (PEEP), permissive hypercapnia, and maintaining a minimum oxygen saturation in order to avoid high oxygen concentrations may be needed. If oxygenation to the required level is not achieved, extracorporeal membrane oxygenation (ECMO) can be considered to bridge the time needed to reduce swelling and blood in the alveoli (see Section 17.3).

8.12.2.3 **LARGE AIRWAY DISRUPTION**

The disruption of the trachea or a major bronchus can be potentially life-threatening. The insertion of a chest tube may open the way for air following the path of least resistance away from the attached lung, thus making ventilation impossible. With an avulsed lung (fallen lung sign on chest X-ray), spontaneous ventilation may be all that keeps the patient alive until the lungs are isolated.

A massive emphysema rising and falling with ventilation should instantly alert to a large airway leak. Lung separation can be achieved by advancing the endotracheal tube beyond the hole, or into the non-disrupted main bronchus. Flexible bronchoscopy may be supportive for identifying where the air leak is. Other options are a DLT or a bronchus blocker. For a large bronchial disruption, a rapid thoracotomy and clamping of the open bronchus can facilitate ventilation.

8.12.2.4 **FLAIL CHEST**

A flail chest can present itself on a scale ranging from an acceptable affliction to a near-death experience where the pain makes breathing impossible. The pain can be treated with morphine, although this may complicate breathing as well; an epidural; and/or ventilation assistance ranging from continuous positive airway pressure (CPAP) to intubation and assisted ventilation. This will depend on concomitant injury. Indications for operative fixation include flail chest, reduction of pain and disability, a chest wall deformity or defect, symptomatic non-union, thoracotomy for other indications, and open fractures. Minimally invasive techniques have been developed and are currently being used.

8.12.2.5 DIAPHRAGMATIC INJURY

Diaphragm rupture is easily missed, especially on the right when covered by the liver. Anaesthetic management will depend on if a thoracic or abdominal approach is chosen. A gastric tube should be inserted to deflate the stomach, and aspiration prevention measures should be utilized for intubation. Nitrous oxide should be avoided. If a thoracic approach is indicated, lung separation is an option to facilitate the operation.

8.12.3 Anaesthetic Management of Thoracic Injury

When presented with a massive thoracic injury, preparation is essential. A guess needs to be made regarding what surgery will be required, and the anaesthesia tailored to accommodate this. Will lung separation be helpful? A DLT makes a surgeon's life easy, but this is only a relative indication. Absolute indications include significant lung bleeding, contamination, overflow from lung abscess, and the inability to ventilate where isolation of the damaged lung is needed. Insert an arterial line for blood gases and large-bore cannulae.

ANAESTHESIOLOGICAL CONSIDERATIONS

- Penetrating trauma is most often treated by chest tubes. Use standard endotracheal tubes for thoracic trauma; DLTs are rarely needed.
- Mark all wounds with metal markers (e.g., a paper clip) before any X-ray or CT scan to show wound track (e.g., to clarify a route in close proximity to the diaphragm).
- Massive air leaks and substantial airway bleeding should initially be treated by endotracheal intubation, preferably below the tracheal injury. A DLT or a bronchial blocker might be considered at a later stage, or a normal tube can be advanced into the right main bronchus if a DLT is not available, for apnoeic surgery on the left lung.
- In the rare event of an emergency room thoracotomy, close communication is necessary in order to evaluate the function and filling of the heart. During suturing on the penetrated heart, low blood pressures are accepted and catecholamines are to be avoided.
- Urgent thoracotomy or sternotomy for pericardial tamponade in the operating theatre in an unstable patient is ideally done with the surgeon ready/prepped and a haemodynamically stable induction (e.g., ketamine 1–2 mg/kg, rocuronium 1.2 mg/kg), a standard endotracheal tube unless familiar with DLTs, fluid bolus, and vasopressors. Expect significant hypotension until the tamponade is relieved, then relative hypertension. In open chest surgery, a visual assessment of the heart can provide information on heart filling and function; is it collapsed, distended, or contracting well?
- Several rib fractures or flail chest might indicate lung contusions with ventilation–perfusion mismatch, shunting, and decreased compliance. Treatment consists of analgesia (consider regional anaesthesia early), restriction of fluids, and ventilatory support (e.g., early non-invasive ventilator support). ECMO might be considered in the extreme cases with persistent hypoxemia after failure of conventional mechanical ventilation.
- Blunt trauma to the heart may lead to a cardiac contusion with arrythmias, ruptures, valvular defects, or intimal tear of the coronary vessels. 12-lead ECG, troponins, and echocardiography are useful for diagnosis.

- Bronchial injuries should initially be treated by intubation with a normal endotracheal tube, preferably below the injury in the trachea, or in the healthy lung. A DLT should only be used as a primary device if the anaesthesiologist is very experienced with these devices and can place the endobronchial lumen without causing further injury.
- In diaphragmatic rupture, a gastric tube should be inserted.
- Consider cell salvage, especially in thoracic injury. Thoracic blood loss may be significant, and it will be non-contaminated blood that can be rehung as full blood, or preferably processed with the cell-saver, then presented as red cell concentrate.
- Autotransfusion may be considered in chest bleeding according to the institution's policy and experience.
- Some centres will undertake early rib fixation.
- Do repeated blood gases to assist in steering lung-protective ventilation.
- Do not forget associated head and cervical spine injuries which may mandate a different approach to the ventilation strategies described above.
- A good pain management strategy may prevent hospital complications such as pneumonia in patients with massive thoracic injury, especially multiple rib fractures. Consider early paravertebral catheters or thoracic epidural analgesia.
- Consider succinctly letting the surgeon know at an appropriate time:
    - Ongoing blood loss
    - Metabolic state (e.g., base deficit or lactate)
    - Vasopressor requirements
    - Overview of coagulation
- Consider asking the surgeon at an appropriate time:
    - Is the patient clotting clinically?
    - How does the perfusion of vital organs look clinically (e.g., bowel)?
    - What are the available treatment options?

LUNG AND HILAR INJURY

- Bleeding can be intrapleural or intrabronchial
    - *Surgeon and anaesthesiologist*: Communicate!
- Hilar injury
    - Risk of converting intrapleural bleeding into intrabronchial bleeding.
- Hilar clamping
    - Can cause acute right heart failure.
    - May require intermittent clamping.

TRACHEOBRONCHIAL INJURY

- 'Cuff beyond the injury'.
- Spontaneous ventilation is maintained until the cuff is below the lesion, if possible!
- Video bronchoscopy increases safety during intubation.

AIR EMBOLISM

- Penetrating chest + profound hypotension or cardiac arrest after intubation and positive-pressure ventilation.
- Trendelenburg's position:
    - Traps air in the apex of the ventricle.
- Hilum of the injured lung quickly controlled.
- Single-lung ventilation should be instituted.
- Needle aspiration is performed to remove air from the cardiac chambers.

- **Cardiac tamponade**
- **Risk** of haemodynamic collapse during induction
- Surgeons gowned and gloved, and the patient prepped and draped before administration of anaesthetic induction agents – may require emergent left anterolateral thoracotomy
- Placement of transcutaneous pacemaker/defibrillator pads for sternotomy incision – risk of arrhythmias

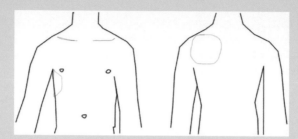

- Placement of transcutaneous pacemaker/defibrillator pads for sternotomy (Source Uptodate)
- **Cardiac arrest**
- Open-heart massage:
  - Two-handed technique.
  - One hand is inserted behind the heart and kept flat, whilst the other lies anteriorly.
  - Compress the heart in a 'clapping' manner from the apex to the superior aspect in an attempt to mimic normal cardiac ejection.
  - 100–120 beats per minute.
- Ventricular fibrillation:
  - Internal defibrillation paddles: 10–50 J shock

REFERENCES AND RECOMMENDED READING

References

1. Mancini M, Smith LM, Nein A, Buechler KJ. Early evacuation of clotted blood and haemothorax using thoracoscopy: case reports. *J Trauma.* 1993 Jan;34(1):144–7. doi: 10.1097/00005373-199301000-00028.

2. Kwan RO, Miraflor E, Yeung L, Strumwasser A, Victorino G. Bedside thoracic ultrasonography of the fourth intercostal space reliably determines safe removal of tube thoracostomy after traumatic injury. *J Trauma Acute Care Surg.* 2012 Dec;**73(6)**:1568–73. doi: 10.1097/TA.0b013e318265fc22.

3. Van As AB, Manganyi R, Brooks A. Treatment of thoracic trauma in children: literature review, Red Cross War Memorial Children's Hospital data analysis, and guidelines for management. *Eur J Pediatr Surg.* 2013 Dec;**23(6)**:434–43. doi: 10.1055/s-0033-1363160. Epub 2013 Dec 10. Review.

4. Kessel B, Dagan J, Swaid F, Ashkenazi I, Olsha O, Peleg K, Givon A. Rib fractures: comparison of associated injuries between pediatric and adult population. *Am J Surg.* 2014 Nov;**208(5)**:831–4. doi: 10.1016/j.amjsurg.2013.10.033. Epub 2014 Mar 26.

5. Lustenberger T, Talving P, Lam L, Inaba K, Mohseni S, Smith JA, et al. Penetrating cardiac trauma in adolescents: a rare injury with excessive mortality. *J Pediatr Surg.* 2013 Apr;**48(4)**:745–9. doi: 10.1016/j.jpedsurg.2012.08.020.

6. Lee LK, Rogers AJ, Ehrlich PF, Kwok M, Sokolove PE, Blumberg S, et al. Occult pneumothoraces in children with blunt torso trauma *Acad Emerg Med.* 2014 Apr;**21(4)**:440–8. doi: 10.1111/acem.12344.

7. Bouhemad B, Zhang M, Lu Q, Rouby JJ. Clinical review: bedside lung ultrasound in critical care practice. *Crit Care.* 2007;**11**:205. Review. doi: 10.1186/cc5668.

8. Advance Trauma Life Support Programme®. In: *Thoracic Skills,* 10th Edn. American College of Surgeons, Chicago, IL, USA. 2018:346–7.

9. Bansal V, Reid CM, Fortlage D, Lee J, Kobayashi L, Doucet J, et al. Determining injuries from posterior and flank stab wounds using computed tomography tractography *Am Surg*. 2014 April;**80(4)**:403–7.

10. O'Connor JV, DuBose JJ, Scalea TM. Damage-control thoracic surgery: Management and outcomes. *J Trauma Acute Care Surg*. 2014 Nov;**77(5)**:660–5. doi: 10.1097/TA.0000000000000451.

11. Goodman M, Lewis J, Guitron J, Reed M, Pritts T, Starnes S. Video-assisted thoracoscopic surgery for acute thoracic trauma. *J Emerg Trauma Shock*. 2013 Apr;**6(2)**:106–9. doi: 10.4103/0974-2700.110757.

12. Patel NJ, Dultz L, Ladhani HA, Cullinane DC, Klein E, McNickle AG, et al. Management of simple and retained hemothorax: a practice management guideline from the Eastern Association for the Surgery of Trauma Practice Guideline *Am J Surg*. 2021 May;**221(5)**:873–84. doi: 10.1016/j.amjsurg.2020.11.032. Epub 2020 Nov 17.

13. Welter S. Repair of tracheobronchial injuries *Thorac Surg Clin*. 2014 Feb;**24(1)**:41–50. doi: 10.1016/j.thorsurg.2013.10.006. Review.

14. Leinicke JA, Elmore L, Freeman BD, Colditz GA. Operative management of rib fractures in the setting of flail chest: a systematic review and meta-analysis. *Ann Surg*. 2013;**258(6)**. doi: 10.1097/SLA.0b013e3182895bb.

15. Cataneo AJM, Cataneo DC, De Oliveira FHS, Arruda KA, El Dib R, de Oliveira Carvalho PE. Surgical versus nonsurgical interventions for flail chest. *Cochrane Database Syst Rev*. 2015 Jul 29;2015**(7)**:CD009919. doi: 10.1002/14651858.CD009919.pub2.

16. Swart E, Laratta J, Slobogean G, Mehta S. Operative treatment of rib fractures in flail chest injuries: a meta-analysis and cost effectiveness analysis. *J Orthop Trauma*. 2017;**31(2)**:64–70(7). doi: 10.1097/BOT.0000000000000750.

17. Brasel KJ, Moore EE, Albrecht RA, deMoya M, Schreiber M, Karmy-Jones R, et al. Western trauma association critical decisions in trauma: management of rib fractures. *J Trauma Acute Care Surg*. 2017;**82(1)**:200–3. doi: 10.1097/TA.0000000000001301.

18. Kasotakis G, Hasenboehler EA, Streib EW, Patel N, Patel MB, Mayur B et al. Open reduction and Internal Fixation of rib fractures. An Eastern Association for the Surgery of Trauma Practice Management Guideline. *J Trauma Acute Care Surg*. 2017 Mar;**82(3)**:618–26. doi: 10.1097/TA.0000000000001350.

19. Mukherjee K, Schubl SD, Tominaga G, Cantrell S, Kim B, Haines KL, et al. Non-surgical management and analgesia strategies for older adults with multiple rib fractures: A systematic review, meta-analysis, and joint practice management guideline from the Eastern Association

for the Surgery of Trauma and the Chest Wall Injury Society. *J Trauma Acute Care Surg*. 2023 Mar 1;**94(3)**:398–407.doi:10.1097/TA.0000000000003830.Epub2022 Nov 15.

20. Yee ES, Verrier ED, Thomas AN. Management of air embolism in blunt and penetrating thoracic trauma. *J Thorac Cardiovasc Surg*. 1983;**85**:661–7.

21. Mattox KL. Approaches to trauma involving the major vessels of the thorax. *Surg Clin N Am*. 1989;**69**:77–91. doi: 10.1016/s0039-6109(16)44737-7.

22. Brown CVR, de Moya M, Brasel KJ, Hartwell JL, Inaba K, Ley EJ, et al. Blunt thoracic aortic injury: a Western Trauma Association critical decisions algorithm. *J Trauma Acute Care Surg*. 2023 Jan 1;**94(1)**:113–16. doi: 10.1097/TA.0000000000003759. Epub 2022 Aug also https://custom.cvent.com/2A7C589629FA4A7181E1D1A892311435/files/a4eaeb3baa984ad181747f704a1108fa.pdf (accessed online September 2023)

23. Kulvatunyou N, Erickson L, Vijayasekaran A, Gries L, Joseph B, Friese RF, et al. Randomized clinical trial of pigtail catheter versus chest tube in injured patients with uncomplicated traumatic pneumothorax. *Br J Surg*. 2014 Jan;**101(2)**:17–22. doi: 10.1002/bjs.9377.

24. Kulvatunyou N, Bauman ZM, Zein Edine SB, de Moya M, Krause C, Mukherjee K, et al. The small (14 Fr) percutaneous catheter (P-CAT) versus large (28–32 Fr) open chest tube for traumatic hemothorax: a multicenter randomized clinical trial. *J Trauma Acute Care Surg*. 2021 Nov 1;**91(5)**:809–13.doi:10.1097/TA.0000000000003180.

25. Morales CH, Mejía C, Roldan LA, Saldarriaga MF, Duque AF. Negative pleural suction in thoracic trauma patients: a randomized controlled trial *J Trauma Acute Care Surg*. 2014 Aug; **77(2)**:251–5. doi: 10.1097/TA.0000000000000281.

26. Nunn A, Prakash P, Inaba K, Escalante A, Maher Z, Yamaguchi S, et al. Occupational exposure during emergency department thoracotomy: a prospective, multi-institution study. *J Trauma Acute Care Surg*. 2018 Jul;**85(1)**:78–84. doi: 10.1097/TA.0000000000001940.

27. Haut ER, Van Arendonk K, Barbosa RR, Chiu WC, et al. An evidence-based approach to patient selection for emergency department thoracotomy: a practice management guideline from the Eastern Association for the Surgery of Trauma. *J Trauma Acute Care Surg*. 2015 Jul;**79(1)**:159–73. doi: 10.1097/TA.0000000000000648.

28. Selesner L, Yorkgitis B, Martin M, Ng G, Mukherjee K, Ignacio R, et al. Emergency department thoracotomy in children: a PTS, WTA, and EAST systematic review and practice management guideline. *J Trauma Acute Care Surg*. 2023 Sep 1;**95(3)**:432–41. doi: 10.1097/TA.0000000000003879. Epub 2023 Mar 11.

29. Burlew CC, Moore EE, Moore FA, Coimbra R, McIntyre RC, Jr, Davis JW, et al. Western trauma association critical decisions in trauma: resuscitative thoracotomy. *J Trauma Acute Care Surg.* 2012;**73(6)**:1359–63. doi: 10.1097/TA.0b013e318270d2df.

30. Western Trauma Association Algorithm for Paediatric Resuscitative Thoracotomy. https://custom.cvent.com/2A7C589629FA4A7181E1D1A892311435/files/1343f0f563a64002ac64c1afce2c9877.pdf (accessed September 2023)

31. Telich-Tarriba JE, Anaya-Ayala JE, Reardon MJ. Surgical repair of right atrial wall rupture after blunt chest trauma. *J Tex Heart Inst.* 2012;**39(4)**:579–81.

32. Lee CN, Leng SA, Sorokin V. Simple and quick repair of cardiac rupture due to blunt chest trauma. *Asian Cardiovasc Thorac Ann.* 2012;**20(1)**:64–5. doi: 10.1177/0218492311421444.

33. Nakajima H, Uwabe K, Asakura T, Yoshida Y, Iguchi A, Niinami H. Emergent surgical repair of left ventricular rupture after blunt chest trauma. *Ann Thorac Surg.* 2014 Aug;**98(2)**:e35–6. doi: 10.1016/j.athoracsur.2014.03.057.

34. Kamiyoshihara M. Igai H, Ibe T, Ohtaki Y, Atsumi J, Nakazawa S, et al. Pulmonary lobar root clamping and stapling technique: return of the "en masse lobectomy". *Gen Thorac Cardiovasc Surg.* 2013 May;**61(5)**:280–91. doi: 10.1007/s11748-012-0159-3. Epub 2012 Sep

Recommended Reading

Burlew CC, Moore EE. Resuscitative Thoracotomy. In: Feliciano DV, Mattox KL, Moore EE. eds. *Trauma*, 9th Edn. McGraw-Hill Education, New York, NY, USA. 2021:299–316.

Ghanta RK, Wall MJ, Mattox KL. Trauma Thoracotomy: Principles and Techniques. In: Feliciano DV, Mattox KL, Moore EE. eds. *Trauma*, 9th Edn. McGraw-Hill Education, New York, NY, USA. 2021:561–6.

Coleman JJ, Pieracci FM, DuBose JJ, Scalea TM, O'Connor JV. Chest Wall and Lung. In: Feliciano DV, Mattox KL, Moore EE. eds. *Trauma*, 9th Edn. McGraw-Hill Education, New York, NY, USA, 2021:567–88.

DuBose JA, Scalea TM, O'Connor JV. Lung, Trachea, Bronchi and Esophagus. In: Feliciano DV, Mattox KL, Moore EE. eds. *Trauma*, 9th Edn. McGraw-Hill Education, New York, NY, USA. 2021:589–98.

Karmy-Jones R, Namias N, Coimbra R, Moore EE, Schreiber M, McIntyre R, Jr, et al. Western trauma association critical decisions in trauma: penetrating chest trauma. *J Trauma Acute Care Surg.* 2014;77(6):994–1002. doi: 10.1097/TA.0000000000000426.

Wall MJ, Ghanta RK, Mattox KL. Heart and Thoracic Vascular Injuries. In: Feliciano DV, Mattox KL, Moore EE. eds. *Trauma*, 9th Edn. McGraw-Hill Education, New York, NY, USA. 2021:599–628.

9.1 The Trauma Laparotomy

9.1.1 Overview

Delayed diagnosis and treatment of abdominal injuries are common causes of preventable death from blunt or penetrating trauma. Approximately 20% of abdominal injuries will require surgery. In the UK, Europe, and Australia, abdominal trauma is predominantly blunt in origin, whilst in the military context, as well as civilian trauma in South Africa, South America, and the larger US cities, it is predominantly penetrating.

The diagnosis of injury following blunt trauma can be difficult, and insight into the mechanism of injury can be helpful. Passenger restraints themselves may cause blunt trauma to the liver, duodenum, or pancreas, and rib fractures are associated with hepatic or splenic injuries. Virtually all penetrating injury to the abdomen should be addressed promptly, especially in the presence of hypotension.

> *Delay to the operating room (OR) of more than 10 minutes, in hypotensive patients with a gunshot wound, increases the risk of mortality by a factor of three.*[1]

Pitfalls

- Blood is not initially a peritoneal irritant, and therefore is not painful, and therefore it may be difficult to assess the presence or quantity of blood present in the abdomen.
- Bowel sounds may remain present for several hours after abdominal injury or may disappear soon after trivial trauma. This sign is therefore particularly unreliable.

Diagnostic modalities depend on the nature of the injury:

- Physical examination
- *Ultrasound*: Focussed abdominal sonography for trauma (FAST)
- Computed tomography (CT) scanning (stable patients only)
- Diagnostic laparoscopy
- Diagnostic peritoneal lavage

Pitfall

Although diagnostic peritoneal aspiration (DPA) is occasionally used, it can be unreliable, as a negative result may be due to no blood in only the area aspirated (false negative) or in an abdominal vessel (false positive).

It is important to appreciate the difference between abdominal surgery as part of the resuscitation process, and the definitive surgical treatment for abdominal trauma:

- *Surgical resuscitation* includes the techniques of 'damage control resuscitation' and 'damage control surgery' and implies only that the surgical procedure is primarily life-saving by stopping bleeding and preventing further contamination, and the patient's physiological derangement precludes definitive repair. (See Chapter 6.)
- *Definitive surgical treatment* implies that the physiological state of the patient allows the definitive surgical repair to take place.

During resuscitation, standard Advanced Trauma Life Support® (ATLS) guidelines should be followed. These should include:

- Standard ABCDE (airway, breathing, circulation, disability, and exposure) priorities

DOI: 10.1201/9781003258124-12

- Nasogastric or orogastric tube
- Urinary catheter

9.1.1.1 DIFFICULT ABDOMINAL INJURY COMPLEXES

There are at least four complex abdominal injury patterns:

- *Aortic and vena caval injuries*: Access to the retroperitoneal great vessels to obtain proximal and distal control is complicated in the presence of a large or enlarging retroperitoneal haematoma. (See Section 9.2.)
- *Major liver injuries*: Management of actively bleeding hepatic injuries may be challenging. Improvement in CT imaging has identified more adult solid organ injury which is managed non-operatively. Unstable patients with major liver injury require urgent laparotomy, which is technically demanding, and the principle of appropriate mobilization and packing is the mainstay of treatment. (See Section 9.5.)
- *Pancreaticoduodenal injuries*: Difficulties in diagnosis and management are often encountered, as the extent of injury to the pancreas and bile ducts, as well as possible retropancreatic vascular injuries, may not be immediately apparent. Missed injuries lead to a significant morbidity and mortality. (See Sections 9.2, 9.4, and 9.6.)
- *Complex pelvic fractures with associated open pelvic injury*: These are particularly difficult to treat and are associated with a high mortality. (See Chapter 10.)

Damage control approaches to these injuries may dramatically improve survival.

9.1.1.2 THE RETROPERITONEUM

The retroperitoneum is divided into:

- A central zone (Zone 1)
- Two lateral zones (Zone 2)
- A pelvic zone (Zone 3)

Injuries to retroperitoneal structures are associated with a high mortality and are often underestimated or missed. Exsanguinating vascular injuries need rapid and efficient access techniques. Large retroperitoneal haematomas often obscure the exact position and extent of the injury. The decision to explore a retroperitoneal haematoma is based on its location and the mechanism of injury, and whether the haematoma is pulsating or rapidly expanding.

Upper midline central retroperitoneal haematomas (Zone 1) *must* be explored, as major abdominal vascular injury, or injury to the pancreas or duodenum, may be present. The retroperitoneum is always approached via a transperitoneal incision, because of the high incidence of intraperitoneal and retroperitoneal injuries occurring simultaneously.

Lateral retroperitoneal haematomas (Zone 2) should not be routinely explored. In both blunt and penetrating trauma, the haematoma should be explored if it is large, expanding, or pulsating, and especially if the patient is unstable. In this case, there is most likely a severe renal or renal artery injury requiring rapid nephrectomy. In all other cases, the Zone 2 haematoma may be left alone, except if a *penetrating* injury is noted to have occurred at or near the hilum of the kidney. CT imaging of such a renal injury guides further management. Peripheral renal penetrating injuries may be left alone and may be managed by non-operative means.[2] (See Section 9.8.)

Non-expanding haematomas related to pelvic fractures (Zone 3) should not be explored. Ongoing bleeding from pelvic fractures is best managed with a combination of external fixation on the pelvis and angiographic embolization. Attempts at ligation of internal iliac vessels are usually unsuccessful. If angio-embolization is not available, expanding pelvic haematomas should be packed. Extraperitoneal pelvic packing is more effective than intraperitoneal pelvic packing and is advocated in unstable patients with pelvic fractures who require surgery for haemodynamic instability. (See Chapter 10.)

9.1.1.3 NON-OPERATIVE MANAGEMENT OP PENETRATING ABDOMINAL INJURY

There is universal agreement that patients with generalized peritonism or haemodynamic instability should undergo urgent laparotomy after penetrating injury to the abdomen. In some institutions with a high volume of penetrating trauma to the abdomen, certain haemodynamically stable patients are managed non-operatively, either through choice or because of the overwhelming volume of cases. (See Section 9.5 on the liver, and Section 9.7 on the spleen, for the non-operative management of solid organ injury.)

It is imperative that serial examination of these patients is undertaken in a meticulous fashion, and that a laparotomy is done if any concerns arise.

Most patients with penetrating abdominal trauma managed non-operatively may be discharged after 24 hours of observation in the presence of a reliable abdominal examination and minimal to no tenderness. In addition, diagnostic laparoscopy may be considered as a tool to evaluate diaphragmatic lacerations and peritoneal penetration to avoid unnecessary laparotomy (see Section 15 on minimally invasive surgery in trauma). If the laparoscopy is positive, one should convert to a full trauma laparotomy to explore the abdominal cavity fully for other injuries.

The Eastern Association for the Surgery of Trauma (EAST) Practice Management Guidelines provide evidence-based guidelines for the management of penetrating abdominal trauma (see **Table 9.1.1**).[3]

9.1.2 **The Trauma Laparotomy**

The trauma laparotomy is not for the faint-hearted; the trauma surgeon should 'be prepared' for the unexpected.

Trauma does not follow guidelines, nor do penetrating injuries follow predictable patterns, so from the outset the surgeon is on a roller-coaster voyage of discovery and needs to be prepared for anything and everything. Therefore, minimizing the decision-making load by having standard setups, equipment, positioning, and additional equipment at hand in a mobile OR trolley is useful.

Preparation of the OR and communication with the OR team prior to surgery are critical, the latter explaining what may be expected and what hazards are likely to be encountered. This sharing of information must include the anaesthetist and scrub nurse at the very least, but preferably the whole OR team. Further information on this can be found in Chapter 2 (on non-technical skills), at the end of this section (in 'Anaesthesiological Considerations'), and in Appendix F ('The Trauma Laparotomy for Scrub Nurses').

The trauma laparotomy contains several essential steps:

- Rapid entry
- Adequate (large) incision

Table 9.1.1 Evidence-Based Guidelines for the Management of Penetrating Injury of the Abdomen	
Level I	There are no level I evidence-based guidelines.
Level II	Patients who are haemodynamically unstable or who have diffused abdominal tenderness after penetrating abdominal trauma should be taken emergently for laparotomy.
	Patients with an unreliable clinical examination (i.e., severe head injury, spinal cord injury, severe intoxication, or need for sedation or intubation) should be explored or further investigation done to determine if there is intraperitoneal injury.
	Others may be selected for initial observation. In these patients: 1. Triple-contrast (oral, intravenous, and rectal contrast) abdominopelvic computed tomography should be strongly considered as a diagnostic tool to facilitate initial management decisions, as this test can accurately predict the need for laparotomy. 2. Serial examinations should be performed, as physical examination is reliable in detecting significant injuries after penetrating trauma to the abdomen. Patients requiring delayed laparotomy will develop abdominal signs. 3. If signs of peritonitis develop, laparotomy should be performed. 4. If there is an unexplained drop in blood pressure or haematocrit, further investigation is warranted.
Level III	Most patients with penetrating abdominal trauma managed non-operatively may be discharged after 24 hours of observation in the presence of a reliable abdominal examination and minimal to no abdominal tenderness.
	Patients with penetrating injury to the right upper quadrant of the abdomen with injury to the right lung, right diaphragm, and liver may be safely observed in the presence of stable vital signs, reliable examination, and minimal to no abdominal tenderness.
	Angiography and investigation for and treatment of diaphragm injury may be necessary as adjuncts to the initial non-operative management of penetrating abdominal trauma.
	Mandatory exploration for all penetrating renal trauma is not necessary.

Table 9.1.2 Practice Management Guidelines for Prophylactic Antibiotic Use in Penetrating Abdominal Trauma

Level I	There are sufficient class I and II data to recommend a single preoperative dose of prophylactic antibiotics with broad-spectrum aerobic and anaerobic coverage as a standard of care for trauma patients sustaining penetrating abdominal wounds. Absence of a hollow viscus injury requires no further administration.
Level II	There are sufficient class I and class II data to recommend continuation of prophylactic antibiotics for only 24 hours in the presence of injury to any hollow viscus.
Level III	There are insufficient clinical data to provide meaningful guidelines for reducing infectious risks in trauma patients with haemorrhagic shock. Vasoconstriction alters the normal distribution of antibiotics, resulting in reduced tissue penetration. To circumvent this problem, the administered dose may be increased two- or threefold and repeated after every 10th unit of blood product transfusion until there is no further blood loss. Once haemodynamic stability has been achieved, antibiotics with excellent activity against obligate and facultative anaerobic bacteria should be continued for periods that depend on the degree of wound contamination. Aminoglycosides have been demonstrated to exhibit suboptimal activity in patients with serious injury, probably due to altered pharmacokinetics of drug distribution.

- Control of massive haemorrhage by:
  - Identification of all injuries
  - Packing
  - Direct control
  - Proximal control (i.e., source control)
- Identification of injuries
- Control of contamination
- Reconstruction (if possible)

9.1.2.1 PREOPERATIVE ADJUNCTS

9.1.2.1.1 Antibiotics[4]

Routine single-dose preoperative intravenous antibiotic prophylaxis should be employed. Subsequent antibiotic policy will depend on the intraoperative findings (**Table 9.1.2**).

The antibiotics commonly recommended include a second-generation cephalosporin, plus metronidazole or, where available, amoxycillin–clavulanate. There is some evidence that aminoglycosides should *not* be used in acute trauma, partly because of the shift in fluids which requires substantially higher doses of aminoglycoside to reach the appropriate minimum inhibitory concentration (MIC), and partly because they work best in an alkaline environment (traumatized tissue is acidic).

The administered dose should be *increased twofold to threefold* and repeated after every 10 units of blood transfusion until there is no further blood loss. If intra-abdominal

bleeding is significant, it may be necessary to give a further dose of antibiotic therapy intraoperatively, due to dilution of the preoperative dose (**Table 9.1.3**).

9.1.2.1.2 Temperature Control[5]

Temperature control is fundamental in preventing complications in the injured patient. Minimizing patient hypothermia by raising the OR temperature to a higher than normal level, and warming the patient with warm air blankets, warmed intravenous fluids, and warmed anaesthetic gases, is very important.

Theatre preparations should, where possible, commence well before the arrival of the patient. These

Table 9.1.3 Antibiotic Prophylaxis and Empiric Therapy in Major Abdominal Injury after First Dose

No pathology found	No further antibiotics
Blood only	No further antibiotics
Small bowel or gastric contamination	Continuation for 24 hours only Copious peritoneal washout
Large bowel, minimal contamination	Continuation for 24 hours only
Large bowel, gross contamination	Copious peritoneal washout 24–72 hours of antibiotics

include warming of the operating theatre, warming of all intravenous fluids, warming of anaesthetic gases, and activating external warming devices such as a Bair Hugger® (3M, St. Paul, MN, USA).

9.1.2.1.3 Blood Collection and Autotransfusion

Preparations must be made for collection of blood in a saline- and heparin-primed drainage system, or a cell-saving device, for autotransfusion if indicated.

9.1.2.2 DRAPING

During the trauma laparotomy, it may become necessary to extend the incision, if required. All patients should therefore be prepared and draped to allow access to the thorax, abdomen, and groins if required (**Figure 9.1.1**).

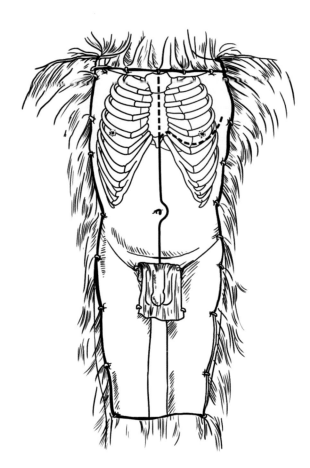

Figure 9.1.1 Exploration of the abdomen, showing extent of skin preparation and draping prior to surgery.

9.1.2.3 INCISION

Once the patient and staff are fully prepared, and the anaesthetist has indicated to the surgical team that all are ready for surgery to commence, the surgeon should waste no time entering the abdomen.

A sharp knife, a profound knowledge of anatomy, and courage are all that are needed in the first 30–60 seconds!

A long, mid-line incision is made with a scalpel, from xiphisternum to pubis, in one sweep of the blade (preferably skirting the umbilicus to the left to avoid the falciform ligament) down to the linea alba. No time is wasted in chasing small bleeders from the wound edges with diathermy. These will stop on their own. Put gauze swabs over them and continue.

The next pass of the knife should be into the linea alba just superior (cranial) to the umbilicus – this being the quickest route to access the peritoneal cavity, as the parietal peritoneum is blended with the anterior abdominal wall at this point due to the umbilical cicatrix. This should obviate the need to pick up the peritoneum as a separate structure.

The peritoneum should be opened last once the entire incision as indicated above has been performed. This is essentially for two reasons: firstly, a closed peritoneum maintains a tampon effect and keeps the incision visible, and secondly, this avoids losing time extending the incision in an abundantly bleeding situation. Usually, the peritoneum can be opened quickly with two fingers or large Mayo's scissors without having to resort to any instrument (which may be dangerous).

Pitfall

- It may not be easy to gain rapid entry to the abdominal cavity where previous surgery has been performed. This is termed a 'hostile abdomen' and may present the surgeon with extreme technical challenges to be able to safely enter the peritoneal space without injuring bowel or other structures adherent to the underlying abdominal scar(s).
- Identification of a hostile abdomen should forewarn the surgeon of difficult access and may be the occasion to resort to left anterior thoracotomy for aortic cross-clamping in the chest, or retrograde endovascular balloon occlusion of the aorta (REBOA) prior to laparotomy, in order to prevent exsanguination during difficult abdominal access.

In patients with gross haemodynamic instability, or who have had significant previous midline surgery, a bilateral subcostal ('clamshell' or 'chevron') incision extending from the anterior axillary line on each side transversely across the midline just superior to the umbilicus may be used.

9.1.2.4 INITIAL PROCEDURE

A quick exploratory 'trauma laparotomy" is performed to identify any other associated injuries:

1. As soon as the abdomen has been opened, large quantities of blood or other fluids may pour out, and a Poole's sucker may usefully be introduced into the abdominal cavity whilst the incision is rapidly extended up and down using large Mayo's scissors to the full extent of the skin incision. Do **not** use fine dissection scissors, such as McIndoe's, for this, as they will be badly blunted by the experience. Scoop out as much blood as possible into a receiver. Do not use a sucker at this time, as it is too slow and will block with clots.

2. Eviscerate the small bowel. Perform a rapid exploration to any obvious site of large-volume (*audible!*) bleeding. Assess the midline structures where packing is inefficient – the aorta, inferior vena cava (IVC), and mesentery – and, if necessary, control with direct pressure or proximal control (e.g., on the aorta). Active bleeding **must** be controlled before proceeding further with exploration.

3. Once access has been achieved, blood and free abdominal contents should be scooped out using a small kidney dish or large gallipot, emptying it out into a large metal washbowl on a stand beside the surgeon. This allows the anaesthetist to view the contents and estimate blood loss; do not use suckers, as they are too slow and will block with clots.

4. Having cleared most of the abdomen of blood and other contaminants into the large washbowl, dry, unfolded packs (for maximum absorption) should be inserted, starting from the places of suspected major bleeding, and working towards those areas which appear less involved. All areas of the abdominal cavity must be packed if injuries are not to be missed.

5. Perform packing as necessary, using large, dry abdominal swabs:
   5.1. Under the left diaphragm
   5.2. In the left paracolic gutter
   5.3. In the pelvis
   5.4. In the right paracolic gutter
   5.5. Into the subhepatic pouch
   5.6. Above and lateral to the liver
   5.7. Directly on any other bleeding area

Pitfalls

- *Use dry swabs throughout*. Dry swabs work better and will not cool the patient further. Pack them open, and loosely, into the above-mentioned anatomical areas. This type of packing is focussed on identifying the origin of bleeding by removing the excess blood from the uninjured parts of the peritoneal cavity.
- *Never pass sharp instruments by hand*. The laparotomy is relatively uncontrolled. **All** sharps (scalpels, needles in needle holders, etc.) **must** be passed into and out of the operative field in a receiver (e.g., a kidney dish) to minimize the risk of a 'needle-stick'.

Packing does not control arterial bleeding.

6. Remove the abdominal packs, one at a time, starting in the area *least* likely to be the site of the bleeding. Then, apply pressure, or compress the organ or area where active bleeding is identified.

7. Once the source of major haemorrhage has been identified – however approximately – the area has been firmly packed, and pressure applied to ensure no further significant bleeding occurs. Having established this,

STOP OPERATING!

8. This is the opportunity for the anaesthetist to catch up with adequate lines, fluid, and transfusion requirements; assess the blood gases, thromboelastogram (TEG), and core temperature; and discuss with the surgical team the likely injuries and options for repair, damage control, or 'bail-out' techniques.
   Deal with lesions in the order of their lethality:
   8.1. Injuries to major blood vessels
   8.2. Major haemorrhage from solid abdominal viscera
   8.3. Haemorrhage from mesentery and hollow organs
   8.4. Retroperitoneal haemorrhage
   8.5. Contamination

Pitfalls

- Resources for possible options must be considered at this point, and if these are severely limited or non-existent, then the absolute minimum should be attempted to simply control bleeding and stop further contamination.
- Heroic surgery accompanied by frantic anaesthesia rarely results in a successful outcome.
- Decisions to transfer to a better-equipped facility, if possible, or a higher-care area to improve the patient's physiology must be made now – not after struggling for another hour or more with a coagulopathic, acidotic, cold patient, whose survival chances lessen by the minute.

It is essential to treat first what kills first.

9.1.2.5 PERFORM THE TRAUMA LAPAROTOMY

Once access had been made into the peritoneal cavity, temporary control of haemorrhage made, and some time given to allow the anaesthetist to address the physiological needs of the patient, the compelling source of bleeding must now be addressed.

Methods of dealing with bleeding vary depending on whether the source is venous or arterial, and if a shunt or repair is required, or whether the vessel can be ligated without major deleterious effects. Similarly, techniques for controlling bleeding are discussed in the relevant chapters.

When the major hazards have been dealt with, a full examination of the abdominal cavity must be made. Routines and patterns vary, but what matters is that the individual surgeon has a routine that he or she follows every time. One way is described here.

Starting from above and moving downwards, the integrity of the diaphragm is checked. It is often forgotten in complex and multi-cavity injuries. Both blunt and penetrating injuries may be responsible for diaphragmatic rupture.

Blunt chest or abdominal trauma may result in a rapid increase in thoracic or abdominal pressure, with traumatic rupture of the diaphragm. This is more common on the left, as the right lobe of the liver protects (to some extent) the right dome of the diaphragm. Nevertheless, if blunt liver trauma of the right lobe is seen (segments VII and VIII especially) and the right triangular and coronary ligaments, along with the falciform ligament, may

need to be divided to properly inspect the dome of the right diaphragm, place high packs, and repair.

Beware a large retrohepatic haematoma in blunt trauma; if it is not expanding, it is best left alone.

The left lobe of the liver is easy to see and mobilize if necessary, to check the diaphragm behind it. Small stab wounds that have entered the lower left chest may easily puncture the diaphragm, leaving the potential for either the stomach or a loop of bowel to be trapped in the defect, and leading to later necrosis of the bowel wall with spillage of gut content into the chest cavity. This may appear in the chest drain effluent and should give a clue as to the diagnosis.

The epigastrium is crowded, and injuries are easy to miss. Specific organ injuries are dealt with in their relevant chapters, and only useful tips will be mentioned here.

Both sides of the stomach must be inspected; even so, it is easy to overlook a small penetrating injury that will store up trouble for the future. If the stomach is deflated, ask the anaesthetist to pass some air into the nasogastric tube, and squeeze the stomach gently, looking for bubbles appearing, or gastric contents, which may be bile-stained. An easy way to inspect the posterior surface of the stomach is by entering the gastro-colic omentum. Usually, this is possible without needing to divide vessels.

Pitfall

With a perforating injury of the anterior wall of the stomach, always inspect for an 'exit wound' posteriorly. If it is not obvious but there is injury posteriorly (e.g., to the diaphragm or the upper pole of the spleen), be prepared to enlarge the anterior hole and inspect from within the stomach itself.

The gall bladder, once decompressed by perforation, may be overlooked. The bile staining present may be assumed to come from the intestine, so care should be taken to carefully inspect the gall bladder for its integrity. (See Section 9.5.)

Little time is spent on trying to preserve the spleen in trauma laparotomies, but there are some occasions when it matters, such as in children. For the most part, trauma to the spleen means splenectomy, which is a quick procedure and should take no more than 10 minutes. This topic is dealt with in Section 9.7.

This approach also gives a view of the superior surface of the pancreas and splenic vessels. It is sometimes possible to view the beginning of the portal vein at its formation from the joining of the splenic and superior mesenteric veins behind the neck of the pancreas. The head of the pancreas is examined by mobilizing the second part of the duodenum and rolling it gently to the left off the IVC, where the head of the pancreas will be seen in the 'C' of the duodenum. The inferior border of the pancreas is best seen by exposing it at the base of the mesentery, lifting the whole small bowel up and to the right. The tail of the pancreas is easily seen at the hilum of the spleen. (See Section 9.6.)

Access to the posterior part of the abdomen.

Be prepared to medially rotate the right and left viscera by dividing the peritoneal reflections.

Having mobilized the duodenal loop by a Kocher manoeuvre, the continuity of the whole small bowel should be assessed, placing Babcock or Duval tissue forceps on points of perforation or division, and rapidly stopping contamination by tying off divided sections with umbilical tapes or the long tags on abdominal swabs or by stapled resection. If several holes are present within a relatively short segment of bowel, they may all be included in the tied-off loop, or it may be rapidly resected with a stapler.

Small perforations where the mesentery meets the bowel wall are difficult to find unless small haematomata there are carefully examined and/or explored. It is helpful to have more than one set of eyes inspecting the bowel; however, the practice of passing it hand-to-hand, from surgeon to assistant, may result in missed injuries (each assumes the other has seen the injury!).

> *Do not be side-tracked whilst making your examination – keep your focus.*
>
> *One pair of hands, two pairs of eyes.*

Once the caecum is reached, a decision may need to be made whether to explore any lateral haematoma in the right flank. If it is the result of blunt trauma and is neither expanding nor pulsatile, it may be left. If there has been penetrating trauma, the safe course of action is to explore it, even if it is neither expanding nor pulsatile. The reason for this is that it is not possible to rule out an injury to the retroperitoneal part of the ascending colon, nor an injury to the urinary tract.[6] If both these injuries are present, then the right kidney should be removed, as an infected urinoma and renal abscess will result. Both a colonic and urinary fistula are likely to occur. However, it is reasonable not to open Gerota's fascia, with a view to managing any concomitant renal injury non-operatively, based on imaging.

The colon is systematically inspected, utilizing full right and left visceral rotations, with care being taken to minimize any faecal contamination. The gastro-colic omentum may need separating from the greater curve of the stomach to visualize the full circumference of the colon.

The rectum is partially retroperitoneal, and pelvic haematomata associated with penetrating trauma require fine judgement in management if further major haemorrhage is to be avoided. Bullet or stab wounds in the buttocks or perineum may well have penetrated either or both bowel and bladder, and each needs full assessment. A urinary catheter should already have been placed so that further drainage at damage control is unnecessary, but if blood has been found on the gloved finger on rectal examination, then a para-rectal corrugated drain may be placed to exit the skin over the ischio-rectal fossa.

At the initial laparotomy, no stoma should be made in a damage control setting. The priority is to minimize time in the OR to the two essentials of stopping bleeding and further contamination – and leaving the reconstructive work to another time when the patient's physiology will withstand more surgery.

Gynaecological organs, unless the patient is pregnant, should not pose a problem, and are unlikely to be a major source of bleeding.

Injuries to the bladder may be difficult to diagnose, as blood in the catheter bag may have come from anywhere along the urinary tract. If the base of the bladder is thought to have been damaged, and no injury is found on initial examination, urethral and suprapubic catheters may be placed, and a bivalve of the bladder made at re-look laparotomy. If the site of injury is still not found, the ureter(s) may have been injured at the point of entry to the bladder and deep to the trigone. Which side – or both – may be identified by asking the anaesthetist to administer a small injection of either methylene blue or furosemide intravenously. Within less than a minute, whilst observing the bladder trigone from within, the ureteric orifices will squirt blue urine, or just a strong jet of normal-coloured urine, demonstrating patency of the ureter on that or both sides.

Bladder, ureteric, and renal repairs can be found in Section 9.8.

9.1.2.5.1 Large Mesenteric Haematoma

The technique for separating the mesenteric root from the retroperitoneum is to mobilize the entire midgut loop, from the transverse colon to the ligament of Treitz. Start by 'Kocherizing' the duodenum, and follow that plane around and behind the hepatic flexure of the colon, down the right paracolic gutter to the caecum. Then turn abruptly upwards (cephalad) again, behind the caecum and in front of the ureter and psoas, along the left-hand edge of the base of the mesenteric root. Continue this dissection, mobilizing the mesenteric root off the IVC and the aorta until the duodeno-jejunal flexure is seen, with the attachment of the ligament of Treitz to its upper surface, passing behind the stomach to the right crus of the diaphragm.

At this point, the entire mid-gut loop may be lifted clear of the abdominal cavity, placed into a sterile bag, and left briefly on the chest of the patient. It is important to warn the anaesthetist about this procedure, as the translocated bowel may rapidly become ischaemic if there is undue traction on the mesenteric base, which will result in a significant acidosis within a very short time, upsetting the smooth running of the anaesthetic and the patient's already disturbed physiology.

Nevertheless, the manoeuvre quickly and clearly demonstrates whether the compelling source of bleeding is from mesenteric vessels or the retroperitoneum.

9.1.2.6 PERFORM DEFINITIVE PACKING

- Use **dry** packs throughout.
- Preferably keep the dry swabs folded, as it is easier to 'layer' them into a cavity or against an organ.
- Do **not** cover them in plastic – they will slip and will be too rigid.
- Packs must exert sufficient force on the organ to tamponade bleeding.
- Packs only work in venous injury (arteries must be controlled directly).
- Arterial perfusion should be preserved.
- Use the least number of packs that will achieve the desired result.

9.1.2.6.1 Liver (See also Section 9.5)

When the initial packs are removed from the right upper quadrant, injury to the liver is assessed. It is prudent at this time to dissect the gastrohepatic ligament at the porta hepatis using blunt and sharp dissection so that a vessel loop (Rumel tourniquet) or vascular clamp can be placed across the portal triad.

The liver is mobilized only if necessary.

Bleeding from the liver may require manual compression. If compression of the liver controls the bleeding, the bleeding is probably venous in nature, and can be arrested with definitive therapeutic liver packing. If not, a Pringle's manoeuvre should be performed. If a Pringle's manoeuvre controls the bleeding, the surgeon should suspect hepatic artery or portal vein injury. Hepatorrhaphy is then performed to control intrahepatic vessels, alone or in combination with packing.

If a Pringle's manoeuvre fails to control bleeding, the likely source is hepatic veins or the IVC. Compression of the liver against the posterior abdominal wall and diaphragm can be useful, and packing should be performed.

9.1.2.6.2 Spleen (See Section 9.7)

When the packs in the left upper quadrant are removed, and if there is associated bleeding from the spleen, a decision should be made on whether the spleen should be preserved or removed.

A vascular clamp placed across the hilum will allow temporary haemorrhage control.

9.1.2.6.3 Pelvis (See Chapter 10)

If the pelvis seems to be a major source of bleeding, intraperitoneal packing should be converted to extraperitoneal pelvic packing once intra-abdominal control has been achieved.

9.1.2.7 SPECIFIC ROUTES OF ACCESS

9.1.2.7.1 Lesser Sac

The stomach is grasped and pulled inferiorly, allowing the operator to identify the lesser curvature and the superior aspect of the pancreas visible through the lesser omentum. The coeliac artery and the body of the pancreas can also be accessed through this approach.

9.1.2.7.2 Greater Sac

The omentum is then grasped and drawn upwards. A window is made in the omentum (via the gastrocolic ligament) and provides access into the lesser sac posterior to the stomach. This allows excellent exposure of the entire body and tail of the pancreas, as well as the posterior aspect of the first part of the duodenum and the medial aspect of the second part. Any injuries to the pancreas can be easily identified. If there is a possibility of an injury to the head of the pancreas, a Kocher manoeuvre should be performed. Additional exposure can be achieved using a right medial visceral rotation.

9.1.2.7.3 Mobilization of the Ascending Colon (Right Hemicolon)

The hepatic flexure is retracted medially, dividing adhesions along its lateral border down to the caecum (**Figure 9.1.2**).

9.1.2.7.4 Kocher Manoeuvre

The Kocher manoeuvre is performed by initially dividing the lateral peritoneal attachment of the duodenum, allowing medial rotation of the duodenum (**Figure 9.1.3**).

The loose areolar tissue around the duodenum is bluntly dissected, and the entire second and third portions of the duodenum are identified and are mobilized medially with a combination of sharp and blunt dissection. This dissection is carried all the way medially to expose the IVC and a portion of the aorta.

The posterior wall of the duodenum can be inspected, together with the right kidney, porta hepatis, and IVC. By reflecting the duodenum and pancreas towards the anterior midline, the posterior surface of the head of the pancreas can be completely exposed (**Figure 9.1.4**). Better inspection of the third part, and inspection of the fourth part, of the duodenum can be achieved by mobilizing the ligament of Treitz and performing a right medial visceral rotation.

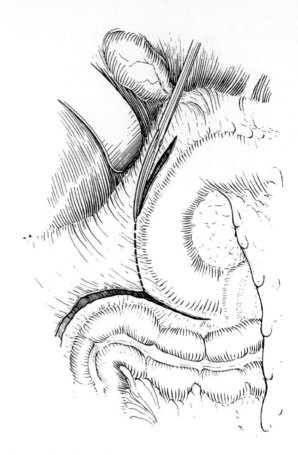

Figure 9.1.3 Kocher manoeuvre.

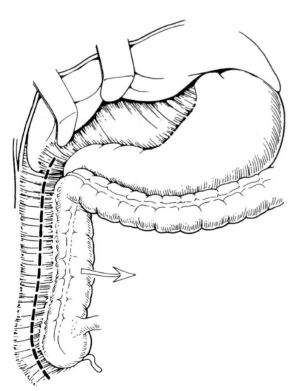

Figure 9.1.2 Mobilization of the right hemicolon.

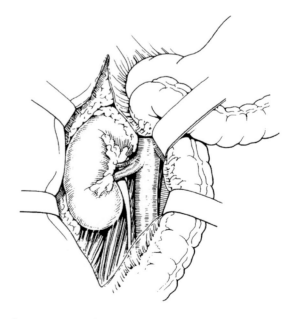

Figure 9.1.4 Reflection of the duodenum and right hemicolon to show the right kidney and inferior vena cava.

9.1.2.7.5 Right Medial Visceral Rotation[7]

This was previously known as the Cattel and Braasch manoeuvre. The small bowel mesentery is mobilized by sharply incising its retroperitoneal attachments from the right lower quadrant to the ligament of Treitz, by progressively lifting the caecum. The entire ascending colon and the caecum are then reflected superiorly towards the left upper quadrant of the abdomen. This will expose the right retroperitoneum. The entire ascending colon and the caecum are then reflected superiorly towards the left upper quadrant of the abdomen.

As the dissection is carried further, the inferior border of the entire pancreas can then be identified and any injuries inspected. Severe oedema, crepitation, or bile staining of the periduodenal tissues implies a duodenal injury until proven otherwise.

> ***Mobilization of the whole duodenum is mandatory for exclusion of duodenal injury.***

These manoeuvres allow for complete exposure of the first, second, third, and fourth parts of the duodenum, along with the head, neck, and proximal body of the pancreas. Access to the vena cava and the renal vessels is also facilitated (**Figure 9.1.5**).

Exposure for repair of the aorta, and the distal body and tail of the pancreas, can be better obtained by performing a left medial visceral rotation.

9.1.2.7.6 Left Medial Visceral Rotation[8]

Medial rotation of the left side of the abdominal contents can be performed by mobilizing the spleen and descending colon, and then displacing the spleen, descending colon, and sigmoid colon to the right (left medial visceral rotation). This allows inspection of the left kidney, retroperitoneum, and tail of the pancreas.

Mobilize the splenorenal ligament and incise the peritoneal reflection in the left paracolic gutter down to the level of the sigmoid colon. The left-sided viscera are then bluntly dissected free of the retroperitoneum and mobilized to the right. Care should be taken to remain in a plane anterior to Gerota's fascia, which covers the kidney. The entire anterior surface of the abdominal aorta and the origins of its branches are exposed by this technique. This includes the coeliac axis, the origin of the superior mesenteric artery, the iliac vessels, and the left renal pedicle (**Figure 9.1.6**). The dense and fibrous superior mesenteric and coeliac nerve plexuses overlie the proximal aorta and need to be sharply dissected in order to identify the renal and superior mesenteric arteries.

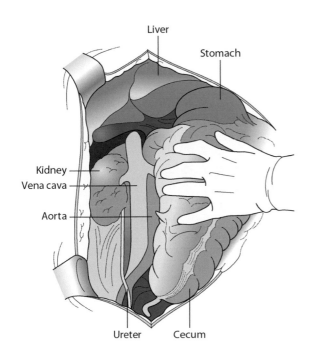

Figure 9.1.5 Right medial visceral rotation.

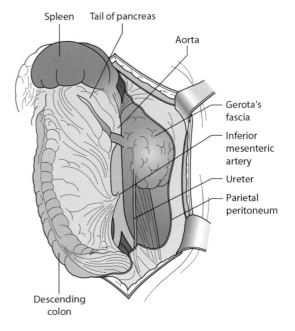

Figure 9.1.6 Left medial visceral rotation.

If vascular access to the kidney is required, Gerota's fascia should be divided on the lateral aspect of the kidney, and the kidney rotated medially to allow access to the renal hilum, as well as the lateral side of the aorta, which can be controlled if necessary.

Pelvic haematomas in the presence of a pelvic fracture should not be explored routinely. In an unstable patient in whom it is suspected that the pelvic bleeding is contributing to haemorrhagic shock, preperitoneal pelvic packing should be done, in combination with external pelvic fixation and, if necessary, angiographic embolization. Attempts at tying the internal iliac vessels are usually unsuccessful.

9.1.2.8 SPECIFIC ORGAN TECHNIQUES

See the sections on specific abdominal organ injuries.

9.1.2.8.1 Hepatic Injury

In severe liver injury, after successful surgical treatment including the removal of devascularized necrotic tissue and resectional debridement in selected cases, the liver is packed, and the injured area compressed with warm pads. After complete exploration of the abdomen and treatment of other injuries and sources of bleeding, the liver packs are removed, and any slight oozing on the surface of the liver can be arrested by sealing with fibrin or haemostatic patches.

> *Fibrin glue cannot, however, compensate for inadequate surgical technique.*

9.1.2.8.2 Splenic Injury

In the *unstable* patient, rapid splenectomy is important, although, when possible in the *stable* patient, the surgeon should consider splenic repair that preserves as much of the damaged spleen as possible, bearing in mind that any delays may have catastrophic consequences due to excessive blood loss. In trauma cases, conservation of the spleen should not take significantly more time than would a splenectomy.

Mesh tamponade is no longer used.

9.1.2.8.3 Pancreatic Injury

When pancreatic injury is suspected, extended exploration of the whole organ is imperative. Parenchymal lacerations that do not involve the pancreatic duct can be sutured when the tissue is not too soft and vulnerable. With or without sutures, a worthwhile option in the treatment of such lacerations is a haemostatic; adequate suction drainage is essential.

9.1.2.8.4 Retroperitoneal Haematoma

Injuries to the retroperitoneal vessels can cause haematomas of varying size, depending on the calibre of the vessels injured and the severity of the injury. Retroperitoneal haematomas can be treated by packing after surgical control of injured vessels and be followed by catheter embolization.

When the patient is stable, the packs may be removed after 24–48 hours. Rebleeding after removal of the packs can necessitate repacking. Slight bleeding can, however, be stopped effectively by spraying on adhesives.

9.1.3 Closure of the Abdomen

9.1.3.1 PRINCIPLES OF ABDOMINAL CLOSURE

On completion of the intra-abdominal procedures, it is important to adequately prepare for closure. This preparation includes:

- Careful evaluation of the adequacy of haemostasis and/or packing.
- Copious lavage and removal of debris within the peritoneum and wound.
- Placement of adequate and appropriate drains, if indicated.
- Ensuring that the instrument and swab counts are completed and correct.

It is important to replace the small intestine in the abdominal cavity with great care at the conclusion of the operation.

9.1.3.2 CHOOSING THE OPTIMAL METHOD OF CLOSURE

Thal and O'Keefe[9] state that the optimal closure technique is chosen based on five principal considerations, and list these as follows:

- The *stability* of the patient (and therefore the need for speed of closure)
- The *amount* of blood loss both prior to and during operation
- The *volume* of intravenous fluid administered
- The *degree* of intraperitoneal and wound contamination
- The *nutritional* status of the patient and possible intercurrent disease

These factors will also dictate the decision to plan for a re-laparotomy, which will naturally influence the method chosen for closure. Other factors that should be taken into consideration are hypothermia, coagulopathy, and acidosis, which are indications to revert to damage control strategies.

9.1.4 Temporary Closure

This is covered in detail elsewhere in this book. (See Chapter 6: 'Damage Control'.)

9.1.5 The Open Abdomen

Advances in trauma care have improved survival after abdominal catastrophes. Nonetheless, patients with open abdomens (OAs) are at risk of increased morbidity. Multiple techniques have been described to manage the OA, including temporary abdominal closure (e.g., the Bogota bag), negative-pressure wound therapy (NPWT), and fascial traction systems (suture traction, Wittmann patch, progressive partial fascial closure, and mesh-mediated fascial traction [MMFT]). Volume removal techniques and complex abdominal reconstruction techniques, including component separation, bridging with biologic prostheses, or placement of synthetic absorbable mesh and eventual skin grafting, have also been described. Despite the variety of options, the optimal treatment remains unclear.

The EAST Practice Management Guidelines on Management of the Open Abdomen were unable to make recommendations regarding the closure of the open abdomen (see **Table 9.1.4**, PICO Format, and **Table 9.1.5** EAST Guidelines).[10]

Table 9.1.4 The PICO Format

P	Patient, Population, or Problem	How would I describe the patient group?
I	Intervention, Prognostic factor, or Exposure	Which main intervention, prognostic factor, or exposure is considered?
C	Comparison or Intervention (if appropriate)	What is the main alternative to compare with the intervention?
O	Outcome you would like to measure or achieve	What can be accomplished, measured, improved, or affected?

Table 9.1.5 Eastern Association for the Surgery of Trauma Practice Management Guidelines for Management of the Open Abdomen

PICO	Recommendation
PICO Question 1	
In haemodynamically normal trauma and emergency general surgery (EGS) patients with OA after DCL in whom intra-abdominal pathology has been addressed and physiology normalized (P), should interventions to reduce visceral oedema (diuresis, hypertonic saline, direct peritoneal resuscitation); (I) versus no interventions (C) be performed to help achieve primary myofascial closure during index admission, reduce ventral herniation after primary myofascial closure during index admission, reduce fascial dehiscence after primary myofascial closure, and reduce incidence of enterocutaneous/atmospheric fistula (ECF) and mortality (O)?	We are unable to make any recommendations regarding the use of techniques to remove visceral oedema in haemodynamically normal trauma and emergency general surgery patients with OAs after DCLs.
PICO Question 2	
In haemodynamically normal trauma and EGS patients with OA after DCL in whom intra-abdominal pathology has been addressed (P), should a fascial traction system be used (I) versus no traction systems (C) to help achieve primary myofascial closure during index admission, reduce ventral herniation after primary myofascial closure during index admission, reduce fascial dehiscence after primary myofascial closure, and reduce incidence of ECF and mortality (O)?	We conditionally recommend the use of a fascial traction system in haemodynamically normal trauma and emergency general surgery patients with OAs after DCL in whom intra-abdominal pathology has been addressed.

9.1.6 **Primary Closure**

Primary closure of the abdominal sheath (or fascia), the subcutaneous tissue, and the skin is obviously the desirable goal and may be achieved when the conditions outlined above are optimal, that is, a stable patient with minimal blood loss and volume replacement, no or minimal contamination, and no significant intercurrent problems, and in whom surgical procedures are deemed to be completed with no anticipated subsequent operation. Should any doubt exist regarding these conditions at the conclusion of operation, it would be prudent to consider a technique of delayed closure.

The most commonly used technique at present is that of *mass closure* of the peritoneum and sheath using a mono-filament suture with a continuous (preferable, since relatively quick) or an interrupted (discontinuous) application. Either absorbable material (e.g., 1 polydioxanone loop) or non-absorbable material (e.g., nylon or polypropylene) may be used. Chromic cargut is not a suitable material.

Whichever method is used, the most important technical point is that of avoiding excessive tension on the tissues of the closure. Remember the 'one centimetre-one centimetre' rule as described by Leaper et al.[11] (the so-called 'Guildford technique'; **Figure 9.1.7**). This uses 4 cm of material for every 1 cm advance. This spacing seems to minimize tension in the tissues, and thus also minimize compromise of the circulation in the area, as well as using the minimum acceptable amount of suture. The use of 0 or 1 looped polydioxanone as a continuous suture is recommended.

Retention sutures should be avoided at all costs.

A wound that is deemed to require these is not suitable for primary closure.

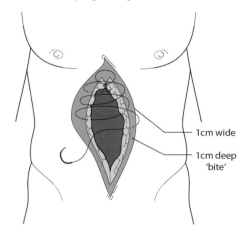

1cm wide

1cm deep 'bite'

Figure 9.1.7 Illustration of the Guildford technique.

Closure of such a wound may result in abdominal compartment syndrome; such a wound should be left open, with a vacuum dressing.

Skin closure as a primary manoeuvre may be done in a case with no or minimal contamination, using monofilament sutures or staples. These latter have the advantage of speed and, whilst being less haemostatic, nevertheless allow for a greater degree of drainage past the skin edges and less tissue reaction.

9.1.7 **Specific Tips and Tricks**

9.1.7.1 **HEADLIGHT**

Even in the most sophisticated of OR suites, clear, well-illuminated vision of the operating field is not optimal. For this reason, the use of a personal, battery-operated headlight of the LED variety is a good addition to the trauma surgeon's armamentarium. In military and austere environments, it is essential, as it may suddenly be the only light available; power cuts are common in Third World countries, and generators fail at the most inappropriate moments. It is a good investment, along with plenty of spare batteries. Do not rely on rechargeable batteries for the reasons given above.

9.1.7.2 **STIRRUPS AND LITHOTOMY POSITION**

The OR scrub nurse should ensure that sterile legging drapes are immediately available should the patient need to be put up into the lithotomy position.

The use of stirrups and lithotomy is not advocated in the initial trauma laparotomy; however, in a complex patient, if the lithotomy position is used, then it is possible to position the scrub nurse (or an assistant) between the patient's legs – perhaps with a small Mayo table over the pubic area. This allows the scrub nurse to see the surgery and anticipate the surgeon's needs, and allows an additional assistant without overcrowding the operative field.

Stirrups should always be in place for injuries that involve – or are suspected of involving – the perineum. For female patients, gynaecological specula and retractors should also be available; and, for both sexes, a good operating sigmoidoscope and light source.

9.1.7.3 **TABLE TILT**

Easy operative access is the aim in all surgery; and just as the senior surgeon, when asked to assist his junior who is struggling, will frequently extend the incision to improve access, so too the use of a table tilt may make all the difference between an uncomfortable operative experience and one that is considerably easier.

A head-down tilt will move the small bowel up out of the pelvis and up under the diaphragm, where it can be held in place by a large roll of gauze. If a head-up tilt is combined with a table tilt to the left, then access to the right lobe of the liver and all the associated biliary anatomy is made easier. A head-up tilt and table tilt to the right will enable access to the spleen and the stomach, though a head-down tilt in this combination is better for repair to the diaphragm itself.

9.1.7.4 BE FLEXIBLE – MOVE!

Trauma surgery requires an open mind – although some knowledge is useful – with no preconceived ideas of exactly what is going to be found, and no rigid operative protocol on how to deal with the situation. This means that the surgeon and the operating team must be prepared to shift positions if unanticipated injury is found, or the procedure could be made technically easier by (for example) standing on the other side of the table or between the legs, raised in lithotomy poles.

The unscrubbed OR personnel should be ready to assist with such moves, along with repositioning of the operating lights. The latter move should not always be delegated to the anaesthetist, who is likely to be busy with resuscitative measures.

9.1.7.5 PERICARDIAL WINDOW

Access to the pericardial sac can be made rapidly and easily from the abdomen by cutting directly backwards into the sac through the diaphragm from the xiphisternum. It is sometimes easier to do this by excising the xiphisternum in an inverted 'V', removing that cartilage in continuity with the backwards incision.

Since the central tendon of the diaphragm and the pericardium share the same embryological origin from the septum transversum, there are no planes to dissect or get lost in. The entry should be immediately into the sac in front of the IVC and below the right atrium, from where it is easy to determine the presence or absence of pericardial tamponade.

9.1.7.6 WASHOUT

The solution to pollution is dilution.

Whether the peritoneal or thoracic cavity is to be washed out, it is a good rule of thumb to consider using at least 6 litres of warm saline – and then doubling it!

There is no advantage to using antiseptic solutions or adding antibiotics to the washouts.

If there has been contamination of the thoracic cavity through a small diaphragmatic hole, and bowel content has entered the thorax, it is wise to extend the diaphragmatic defect in a radial direction (to avoid the phrenic nerve and blood supply), allowing the passage of a hand into the thoracic cavity. This will allow a much more thorough lavage of the thorax, using the hand as a paddle, and less likelihood of retained bowel content and subsequent abscess formation. Always place a large-bore intercostal basal drain, passed up *behind* the hilum of the lung in such cases, before closing the diaphragmatic defect.

Similarly, it is important to make sure that all peritoneal and retroperitoneal recesses are fully irrigated and washed out, though the bare area of the liver and the right suprahepatic space do not need to be disturbed if the right coronary ligament has not been transgressed.

If there have been through-and-through injuries to the liver, it is not a good idea to wash these out if they are not bleeding. (See Section 9.5 on hepatic injury.)

Gross contamination with colonic contents within the peritoneum will require a second look and further washout in 24 hours if the patient's physiology is robust enough.

9.1.7.7 DRAINS

There is no place for drains in the acute damage control laparotomy – with one exception: to the pancreas and duodenum.

Digestive enzymes free in the peritoneum are poor partners to a smooth recovery. Suction drains are recommended.

9.1.7.8 STOMAS

There is no place for stoma formation, either temporary or permanent, in an initial damage control laparotomy. At the first procedure, a temporary closure will have been used, and any divided bowel ends will have been sealed by one means or another ('clip/tie/staple and drop'). Even if the ends are ischaemic, they will not cause leakage for at least 48–72 hours, by which time a second-look laparotomy should have been performed.

Temporary stomas may be formed if the patient's physiology is still precarious at second look, in preference to anastomosis, which is highly risky in the presence of persistent hypotension, or during the administration of inotropes. This may necessitate the formation of the 'split stoma', where both ends of what will become an anastomosis are brought out separately at different sites on the abdominal wall.

It is important to give thought to the main priority for their maintenance (i.e., ease of nursing care). Thus, allow enough space around the stoma for the application of adhesive bags and the cleaning of the surgical wounds. Place stomas more laterally, higher (cranial direction) than normal.

Where a wound of the lower recto-sigmoid has necessitated local excision, it is wise not to oversew the rectal stump, as this creates a blind loop. Then, if the patient later exhibits signs of further sepsis in the ward or intensive care unit (ICU), it will be very difficult to know whether an injury has been missed, the rectal stump has 'blown', or some other site of sepsis is responsible for the patient's decline. In the postoperative abdomen, it is virtually impossible to know – even on CT scanning – if the rectal stump is intact or not, as there will inevitably be murky fluid and postoperative exudate in the peritoneal cavity and pelvis.

It is therefore a good idea to bring up the rectal stump, open, into the lower extent of the laparotomy incision as a mucous fistula. This may require a little mobilization of the rectum to achieve, but it is a safer procedure than leaving a viable, peristaltic, blind-ended time-bomb in the pelvis of a critically ill patient. A tube or corrugated drain can be left coming out of the anus and sutured to the skin of the buttock for safety.

Another advantage of forming a rectal mucous fistula is that it makes the subsequent anastomosis of the colon to the rectum very easy, as the rectal stump is readily available to the surgeon, who does not then have to delve into matted pelvic adhesions to discover its whereabouts, risking further bowel perforation.

9.1.8 Two Catheters: Bladder Injury

(See also Section 9.8 on urological injury.)

Where there has been a bladder injury needing repair, it is a good idea to open the bladder by bivalving it in the sagittal plane (to avoid damaging its blood supply), so that the injury can be seen from both sides. This enables a sound repair to be performed that will include the bladder mucosa. (Like the oesophagus, the integrity

of a bladder repair hinges mainly on good mucosal apposition.)

Once this has been achieved, in male patients, positioning both a suprapubic and a silicon urethral catheter allows both greater safety in management, and more control.

The suprapubic catheter should not be brought out through the bivalve incision into the bladder, as this will almost certainly create a urinary fistula, so it should be brought out of the bladder wall via a separate stab incision into the dome of the bladder and secured by a purse-string suture with absorbable material. It should then be brought out through another stab incision in the abdominal wall, away from the laparotomy incision, and again secured to the skin.

It is not necessary to routinely use suprapubic catheterization in most patients after bladder repair, and placing a large-bore silastic catheter (in lieu of a latex catheter) in the urethra will suffice in most cases. The avoidance of routine suprapubic catheterization has been shown to be associated with lower morbidity and shorter hospital stay. If the urethral catheter should become blocked by blood clots in the postoperative period, it can simply be irrigated or replaced if necessary.

A suprapubic catheter, however, allows the surgeon to assess the patient's voiding ability – once withdrawn – without compromising the bladder repair's integrity. In this way, if the patient is unable to void, the suprapubic catheter acts as a safety valve, and can be released, having been clamped for 'trial-without-catheter' (TWoC). Usually, a few more days with suprapubic drainage are all that is required for the bladder to settle down, and the normal urethral mechanism to resume function.

Once the patient is again voiding good volumes and has a post-micturition sonar confirmation of an empty bladder, the suprapubic catheter may be removed with confidence.

9.1.9 Early Tracheostomy

In damage control situations, it is important to anticipate physiological needs. Patients are in critical condition and do not tolerate multiple surgical insults easily. Surgery in trauma – albeit (hopefully) controlled – constitutes second, third, and even fourth 'hits' on the patient's physiology, so anticipation of future physiological need is necessary from the outset.

Within this remit, ventilatory support is a vital component, and the need for ongoing airway management via the formation of a tracheostomy in the future should be discussed at the first damage control laparotomy, or the second-look at the latest: that is the case if the tracheostomy is to be performed in the OR by the surgical team. Transcutaneous, Seldinger-type tracheostomies may now be performed quite easily in the ICU if required.

Pitfall

This procedure needs to be anticipated early on, and not postponed until the patient has gross retained bronchial secretions and is tipping into respiratory failure which may then demand that regular bronchoscopy be performed until adequate bronchial toilet is achieved, and blood gases are returned to normal.

9.1.10 Briefing for Operating Room Scrub Nurses

A separate briefing for OR scrub nurses comprises Appendix F of this manual.

9.1.11 Summary

Think ahead.
This is the mantra for all on the trauma team, and means:
'Be ready for anything – because it will happen'.

The trauma laparotomy is a team event:
The anaesthesiologist and scrub staff must
all be fully involved and informed of all decision-making.

ANAESTHESIOLOGICAL CONSIDERATIONS

- The trauma laparotomy may be performed for a myriad of reasons. Central in the decision-making, however, is the evolution of physiological derangement. Uncontrolled bleeding mandates immediate transportation to the OR. Hollow viscus injury may allow for extensive time-consuming investigations. Solid organ injuries can be managed non-operatively in the patient who can be stabilized.
- In the physiologically unstable patient, the team should realize that the investigations very often can be performed after the trauma laparotomy. This allows time to contain the bleeding, restore some measure of physiology, and proceed to more sophisticated injury-focussed investigations and procedures. The patient's physiology also influences choices such as choosing for non-operative management, a laparoscopic intervention, or interventional radiology.
- Anaesthesia for the trauma laparotomy consists of essential procedures and secondary procedures. Essential procedures include a definitive airway, two large-bore intravenous cannulae, a gastric tube to guide surgery, and a urine catheter, followed by an arterial and central lines and other monitors. These can be placed during the procedure and should be anticipated in the positioning of the patient and drapes. A rapid infuser is mandatory, if available, with the availability of large-bore lines. A device to warm and rapidly infuse blood and blood products is mandatory.
- The fluid management should be a balance between the safety margin needed to maintain safe circulation parameters (the more blood is lost and the faster it is lost, the more margin you will need) and overfilling, resulting in abdominal compartment syndrome (amongst other things!).
- Initiation of the massive haemorrhage (massive transfusion) protocol (MHP/MTP) in severe injury should be early.
- The anaesthesiologist should monitor physiology and coagulation profiles and communicate results with the team. Usually deep muscle relaxation is maintained (the patient is typically not going to be extubated early). **Early contact with ICU is mandatory, and handover is physician to physician.**
- Monitor safety in the surgical operation area: blood lost, whether haemostasis has been achieved, the timing of the damage control procedure, does the surgeon stick to damage control; and, when safely able to do so, organize the next steps in the treatment sequence.

- The trauma laparotomy influences anaesthesia. Importantly, opening the abdomen can release a torrential bleeding from a previously compressed vessel. Proximal and distal control of the aorta or the IVC or strangulation of the mesenteric blood flow can have profound effects on the circulation. Liver packing on to the diaphragm and the Pringle's manoeuvre may obstruct venous return. A tear in the diaphragm with displacement of intra-abdominal organs into the chest cavity impairs normal ventilation.

The laparotomy in trauma needs to be performed in a systematic fashion. The ease with which injuries can be missed, and the potentially catastrophic consequences of a missed injury, mandate that extreme care is taken to exclude injuries, based on the injury complexes, and the way in which the laparotomy is approached. Careful examination of each organ is essential.

REFERENCES AND FURTHER READING

References

1. Meizoso JP, Rattan R, Namias NJ. Delays to the operating room increase mortality in sick trauma patients. *J Trauma Acute Care Surg*. 2017 Oct;**83(4)**:747. doi:10.1097/TA.0000000000001512

2. Santucci RA, Fisher MB. The literature increasingly supports expectant (conservative) management of renal trauma–a systematic review. *J Trauma*. 2005 Aug;59(2):493–503. doi: 10.1097/01.ta.0000179956.55078.c0.

3. Como JJ, Bokhari F, Chiu WC, Duane T, Holevar MR, Tandoh MA, et al. Practice management guidelines for selective nonoperative management of penetrating abdominal trauma. *J Trauma*. 2010 Mar;**68(3)**:721–33. doi: 10.1097/TA.0b013e3181cf7d07.

4. Goldberg SR, Anand RJ, Como JJ, Dechert T, Dente C, Luchette FA, Prophylactic antibiotic use in penetrating abdominal trauma: an Eastern Association for the Surgery of Trauma practice management guideline. *J Trauma Acute Care Surg*. 2012 Nov;**73(5 Suppl. 4)**:S321–5. doi: 10.1097/TA.0b013e3182701902.

5. Hardcastle TC, M Stander M, Kalafatis N, Hodgson RE, Gopalan D. External patient temperature control in emergency centres, trauma centres, intensive care units and operating theatres: A multi-society literature review. *S Afr Med J*. 2013 Aug 6;**103(9)**:609–11. doi: 10.7196/samj.7327.

6. Oosthuizen GV, Weale R, Kong VY, Bruce JL, Urry RJ, Laing GL, et al. The effect of a concomitant renal injury on the outcome of colonic trauma. *Am J Surg*. 2018 Aug;**216(2)**:230–4. doi: 10.1016/j.amjsurg.2017.11.036.

7. Cattell RB, Braasch RW. A technique for the exposure of the third and fourth parts of the duodenum. *Surg Gynaecol Obstet*. 1960;**111**:379–85.

8. Mattox KL, McCollum WB, Jordan GL Jr, Beall AC Jr, DeBakey ME. Management of upper abdominal vascular trauma. *Am J Surg*. 1974 Dec;**128(6)**:823–8.

9. Thal ER, O'Keefe T. Operative exposure of abdominal injuries and closure of the abdomen. In *ACS Surgery: Principles and Practice*. New York: Web MD, 2007: Section 7 Chapter 9.

10. Mahoney EJ, Bugaev N, Appelbaum R, Goldenberg-Sandau A, Baltazar GA, Posluszny J, et al. Management of the open abdomen: A systematic review with meta-analysis and practice management guideline from the Eastern Association for the Surgery of Trauma. *J Trauma*. 2022 Sept;**93(3)**:e110–8. doi: 10.1097/TA.0000000000003683. Epub 2022 May 12.

11. Leaper DJ, Pollock AV, Evans M. Abdominal wound closure: a trial of nylon, polyglycolic acid and steel sutures. *Br J Surg* 1977 Aug;**64(8)**:603–6. doi: 10.1002/bjs.1800640822.

Recommended Reading

Hirshberg A. Mattox KL. *Top Knife: The Art and Craft of Trauma Surgery*. Harley, United Kingdom: TFM Publishing Ltd, 2005.

Ogura T, Lefor AT, Nakano M, Izawa Y, Morita H. Nonoperative management of hemodynamically unstable abdominal trauma patients with angioembolization and resuscitative endovascular balloon occlusion of the aorta. *J Trauma Acute Care Surg*. 2015;**78(1)**:132–5. doi: 10.1097/TA.0000000000000473.

2017 update of the WSES guidelines for emergency repair of complicated abdominal wall hernias https://wjes.biomedcentral.com/articles/10.1186/s13017-017-0149-y

Western Trauma Association Guidelines (http://www.westerntrauma.org)

Martin M, Brown CVR, Shatz DV, Alam HB, Brasel KJ, Hauser CJ, et al. Evaluation and management of abdominal stab wounds: A Western Trauma Association critical decisions algorithm. *J Trauma Acute Care Surg.* 2018 Nov;**85(5)**:1007–15. doi: 10.1097/TA.0000000000001930.

Martin MJ, Brown CVR, Shatz DV, Alam H, Brasel K, Hauser CJ, et al. Evaluation and management of abdominal gunshot wounds: A Western Trauma Association critical decisions algorithm. *J Trauma Acute Care Surg.* 2019 Nov;**87(5)**: 1220–27. doi: 10.1097/TA.0000000000002410.

Sava J, Alam, HB, Vercruysse G, Martin M, Brown C, Brasel K, et al. Management of the open abdomen after damage control surgery. *J Trauma Acute Care Surg.* 2019 Nov;87(5):1232–8. doi: 10.1097/TA.0000000000002389

9.2 Abdominal Vascular Injury

9.2.1 **Overview**

Abdominal vascular injury presents a serious threat to life, where preparedness and anticipation are vital to a successful outcome. Consideration of both the possible injuries and the surgical approach to manage them is crucial. Adequate preparation is essential; an adequate incision will be required.

It is helpful to have available all the apparatus for massive transfusion, with activation of the massive transfusion protocol, ensuring rapid mobilization of packed cells, plasma, and platelets to the emergency department and operating room.

Major vessel injuries within the abdominal cavity primarily present as haemorrhagic shock that does not respond to resuscitation; thus, immediate surgery becomes a part of the resuscitative effort. In penetrating injury, this may necessitate an emergency department thoracotomy (EDT) and aortic cross-clamp. Consideration should also be given to resuscitative endovascular balloon occlusion of the aorta (REBOA; see Section 15.3), which has a role in controlling abdominal and pelvic haemorrhage in a similar but less invasive manner to that of EDT (see Section 8.9).[1]

The emergency department thoracotomy (EDT) is usually not indicated in the severely shocked patient with blunt abdominal trauma, as the survival rate is close to zero.

With an expanding haematoma, source control with direct or proximal control of the vessel is mandatory for success, where the surgeon should anticipate gaining control above the level of the injury. The steps in decision-making can be iterated thus:

1. **Is the patient's condition so parlous that immediate aortic cross-clamping must be undertaken via a thoracotomy?**

   Typically, this is the patient who has lost cardiac output (loss of palpable central pulse) immediately prior to reception in the resuscitation bay or is about to do so (drop in Glasgow Coma Scale [GCS] score, drop in end-tidal CO_2, bradycardia). The cross-clamping will cut off the arterial bleeding distally and preserve blood flow to the brain and coronary vessels.

   In patients with pending arrest (or very low systolic pressure of thin palpated pulses), the use of partial REBOA might have some positive effect, as seen by the ABOtrauma registry and AORTA registry recently. Survival is very low, but there are survivors. If the patient does not respond to REBOA (REBOA non-responder), the survival rate is zero.

2. **Does the patient's condition permit expedited transfer to the operating room for definitive haemorrhage control?**

   This is the patient in whom ongoing volume resuscitation is needed to maintain a coherent circulatory output and the threat of decompensation is ever-present.

3. **Does the patient's condition permit computed tomography (CT) scan as a prelude to definitive operative repair (or transfer to the interventional radiology [IR] suite for embolization of amenable injury patterns)?**

This patient will have responded to initial resuscitation such that they can withstand a 10–15-minute period of transfer and CT scanning. With the use of a hybrid emergency room and gantry CT, this might be a very fast procedure that is possible to do, but **CT should not cause treatment delay**.

Pitfall

Step 3 must not be exploited as a means of deferring surgical control by those who are unfamiliar with, and therefore anxious about executing, the surgical interventions described in this chapter.

9.2.2 Retroperitoneal Haematoma

Haematomas are:

- Central (Zone 1)
- Lateral (Zone 2)
- Pelvic (Zone 3)

9.2.2.1 CENTRAL HAEMATOMA

Central haematomas can be further classified according to whether the apex lies in the *supracolic* or *infracolic* portion of the abdomen, as judged by whether the apex is positioned with respect to the mesentery of the transverse colon. Haematomas that lie largely inferior (caudal) to this landmark involve the aortic bifurcation or the inferior mesenteric artery (IMA)-bearing portion and are exposed by transperitoneal or left medial visceral rotation that may not need splenic, renal, or pancreatic mobilization. Haematomas that lie above (cranial) are due to the more challenging injuries of the juxta-renal and suprarenal aorta or injury to the superior mesenteric artery (SMA)–bearing or coeliac artery–bearing portions.

- If the apex of the central haematoma is to the *right* side of the midline, and observed bleeding is primarily venous in nature, the right colon should be mobilized to the midline, including the duodenum and head of the pancreas (right medial visceral rotation).

This will expose the infrarenal cava and infrarenal aorta. It will also facilitate access to the portal vein.

- If the apex of the central haematoma is on the *left* side of the midline, and observed bleeding is primarily arterial in nature, it is best to approach the injury from the left. Left medial visceral rotation provides access to the aorta, the coeliac axis, the superior mesenteric artery, the splenic artery and vein, and the left renal artery and vein. In order to reach the posterior wall of the aorta, the kidney should be mobilized as well and rotated medially on its pedicle, taking great care not to cause further injury.

9.2.2.2 LATERAL HAEMATOMA

If these are not expanding or pulsatile, blunt injuries are best left alone, as the damage is usually renal. Renal injuries can generally be managed non-operatively including the use of selective embolization. However, with penetrating injury, because of the risk of damage to adjacent structures such as the ureter, it is safer to explore lateral haematomas. The surgeon must also be confident that there is no perforation of the posterior part of the colon in the paracolic gutters on either side.

9.2.2.3 PELVIC HAEMATOMA

If the patient is stable, contrast-enhanced CT in the emergency situation may demonstrate a large pelvic haematoma with a vascular 'blush' indicating ongoing arterial bleeding. In this case, it may be more appropriate to transfer the patient for immediate embolization.

- Pelvic haematomas discovered at laparotomy should be considered in terms of patient stability.
  - Non-expanding haematomas in the context of a physiologically stable or improving patient are best left alone.
  - Expanding haematomas with patient instability must be dealt with.

9.2.2.3.1 Extraperitoneal Pelvic Packing (EPP)

In the context of blunt trauma (fractured pelvis), the first concern should be to ensure that a pelvic binder is correctly positioned to reduce pelvic volume. The next is to perform extraperitoneal pelvic packing (EPP).[2] Haemostats are applied to the incised peritoneal edge, located on either side of the lower 25% of the laparotomy full-length incision. The pre-peritoneal plane is then developed laterally such that the haematoma is entered, and the clot is evacuated manually. It is important that the plane posterior to the rectum is fully developed before tightly packing this space with 2–3 large swabs. The manoeuvre should be repeated for the opposite side. If the packs remain dry, then no further adjunctive manoeuvres are required. If strike-through occurs, then re-pack again. If strike-through occurs despite this, then the relevant internal iliac artery should be ligated. Even if EPP controls the bleeding, the patient should be transferred to the IR suite for angiography, interrogation of vascular integrity, and selective embolization at the completion of the damage control laparotomy. Once haemostasis is fully secured in this manner, and the patient's haemodynamic state is more stable, consideration can be given to loosening of the pelvic binder in order to prevent pressure sores. Stabilization of the pelvis using external fixators or a C-clamp in the operating room can be considered, but this does not always provide adequate posterior fixation and is secondary to effective pelvic packing and embolization, or the EVTM (endovascular resuscitation and trauma management) concept.

9.2.3 Surgical Approach to Major Abdominal Vessels

9.2.3.1 INCISION

The patient must be prepared 'from sternal notch to knee'. It is critical to gain proximal and distal control, and patient preparation should include the need to extend to a left lateral thoracotomy to gain access to the thoracic aorta, a median sternotomy to control the intracardiac inferior vena cava (IVC), and groin incisions to gain control of the iliac vessels.

9.2.3.2 MEDIAL VISCERAL ROTATIONS

See Section 9.1.2.7, particularly Subsections 9.1.2.7.5 and 9.1.2.7.6.

9.2.3.3 AORTA

Control of the aorta can be achieved at several different levels, depending on the site of injury.

(For indications and use of REBOA, see Section 15.3.)

The supracoeliac aorta can be exposed by the following steps:

a. Retracting the left lobe of the liver towards the patient's right shoulder.

b. Retracting the body of the stomach towards the left hip.

c. Making a window in the lesser omentum.

d. Visualizing the peritoneum covering the crus of the diaphragm.

e. Sharply incising the peritoneum to expose the muscle fibres of the crus.

f. Splitting the fibres longitudinally, such that the pearly white adventitia of the aorta is seen.

g. Developing the plane on either side of the aorta to admit the jaws of a straight vascular clamp (**Figure 9.2.1**)

Pitfall

Clamping the oesophagus rather than the aorta. Identification of the oesophagus which lies to the left of the aorta is aided by the prior placement of a nasogastric tube.

Exposure of the suprarenal aorta is difficult from the anterior approach, especially in the context of a supracolic haematoma overlying the coeliac and superior mesenteric artery regions. Exposure can be obtained by performing a left medial visceral rotation procedure. The

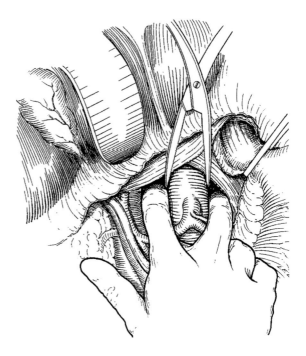

Figure 9.2.1 Control of the aorta by cross-clamping at the crura of the diaphragm.

entire abdominal aorta and the origins of its branches are exposed by this technique. This includes the coeliac axis, the origin of the superior mesenteric artery, the iliac vessels, and the left renal pedicle. The dense and fibrous superior mesenteric and coeliac nerve plexuses, however, overlie the proximal aorta and need to be sharply dissected in order to identify the renal and superior mesenteric arteries.[3]

Pitfall

Dissecting out the coeliac and superior mesenteric arteries is challenging due to dense ganglionic tissues. It is strongly recommended that the supracoeliac aorta is controlled before entering the supracolic central haematoma. This can be done via two ways: transperitoneal (see below) either via the lesser omentum or via the retroperitoneum. The latter route involves the fullest possible left medial visceral rotation (including the kidney, spleen, and pancreas) with division of the left crus from the lateral aspect.

The distal aorta can be approached transperitoneally by retracting the small bowel to the right, the transverse colon superiorly, and the descending colon to the left. The aorta below the left renal vein can be accessed by incising the peritoneum over it and mobilizing the third and fourth parts of the duodenum superiorly. Both iliac vessels can be exposed by distal continuation of the dissection. The ureters should be identified and carefully preserved, especially in the region of the bifurcation of the iliac vessels.

Treatment of aortic or caval injuries is usually straightforward. Extensive lacerations are not compatible with survival, and it is uncommon to require graft material to repair the aorta. Caval injuries below the renal veins, if extensive, can be ligated, although lateral repair is preferred. Injuries above the renal veins in the cava should be repaired, if possible (suture repair, patching, or inlay segmental grafting), as ligation at this level is usually not survivable.

9.2.3.4 COELIAC AXIS

The left colon is reflected to the right, together with the spleen and the tail of the pancreas, to display the aorta and its branches. The coeliac trunk lies behind and inferior to the gastro-oesophageal junction. Injuries to this area are commonly missed, particularly in patients with stab wounds. Major vascular injury is particularly likely if there is a central retroperitoneal haematoma. In this situation, proximal vascular control prior to entering the haematoma is essential, either locally in the abdomen or via a left lateral thoracotomy. Division of the left triangular ligament and mobilization of the lateral segment of the left lobe of the liver are also helpful.

It is difficult to 'repair' the coeliac axis, as it is a short trunk-like vessel where access is by adherent ganglionic tissues and the branching origins of the left gastric, common hepatic, and splenic vessels. Bleeding from this structure is more akin to haemorrhage from a direct injury to the front of the aorta, and surgical control approximates to direct oversewing of an identifiable haemorrhage point with 3-0 Prolene® (Johnson & Johnson, New Brunswick, NJ, USA) with a secondary goal of maintenance of perfusion of its branches. End-organ ischaemia is not a likelihood, assuming that the superior mesenteric artery and inferior mesenteric artery remain intact.

The left gastric and splenic arteries can be ligated. The common hepatic artery can be safely tied provided that the injury is proximal to the gastroduodenal artery.

9.2.3.5 SUPERIOR MESENTERIC ARTERY[4]

The superior mesenteric artery is a vital artery for the viability of the small bowel, and it should always be repaired, using conventional techniques. Proximally, the artery is accessible from the aorta at the level of the renal arteries and is best approached with a left medial visceral rotation (**Figure 9.2.2**). More distally, the artery is accessed at the root of the small bowel mesentery.

If a period of ischaemia has elapsed, or the surgery is part of a damage control procedure, the artery should be shunted, using a plastic vascular shunt (e.g., a Javid™ shunt, Bard, Tempe, AZ, USA), until repair can be affected.[5]

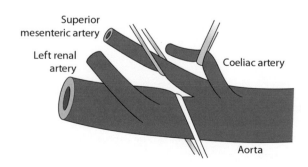

Figure 9.2.2 Anatomy of the superior mesenteric artery.

If repair is not possible, and replacement of the artery with a graft is required, it is best to place the graft on the infrarenal aorta, away from the pancreas and areas of potential leak.[6] Placement of the proximal end of the graft too high can result in kinking and subsequent occlusion of the graft when the bowel is returned to the abdominal cavity. The graft must be tailored so that there is no tension, and the aortic suture line must be covered to prevent an aorto-enteric fistula (**Figure 9.2.2**).

The survival rate with penetrating injuries of the superior mesenteric artery is approximately 58%, falling to 22% if a complex repair is required.[6,7]

The superior mesenteric vein can be either shunted or simply ligated.[8]

9.2.3.6 INFERIOR MESENTERIC ARTERY

Injuries to the inferior mesenteric artery are uncommon, and the artery can generally be tied off. The viability of the colon should be checked before closure, with planned reoperation to evaluate viability of the colon.

9.2.3.7 RENAL ARTERIES

Preliminary vascular control is best obtained by accessing the renal arteries on the aorta using a standard infrarenal aortic approach. Access can also be obtained by mobilizing the viscera medially.

Repair is done using standard vascular techniques. However, the kidney tolerates warm ischaemia poorly, with 45 minutes of clamp time usually associated with permanent loss of function. Therefore, if there has been complete transection of the artery, and the kidney is of doubtful viability, preservation may not be in the best interest of the patient and an early nephrectomy considered.

9.2.3.8 ILIAC VESSELS

Proximal and distal control may be required, and distal control via a separate groin incision should be considered.

The iliac vessels are exposed by lifting the small bowel upwards, out of the pelvis. On the left, the sigmoid colon and its mesentery can be mobilized, and on the right, division of the peritoneal attachments over the caecum and mobilization of the caecum to the midline will aid exposure of the vessels.

The ureters must be formally identified, as they cross the iliac bifurcation.

Pitfall

The common iliac veins are often strongly adherent to the back wall of the common iliac artery and attempts to 'sling' or encircle the arteries, or to mobilize the vein off the back of the artery, for purposes of control may result in torrential bleeding. A 'just enough' policy to dissection is advisable, with the operator gaining enough access to the front and sides of the common iliac artery and vein (CIA/CIV) to allow room for a clamp above and below the injury zone; sometimes a side-biting clamp (e.g., a Satinsky clamp) is sufficient.

9.2.3.9 INFERIOR VENA CAVA (IVC)[9]

Suprahepatic IVC (see Section 9.4.8)

This is usually required for injuries affecting the retrohepatic IVC or hepatic veins. A frequently fatal injury complex is heralded by profuse venous bleeding that emanates from the back of the liver, not controlled by clamping of the portal triad but only controllable by direct downward pressure over the front of the liver such that the cava is firmly compressed.

Following exposure and clamping of the IVC above the renal vessels (see below) and whilst maintaining downward pressure on the liver, the coronary ligaments must be divided such that the liver can be displaced inferior-medially and the suprahepatic IVC seen. This manoeuvre is helped by splitting the central tendon of the diaphragm such that the portion of the IVC traversing the pericardium and diaphragm is revealed. The laparotomy incision can be extended across the costal margin into the right chest as a further adjunct. Alternatively, access to the suprahepatic IVC can be obtained from within the chest by performing a median sternotomy and opening the pericardium. Alternatively, the surgeon must fully mobilize the liver by incising the central tendon of the diaphragm, or by performing a median sternotomy and opening the pericardium.

The above-described procedure is best attempted by surgeons experienced with the technique. It may be safer to attempt restoring containment of the retrohepatic space/bare area of the liver by packing, and the use of vena cava REBOA (REBOAVC).

Infrahepatic IVC

The infrahepatic vena cava can be exposed by means of a right medial visceral rotation (**Figure 9.2.3**).

(See also right medial visceral rotation in Section 9.1.2.5.)

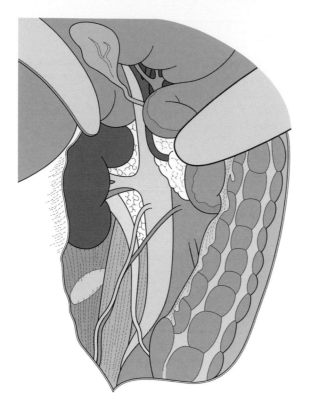

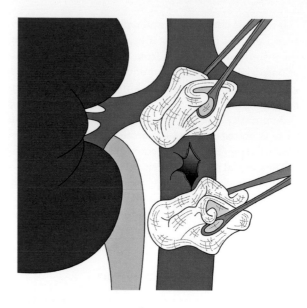

Figure 9.2.4 Control of the inferior vena cava using swab pressure.

Figure 9.2.3 Right medial visceral rotation to expose the inferior vena cava.

The right colon is mobilized by taking down the hepatic flexure and incising the peritoneal reflection down the length of the right paracolic gutter. The colon is then reflected medially in a plane anterior to Gerota's fascia. If more exposure is required, the root of the mesentery can be mobilized by dividing the inferior mesenteric vein. Performance of a Kocher manoeuvre and medial mobilization of the duodenum and head of the pancreas will reveal the segment of vena cava immediately below the liver and provide excellent exposure of the right renovascular pedicle.

Control is best achieved by direct pressure on the IVC above and below the injury, utilizing swabs (**Figure 9.2.4**).

If more definitive control is required, a combination of vascular clamps to the renal arteries and Rumel[10] tourniquets placed above the renal vessels (suprarenal), or above and below the injury, should be used (**Figure 9.2.5**).

Injuries to the posterior part of the IVC should always be expected with penetrating injury to the anterior part

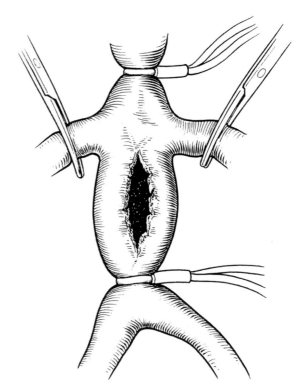

Figure 9.2.5 Control of the inferior vena cava with clamps and two Rumel tourniquets.

of the IVC. Not all bleeding posterior wounds need to be repaired.

It is very difficult to 'roll' the IVC to approach it posteriorly, due to multiple lumbar veins, so all injuries should be approached transcavally. Not all non-bleeding posterior wounds require repair.

Provided it is infrarenal, ligation of the IVC is acceptable.

9.2.3.10 **PORTAL VEIN**[11]

The portal vein lies in the free edge of the lesser omentum, together with the common bile duct and the hepatic artery (**Figure 9.2.6**).

The portal vein generally can be controlled with a Pringle's manoeuvre. If the injury is more proximal, it may be necessary to reflect the duodenum medially, or divide the pancreas.

The portal vein should be shunted early to avoid venous hypertension of the bowel, which will make access to the area increasingly difficult. The stent can be left in place as part of a damage control procedure or repaired. Portocaval shunting is a possibility, with ligation as a last resort which, however, carries a high mortality.

9.2.4 **Shunting**

If repair is not possible, or the procedure is being abbreviated, vascular shunting will restore circulation. It can be performed atraumatically and rapidly.

If a Javid™ or other proprietary shunts are available, these can be used. However, if they are not, a shunt can be fashioned from a suitable size of plastic tube, for example nasogastric tube, endotracheal tube, chest tube, or the like:

- The length required is three times the length of the defect.
- The diameter should be two-thirds of the diameter of the vessel to be shunted.

The shunt is fashioned as follows (**Figure 9.2.7**):

- Choose a plastic tube with the correct diameter.
- Cut the tube to length, as described above, bevelling the edges so that they can be passed into the vessel.
- Tie a length of silk around the tube, dividing it into a one-third to two-thirds ratio.

Once the vessel has been controlled, using either clamps or Rumel tourniquets:

- Clamp one end of the shunt to prevent leakage.

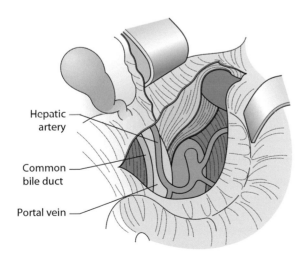

Figure 9.2.6 Access to the portal vein.

Hepatic artery

Common bile duct

Portal vein

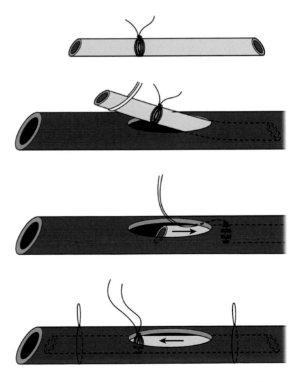

Figure 9.2.7 Diagrammatic representation of the 'manufacture' and placement of a vascular shunt.

- Pass the 'long' (two-thirds) end of the shunt up the vessel until the shunt is lying inside the vessel lumen or proximally, releasing the tourniquet to allow it to pass through.
- Using the silk as a 'handle', pull the shunt distally into the other end of the vessel.
- Secure it with ties.

There is no need for anticoagulation, as the patients are often coagulopathic and the rate of flow itself should prevent clot formation. The shunt can be left in place for 48–72 hours.

REFERENCES

1. Brenner ML, Moore LJ, DuBose JJ, Tyson GH, McNutt MK, Albarado RP, et al. A clinical series of resuscitative endovascular balloon occlusion of the aorta for hemorrhage control and resuscitation. *J Trauma Acute Care Surg*. 2013 Sep;**75(3)**:506–11. doi: 10.1097/TA.0b013e31829e5416.2.
2. Smith WR, Moore EE, Osborn P, Agudelo JF, Morgan SJ, Parekh AA, et al. Retroperitoneal packing as a resuscitation technique for haemodynamically unstable patients with pelvic fractures: report of two representative cases and a description of technique. *J Trauma*. 2005 Dec;**59(6)**:1510–14. doi: 10.1097/01.ta.0000197330.81352.94.
3. Accola KD, Feliciano DV, Mattox KL, Bitondo CG, Burch JM, Beall AC Jr, Jordan GL Jr. Management of injuries to the suprarenal aorta. *Am J Surg*. 1987 Dec;**154(6)**:613–8. doi: 10.1016/0002-9610(87)90227-3.
4. Asensio JA, Berne JD, Chahwan S, Hanpeter D, Demetriades D, Marengo J, et al. Traumatic injury to the superior mesenteric artery. *Am J Surg*. 1999 Sep;**178(3)**:235–9. doi: 10.1016/s0002-9610(99)00166-x.
5. Reilly PM, Rotondo MF, Carpenter JP, Sherr SA, Schwab CW. Temporary vascular continuity during damage control: intraluminal shunting for proximal superior mesenteric artery injury. *J Trauma*. 1995 Oct;**39(4)**:757–60. doi: 10.1097/00005373-199510000-00028.
6. Accola KD, Feliciano DV, Mattox KL, Burch JM, Beall AC Jr, Jordan GL Jr. Management of injuries to the superior mesenteric artery. *J Trauma*. 1986 Apr;**26(4)**:313–19. doi: 10.1097/00005373-198604000-00002.
7. Asensio JA, Britt LD, Borzotta A, Peitzman A, Miller FB, Mackersie RC, et al. Multi-institutional experience with the management of superior mesenteric artery injuries. *J Am Coll Surg*. 2001 Dec;**193(6)**:354–65; discussion 365–6. doi: 10.1016/s1072-7515(01)01044-4.
8. Donahue TK, Strauch GO. Ligation as definitive management of injury to the superior mesenteric vein. *J Trauma*. 1988 Apr;**28(4)**:541–3. doi: 10.1097/00005373-198804000-00023.
9. Feliciano DV, Burch JM, Mattox K, Edelman M. Injuries of the inferior vena cava. *Am J Surg*. 1988 Dec;**156(6)**:548–52. doi: 10.1016/s0002-9610(88)80550-6.
10. Welling DR, Rich NM, Burris DG, Boffard KD, Devries WC. Who was William Ray Rumel? *World J Surg*. 2008 Sep;**32(9)**:2122–5. doi: 10.1007/s00268-008-9599-4.
11. Stone HH, Fabian TC, Turkleson ML. Wounds of the portal venous system. *World J Surg*. 1982;**6**:335–41. doi: 10.1016/0002-9610(82)90074-5.

9.3 Bowel, Rectum, and Diaphragm

9.3.1 Overview

The surgeon must always bear in mind the three-dimensional nature of wound tracks in penetrating injury. An odd number of bowel enterotomies should prompt a second look for missed injury.

In all patients who are subjected to laparotomy after injury, the entire length of bowel, from the oesophagogastric junction to the stomach, the small bowel from the ligament of Treitz, the ileo-caecal valve, and the large bowel from the caecum to the rectum, and their mesenteries, should be inspected. (See Section 9.1: 'The Trauma Laparotomy'.)

Pitfall

Failure to inspect the diaphragm, especially in the presence of penetrating injury, especially if below the 5th intercostal space.

Both the surgeon and the assistant independently inspect the same segment at the same time. Ideally, only one operator handles the bowel at any time, as otherwise each operator thinks that the other is doing the inspection.

Two hands, but four eyes.

The commonest sites of missed organ injury in the abdomen are:

- Diaphragm
- Oesophago-gastric junction
- Along the lesser or greater curvature of the stomach (a penetrating injury can be obscured by the fatty envelope of the vessels in these locations)
- The posterior aspect of the stomach and adjacent pancreas (in the lesser sac; a missed injury here led to the death of President McKinley in 1902)[1]
- Small bowel (a small penetrating injury to the small bowel can be easy to miss)
- Retroperitoneal colon and rectum

9.3.2 **Diaphragm**

The diaphragm divides the torso into thoracic and abdominal components. Particularly with penetrating injury, the penetration may go through the diaphragm and give misleading signs. For example, a stab wound of the lower chest with a haemothorax may reflect an intra-abdominal injury to the liver, spleen, or kidney, with blood draining through the diaphragm into the chest. All diaphragmatic injuries benefit from early diagnosis and repair. The presence of a defect poses significant risk of herniation of abdominal contents (most commonly, stomach or colon) into the chest because the thoracic cavity is at negative pressure compared to the abdominal cavity. Herniation may occur during the acute trauma phase or may be delayed by months to years, and it may be acutely life-threatening due to strangulation and/or tension gastrothorax or colothorax.

Diagnosis of a diaphragmatic defect is not possible with imaging unless *herniation has occurred*. In the case of herniation, chest X-ray may demonstrate the appearance of a raised hemidiaphragm or the presence of a hollow viscus in the chest. Passage of a nasogastric tube prior to performing a chest X-ray will show the presence of a herniated stomach in the left thoracic cavity. CT is helpful to demonstrate hollow as well as solid viscera in the chest. In the event of blunt trauma with acute herniation through the left hemidiaphragm, it is important to rule out an oesophageal blow-out injury (i.e. look for gas in the posterior mediastinum in the vicinity of the thoracic or oesophageal). Although rare, missing this injury is potentially life-threatening.

When herniation has not occurred through a diaphragmatic injury, the only way to diagnose it is by *direct inspection*. Penetrating trauma to the *left* thoraco-abdominal region (the ribcage below the fifth intercostal space) may be associated with as high as 40% likelihood of a diaphragmatic defect.[1] If such a patient is stable and has no indication for laparotomy, laparoscopy or video-assisted thoracoscopy (VATS) is helpful for inspection of the diaphragm. VATS is useful in patients who may benefit from the simultaneous management of a pleural collection; otherwise, many surgeons prefer laparoscopy. However, if an indication for laparotomy exists, it remains preferable to laparoscopy (see Chapter 15). Laparoscopic or thoracoscopic repair of the diaphragm is indicated if a defect is found, regardless of the size of the defect.

The Eastern Association for the Surgery of Trauma (EAST) PICO (population, intervention, comparison, and outcome) guidelines may be helpful as shown in **Tables 9.3.1** and **9.3.2**.[2]

Note that penetrating injury to the *right* thoraco-abdominal region does not routinely require the above-mentioned approach, since the liver tends to act as a barrier, and herniation on this side is uncommon.

Herniation through the diaphragm mandates exploratory laparotomy in most cases, to exclude subdiaphragmatic visceral injuries.

Repair of the diaphragm at laparotomy is relatively straightforward. It is crucial to hold the laceration at its apices with two Littlewoods or Allis tissue forceps and to *pull the diaphragm out towards oneself*. This greatly facilitates repair, as opposed to struggling in the depths of the abdomen. The laceration can be sutured in a continuous fashion

Table 9.3.1 PICO Format for Recommendations

P	Patient, Population, or Problem	How would I describe the patient group?
I	Intervention, Prognostic factor, or Exposure	Which main intervention, prognostic factor, or exposure is considered?
C	Comparison or Intervention (if appropriate)	What is the main alternative to compare with the intervention?
O	Outcome you would like to measure or achieve	What can be accomplished, measured, improved, or affected?

Table 9.3.2 PICO Recommendation for Diaphragmatic Injury

PICO	Question	Guidelines
1	In left-sided thoracoabdominal stab wound patients who are haemodynamically stable and without peritonitis (P), should laparoscopy (I) or computed tomography (C) be performed to decrease the incidence of missed diaphragmatic injury (O)?	In left thoracoabdominal stab wound patients who are haemodynamically stable and without peritonitis (P), we **conditionally recommend** laparoscopy (I) rather than computed tomography (C) to decrease the incidence of missed diaphragmatic injury (O).
2	In penetrating thoracoabdominal trauma patients who are haemodynamically stable without peritonitis and in whom a right diaphragm injury is confirmed or suspected (P), should operative (I) or non-operative (C) management be undertaken to minimize both the need for delayed operation for diaphragmatic hernia and the risk of surgical morbidity (procedural complications, LOS, surgical site infection, and empyema) (O)?	In penetrating thoracoabdominal trauma patients in whom a right diaphragm injury is confirmed or suspected, and who are haemodynamically stable without peritonitis (P), we **conditionally recommend** non-operative (I) over operative (O) management in weighing the risks of delayed herniation, missed thoracoabdominal organ injury, and surgical morbidity (procedural complications, LOS, surgical site infection, and empyema) (O).
3	In haemodynamically stable trauma patients with acute diaphragm injuries (P), should the abdominal (I) or thoracic (C) approach be used to repair the diaphragm to decrease mortality, delayed herniation, missed thoracoabdominal organ injury, and surgical approach–associated morbidity (procedural complications, LOS, surgical site infection, and empyema) (O)?	In haemodynamically stable trauma patients with acute diaphragm injuries, we **conditionally recommend** (P) the abdominal (I) rather than the thoracic (C) approach to repair the diaphragm to decrease mortality, delayed herniation, missed thoracoabdominal organ injury, and surgical approach–associated morbidity (procedural complications, LOS, surgical site infection, and empyema) (O).
4	In patients who present with delayed visceral herniation through a traumatic diaphragmatic injury (P), should the abdominal (I) or thoracic (C) approach be used to decrease mortality and surgical approach–related morbidity (procedural complications, surgical site infection, LOS, and empyema) (O)?	In patients who present with delayed visceral herniation through a traumatic diaphragmatic injury (P), **we make no recommendation** in regard to the routine surgical approach, abdominal (I) or thoracic (O), to decrease mortality and surgical approach–related morbidity (procedural complications, surgical site infection, LOS, and empyema) (O).
5	In patients with acute penetrating diaphragmatic injuries without concern for other intra-abdominal injuries (P), should laparoscopic (I) or open (C) repair be performed to decrease mortality, delayed herniation, missed thoracoabdominal organ injury, and surgical approach–associated morbidity (procedural complications, LOS, surgical site infection, and empyema) (O)?	In patients with acute penetrating diaphragmatic injuries without concern for other intra-abdominal injuries (P), we **conditionally recommend** laparoscopic (I) over open (C) repair in weighing the risks of mortality, delayed herniation, missed thoracoabdominal organ, and surgical approach–associated morbidity (procedural complications, LOS, surgical site infection, and empyema) (O).

Note: As it is generally accepted that penetrating injuries to the left diaphragm require repair, no PICO question was formulated to study this topic.

using a non-absorbable suture. There is **no** evidence that a braided suture or interrupted sutures make much difference; however, interrupted sutures may be helpful when dealing with a jagged laceration or a blown-out laceration which stretches in two or three directions. The use of synthetic material to close large defects from high-velocity missile or shotgun injuries is only rarely indicated. If the defect is so large that the edges cannot be opposed, it can be closed with a patch, such as polytetrafluoroethylene (PTFE). Ideally, this is done using a transthoracic approach.

If the laceration is close to the pericardium,
extra care must be taken not to inadvertently
include the pericardium in the suture.

If there is major contamination of the abdominal cavity, then the thoracic cavity must be thoroughly washed out as well, using copious amounts of normal saline, and a chest drain placed. It may be necessary to enlarge the diaphragmatic defect in order to facilitate adequate chest washout. The laceration can be enlarged radially towards the chest wall (cutting the diaphragm transversely may divide branches of the phrenic nerve); or, if the injury is peripheral, the defect may be enlarged transversely along the chest wall. The diaphragmatic defect should be closed prior to washing out the abdominal cavity to avoid further contamination.

The complications of injuries to the diaphragm are primarily related to late diagnosis with hernia formation and incarceration. Phrenic nerve palsy is another complication, but this is uncommon after penetrating trauma.

9.3.3 **Stomach**

The stomach is lifted and pulled caudally, using two Babcock forceps, and the anterior surface inspected. It is helpful if there is a nasogastric tube in place – place the forceps around the tube, forming a useful gastric retractor. The lesser sac should be entered through the greater omentum, and the stomach can then be lifted to allow inspection of its posterior surface (as well as the body and tail of the pancreas).

The stomach is highly vascular, and in all injuries, life-threatening bleeding can result. All holes should be repaired using a continuous, full-thickness 2/0 or 3/0 monofilament suture. Simple gastric injuries can be minimally debrided and closed; more complex gastric injuries should be controlled by non-anatomic resection, with reconstruction deferred to the re-look laparotomy.

Pitfall

In all penetrating injuries in which a hole is found on the anterior surface of the stomach, it is important to seek the corresponding hole on the posterior wall of the stomach. If this cannot be found, enlarge the anterior hole, and inspect the stomach from within: 'Penetrating holes generally go in pairs – one in, one out'. Carefully inspect the lesser and greater curvatures where a small defect may be obscured by the fatty envelopes of the gastric vasculature.

9.3.4 **The Duodenum**

The duodenum must be carefully inspected from the pylorus to the ligament of Treitz. If there is a haematoma on the duodenum, it is mandatory to perform a Kocher manoeuvre and inspect the posterior surface of the duodenum. A Duval forceps is useful in providing the gentle retraction needed when working with duodenum. See Section 9.4.

9.3.5 **Small Bowel**

The fundamental decision to be made on every patient is: damage control or definitive surgery.

The decision will depend on the context: the injury pattern, the physiological status of the patient, and the nature and volume of other patients waiting. If the decision is made to 'damage control' the patient, then management of visceral injury is usually simple. The stomach will require haemostatic sutured closure; the rest of the bowel will usually be dealt with by resecting damaged gut and leaving it stapled or tied off in discontinuity ('clip-and-drop'). Definitive intestinal surgery can be undertaken at re-look surgery, when the patient should be in a better physiological state.

Starting at the ligament of Treitz, each segment of the small bowel is inspected and then flipped over to examine the opposite side. The mesentery is carefully inspected as well. If the bowel is accidentally dropped, start again at the ligament of Treitz!

9.3.5.1 THE STABLE PATIENT

Small bowel injuries should be closed, with primary repair or resection and primary anastomosis as appropriate. Consider one resection and anastomosis when several wounds are localized close to each other. Be mindful, however, that bowel should be preserved wherever possible.

When multiple small wounds are present (e.g., following a shotgun injury), a skin stapler (35W) can be used to close individual holes safely.

9.3.5.2 THE UNSTABLE PATIENT

If the patient is haemodynamically unstable, damage control is likely, and bowel injuries should be treated using damage control procedures. The priority is to treat the haemorrhage, and then to control contamination.

Small wounds can be closed rapidly, using a 35W skin stapler or with mass closure. In patients with more extensive injuries requiring damage control, simple proximal and distal closure of the injured bowel using a GIA-type stapler or umbilical tape (with rapid resection of the injured segment) is the best way to prevent ongoing soiling.

Neither any anastomosis nor any stoma should be performed at this stage, as these can be time-consuming, the tissue viability is uncertain, and the leak rate is much higher, especially in the presence of concomitant contamination. At the time of re-look laparotomy, the feasibility of anastomosis versus the need for ileostomy or colostomy is assessed.

Pitfall

In wounds caused by small penetrating missiles, for example with a shotgun, it is easy to miss multiple holes, which are often less than 2 mm in diameter. It is recommended that, in these cases, the bowel be passed through a bowl of water, so that any air leak will show itself as bubbles. All such injuries should be re-inspected at 36–48 hours, and the procedure repeated.

9.3.6 Large Bowel[3,4]

The World War II experience of poor outcomes following complications of repair or anastomosis after colonic injury led to a policy of mandatory colostomy for colon injury that continued into civilian practice in the postwar years. In 1979, a randomized trial found that primary repair was associated with fewer complications than diversion; however, throughout the trial,

approximately half of the total patients with colonic injury were excluded from randomization and had a mandatory colostomy due to the presence of factors assumed to increase risk of complications (shock, extensive faecal contamination, prolonged delay from injury to operation, destructive colonic injury, or multiple associated injuries). Subsequent trials and a meta-analysis confirmed mortality was not significantly different between diversion and repair; however, morbidity was significantly less with primary repair. A further important consideration when considering optimal primary surgery is the morbidity inherent in colostomy reversal; complications following closure after colon injury have been reported to occur in up to half of patients.

In a civilian major trauma centre, primary repair appears safe even when the colonic injury is severe; however, a multicentre prospective study on destructive colon wounds confirmed that abdominal complications are more likely if the patient was critically injured, and the transfusion requirement was ≥4 units of blood or there was severe faecal contamination associated with the bowel injury. Importantly, the actual surgical method of colon wound management (colostomy or repair/anastomosis) made no difference.

Pragmatic recommendations for the management of patients with colonic injury were produced in the early years of the 21st century: patients with non-destructive injuries should undergo minimal debridement of the colonic injury and primary repair; patients with destructive wounds of the colon but without co-existent serious injury, comorbidities, or large transfusion requirement should undergo resection and anastomosis; whilst patients with destructive wounds, co-existing critical injury, significant medical illness, or transfusion requirements of >6 units should undergo faecal diversion. Utilizing these guidelines led to colostomy being undertaken for <10% of all colon wounds with acceptable morbidity.

9.3.6.1 THE STABLE PATIENT

For colonic injuries, indications for colostomy are still debated. Time from injury, haemodynamic status, comorbid conditions, and degree of contamination will influence the decision. More primary repairs and primary anastomoses are being performed, with fewer colostomies. Simple colonic injuries can be treated in much the same way as a simple small bowel injury, with local debridement and primary repair. When there are multiple small and large bowel lacerations, a protective ileostomy can be helpful.

9.3.6.2 THE UNSTABLE PATIENT

In the unstable patient undergoing a damage control procedure, small wounds can simply be sutured using a 2/0 or 3/0 monofilament suture. The wounds can be re-inspected at the re-look procedure.

Larger wounds should be excluded in the same manner as with the small bowel. All macroscopic contamination should be washed out using copious amounts of warmed saline before (temporary) closure. This wash-out may serve the added purpose of core rewarming if necessary.

Destructive colonic injuries should be treated with resection and stapling or tying off in discontinuity. The decision to restore continuity by anastomosis or divert is made at re-look laparotomy. In a recent series, up to 75% of patients with colon injury undergoing damage control laparotomy had anastomosis at subsequent laparotomy with acceptable rates of complications. If a damage control patient remains critically unwell at time of first re-look (typically at 48 hours) with inotropes still required, if they have a large burden of injury, or if they have had a massive transfusion, it is advisable to avoid a colonic anastomosis and opt for colostomy at the final procedure when definitive closure was intended. If a stoma is considered the most appropriate management for the patient, surgeons should be aware that early colostomy closure can be achieved safely.

Pitfalls

- No stomas should be performed in the unstable patient, as this prolongs the surgical time and may make things more complex in the presence of competing injury.
- Stomas should be performed only at the last damage control procedure.
- Stomas should be placed more laterally (away from the skin edge), and at the level of the umbilicus.

9.3.7 Rectum[5]

Surgeons consider the rectum in distinct parts: the intraperitoneal upper third and the extraperitoneal lower two-thirds. Diagnosis of rectal injury can be difficult and, as low rectal injuries are, by definition, not within the peritoneal cavity, they can easily be missed. Any penetrating injury at the level of the lower abdomen, hips, or thighs (such as penetrating injury to the buttocks) may be associated with a rectal injury. Major pelvic fracture can also cause injury to the rectal muscle tube.

Suspicion of rectal injury mandates specific investigation; luminal examination with a flexible sigmoidoscope is much more likely to identify a rectal injury than a rigid sigmoidoscopy, which can have a high false-negative rate. Preoperative CT (in a stable patient) may be helpful in delineating a bullet track and/or suggesting the likelihood of rectal injury in the form of perirectal gas and/or extravasation of rectal contrast. CT in this setting has the added benefit of demonstrating injuries to other pelvic structures such as the ureters, bladder, blood vessels, and internal female structures – invaluable for preoperative planning.

An intraperitoneal rectal injury should be debrided and repaired, and should best be covered by proximal diversion (loop sigmoid colostomy).

An extraperitoneal rectal injury is usually inaccessible and is treated by proximal diversion only.

Pitfall

Do not use routine presacral drainage or distal rectal washout. This will increase the risk of contamination, or secondary infection.

See **Table 9.3.3**

9.3.8 Mesentery

Arterial bleeders should be tied off. Do not extend mesenteric lacerations, and if necessary, oversew bleeding wounds. Watch for bowel ischaemia once the mesentery has been dealt with in this manner.

9.3.9 Adjuncts

9.3.9.1 ANTIBIOTICS

Practice management guidelines for prophylactic antibiotic use in penetrating abdominal trauma are given in Section 9.1.2.

Table 9.3.3 Management of Penetrating Extraperitoneal Rectal Injuries: An Eastern Association for the Surgery of Trauma (EAST) Practice Management Guideline

PICO	Question	Guidelines
1	In patients with non-destructive penetrating extraperitoneal rectal injuries (P), should proximal diversion (I) be performed versus no proximal diversion with primary repair (if feasible) (C) to decrease the incidence of complications (O)?	Despite the overall quality of evidence being very low, the panel considered that most patients would place a high value on avoidance of mortality and infectious complications. All of these factors resulted in the formulation of a conditional recommendation by the committee. The committee concludes that the desirable effects of adherence to a recommendation probably outweigh the undesirable effects. Thus, in patients with non-destructive penetrating extraperitoneal rectal injuries, we **conditionally recommend** proximal diversion (vs. non-diversion).
2	In patients with non-destructive penetrating extraperitoneal rectal injuries (P), should presacral drainage (I) versus no presacral drainage (C) be performed to decrease the incidence of complications (O)?	In patients with non-destructive extraperitoneal rectal injuries, we **conditionally recommend against** the routine use of presacral drains.
3	In patients with non-destructive penetrating extraperitoneal rectal injuries (P), should distal rectal washout be performed (I) versus no distal rectal washout (C) to decrease the incidence of complications (O)?	In patients with non-destructive penetrating extraperitoneal rectal injuries, **we conditionally recommend not performing** distal rectal washout (vs. performance of distal rectal washout).

REFERENCES AND SELECTED READINGS

References

1. Mjoli M, Oosthuizen G, Clarke D, Madiba T. Laparoscopy in the diagnosis and repair of diaphragmatic injuries in left-sided penetrating thoracoabdominal trauma: laparoscopy in trauma. *Surg Endosc.* 2015;**29(3)**:747–52. doi: 10.1007/s00464-014-3710-8.

2. McDonald, AA, Robinson Bryce RH, Alarcon L, Bosarge PL, Dorion, H. Evaluation and management of traumatic diaphragmatic injuries: a Practice Management Guideline from the Eastern Association for the Surgery of Trauma. *J Trauma Acute Care Surg.* 2018 Jul;**85(1)**:198–207. doi: 10.1097/TA.0000000000001924.

3. Sharpe JP, Magnotti LJ, Fabian TC. Evolution of the operative management of colon trauma. *Trauma Surg Acute Care Open.* 2017;2:e000092. doi: 10.1136/tsaco-2017-000092.

4. Berne JD, Velmahos GC, Chan LS, Asensio JA, Demetriades D. The high morbidity of colostomy closure after trauma: further support for the primary repair of colon injuries. *Surgery.* 1998 Feb;**123(2)**:157–64.

5. Bosarge PL, Como JJ, Fox N, Falck-Ytter Y, Haut ER, Dorion HA, et al. Management of penetrating extraperitoneal rectal injuries: an Eastern Association for the Surgery of Trauma practice management guideline. *J Trauma Acute Care Surg.* 2016 Mar;**80(3)**:546–51. doi: 10.1097/TA.0000000000000953.

Selected Readings

Trust MD, Brown CVR. Penetrating injuries to the colon and rectum. *Curr Trauma Rep.* 2015;**1(2)**:113–18. doi: 10.1007/s40719-015-0013-z.

Weinberg JA, Croce MA. Penetrating injuries to the stomach, duodenum, and small bowel. *Curr Trauma Rep.* 2015;**1(2)**:107–12. doi: 10.1007/s40719-015-0010-2.

9.4 The Duodenum

9.4.1 **Overview**

Duodenal injuries can pose a formidable challenge to the surgeon, and failure to manage them properly can have devastating results. The total amount of fluid passing through the duodenum exceeds 6 L per day, and a fistula in this area can cause serious fluid and electrolyte imbalance. A large amount of activated enzymes liberated into a combination of the retroperitoneal space and the peritoneal cavity can be life-threatening.

Both the pancreas and the duodenum are well protected in the superior retroperitoneum deep within the abdomen. Since these organs are in the retroperitoneum, they usually do not present with peritonitis, and are delayed in their presentation. Therefore, in order to sustain an injury to either one of them, there must be other associated injuries. If there is an anterior penetrating injury, the stomach, small bowel, transverse colon, liver, spleen, or kidneys are frequently also involved; whereas there needs to be a high index of suspicion with penetrating injury to the back which can injure the duodenum, leading to retroperitoneal contamination without peritonitis. If there is a blunt traumatic injury, there are frequently fractures of the lower thoracic or upper lumbar vertebrae. It requires a high level of suspicion and significant clinical acumen as well as aggressive radiographic imaging to identify an injury to these organs this early in the presentation.

Preoperative diagnosis of isolated duodenal injury can be very difficult to make, and there is no single method of duodenal repair that eliminates the potential for dehiscence of the duodenal suture line. As a result, the surgeon is frequently confronted with the dilemma of choosing between several preoperative investigations and many surgical procedures. A detailed knowledge of the available operative choices and when each one of them is preferably applied is important for the patient's benefit.[1]

9.4.2 **Mechanism of Injury**

9.4.2.1 **PENETRATING TRAUMA**

Penetrating trauma is the leading cause of duodenal injuries in countries with a high incidence of civilian violence. Because of the retroperitoneal location of the duodenum, and its proximity to several other visceral and major vascular structures, isolated penetrating injuries of the duodenum are infrequent. The need for abdominal exploration is usually dictated by associated injuries, and the diagnosis of duodenal injury is usually made in the operating room.

9.4.2.2 **BLUNT TRAUMA**

Blunt injuries to the duodenum are both less common and more difficult to diagnose than penetrating injuries, and they can occur in isolation or with pancreatic injury. These usually occur when crushing the duodenum between the spine and a steering wheel or handlebar, or when some other force is applied to the duodenum. These injuries can be associated with flexion/distraction fractures of the L1–L2 vertebrae – the 'chance type' fracture. 'Stomping' and striking the mid-epigastrium are common. Less common in deceleration injury patterns are tears at the junction of the third and fourth parts of the duodenum. These injuries occur at the junction of free (intraperitoneal) parts of the duodenum with fixed (retroperitoneal) parts. A high index of suspicion based on the mechanism of injury and physical examination findings may lead to further diagnostic studies.

9.4.2.3 **PAEDIATRIC CONSIDERATIONS**

A recent multi-institutional investigation found that child abuse was consistently associated with duodenal injuries in children younger than 2 years; also, the most common mechanism causing duodenal injuries in children younger than 5 years was non-accidental trauma.

9.4.3 **Diagnosis**

9.4.3.1 **CLINICAL PRESENTATION**

The clinical changes in isolated duodenal injuries may be extremely subtle until severe, life-threatening peritonitis develops. In most of the retroperitoneal perforations, there is initially only mild upper abdominal tenderness with a progressive rise in temperature, tachycardia, and occasionally vomiting. After several hours, the duodenal contents may extravasate into the peritoneal cavity, with the development of peritonitis, or, with posterior stab wounds, leak enteric contents from the wound. If the duodenal contents spill into the lesser sac, they are usually 'walled off' and localized, although they can occasionally leak into the general peritoneal cavity via the foramen of Winslow, with resultant generalized peritonitis.[2]

9.4.3.2 SERUM AMYLASE AND SERUM LIPASE

Theoretically, duodenal perforations are associated with a leak of amylase and other digestive enzymes, and it has been suggested that determination of the serum amylase concentration might be helpful in the diagnosis of blunt duodenal injury. However, the test lacks sensitivity. The duodenum is retroperitoneal, the concentration of amylase in the fluid that leaks is variable, and amylase concentrations often take hours to days to increase after injury. Although serial determinations of serum amylase are better than a single, isolated determination on admission, sensitivity is still poor, and necessary delays are inherent in serial determinations. If the serum amylase level is elevated on admission, a diligent search for duodenal rupture is warranted. The presence of a normal amylase level, however, does not exclude duodenal injury.[3]

Many institutions now use lipase as the marker of pancreatic injury, and studies suggest that it may be a more sensitive marker of pancreatic injury and abdominal injury than amylase, although its role in duodenal injury is unclear.

9.4.3.3 DIAGNOSTIC PERITONEAL LAVAGE/ ULTRASOUND

The duodenum, like the pancreas, lies in the retroperitoneum, so that neither ultrasound nor diagnostic peritoneal lavage (DPL) will be reliable. If performed, the amylase level in the lavage fluid should be measured.

9.4.3.4 RADIOLOGICAL INVESTIGATION

9.4.3.4.1 Computed Tomography

Computed tomography (CT) scan is the imaging technique of choice for the investigation of subtle duodenal injuries.[4] It is very sensitive to the presence of small amounts of retroperitoneal air, blood, or extravasated contrast from the injured duodenum, especially in children,[5] although in adults its reliability is more

controversial. The presence of periduodenal wall thickening or haematoma without extravasation of contrast material should be investigated with a gastrointestinal study with diatrizoate meglumine (Gastrografin). If the result is normal, it should be followed by a barium contrast study, if the patient's condition allows this.

9.4.3.4.2 Radiological Contrast Studies

An upper gastrointestinal series using water-soluble contrast material can provide positive results in 50% of patients with duodenal perforations. Gastrografin should be administered, and the study should be done under fluoroscopic control with the patient in the right lateral position. If no leak is observed, the investigation continues with the patient in the supine and left lateral positions. If the Gastrografin study is negative, it should be followed by administration of barium to allow the detection of small perforations more readily. Upper gastrointestinal studies with contrast are also indicated in patients with a suspected intramural haematoma of the duodenum (see Section 9.4.6.1) because they may demonstrate the classic 'coiled-spring' appearance of complete obstruction by the haematoma.[6]

9.4.3.5 DIAGNOSTIC LAPAROSCOPY

Unfortunately, diagnostic laparoscopy does not confer any improvement over more traditional methods in the investigation of the duodenum. In fact, because of its anatomical position, diagnostic laparoscopy is a poor modality to determine organ injury in these cases.[7]

9.4.4 Duodenal Injury Scale

Grading systems have been devised to characterize duodenal injuries (**Table 9.4.1**).[8]

9.4.5 Management[9]

Management can be very complicated with significant risk (**Figure 9.4.1**). Exploratory laparotomy remains the ultimate diagnostic test if a high suspicion of duodenal injury continues in the face of absent or equivocal radiographic signs.[10]

Most duodenal injuries can be managed by simple repair. More complicated injuries may require more sophisticated techniques. 'High-risk' duodenal injuries

Table 9.4.1 Duodenum Injury Scale

Grade*	Type of Injury	Description of Injury
I	Haematoma Laceration	Involving a single portion of duodenum Partial thickness, no perforation
II	Haematoma Laceration	Involving more than one portion Disruption < 50% of circumference
III	Laceration	Disruption 50%–75% of circumference of D2 Disruption 50%–100% of circumference of D1, D3, or D4
IV	Laceration	Disruption > 75% of circumference of D2 Involving the ampulla or distal common bile duct
V	Laceration Vascular	Massive disruption of the duodenopancreatic complex Devascularization of duodenum

*Advance one grade for multiple injuries up to grade III.

Note: See also Appendix B, 'Trauma Scores and Scoring Systems'.

D1, first portion of duodenum.
D2, second portion of duodenum.
D3, third portion of duodenum.
D4, fourth portion of duodenum.

are followed by a high incidence of suture line dehiscence, and their treatment should include duodenal diversion. The management of all full-thickness duodenal lacerations should include adequate external periduodenal drainage. Pancreaticoduodenectomy is practised only if no alternative is available. 'Damage control' should precede the definitive reconstruction.

9.4.6 **Surgical Approach**

Although useful for research purposes, the specifics of the grading systems are less important than several simple aspects of the duodenal injuries:

- The anatomical relation to the ampulla of Vater.
- The characteristics of the injury (simple laceration versus destruction of duodenal wall).
- The circumference of the duodenum involved.
- Associated injuries to the biliary tract or pancreas, or major vascular injuries.

Timing of the operation is also very important, as mortality rises from 11% to 40% if the time interval between injury and operation is more than 24 hours. (See also Section 9.6.7 on the surgical approach to the pancreas.)

In addition to the Kocher manoeuvre to visualize the second part of the duodenum, a medial visceral rotation can be used to expose the entire transverse part of the duodenum. Alternatively, the fourth part of the duodenum can be mobilized by dividing the ligament of Treitz and gently dissecting with right index finger in the avascular plane behind the transverse duodenum. Combining this with the Kocher manoeuvre allows the index fingers to be brought together from both sides and thereby to exclude a posterior perforation of the transverse part of the duodenum.

From a practical point of view, the duodenum can be divided into one 'upper' portion that includes the first and second parts, and another 'lower' portion that includes the third and fourth parts. The 'upper' portion has complex anatomical structures within it (the common bile duct and the sphincter) and the pylorus. It requires distinct manoeuvres to diagnose injury (cholangiogram and direct visual inspection) and complex techniques to repair them. The first and second parts of the duodenum are densely adherent and dependent for their blood supply on the head of the pancreas; therefore, the diagnosis and management of any injury are complex, and resection, unless involving the entire 'C' loop and pancreatic head, is impossible. The 'lower' portion involving the third and fourth parts of the duodenum can generally be treated like the small bowel, and the diagnosis and management of injury are relatively simple, including debridement, closure, resection, and anastomosis.

9.4.6.1 **INTRAMURAL HAEMATOMA**

This is a rare injury of the duodenum specific to patients with blunt trauma. It is most common in children with isolated force to the upper abdomen, possibly because of the relatively flexible and pliable musculature of the child's abdominal wall, and half of the cases can be attributed to child abuse.

The haematoma develops in the submucosal or subserosal layers of the duodenum. The duodenum is *not* perforated. Such haematomas can lead to obstruction. The symptoms of gastric outlet obstruction can take up to 48 hours to present. This is due to the gradual increase of

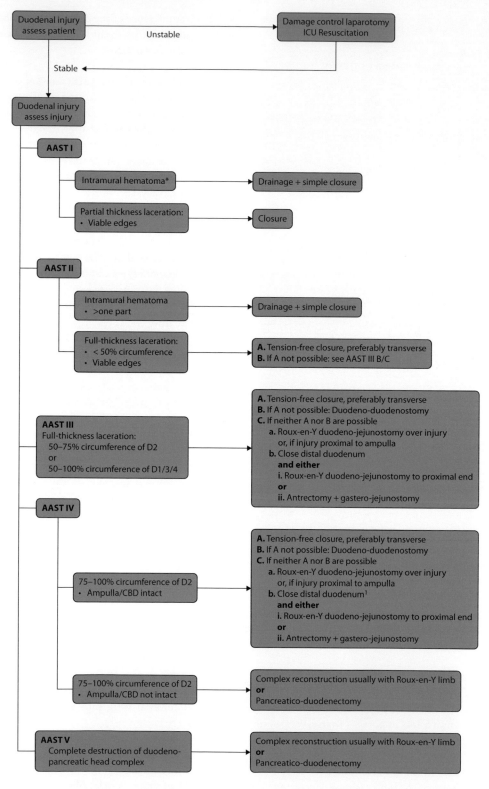

Figure 9.4.1 Western Trauma Association (WTA) algorithm for duodenal injuries.

the size of a haematoma as the breakdown of the haemo-globin makes it hyperosmotic, with resultant fluid shifts into it. The diagnosis can be made by double-contrast CT scan or upper gastrointestinal contrast studies that show the 'coiled-spring' or 'stacked-coin' sign.[6]

Management of the injury is usually considered non-surgical, and if associated injuries can be ruled out, best results are obtained by conservative treatment.[11] Gastric residual volume will slowly decrease, eventually allowing normal feeding. If there is no improvement, the patient should undergo laparotomy to rule out the presence of duodenal perforation or injury of the head of the pancreas, which may be an alternative cause of duodenal obstruction.

The treatment of an intramural haematoma that is found at early laparotomy is controversial. One option is to open the serosa, evacuate the haematoma without violation of the mucosa, and carefully repair the wall of the bowel. The concern is that this may convert a partial tear to a full-thickness tear of the duodenal wall. Another option is to carefully explore the duodenum to exclude a perforation, leaving the intramural haematoma intact and planning nasogastric decompression postoperatively.

9.4.6.2 DUODENAL LACERATION

The great majority of duodenal perforations and lacerations can be managed with simple surgical procedures. This is particularly true with penetrating injuries, when the time interval between injury and operation is normally short. On the other hand, the minority are 'high risk', for example with increased risk of dehiscence of the duodenal repair, increased morbidity, and sometimes increased mortality. These injuries are related to associated pancreatic injury, blunt or missile injury, involvement of more than 75% of the duodenal wall, injury of the first or second part of the duodenum, a time interval of more than 24 hours between injury and repair, and associated common bile duct injury. In these high-risk injuries, several adjunctive operative procedures have been proposed to reduce the incidence of dehiscence of the duodenal suture line.

Pitfall

Iatrogenic perforations of the duodenum are occasionally seen during and after ERCP (endoscopic retrograde of cholangiopancreatography); prompt recognition and repair are paramount for a good prognosis, but most cases are diagnosed after the procedure, hours or days later, and the repair constitutes a surgical challenge.[12]

Recently, further evidence has supported a more simplified surgical approach to these injuries with improved outcomes compared to complex technical solutions.[11] Methods of repair of the duodenal trauma as well as 'supportive' procedures against dehiscence are described below.

9.4.6.3 REPAIR OF THE PERFORATION

Most injuries of the duodenum can be repaired by primary closure in one or two layers. The closure should be oriented transversely, if possible, to avoid luminal compromise. Excessive inversion should be avoided. Longitudinal duodenotomies can usually be closed transversely if the length of the duodenal injury is less than 50% of the circumference of the duodenum.

If primary closure would compromise the lumen of the duodenum, several alternatives have been recommended. Pedicled mucosal graft, as a method of closing large duodenal defects, has been suggested, using a segment of jejunum or a gastric island flap from the body of the stomach. An alternative to that is the use of a jejunal serosal patch to close the duodenal defect. The serosa of the loop of the jejunum is sutured to the edges of the duodenal defect. Although encouraging in experimental studies, the clinical application of both methods has been limited, without beneficial results, and suture line leaks have been reported.[13]

9.4.6.4 COMPLETE TRANSECTION OF THE DUODENUM

The preferred method of repair is usually primary anastomosis of the two ends after appropriate debridement and mobilization of the duodenum. This is frequently the case with injuries of the first, third, or fourth part of the duodenum, where mobilization is technically not difficult. However, if a large amount of tissue is lost, approximation of the duodenum may not be possible without producing undue tension on the suture line. If this is the case and complete transection occurs in the first part of the duodenum, it is advisable to perform an antrectomy with closure of the duodenal stump and a Bilroth II gastrojejunostomy. When such injury occurs distal to the ampulla of Vater, closure of the distal duodenum and Roux-en-Y duodenojejunal anastomosis are appropriate.

Mobilization of the second part of the duodenum is limited by its shared blood supply with the head of the pancreas. A direct anastomosis to a Roux-en-Y loop sutured over the duodenal defect in an end-to-side fashion is the procedure of choice. This also can be applied as an alternative method of operative management of extensive defects to the other parts of the duodenum when primary anastomosis is not feasible.

External drainage should be provided in all duodenal injuries, because it affords early detection and control of the duodenal fistula. The drain is preferably a simple, soft silicone rubber, closed system placed adjacent to the repair.

9.4.6.5 DUODENAL DIVERSION

In high-risk duodenal injuries, duodenal repair is followed by a high incidence of suture line dehiscence. In order to protect the duodenal repair, the gastrointestinal contents – with their proteolytic enzymes – can be diverted with a gastrojejunostomy, a practice that would also make the management of a potential duodenal fistula easier. The evidence for this procedure is equivocal, although there remains a role in selected cases.

9.4.6.6 DUODENAL DIVERTICULATION

This includes a distal Bilroth II gastrectomy, closure of the duodenal wound, placement of a decompressive catheter into the duodenum, and generous drainage of the duodenal repair. Truncal vagotomy and biliary drainage could be added. Resection of a normal distal stomach cannot be beneficial to the patient. This procedure is not recommended and should not be considered unless there is a large amount of destruction and tissue loss, and no other course is possible.

9.4.6.7 PYLORIC EXCLUSION

Pyloric exclusion is rarely used. (See within Section 9.6.7.2 on pancreatic surgery.)

9.4.6.8 PANCREATICODUODENECTOMY (WHIPPLE'S PROCEDURE) (SEE SECTION 9.6.7 ON PANCREATIC SURGERY)

This is a major procedure to be practised in trauma only if no alternative is available. Damage control with control of bleeding and of bowel contamination, and ligation of the common bile and pancreatic ducts, should

be the rule.[14] Reconstruction should take place within 48 hours or when the patient is stable.

Extensive local damage of the intraduodenal or intrapancreatic bile duct injuries frequently necessitates a staged pancreaticoduodenectomy. Less extensive local injuries can be managed by intraluminal stenting, sphincteroplasty, or reimplantation of the ampulla of Vater.

REFERENCES AND RECOMMENDED READING

References

1. Neal MD, Britt LD, Watson G, Murdock A, Peitzman AB. Abdominal injury – duodenum and pancreas. In Peitzman AB, Rhodes M, Schwab SW, Yealy DM, Fabian TC, eds. *The Trauma Manual: Trauma and Acute Care Surgery*. 4th ed. Philadelphia: Lippincott Williams and Wilkins, 2013: 374–62.

2. Carrillo EH, Richardson JD, Miller FB. Evolution in the management of duodenal injuries. *J Trauma*. 1996 Jun;**40(6)**:1037–45; discussion 1045–6. Review. doi: 10.1097/00005373-199606000-00035.

3. Takishima T, Sugimoto K, Hirata M, Asari Y, Ohwada T, Katika A. Serum amylase level on admission in the diagnosis of blunt injury to the pancreas: its significance and limitations. *Ann Surg*. 1997 Jul;**226**:70–6. doi: 10.1097/00000658-199707000-00010.

4. Kunin JR, Korobkin M, Ellis JH, Francis IR, Kane NM, Siegel SE. Duodenal injuries caused by blunt abdominal trauma: value of CT in differentiating perforation from haematoma. *Am J Roentgenol*. 1993 June;**160(6)**:1221–3. doi: 10.2214/ajr.160.6.8498221.

5. Shilyansky J, Pearl RH, Kreller M, Sena LM, Babyn PS. Diagnosis and management of duodenal injuries in children. *J Paed Surg*. 1997 June;**32**:229–32. doi: 10.1016/s0022-3468(97)90642-4.

6. Kadell BM, Zimmerman PT, Lu DSK. Radiology of the abdomen. In Zimmer MJ, Schwartz SI, Ellis H, eds. *Maingot's Abdominal Operations*. Stanford, CT: Appleton & Lange, 1997: 3–116.

7. Brooks AJ, Boffard KD. Current technology: laparoscopic surgery in trauma. *Trauma*. 1999;**1**:53–60.

8. Moore EE, Cogbill TH, Malangoni MA, Jurkovich GJ, Shackford SR, Champion HR, et al. Organ injury scaling, II: pancreas, duodenum, small bowel, colon, and rectum. *J Trauma*. 1990 Nov;**30(11)**:1427–9.

9. Malhotra A, Biffl WL, Moore EE, Schreiber M, Albrecht RA, Cohen M, et al. Western trauma association critical decisions in trauma: diagnosis and management of duodenal injuries. *J Trauma Acute Care Surg.* 2015 Dec;**79(6)**:1096–101. doi: 10.1097/TA.0000000000000870.

10. Degiannis E, Boffard K. Duodenal injuries. *Br J Surg.* 2000 Nov;**87(11)**:1473–9. Review. doi: 10.1046/j.1365-2168.2000.01594.x.

11. Touloukian RJ. Protocol for the nonoperative treatment of obstructing intramural duodenal haematoma during childhood. *Am J Surg.* 1983 Mar;**145**:330–4. doi: 10.1016/0002-9610(83)90193-9.

12. Ordoñez C, García A, Parra MW, Scavo D, Pino LF, Millán M, et al. Complex penetrating duodenal injuries: less is better. *J Trauma Acute Care Surg.* 2014;**76**:1177–83. doi: 10.1097/TA.0000000000000214.

13. Ivatury RR, Gaudino J, Ascer E, Nallathambi M, Ramirez-Schon G, Stahl WM, et al. Treatment of penetrating duodenal injuries. *J Trauma.* 1985 Apr;**25**:337–41.

14. Kauder DR, Schwab SW, Rotondo MF. Damage control. In Ivantury RR, Cayten CG, eds. *The Textbook of Penetrating Trauma.* Baltimore: Williams & Wilkins, 1996: 717–25.

Recommended Reading

Asensio JA, Demetriades D, Berne JD. A unified approach to surgical exposure of pancreatic and duodenal injuries. *Am J Surg.* 1997 July;**174(1)**:54–60. doi: 10.1016/S0002-9610(97)00029-9.

Phillips B, Turco L, McDonald D, Mause A, Walters RW. Penetrating injuries to the duodenum: An analysis of 879 patients from the National Trauma Data Bank, 2010 to 2014. *J Trauma Acute Care Surg.* 2017 Nov;**83(5)**:810–17. doi: 10.1097/TA.0000000000001604.

Ivatury RR, Nassoura ZE, Simon RJ, Simon RJ. Complex duodenal injuries. *Surg Clin North Am.* 1996 Aug;**76(4)**:797–812. Review. doi: 10.1016/s0039-6109(05)70481-3.

9.5 The Liver and Biliary System

9.5.1 **Overview**

Most liver injuries are diagnosed on the trauma computed tomography (CT), relatively asymptomatic, and low grade, and do not require surgical intervention. Operative management of high-grade hepatic lacerations is technically very challenging and can be a devastating experience! Exquisite decision-making; thorough understanding of hepatic anatomy including the arterial supply, portal venous supply, and hepatic venous drainage; and advanced operative techniques are essential. The evolution in management of hepatic injury has evolved since packing was first described over 100 years ago, through aggressive surgery, to refinement of techniques, and the increasing role of non-operative management (NOM) of most injuries.[1]

More recently, Gaarder concluded that the changes to haemostatic resuscitation and treatment protocols were associated with a further decrease in laparotomy and embolization rates as well as improved overall mortality. They found that NOM was safe in 70% of patients with high-grade Organ Injury Scale (OIS) injuries (grades 4 and 5), in contrast to the critically ill significantly unstable 30% that require surgery who still have high mortality.[2]

Richardson and co-workers managed approximately 1200 blunt hepatic injuries over a 25-year period. NOM was used in up to 80% of cases. Deaths secondary to injury dropped from 8% to 2%.[3]

The key to success is the appreciation of the patient's physiology, as this is the fundamental deciding factor between operative and non-operative approaches, rather than anatomical injury grading.

The liver is composed of a right and a left half, defined by Cantlie's line separating the two. Cantlie's line runs from the gallbladder fossa to the inferior vena cava (IVC). The liver is divided into eight Couinaud's segments. Segment I is the caudate lobe, segments II–IV make up the left hemi-liver, and the right hemi-liver comprises segments V–VIII (see **Figure 9.5.1**).

Whilst management of liver trauma does not require an in-depth knowledge of the liver segmental anatomy, there are key anatomical factors to consider that can guide management. The structures within the porta hepatis include the hepatic artery, portal vein, and bile duct. The portal triad is encased in an extension of

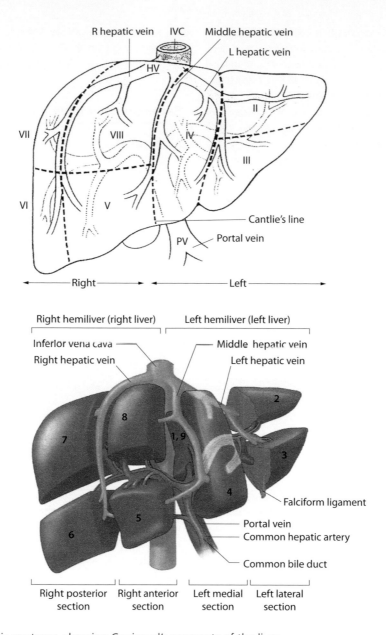

Figure 9.5.1 Hepatic anatomy, showing Couinaud's segments of the liver.

Glisson's capsule, and thus relatively resistant to blunt injury. The portal triad runs *within* the segments of the liver. The major hepatic veins (right, left, and middle) have no valves; are thin, delicate structures, not protected by an extension of Glisson's capsule; run *between* the segments of the liver; and drain directly into the IVC within 1–2 cm of the right atrium. Logically in blunt trauma, especially the hepatic veins are the most likely to be injured, whilst the thicker-walled hepatic arteries within Glisson's capsule are the most protected. Equally,

if imaging demonstrates hepatic artery involvement, then there will inevitably be bile duct injury.

Difficult-to-control, life-threatening haemorrhage in the operating room (OR) is generally related to major hepatic vein or retrohepatic IVC injury. The liver generally encases a portion of the retrohepatic cava, at times circumferentially. Full mobilization of the liver to expose the retrohepatic IVC requires division of this attachment. The major hepatic veins are 8–12 cm in length, the majority of which is intrahepatic. Injury to the major hepatic veins is generally to this portion of the veins and can initially be controlled by compression, but at times may require suture ligation. The extrahepatic segments of the major hepatic veins are < 2 cm in length and are less commonly injured. Injury to the extrahepatic portion of the major hepatic veins generally presents as exsanguinating haemorrhage and carries a high mortality. In addition, 3–11 short hepatic veins run directly from the liver to the IVC; they can also be a source of haemorrhage, especially in blunt deceleration injury, and must be identified and controlled if liver resection is necessary. The short hepatic veins can be large, especially if the right hepatic vein is found to be diminutive. Finally, the liver parenchyma will tolerate ligation or embolization of hepatic artery branches, but the bile ducts will not. The bile ducts depend on the hepatic artery for their blood supply (**Figure 9.5.2**), which needs to be considered when considering embolization as a definitive management.[4]

Segmental anatomical resection has been well documented but is usually not applicable to trauma.

The forces from blunt injury are direct compressive forces or shear forces. The elastic tissue within arterial blood vessels makes them less susceptible to tearing than other structures within the liver. Venous and biliary ductal tissue are moderately resistant to shear forces, whereas the liver parenchyma is not. Thus, fractures within the liver parenchyma tend to occur along segmental fissures (*remember*: this is where the major hepatic veins course) or directly in the parenchyma. This causes shearing of branches emanating from the major hepatic and portal veins. With severe deceleration injury and traction injury, the origin of the short retrohepatic veins may be ripped from the cava, causing devastating haemorrhage (these

veins may be as large as 1 cm in diameter). Similarly, the small branches from the caudate lobe entering directly into the cava are at high risk for shearing with linear tears on the caval surface. Direct compressive forces usually cause tearing between segmental fissures in an anterior–posterior vector. Horizontal fracture lines into the parenchyma give the characteristic burst pattern to such liver injuries. If the fracture lines are parallel, these have been dubbed 'bear claw'-type injuries and probably represent where the ribs have been compressed directly into the parenchyma. This can cause massive haemorrhage if there is direct extension or continuity with the peritoneal cavity.

Appropriate decision-making is critical to a good outcome:

- The patient's physiology drives decision-making – unstable physiology requires surgery, whereas stable physiology does not, regardless of grade of liver injury.
- Patients actively bleeding from major liver injury must be taken to the OR promptly, with rapid haemorrhage control and ongoing haemostatic resuscitation. Any delay in doing so increases risks of coagulopathy and mortality.
- If surgery is indicated, the simplest, quickest technique that can restore haemostasis is the most appropriate. Eighty per cent of liver injuries that require surgery can be successfully managed with correct liver packing.

Be a minimalist – if you have controlled the liver bleeding in an unstable patient: STOP – PACK – LEAVE THE OR.

- Do **not** abort the operation and leave the OR if surgical bleeding is not controlled. Damage control and truncating the operation are indicated for medical bleeding (coagulopathy).
- If simple manoeuvres fail to control haemorrhage, the decision to proceed with hepatorrhaphy or resectional debridement must be made quickly, and surgeons must equip themselves with the appropriate skills to undertake this.

9.5.2 **Resuscitation**

The haemodynamically *stable* patient without signs of peritonitis or another indication for operation is

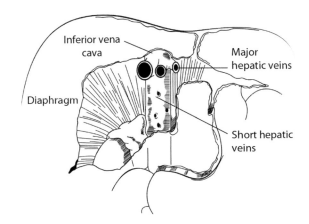

Figure 9.5.2 Retrohepatic anatomy of the liver. The major hepatic veins and short hepatic veins are shown.

generally managed non-operatively (> 80% of blunt liver injuries).

The haemodynamically *unstable* patient with liver injuries requires immediate surgical exploration to achieve haemostasis and exclude other sources of bleeding. The patient in whom a surgical approach is decided upon or is mandated by haemodynamic instability should be transferred to the OR as rapidly as possible after the following are completed:

Consider early damage control and packing before the coagulopathy is established!

Once the patient is cold, coagulopathic, and in irreversible shock, the battle usually is lost.

Call for senior help early in the operation.

Pitfall

Resuscitative endovascular balloon occlusion of the aorta (REBOA) should be considered with huge caution in severe liver injury, as Zone 1 REBOA may simply increase the risk of hepatic venous bleeding whilst delaying transfer to the OR.

9.5.3 Diagnosis

Control of bleeding takes priority over any diagnostic procedure (including CT).

Any delay to control of bleeding will increase mortality. Surgery should not be delayed by multiple emergency department procedures such as limb X-rays, unnecessary ultrasonography, and vascular access procedures. CT of the brain should be delayed until the patient is stable. Hypotension significantly increases mortality for traumatic brain injury. The anaesthesiologist can continue resuscitation in the OR.

In the patient with blunt injury, there may be an absence of clear clinical signs such as rigidity, distension, or unstable vital signs. Up to 40% of patients with significant haemoperitoneum have no obvious abdominal signs. CT is the investigation of choice for all but the most unstable patients, and it will demonstrate the liver injury, but unless there is associated bowel injury necessitating laparotomy, the decision on the need for operative management is based on the patient's physiology. Focussed assessment with sonography for trauma (FAST) may be useful in the setting of blunt injury and haemodynamic instability, since the presence of free fluid in the abdominal cavity will direct you quickly to the OR in a hypotensive patient. With a haemodynamically stable patient, diagnostic peritoneal lavage is rarely required these days due to the availability of FAST, but if available in the blunt trauma setting it may be useful, particularly when CT support services are inadequate or unavailable.

The purpose of diagnostic investigations in a stable patient is to better understand who can be safely managed non-operatively, to assist decision-making in NOM, and to act as a baseline for comparison in future imaging studies. Contrast-enhanced high-resolution CT enables an accurate diagnosis of liver injuries.

Penetrating wounds of the liver usually do not present a diagnostic problem, as most surgeons would still advocate laparotomy, although there are series of non-operatively managed penetrating liver injury. CT scan can be useful in very select circumstances—such as in the haemodynamically stable patient who is suspected to have an injury of the right upper quadrant, isolated to the liver only. In this setting, trajectory of the injury can be confirmed, vascular viability can be delineated, and assistance can be provided with the decision of whether to manage the injury non-operatively (NOM) versus operatively, with or without embolization.

9.5.4 Liver Injury Scale[5]

The American Association for the Surgery of Trauma's (AAST) Committee on Organ Injury Scaling has developed a liver injury scale (**Table 9.5.1**) and a grading system (**Table 9.5.2**) for classifying injuries to the liver.

Hepatic injuries are graded on a scale of I to VI, with grade I representing superficial lacerations and small subcapsular haematomas and VI representing avulsion of the liver from the vena cava. Isolated injuries that are not extensive (grades I to III) are usually managed non-operatively; however, extensive parenchymal injuries and those involving the juxtahepatic veins (grades IV and V) may require surgical manoeuvres for successful treatment. Hepatic avulsion (grade VI) is generally lethal.

Eighty percent of blunt liver injuries are grade I–III. Grades IV and V comprise 15%–20% of blunt liver injuries, and these are the patients who are unstable and require immediate laparotomy for control of haemorrhage. In general, if the patient with blunt liver injury is stable enough for CT, the patient can be managed non-operatively. Truly stable patients without signs of active bleeding,

Table 9.5.1 Liver Injury Scale, 2018 Revision

AAST Grade*	AIS Severity	Imaging Criteria (CT Findings)	Operative Goals	Pathologic Criteria
I	2	**Haematoma** Subcapsular haematoma < 10% surface area **Laceration** Parenchymal laceration < 1 cm in depth	**Haematoma** Subcapsular haematoma < 10% surface area **Laceration** Parenchymal laceration < 1 cm in depth Capsular tear	**Haematoma** Subcapsular haematoma < 10% surface area **Laceration** Parenchymal laceration < 1 cm Capsular tear
II	2	**Haematoma** Subcapsular haematoma 10%–50% surface area Intraparenchymal haematoma < 10 cm in diameter **Laceration** Laceration 1–3 cm in depth and < 10 cm length	**Haematoma** Subcapsular haematoma 10%–50% surface area Intraparenchymal haematoma < 10 cm in diameter **Laceration** Laceration 1–3 cm in depth and > 10 cm length	**Haematoma** Subcapsular haematoma 10%–50% surface area Intraparenchymal haematoma < 10 cm in diameter **Laceration** Laceration 1–3 cm in depth and > 10 cm length
III	3	**Haematoma** Subcapsular haematoma > 50% surface area Ruptured subcapsular or parenchymal haematoma Intraparenchymal haematoma > 10 cm **Laceration** Laceration > 3 in cm depth Any injury in the presence of a liver vascular injury or active bleeding contained within liver parenchyma	**Haematoma** Subcapsular haematoma > 50% surface area or expanding Ruptured subcapsular or parenchymal haematoma Intraparenchymal haematoma > 10 cm **Laceration** Laceration 3 cm in depth	**Disruption** Parenchymal disruption involving 25%–75% of a hepatic lobe
IV	4	**Disruption** Parenchymal disruption involving 25%–75% of a hepatic lobe **Vascular injury** Active bleeding extending beyond the liver parenchyma into the peritoneum	**Disruption** Parenchymal disruption involving 25%–75% of a hepatic lobe or 1–3 Couinaud's segments within a single lobe	**Disruption** Parenchymal disruption involving >75% of a hepatic lobe
V	5	**Disruption** Parenchymal disruption involving > 75% of a hepatic lobe	**Disruption** Parenchymal disruption involving > 75% of a hepatic lobe or > 3 Couinaud's segments within a single lobe	**Vascular injury** Juxtahepatic venous injury to include retrohepatic vena cava and central major hepatic veins

(Continued)

Table 9.5.1 (Continued) Liver Injury Scale, 2018 Revision

AAST Grade*	AIS Severity	Imaging Criteria (CT Findings)	Operative Goals	Pathologic Criteria
		Vascular injury Juxtahepatic venous injury to include retrohepatic vena cava and central major hepatic veins	**Vascular injury** Juxtahepatic venous injury to include retrohepatic vena cava and central major hepatic veins	
VI	6	Hepatic avulsion		

Note: Vascular injury is defined as a pseudoaneurysm or arteriovenous fistula and appears as a focal collection of vascular contrast that decreases in attenuation with delayed imaging. Active bleeding from a vascular injury presents as vascular contrast, focal or diffuse, that increases in size or attenuation in the delayed phase. Vascular thrombosis can lead to organ infarction.

*Grade based on the highest grade assessment made on imaging, at operation, or on pathologic specimen. More than one grade of liver injury may be present and should be classified by the higher grade of injury. Advance one grade for multiple injuries up to a grade III.

irrespective of the grade of liver injury or amount of haemoperitoneum, are good candidates for NOM.

9.5.5 Management

Traditionally, discussion of liver injuries differentiates between those arising from blunt and those arising from penetrating trauma. In general, blunt hepatic injury carries a higher mortality rate than penetrating liver injury due to the magnitude of parenchymal injury. Most stab wounds to the liver cause relatively minor injury unless a critical structure such as the hepatic vein, the intrahepatic cava, or the portal structures is injured. In contrast, gunshot wounds, particularly high-energy injuries, and shotgun blasts can be devastating. High-grade parenchymal liver injury (grades IV and V) and juxtahepatic caval injury from severe blunt trauma carry high mortality rates and continue to be the most challenging for the surgeon.

Table 9.5.2 Liver Trauma Grading

Severity	WSES Grade	AAST	Haemodynamic
Minor	WSES grade I	I–II	Stable
Moderate	WSES grade II	III	Stable
Severe	WSES grade III	IV–V	Stable
	WSES grade IV	I–VI	Unstable

The World Society of Emergency Surgery (WSES) revised guidelines (2020) can be helpful (see **Table 9.5.3**).[6]

9.5.5.1 NON-OPERATIVE MANAGEMENT (NOM)[7,8]

Nearly all children and up to 80% of adults with blunt hepatic injuries can be treated without laparotomy. This change in approach has been occasioned by the increasing availability of rapid ultrasound, helical CT, and interventional radiology (see **Table 9.5.4**).

The primary requirement for non-operative therapy is haemodynamic stability. To confirm stability, frequent assessment of vital signs and monitoring of the haematocrit and lactate or base deficit are necessary, in conjunction with CT. Continued haemorrhage is rare and occurs in 1%–4% of patients. Hypotension may develop, usually within the first 24 hours after hepatic injury, but sometimes several days later. Failure rates from NOM in well-selected patients are extremely low (1%).

The presence of extravasation of contrast on CT denotes active bleeding, depending on the phase of the scan. The hepatic arteries are relatively protected by Glisson's capsule, and although they can be injured in isolation in penetrating trauma, in blunt injury there is likely to be associated hepatic venous and portal venous bleeding. In isolated arterial haemorrhage following blunt trauma, therapeutic angiography with embolization should be applied early; otherwise, operative intervention will become necessary, but consider whether further management of the other structures

Table 9.5.3 World Society of Emergency Surgery (WSES) Guidelines for the Management of Liver Injury[6]

Diagnostic procedures	• The diagnostic methods on admission are determined by the haemodynamic status (GoR 1A). • eFAST is rapid in detecting intra-abdominal free fluid (GoR 1A). • CT scan with intravenous contrast is the gold standard in haemodynamically stable trauma patients (GoR 1A).
Non-operative management (NOM)	• NOM should be the treatment of choice for all haemodynamically stable minor (WSES I and AAST I–II), moderate (WSES II and AAST III), and severe (WSES III and AAST IV–V) injuries in the absence of other internal injuries requiring surgery (GoR 2A). • In patients considered transient responders with moderate (WSES II and AAST III) and severe (WSES III and AAST IV–V) injuries, NOM should be considered only in selected settings, provided the immediate availability of trained surgeons; an operating room; continuous monitoring, ideally in an ICU or ER setting; and access to angiography, angioembolization, blood, and blood products; and in locations where a system exists to quickly transfer such patients to higher level-of-care facilities (GoR 2B). • A CT scan with intravenous contrast should always be performed in patients being considered for NOM (GoR 2A). • AG/AE may be considered as a first-line intervention in haemodynamically stable patients with arterial blush on CT scan (GoR 2B). • In haemodynamically stable children, the presence of contrast blush on CT scan is not an absolute indication for AG/AE (GoR 2B). • Serial clinical evaluations (physical exams and laboratory testing) must be performed to detect a change in clinical status during NOM (GoR 2A). • NOM should be attempted in the setting of concomitant head trauma and/or spinal cord injuries with reliable clinical exam, unless the patient could not achieve specific haemodynamic goals for the neurotrauma and the instability might be due to intra-abdominal bleeding (GoR 2B). • ICU admission in isolated liver injury may be required only for moderate (WSES II and AAST III) and severe (WSES III and AAST IV–V) lesions (GoR 2B). • In selected cases where an intra-abdominal injury is suspected in the days after the initial trauma, interval laparoscopic exploration may be considered as an extension of NOM and a means to plan patient management in a step-up treatment strategy (GoR 2C). • In low-resource settings, NOM could be considered in patients with haemodynamic stability without evidence of associated injuries, with negative serial physical examinations and negative imaging and blood tests (GoR 2C).
Operative management (OM)	• Haemodynamically unstable and non-responder patients (WSES IV) should undergo OM (GoR 2A). • Primary surgical intervention should be to control the haemorrhage and bile leak, and for initiation of damage control resuscitation, as soon as possible (GoR 2A). • Major hepatic resections should be avoided at first and only considered in subsequent operations, in a resectional debridement fashion in cases of large areas of devitalized liver tissue, done by experienced surgeons (GoR 2B). • Angioembolization is a useful tool in cases of persistent arterial bleeding after non-haemostatic or damage control procedures (GoR 2A). • Resuscitative endovascular balloon occlusion of the aorta (i.e. REBOA) may be used in haemodynamically unstable patients as a bridge to other, more definitive procedures for haemorrhage control (GoR 2B).

(Continued)

Table 9.5.3 (*Continued*) World Society of Emergency Surgery (WSES) Guidelines for the Management of Liver Injury[6]

Short- and long-term follow-up	• Intrahepatic abscesses may be successfully treated with percutaneous drainage (GoR 2A). • Delayed haemorrhage without severe haemodynamic compromise may be managed at first with AG/AE (GoR 2A). • Hepatic artery pseudoaneurysm should be managed with AG/AE to prevent rupture (GoR 2A). • Symptomatic or infected bilomas should be managed with percutaneous drainage (GoR 2A). • A combination of percutaneous drainage and endoscopic techniques may be considered in managing post-traumatic biliary complications not suitable for percutaneous management alone (GoR 2B). • Lavage/drainage and endoscopic stenting may be considered as the first approach in delayed post-traumatic biliary fistula without any other indication for laparotomy (GoR 2B). • Laparoscopy as an initial approach should be considered in cases of delayed surgery, so as to minimize the invasiveness of surgical intervention and to tailor the procedure to the lesion (GoR 2B).
Thrombo-prophylaxis, feeding, and mobilization	• Mechanical prophylaxis is safe and should be considered in all patients with no absolute contraindication (GoR 2A). • LMWH-based prophylaxis should be started as soon as possible following trauma and may be safe in selected patients with liver injury treated with NOM (GoR 2B). • In those patients taking anticoagulants, individualization of the risk–benefit balance of anticoagulant reversal is suggested (GoR 1C). • Early mobilization should be achieved in stable patients (GoR 2A). • In the absence of contraindications, enteral feeding should be started as soon as possible (GoR 2A).

AAST, American Association for the Surgery of Trauma
AE, angioembolization
AG, angiography
CT, computed tomography
eFAST, extended focussed assessment with sonography for trauma
GoR, Grade of recommendation
LMWH, low-molecular-weight heparin
NOM, non-operative management
OM, operative management
REBOA, resuscitative endovascular balloon occlusion of the aorta
WSES, World Society of Emergency Surgery

Table 9.5.4 American Association for the Surgery of Trauma (AAST) Evidence-Based Guidelines for Selective Non-Operative Management of Hepatic Injury

Level of Evidence	Recommendation
I	Patients who have diffuse peritonitis or who are haemodynamically unstable after blunt abdominal trauma should be taken urgently for laparotomy.
II	1. A routine laparotomy is not indicated in the haemodynamically stable patient without peritonitis presenting with an isolated blunt hepatic injury. 2. In the haemodynamically stable blunt abdominal trauma patient without peritonitis, an abdominal computed tomography (CT) with intravenous contrast should be performed to identify and assess the severity of injury to the liver. 3. The severity of hepatic injury (as suggested by CT grade or degree of haemoperitoneum), neurologic status, age > 55, and/or the presence of associated injuries are not contraindications to a trial of non-operative management in a haemodynamically stable patient. 4. Angiography with embolization should be considered in a haemodynamically stable patient with evidence of active extravasation (a contrast blush) on abdominal CT. 5. Nonoperative management of hepatic injuries should only be considered in an environment that provides capabilities for monitoring, serial clinical evaluations, and an operating room available for urgent laparotomy.

Table 9.5.4 (*Continued*) American Association for the Surgery of Trauma (AAST) Evidence-Based Guidelines for Selective Non-Operative Management of Hepatic Injury

Level of Evidence	Recommendation
III	1. After blunt hepatic injury, clinical factors such as a persistent systemic inflammatory response, increasing/persistent abdominal pain, or an otherwise unexplained drop in haemoglobin should prompt re-evaluation by CT. 2. Interventional modalities such as endoscopic retrograde cholangiopancreatography (ERCP), angiography, laparoscopy, or percutaneous drainage may be required to manage complications (bile leak, biloma, bile peritonitis, hepatic abscess, bilious ascites, and haemobilia) that arise as a result of non-operative management of blunt hepatic injury. This is most likely to be necessary in grade IV and V hepatic injuries. 3. Pharmacologic prophylaxis to prevent venous thromboembolism can be used for patients with isolated blunt hepatic injuries without increasing the failure rate of non-operative management, although the optimal timing of safe initiation has not been determined.
Unanswered questions	1. Frequency of haemoglobin measurements 2. Intensity and duration of monitoring 3. Duration and intensity of restricted activity (both in hospital and after discharge) 4. Optimum length of stay for both the intensive care unit and the hospital

such as drainage for a bile duct injury will be required. Angiography/embolization may also be used postoperatively as a component of damage control for major liver injury.

A persistently falling haematocrit requires transfusion, angioembolization, and/or surgical response.

9.5.5.2 SUBCAPSULAR HAEMATOMA

An uncommon but troublesome hepatic injury is subcapsular haematoma, which arises when the parenchyma of the liver is disrupted by blunt trauma, but Glisson's capsule remains intact. Subcapsular haematomas range in severity from minor blisters on the surface of the liver to ruptured central haematomas accompanied by severe haemorrhage. They may be recognized either at the time of the operation or in the course of CT scanning. If a grade I or II subcapsular haematoma (i.e. a haematoma involving less than 50% of the surface of the liver that is not expanding and is not ruptured) is discovered during an exploratory laparotomy, **it should be left alone**. If the haematoma is explored, meatotomy with selective ligation may be required to control bleeding vessels. Even if effective, one must still contend with diffuse haemorrhage from the large, denuded surface, and packing may also be required. **A haematoma that is expanding during operation (grade III) may have to be explored.**

Such lesions are often the result of uncontrolled arterial haemorrhage, and packing alone may not be successful. An alternative strategy is to pack the liver to control venous haemorrhage, close the abdomen, and perform hepatic arteriography and embolization of the bleeding vessels. **Ruptured grades III and IV haematomas are treated with exploration and selective ligation, with or without packing (Figure 9.5.3).**

9.5.5.3 OPERATIVE (SURGICAL) MANAGEMENT

Eighty per cent of liver injuries requiring surgical intervention are managed simply by evacuating the intraperitoneal blood and appropriately packing the liver, followed by a re-look laparotomy at 24–48 hours. However, 20% of liver injuries requiring surgical intervention require direct control of more major hepatic bleeding. Tissue sealants may be a useful adjunct.[9] Caution must be exercised, since bile within the peritoneal cavity is not always well tolerated, and closed suction drainage should be routine in these patients.

9.5.6 Surgical Approach[10–12]

During treatment of a major hepatic injury, ongoing haemorrhage may pose an immediate threat to the

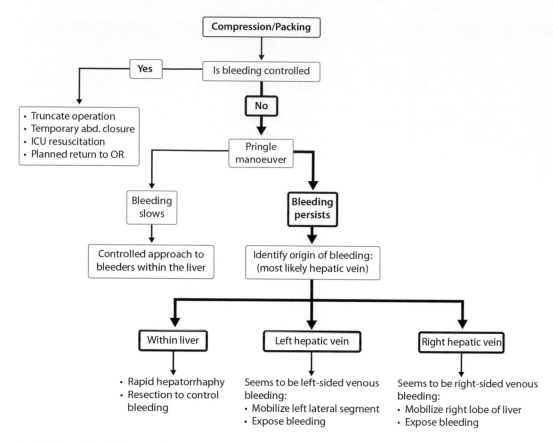

Figure 9.5.3 Surgical decision-making algorithm in major hepatic trauma.

patient's life, and temporary control will give the anaesthesiologist time to restore the circulating volume before further blood loss occurs. This is best achieved immediately upon entry into the abdomen by direct manual compression of the liver. The goal is to restore the normal anatomy by manual compression and then maintain it with packing. Compress right and left halves of the liver back to normal anatomy, and simultaneously push the liver posteriorly to tamponade potential retrohepatic venous bleeding.

In addition, multiple bleeding sites beyond the liver are common with both blunt and penetrating trauma. Even if the liver is not the highest priority, temporary control of hepatic bleeding allows repair of other injuries without unnecessary blood loss. As always, the most active/life-threatening bleeding must be controlled first.

- Perihepatic packing
- Pringle manoeuvre
- Tourniquet or liver clamp application

- Electrocautery, Aquamantys® bipolar sealer (Medtronic, Minneapolis, MN, USA), or argon beam coagulator
- Haemostatic agents and glues (FloSeal® Hemopatch® patch, Baxter, Deerfield, IL, USA)
- Hepatic suture
- Hepatorrhaphy and non-anatomic resection (resectional debridement)

9.5.6.1 INCISION

The patient is placed in the supine position.

- Warming devices are placed around the upper body and lower limbs.
- The chest and abdomen are surgically prepared and draped. Prep the patient from chin to mid-thighs, and table-to-table laterally.
- The instruments necessary to extend the incision into a sternotomy or thoracotomy must be available.

- A generous midline incision from xiphisternum to pubis is the standard incision required. On rare occasion, for the patient *in extremis*, a combined sternotomy and midline laparotomy approach is recommended from the outset to allow access for internal cardiac massage and vena caval vascular control. Supradiaphragmatic intrapericardial IVC control is often easier than abdominal control adjacent to a severe injury. However, this opens another body cavity and is uncommonly necessary.
- Do not hesitate to extend the midline incision with a right subcostal incision if there is difficulty exposing the IVC, hepatic veins, or right lobe of the liver.
- A table-mounted retractor, such as the Omnitract®- or Bookwalter®-type automatic retractor, greatly facilitates access. Apply the retractor to pull the ribcage cephalad and anteriorly to optimize exposure.

9.5.6.2 INITIAL ACTIONS

Once the abdomen has been opened, intraperitoneal blood is evacuated, and if there is evidence of hepatic bleeding, the liver should be initially packed, and the abdomen rapidly examined to exclude extrahepatic sites of blood loss. Autotransfusion should be considered. If this controls the bleeding, the anaesthetist has had an opportunity to restore intravascular volume, and haemostasis achieved for any extrahepatic injury, the liver injury then can be approached. If initial manual compression and/or packing does not control the liver bleeding then the liver injury should be addressed without delay.

In dealing with liver injury, be a minimalist – if the lesion has ceased bleeding, nothing more needs to be done in most cases and, above all, the non-bleeding lesion should not be explored further. If further surgery is required, adequate exposure and mobilization of the liver are necessary. Most injuries do not require formal mobilization of the injured lobe to permit repair or packing. Mobilize only enough to allow appropriate packing or control.

'Perfection is the enemy of good!'

The non-bleeding liver should not be explored further.

Call early for senior help for complex liver injuries which continue to bleed.

9.5.6.3 TECHNIQUES FOR TEMPORARY CONTROL OF HAEMORRHAGE

- Perihepatic packing
- Hepatic 'tourniquet'
- Tract tamponade balloons
- Pringle manoeuvre
- Tractotomy, direct suture ligation, or hepatic resection
- Hepatic artery ligation
- Hepatic vascular isolation
- Techniques to control retrohepatic caval bleeding
  - Moore–Pilcher balloon
  - Veno-venous bypass (uncommonly needed)

Perihepatic packing

The philosophy of packing has altered, and packs are used to restore the anatomical relationship of the components, and secondarily to act as a gentle compressive agent aimed to overcome portal and hepatic venous pressure.

Pitfall

Packs for a liver wound should **not** be pushed into the wound itself, as this worsens the injury and causes further bleeding.

Liver packing is often the definitive treatment, particularly with bilobar injury, or it buys time if the patient develops coagulopathy or hypothermia, or if there are no blood resources. Liver packing is the method of choice in the first instance. If packing is successful, and the bleeding is controlled, no further action may be required – this decision must be made early in the operation before the patient has received large numbers of red blood cells (RBCs) in transfusion. If simple actions fail to control bleeding, then a more complex operation will be necessary. Furthermore, surgical expertise and speed are essential to rapidly controlling the bleeding.

Pitfall

It is usually not necessary to mobilize the liver. If necessary, the liver can be mobilized by division of the hepatic ligaments (see below) until the bleeding has been controlled. Just sufficient mobilization of the liver is needed to allow pack placement, and restoration of the liver shape is required. Be aware of further opening liver injury through the placement of packs.

Blood loss, not time, is your 'clock' when dealing with major hepatic injury.

Packing is initially performed using large **dry** flat abdominal packs, placed laterally, inferiorly, medially, and around the liver, restoring the anatomical shape and providing radial compressive forces, while avoiding direct compression of the IVC. Ideally, it is **not** necessary to unfold these. Careful placement of packs is capable of controlling haemorrhage from most hepatic venous injuries.

Restore the anatomy of the liver by direct manual compression (**Figure 9.5.4a**).

The best packing will compress the liver laterally (against the lateral abdominal wall) and posteriorly (against the posterior abdominal wall), not upwards to the dome of the diaphragm. The liver is then packed posteriorly, without compressing the IVC.

- Place the first pack(s) across the injury to stabilize the damaged tissue.
- Ideally, place only one pack between the liver and the lateral abdominal wall.
- Pack the infero-medial surface of the liver from the porta hepatis laterally. This moves the right lobe of the liver laterally (**Figure 9.5.4b**) and avoids posterior compression on the IVC.
- Pack the anterior liver space between the anterior subcostal margin in the liver, compressing the liver posteriorly. Packs may be placed between the liver and the diaphragm, posteriorly and laterally, and between the liver and the anterior chest wall. The liver should not be packed so tightly as to cause compression of the vena cava which will reduce venous return.
- **There is no benefit in placing multiple packs between the dome of the liver and the diaphragm, which will only have the effect of raising the diaphragm.**

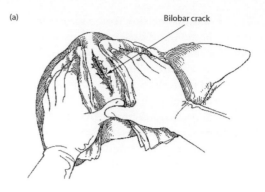

(a)   Bilobar crack

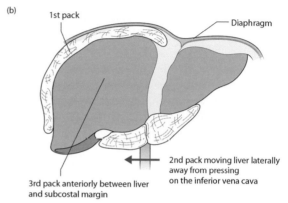

(b)   1st pack   Diaphragm

2nd pack moving liver laterally away from pressing on the inferior vena cava

3rd pack anteriorly between liver and subcostal margin

Figure 9.5.4 Diagram showing packing of the liver. (a) Manual use of swabs for the restoration of anatomy of the liver. (b) Final packing.

Rarely are more than five packs required if correctly placed. If this is not effective, more definitive management is required, and this decision needs to be made early or outcome will be poor. The minimum number of packs to achieve haemostasis should be used.

Pitfall

Packing is not as effective for injuries of the left lobe, because with the abdomen open, there is insufficient abdominal and thoracic wall anterior to the left lobe to provide adequate counter-compression. Fortunately, haemorrhage from the left lobe can be controlled by dividing the left triangular and coronary ligaments and compressing the lobe between the hands— segments II and III can be resected rapidly if needed.

Key factors for success in packing the liver are:

- Use dry abdominal swabs. (Wet swabs are less absorbent and exacerbate hypothermia.)

- Use them 'folded', as it is easier to layer them for even pressure.
- Ensure that they have radiopaque markers included in their manufacture.
- Do *not* cover them with plastic, as they will not hold position.
- Ongoing bleeding despite initial packing mandates repacking or another haemostatic procedure, and consideration of embolization.

During the period when the packs are placed, it is important to establish more intravenous access lines and other monitoring devices as needed. Hypothermia should be anticipated, and corrective measures taken. After haemodynamic stability has been achieved, the packs are removed, and the injury to the liver is rapidly assessed. The control of haemorrhage is the first consideration, followed by control of contamination. If the bleeding has stopped, nothing further may be required.

If in doubt, apply damage control techniques, with definitive packing of the liver.

- Packing will not control arterial injury.
- Consider angiography and embolization following damage control surgery.
- Packs should preferably be removed within 24–72 hours. If removed too early, bleeding may recur. A higher risk of perihepatic infection results from packs remaining longer than 72 hours.
- The packs should be carefully removed to avoid precipitating further bleeding.
- Packs are removed in the reverse order to insertion. **Last in, first out.**
- 'Roll' the packs off, using warmed normal saline if required.
- If there is no bleeding, the packs can be left out, and closed suction drains placed.
- Necrotic tissue should be resected.

Two complications may be encountered with the packing of hepatic injuries. First, tight packing compresses the IVC, decreases venous return, and reduces right ventricular filling; hypovolaemic patients may not tolerate the resultant decrease in cardiac output. Second, perihepatic packing forces the right diaphragm to move superiorly and impairs its motion; this may lead to increased airway pressures and decreased tidal volume.

If compression and packing are unsuccessful, then it will be necessary to achieve direct access to the bleeding vessel and direct suture ligation. This will often necessitate extension of the wound to gain access and view the bleeding point. During this direct access, bleeding can be temporarily controlled by direct compression, which requires a capable assistant. Temporary clamping of the porta hepatis (Pringle manoeuvre) is also a useful adjunctive measure. Other adjunctive measures include interruption of the venous or arterial inflow to a segment or lobe (used in less than 1% of all liver injuries), haemostatic agents such as crystallized bovine collagen, fibrin adhesives, gel foam, and use of an argon laser or harmonic scalpel.

Segments II and III

When faced with bleeding from the left lobe of the liver, it is easier to suture the actively bleeding liver. If this is not possible, once the bleeding lobe has been mobilized, gentle compression can be applied, usually with success. Bleeding from the left lateral segment can be definitively and rapidly controlled with resection using stapling devices.

'Hepatic tourniquets' are historical as they are difficult to use, and they tend to slip off or tear through the parenchyma if placed over an injured area.

Track tamponade balloons[13]

These can be useful in haemostasis of a track from a stab or gunshot wound. The balloon is threaded down the track and inflated to tamponade the bleeding from the inside out. The balloon can be manufactured by the surgeon using either Penrose rubber tubing, or even a condom and a nasogastric tube. A Sengstaken–Blakemore tube for tamponade of oesophageal varices is ideal.

Pringle manoeuvre

If there is ongoing bleeding, the Pringle manoeuvre is often used as an adjunct to liver packing, for the temporary control of haemorrhage. When encountering life-threatening haemorrhage from the liver, the hepatic pedicle should be compressed manually. The compression of the hepatic pedicle via the foramen of Winslow is known as the Pringle manoeuvre. The liver then should be packed, as described in Section 9.5.6.3.1. The hepatic pedicle is best clamped from the left side of the patient, by digitally dissecting a small hole in the lesser omentum, near the pedicle, and then placing a soft clamp over the pedicle from the left-hand side, through the foramen of Winslow. The advantage of this approach is the avoidance of injury to the structures within the hepatic pedicle, and the assurance that the clamp will be properly placed the first time. The pedicle can be left clamped for up to an hour. However, this is probably true only in the haemodynamically stable patient. In the hypotensive patient, intermittent clamping produces less ischaemia than continuous clamping; leave the clamp on for 10 minutes at a time, then allow 5 minutes of reperfusion before replacement of the clamp. The clamp should be replaced as soon as possible with a Rumel vascular sling.

The Pringle manoeuvre is both therapeutic and diagnostic. If bleeding within the liver stops with the Pringle manoeuvre, haemorrhage is from branches of the hepatic artery or the portal vein—these bleeding sites should be controlled. If haemorrhage persists with the clamp on the porta hepatis, the source of bleeding is generally from the hepatic veins or the retrohepatic vena cava, or, less commonly, aberrant extrapedicular arterial supply to the left or right lobe.

Getting access to deeper bleeding within the liver

At times, extension of the liver injury may be needed to gain access to deeper bleeding, preferably using the 'finger fracture' technique. Remember that as you proceed more deeply within the liver, the vessels become larger.

Finger fracture

To provide the above access, 'finger fracture' through normal liver tissue to get to the injured vessels deep in the parenchyma. The normal capsule is 'scored' using a diathermy or scalpel. Then the normal liver tissue is gently compressed between thumb and forefinger, rubbing the normal parenchymal tissue away, leaving just the intact vessels for ligation or clipping. Avoid forceful pinching or crushing of the liver tissue, as this may disrupt the hepatic vasculature, increasing the haemorrhage.

Stapling devices

Stapling devices provide an even rapider method to resect/divide liver parenchyma. Crushing staples with a vascular load are best. The LigaSure® (Medtronic) or equivalent may also be used to quickly divide liver parenchyma.

As with any liver surgery, be certain to protect normal/non-insured vasculature and bile ducts as you perform these manoeuvres. Knowledge of hepatic anatomy is critical.

Do not cross Cantlie's line as you resect a lobe or segment.

Hepatic suture

Suturing of the hepatic parenchyma is not routinely recommended to control more superficial lacerations, as these are best controlled with packing. If, however, the capsule of the liver has been stripped away by the injury, sutures which are tied over the capsule are far less effective.

The liver is usually sutured using a large, curved, blunt-nosed needle with 0 or 2/0 resorbable sutures. The large diameter prevents the suture from pulling through Glisson's capsule. At times, this may be life-saving. On the other hand, deeper injury may be present with resultant haemorrhage, abscess, or biloma. For shallow lacerations, a simple continuous suture may be used to approximate the edges of the laceration. For deeper lacerations, interrupted horizontal mattress sutures may be placed parallel to the edges, and tied over the capsule. The danger of suturing is that sutures tied too tightly may cut off the blood supply to viable liver parenchyma, resulting in necrosis.

Most sources of venous haemorrhage can be managed with intraparenchymal sutures.

Pitfall

The best way of ensuring haemostasis is to ensure that the damaged liver anatomy is 'reconstituted' and that the injured surfaces are in contact with one another. This is best treated by meticulous packing.

Hepatic resection[9,14]

In elective circumstances, anatomic resection produces good results, but in the uncontrolled circumstances of trauma, mortality has been recorded at rates of more than 50%. Liver resection should be reserved for:

- Delayed lobectomy in patients where packing initially controls the haemorrhage, but where there is a segment of the liver that is non-viable
- Almost free segments of liver
- Devitalized liver at the time of pack removal

Hepatic shunts

The atriocaval shunt was designed to achieve hepatic vascular isolation whilst still permitting some venous blood from below the diaphragm to flow through the shunt into the right atrium. A shunt can be introduced from above via the left atrial appendage, or from below via the sapheno-femoral junction.

The mortality rate remains high with this approach, and it is no longer in use.

9.5.6.4 MOBILIZATION OF THE LIVER

In general, and for most injuries, it is *not* necessary to mobilize the liver; injuries can be managed without resorting to full mobilization, whilst only a degree of mobilization may be required to allow successful packing. However, in some situations, particularly with injury to the superior or posterior aspects, mobilization is necessary.

Ensure that the table-mounted self-retaining retractor (Omnitract, Bookwalter, Rochard®, etc.) is lifting the costal margin in both a cephalad and anterior direction. Lifting the ribcage anteriorly (away from the table) is critical for adequate exposure. Access to the right lobe of the liver is restricted due to the right subcostal margin and the posterior attachments. If a self-retaining retractor is not immediately available, the costal margin can be elevated, initially with a Morris retractor, and then with a Kelly or Deaver retractor. The right triangular and coronary ligaments are divided with scissors or cautery. Avoid entering the diaphragm or liver parenchyma as you do so. This usually can be done under vision, but in the larger subject it can be accomplished blindly from the patient's left side. The superior coronary ligament is divided, avoiding the lateral wall of the right hepatic vein. The inferior coronary ligament is divided, taking care not to injure the right adrenal gland (which is vulnerable because it lies directly beneath the peritoneal reflection) or the retrohepatic vena cava. When the ligaments have been divided, the right lobe of the liver can be rotated medially into the surgical field. Sudden onset or aggravation of bleeding during mobilization of the right liver attests to hepatic vein or retrohepatic caval injury and mandates immediate replacement of the mobilized liver and damage control packing.

The left lobe can be easily mobilized by dividing the left triangular ligament under vision, avoiding injury to the left inferior phrenic vein and the left hepatic vein.

Pitfall

In the event of a retrohepatic haematoma being evident, rotation of the right lobe of the liver should be avoided unless strong indications are present, and adequate expertise is available. Packing and transport to a higher-level centre may be a safer option!

If exposure of the junction of the hepatic veins and the retrohepatic vena cava is necessary, the midline abdominal incision can be extended by means of a median sternotomy, or a lateral subcostal extension. The pericardium and the diaphragm then can be divided in the direction of the IVC. In an unstable patient, a more rapid means to access the suprahepatic IVC is via the abdomen through the central diaphragm/pericardium, and approach via the intracardiac route.

9.5.6.5 HEPATIC ISOLATION

Hepatic vascular isolation is accomplished by occlusion of the blood vessel access to the liver:

- Clamping the aorta at the diaphragm
- Executing a Pringle manoeuvre
- Clamping the IVC above the right kidney (infrahepatic and suprarenal)
- Clamping the IVC above the liver (suprahepatic)

The time limit for isolation is about 30 minutes. The technique is not straightforward and is best achieved by those experienced in its use. In patients scheduled for elective procedures, this technique has enjoyed nearly uniform success, but in trauma patients, the results have been disappointing.

Access to the suprarenal, infrahepatic IVC is through a Kocher rotation of the duodenum, and then clamping the IVC under direct vision.

Access to the suprahepatic, infradiaphragmatic IVC is obtained via mobilization of the suspensory ligaments, gently pulling the right lobe of the liver caudally and anteromedially, then applying a curved vascular clamp over the dome of the liver on the right and clamping the IVC at the diaphragmatic hiatus. A headlight may be useful.

In certain circumstances, it is easier to control the suprahepatic IVC *above* the diaphragm.

9.5.6.5.1 Intrapericardial Control of the Inferior Vena Cava

A small hole is made in the diaphragmatic pericardium as superiorly as possible. Be careful to avoid injury to the heart with this manoeuvre (**Figure 9.5.5a**). The pericardium is bluntly dissected from the posterior aspect of the sternum. With a clamp or finger protecting the heart, electrocautery or scissors are used to split the central diaphragm posteriorly. Curve towards the patient's right as you approach entry of the IVC into the

(a)

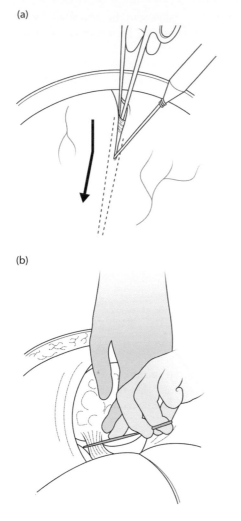

(b)

Figure 9.5.5 (a) Splitting of the diaphragm. (b) Clamping of the suprahepatic inferior vena cava above the diaphragm.

pericardium. The heart is lifted cephalad and anteriorly with your left hand; a vascular clamp is placed on the IVC[9] (**Figure 9.5.5b**).

9.5.7 **Perihepatic Drainage**

Several prospective and retrospective studies have demonstrated that the use of either Penrose or sump drains carries a higher risk of intra-abdominal infection than the use of either closed suction drains or no drains at all. If drains are to be used, closed suction devices are preferred.

Pitfall

Patients who are initially treated with perihepatic packing may also require drainage; however, drainage is not indicated at the initial damage control procedure, given that the patient will be returned to the OR within the next 36–48 hours.

Subsequently, the primary function is to drain bile, not blood.

The best treatment for a postoperative bile leak is prevention, although biliary injuries frequently leak despite attempts to suture them. Haemostatic patches are also valuable adjuncts to seal bile leaks.

9.5.8 **Complications**

Overall mortality for patients with hepatic injuries is approximately 10%. The most common cause of death is exsanguination, followed by multiple organ dysfunction syndrome (MODS) and intracranial injury.

- Morbidity and mortality increase in proportion to the injury grade and to the complexity of repair.
- Hepatic injuries caused by blunt trauma carry a higher mortality than those caused by penetrating trauma.
- Infectious complications occur more often with penetrating trauma.

Postoperative haemorrhage occurs in a small percentage of patients with hepatic injury. The source may be either a coagulopathy or a missed vascular injury (usually to an artery). In most instances of persistent postoperative haemorrhage, the patient is best served by return to the OR. Arteriography with embolization may be considered in selected patients. If coagulation studies indicate that a coagulopathy is the likely cause of postoperative haemorrhage, then correction of the coagulopathy must be a critical part of the strategy.

Perihepatic infections occur in fewer than 5% of patients with significant hepatic injury. They develop more often in patients with penetrating injuries than in patients with blunt injuries, presumably because of the greater frequency of enteric contamination. An elevated temperature and a rising white blood cell count should prompt a search for intra-abdominal infection. In the absence of pneumonia, an infected line, or urinary tract infection, an abdominal CT with intravenous and upper gastrointestinal contrast should be obtained.

Many perihepatic infections (but not necrotic liver) can be treated with CT or ultrasound-guided drainage.

Bilomas are loculated collections of bile that may become infected. They are best drained percutaneously under radiological guidance. If a biloma is infected, it should be treated as an abscess and drained; if it is sterile, it will eventually be resorbed.

Biliary ascites is caused by disruption of a major bile duct and requires reoperation and the establishment of appropriate drainage. Even if the source of the leaking bile can be identified, primary repair of the injured duct can be difficult to achieve. It is best to wait until a firm fistulous communication is established with adequate drainage. Adjunctive, transduodenal drainage by endoscopic retrograde cholangiopancreatography (ERCP) and papillotomy (ductotomy), or stent placement, may be of benefit in selected cases. Secondary infection of biliary ascites may lead to biliary peritonitis, which may require urgent drainage by laparotomy or laparoscopy with appropriate use of antibiotics.

Biliary fistulas occur in up to 15% of patients with major hepatic injury. They are usually of little consequence and generally close without specific treatment. In rare instances, a fistulous communication with intrathoracic structures forms in patients with associated diaphragmatic injuries, resulting in a bronchobiliary or pleurobiliary fistula. Because of the pressure differential between the biliary tract and the thoracic cavity, most of these fistulas must be closed operatively.

Haemorrhage from hepatic injuries is often treated without identifying and controlling each bleeding vessel individually, and arterial pseudoaneurysms may develop. As the pseudoaneurysm enlarges, it may rupture into the parenchyma of the liver, into a bile duct, or into an adjacent branch of the portal vein. Rupture into a bile duct results in haemobilia, which is characterized by intermittent episodes of right upper quadrant pain, upper gastrointestinal haemorrhage, and jaundice; rupture into a portal vein may result in portal vein hypertension with bleeding varices. Both complications are rare and are best managed with hepatic arteriography and embolization.

9.5.9 **Injury to the Retrohepatic Vena Cava**

Approximately 2% of all liver injuries are complex and represent injuries to major hepatic venous structures, the portal triad, and the intrahepatic cava; the injuries are bilobar or are difficult to control because of hypothermia and coagulopathy. Injuries to the hepatic vein or retrohepatic cava can be approached in the following ways:

- Direct compression (may require extension of the laceration).
- Direct suture after mobilization.
- Packing.
- Temporary clamping of the porta hepatis, suprarenal cava, and suprahepatic cava (vascular isolation – see Section 9.5.6.5).
- Veno-venous bypass (Heaney technique).
- Atriocaval shunt is rarely successful.

Direct compression and control of hepatic venous injuries can be accomplished in some patients. Major liver injury requires manual compression and simultaneous mobilization, using medial rotation and retraction – a difficult manoeuvre. Ideally, two experienced surgeons are now in the OR. In such a situation, the most senior surgeon should be the one doing the direct compression, and the assistant should do the actual suturing of the hepatic vein or cava.

Adequate exposure, experienced surgeons, good anaesthesia help, and a deep blood bank are essential in salvaging these patients.

However, in many cases, especially with blunt injury, packing the liver against the cava secures haemostasis as part of damage control, and the definitive care can take place later.

Hepatic vascular isolation, by clamping of the porta hepatis, suprarenal cava, and suprahepatic cava, can be done on a temporary basis (see Section 9.5.6.5). This requires considerable experience by the anaesthesiologist and a surgeon capable of dealing with the problems rapidly.

Veno-venous bypass has been used successfully in liver transplant surgery and, with new heparin-free pumps and tubing, may have a place in the treatment of trauma patients, but it is unlikely to be available.

Liver packing is the method of choice when expertise in more sophisticated techniques is not available, or when it is therapeutic in controlling the bleeding.

9.5.10 **Injury to the Porta Hepatis[15]**

If there is a haematoma in the porta hepatis, there is a high probability of injury to the vessels of the portal triad, often in association with injury to the common bile duct (CBD).

The key is to obtain source control.

- Before entering the haematoma, perform a Pringle manoeuvre, preferably with a Rumel tourniquet. *Isolate proximally and distally.*
- Control bleeding vessels in the porta, initially with finger compression, and subsequently with vascular clamps. *Do not clamp blindly!*
- Do **not** place sutures or ties until the CBD has been identified.
- When in doubt, *shunt* the portal vein.
- The hepatic artery can be ligated if necessary.

Injuries to the porta hepatis can be exsanguinating. Common hepatic and right and left hepatic arteries usually can be managed by simple ligation. Remember that hepatic artery ligation or embolization is well tolerated by the liver parenchyma (via portal vein flow) but not by the bile ducts (which depend on arterial flow).

Injury to the left or right portal vein can be ligated if necessary. Ligation of the main portal vein has been reported to be successful; however, shunting as part of damage control, and subsequent repair, are recommended whenever possible.

9.5.11 Removal of Packs (Aim for 36–49 Hours)

Packing should be removed in the standard damage control sequence (when the patient is warm, appropriately transfused, and haemodynamic, and respiratory parameters have been normalized). It is recommended that lateral and medial suction drains be placed after packs have been removed, as biliary leak is relatively common.

Pack removal: Last in, first out.

Do not 'pull' the packs out. Roll them off from one corner, one at a time.

Use irrigation to release them if required (though they will usually be damp enough).

9.5.12 Injury to the Bile Ducts and Gallbladder[16–18]

Injuries to the extrahepatic bile ducts, although rare, can be caused by either penetrating or blunt trauma. The diagnosis is usually made by noting the accumulation of bile in the upper quadrant during laparotomy for treatment of associated injuries.

Bile duct injuries can be divided into those below the confluence of the cystic duct and common duct and those above the cystic duct. Treatment of CBD injuries after external trauma is complicated by the small size and thin wall of the normal duct.

For the lower ductal injuries (those injuries below the cystic duct), when the tissue loss is minimal, the lesion can be closed over a T-tube (as with exploration of the CBD for stones), or by initial simple gravity drainage followed by subsequent ERCP-guided stent placement. If the duct has completely transected, it is best treated with Roux-en-Y hepaticojejunostomy.

In higher ductal injuries between the confluence of the cystic duct and the common duct and the hepatic parenchyma, a hepaticojejunostomy is recommended. An adjunctive measure is to bring the Roux-en-Y end to the subcutaneous tissue so that access can be gained later if a stricture develops. Percutaneous intubation of the Roux-en-Y limb is then possible with dilatation of the anastomosis.

Treatment of injury to the left or right hepatic duct is even more difficult. If only one hepatic duct is injured, a reasonable approach is to ligate it and deal with any infections or atrophy of the lobe rather than to attempt repair. If both ducts are injured, each should be intubated with a small catheter brought through the abdominal wall. Once the patient has recovered sufficiently, delayed repair is performed under elective conditions with a Roux-en-Y hepaticojejunostomy.

ANAESTHESIOLOGICAL CONSIDERATIONS

- Establish adequate upper limb large-bore vascular access, and initiate resuscitation fluids. Infuse blood products early and preferentially if the patient is profoundly hypotensive. Monitor haemostasis, and correct accordingly. Avoid excessive (any) crystalloid/colloid infusion.
- **Avoid IV access below the diaphragm**, as this may exacerbate bleeding from the liver or IVC.
- Initiation of the massive haemorrhage (massive transfusion) protocol must be early in severe liver injuries.

- Patients actively bleeding from major liver injury must be taken to the OR promptly, with rapid haemorrhage control. Any delay in doing so increases the risks of coagulopathy and mortality.
- Resuscitation of patients with liver injury is best done simultaneously with the surgery.
- When the surgeon is packing the liver, monitor venous return to avoid occlusion of the IVC by the packing. Judicious use of principles of 'low-CVP' (central venous pressure) anaesthesia from elective liver resection surgery may be used with caution in the trauma setting. Liver bleeding is largely venous and will benefit from reduced portal venous pressure. Keep in mind that trauma patients will typically have less reserve than elective surgical patients and will tend to high systemic vascular resistance (SVR) states, meaning that central perfusion is more at risk.
- The patient's physiology drives decision-making: unstable physiology requires surgery, whereas stable physiology does not, regardless of grade of liver injury.
- The use of REBOA is a joint surgical–anaesthesiological decision.
- REBOA should be considered with **huge caution** in severe liver injury, as Zone I REBOA may simply increase the risk of hepatic venous bleeding whilst delaying transfer to the OR.

REFERENCES AND RECOMMENDED READING

References

1. Brooks A, Reilly JJ, Hope C, Navarro A, Naess PA, Gaarder C. Evolution of non-operative management of liver trauma. *Trauma Surg Acute Care Open.* 2020 Nov 3;**5(1)**:e000551. doi: 10.1136/tsaco-2020-000551.

2. Gaski IA, Skattum J, Brooks A, Koyama T, Eken T, Naess PA, Gaarder C. Decreased mortality, laparotomy, and embolization rates for liver injuries during a 13-year period in a major Scandinavian trauma center. *Trauma Surg Acute Care Open.* 2018 Nov 5;**3(1)**:e000205. doi: 10.1136/tsaco-2018-000205.

3. Richardson JD, Franklin GA, Lukan JK, Carrillo EH, Spain DA, Miller FB, et al. Evolution in the management of hepatic trauma: a 25-year perspective. *Ann Surg.* 2000 Sep;**232(3)**:324–30. doi: 10.1097/00000658-200009000-00004.

4. Buckman RF Jr, Miraliakbari R, Badellino MM. Juxtahepatic venous injuries: a critical review of reported management strategies. *J Trauma.* 2000 May;**48(5)**:978–84. doi: 10.1097/00005373-200005000-00030.

5. Kozar RA, Crandall M, Shanmuganathan K, Zarzaur B, Coburn M, Cribari C, et al. Organ injury scaling 2018 update: spleen, liver, and kidney. *J Trauma Acute Care Surg.* 2018 Dec;**85(6)**:1119–22. doi: 10.1097/TA.0000000000002058.

6. Coccolini, F, Coimbra, R, Ordonez, C, Kluger Y, Vega F, Moore EE, et al. Liver trauma: WSES 2020 guidelines. *World J Emerg Surg.* 2020 Mar 30;**15(1)**:24. doi: 10.1186/s13017-020-00302-7.

7. Stassen NA, Bhullar I, Cheng JD, Crandall M, Friese R, Guillamondegui O, et al. A Non-operative management of blunt hepatic injury: an Eastern Association for the Surgery of Trauma Practice Management Guideline. *J Trauma Acute Care Surg.* 2012 Nov,**73(5 Suppl 4)**.S288–93. doi. 10.1097/TA.0b013e318270160d Supplement 4: S289–300 In: Trauma Practice Management Guidelines. Eastern Association for the Surgery of Trauma. http://www.east.org. Online. Doi:10.1097/TA.0b013e318270160d. Accessed January 2015.

8. Polanco PM, Brown JB, Puyana JC, Billiar TR, Peitzman AB, Sperry JL. The swinging pendulum: a national perspective of nonoperative management in severe blunt liver injury. *J Trauma Acute Care Surg.* 2013 Oct;**75(4)**:590–5. doi: 10.1097/TA.0b013e3182a53a3e.

9. Ochsner MG, Maniscalco-Theberge ME, Champion HR. Fibrin glue as a haemostatic agent in hepatic and splenic trauma. *J Trauma.* 1990 July;**30(7)**:884–7. doi: 10.1097/00005373-199007000-00020.

10. Peitzman AB, Marsh JW. Advanced operative techniques in the management of complex liver injury. *J Trauma Acute Care Surg.* 2012 Sep;**73(3)**:765–70. doi: 10.1097/TA.0b013e318265cef5.

11. Kozar RA, Feliciano DV, Moore EE, Moore FA, Cocanour CS, West MA, et al. Western Trauma Association/Critical decision in trauma: operative management of blunt hepatic injury. *J Trauma.* 2011 Jul; **71(1)**:1–5. doi: 10.1097/TA.0b013e318220b192.

12. American College of Surgeons. *Operative Exposure in Abdominal Trauma: Exposure of Liver Injuries.* ASSET: Advanced Operative Skills for Exposure in Trauma, Chicago. 2019.

13. Poggetti RS, Moore EE, Moore FA, Mitchell MB, Read RA. Balloon tamponade for bilobar transfixing hepatic gunshot wounds. *J Trauma*. 1992 Nov;**33(5)**:694–7. Review. doi: 10.1097/00005373-199211000-00018.

14. Polanco P, Leon S, Pineda J, Puyana JC, Ochoa JB, Alarcon L, et al. Hepatic resection in the management of complex injury to the liver. *J Trauma*. 2008 Dec;**65(6)**:1264–9; discussion 1269–70. doi: 10.1097/TA.0b013e3181904749.

15. Sheldon GF, Lim RC, Yee ES, Petersen SR. Management of injuries to the porta hepatis. *Ann Surg*. 1985 Nov;**202**(5):539–45. doi: 10.1097/00000658-198511000-00002.

16. Bade PG, Thomson SR, Hirshberg A, Robbs JV. Surgical options in traumatic injury to the extrahepatic biliary tract. *Br J Surg*. 1989 Mar;**76(3)**:256–8. doi: 10.1002/bjs.1800760314.

17. Feliciano DV, Bitondo CG, Burch JM, Mattox KL, Beall AC Jr, Jordan GL Jr. Management of traumatic injuries to the extrahepatic biliary ducts. *Am J Surg*. 1985 Dec;**150(6)**:705–9.

18. Posner MC, Moore EE. Extrahepatic biliary tract injury: operative management plan. *J Trauma*. 1985 Sep;**25(9)**:833–7. doi: 10.1097/00005373-198509000-00004.

Recommended Reading

Ivatury RR ed. *Operative Techniques for Severe Liver Injury*. Springer, New York. 2015.

Pachter HL. Prometheus bound: Evolution in the management of hepatic trauma- from myth to reality. 2011 Fitts Oration. *J Trauma Acute Care Surg*. 2012 Feb;**72(2)**:321–9. doi: 10.1097/TA.0b013e31824b15a7.

9.6 Pancreas

9.6.1 Overview

Pancreatic and combined pancreaticoduodenal injuries remain a dilemma for most surgeons, and, despite advances and complex technical solutions, they still carry a high morbidity and mortality. The increase in penetrating injuries throughout the world, and the increase in wounding energy from gunshots, have made the incidence of pancreatic injury more common. Pancreatic injury must be suspected in all patients with abdominal injuries, even those who initially have few signs. Since the pancreas is retroperitoneal, it usually does not present with peritonitis. It requires a high level of suspicion and significant clinical acumen, as well as aggressive radiographic imaging, to identify an injury early.

The pancreas and duodenum are difficult areas for surgical exposure and represent a major challenge for the operating surgeon when these organs are substantially injured. The retroperitoneal location of the pancreas also contributes to the difficulty in diagnosis as the organ is concealed, resulting in delay in diagnosis, with an attendant increase in morbidity.

Management varies from simple drainage to highly challenging procedures, depending on the severity, the site of the injury, and the integrity of the duct. Accurate intraoperative investigation of the pancreatic duct is particularly challenging. To compound this, pancreatic trauma is associated with a high incidence of injury to adjoining organs (duodenum, kidney, and liver) and major vascular structures, which adds to the high morbidity and mortality.[1]

> *The surgeon must always be critically aware of the patient's changing physiological state and be prepared to forsake the technical challenge of definitive repair for life-saving damage control.*

9.6.2 Anatomy

The pancreas lies at the level of the pylorus and crosses the first and second lumbar vertebrae. It is about 15 cm long from the duodenum to the hilum of the spleen, 3 cm wide, and up to 1.5 cm thick. The head lies within the concavity formed by the duodenum, with which it shares its blood supply through the pancreaticoduodenal arcades.

The pancreas has an intimate anatomical relationship with the upper abdominal vessels. It overlies the inferior vena cava, the right renal vessels, and the left renal vein. The uncinate process encircles the superior mesenteric artery and vein, whilst the body covers the suprarenal aorta and left renal vessels. The tail is closely related to the splenic hilum and left kidney, and overlies the splenic artery and vein, with the artery marking a tortuous path at the superior border of the pancreas.

There are several named arterial branches to the head, body, and tail that must be ligated in spleen-sparing procedures. Studies have shown that between seven and 10 branches of the splenic artery, and 13 to 22 branches of the splenic vein, run into the pancreas.

9.6.3 Mechanisms of Injury

9.6.3.1 BLUNT TRAUMA

The relatively protected location of the pancreas means that a high-energy force is required to damage it. Most injuries result from motor vehicle accidents in which the energy of the impact is directed to the upper abdomen – epigastrium or hypochondrium – commonly through the steering wheel of an automobile. This force results in crushing of the retroperitoneal structures against the vertebral column, which can lead to a spectrum of injury from contusion to complete transection of the body of the pancreas.

9.6.3.2 PENETRATING TRAUMA

The rising incidence of penetrating trauma has increased the incidence of injury to the pancreas. A stab wound damages tissue only along the track of the knife, but in gunshot wounds the passage of the missile and its pressure wave will result in injury to a wider region. Consequently, the pancreas and its duct must be fully assessed for damage in any penetrating wound that approaches the substance of the gland. Injuries to the pancreatic duct occur in 15% of cases of pancreatic trauma and are usually a consequence of penetrating trauma.

9.6.4 Diagnosis

The central retroperitoneal location of the pancreas makes the investigation of pancreatic trauma a diagnostic challenge: the specific diagnosis is often unsuspected, until laparotomy, especially if there are competing life-threatening vascular and other intra-abdominal organ injuries. In recent years, there has been debate about the need for accurate assessment of the integrity of the main pancreatic duct. Bradley[2] showed that mortality and morbidity were increased when there was failure or delay in recognizing ductal injury. When these results are reviewed in conjunction with earlier work, which showed an increase in late complications if ductal injuries were missed,[3] the importance of evaluating the duct is evident.

9.6.4.1 CLINICAL EVALUATION

In a patient with an isolated pancreatic injury, even ductal transection may be initially asymptomatic or have only minor signs, and this possibility must be kept in mind. Clinical examination is notoriously *unreliable*.

9.6.4.2 SERUM AMYLASE AND SERUM LIPASE

The levels of the serum amylase and serum lipase are not related to pancreatic injury in either blunt or penetrating trauma. A summary on serum amylase in blunt abdominal trauma by Biffl[4] showed a positive predictive value of 10% and a negative predictive value of 95% for pancreatic injury, although more recent work has suggested that accuracy may be improved when the activity is measured more than 3 hours after injury.[5] At present, serum amylase has little value in the initial evaluation of pancreatic injury. There is increasing interest in the value of lipase in trauma, but to date there remain little data to support this, and neither should be relied upon to rule out pancreatic injury.

9.6.4.3 ULTRASOUND

The posterior position of the pancreas almost completely masks it from diagnostic ultrasound.

9.6.4.4 DIAGNOSTIC PERITONEAL LAVAGE (DPL)

DPL has been largely superseded. The retroperitoneal location of the pancreas renders DPL inaccurate in the prediction of isolated pancreatic injury. However, the numerous associated injuries that may occur with pancreatic injury may make the lavage diagnostic if the level of amylase in the lavage fluid is checked.

9.6.4.5 COMPUTED TOMOGRAPHY (CT)

CT scan has been advocated as the best investigation for evaluation of the retroperitoneum. In a haemodynamically stable patient, CT scanning with contrast enhancement has a sensitivity and specificity as high as 80%. However, particularly in the initial phase, CT scanning may miss or underestimate the severity of a pancreatic injury,[6] so normal findings on the initial scan do not exclude appreciable pancreatic injury, and a repeat scan in the light of continuing symptoms may improve its diagnostic ability.

9.6.4.6 ENDOSCOPIC RETROGRADE CHOLANGIOPANCREATOGRAPHY (ERCP)

There are two phases in the investigation of pancreatic injury in which ERCP may have a role.[7]

9.6.4.6.1 Acute Presentation

A very small number of patients with isolated pancreatic trauma occasionally have initially benign clinical findings. ERCP has no practical role in the investigation of pancreatic duct injury in the acute phase, as most patients will not be stable enough and their injuries will not allow positioning for ERCP. In those patients who do not settle with conservative management and there is suspicion of ductal injury, ERCP will give detailed information about the ductal system, although cannulation of the pancreatic duct can itself cause pancreatitis. There is increasing discussion of the role of ERCP-placed pancreatic duct stents for ductal injury; however, there is limited literature to support this.

9.6.4.6.2 Delayed Presentation

A small number of patients present with symptoms months to years after the initial injury, potentially with a retroperitoneal collection or pancreatic fistula. Magnetic resonance cholangiopancreatography (MRCP; see below) is likely to be the initial investigation; however, ERCP can be used to assess the integrity of the duct and consider pancreatic duct stenting.

9.6.4.7 MAGNETIC RESONANCE CHOLANGIOPANCREATOGRAPHY (MRCP)

MRCP is the mainstay of evaluation of the pancreaticobiliary tree in the non-acute setting. It has no role in the *initial* evaluation of the injured patient, but it has value in the assessment for ductal injury in those patients who have developed a complication such as a pseudocyst or pancreatic fistula.[8]

MRCP can allow better selection of patients with suspected injuries than can ERCP, because patients with an intact pancreatic duct or minor injury can be successfully treated conservatively. Some authors believe that it will have an increasing role in identifying patients who are unlikely to benefit from endoscopic intervention, those with an intact pancreatic duct (or very minor injury), and those with severe duct strictures or obstruction.

9.6.4.8 INTRAOPERATIVE PANCREATOGRAPHY

Intraoperative visualization of the pancreatic duct has been advocated in the investigation of the duct, particularly when it is not possible to assess its integrity by examination. Nevertheless, in the opinion of several authors, simple examination of the area of injury for several minutes with loupe magnification reveals clear pancreatic fluid leakage in most injuries that involve the pancreatic duct.[9] An accurate assessment of the degree of injury to the duct will reduce the complication rate, indicate the most appropriate operation, and, when no involvement is found, allow a less aggressive procedure to be undertaken. However, the ductal system frequently cannot be found due to its small size in previously normal patients. Intraoperative investigation by transduodenal pancreatic duct catheterization or distal cannulation of the duct in the tail through a pancreatic incision is not recommended. A cholecystocholangiogram using methylene blue may be helpful in some cases.

Intraoperative ultrasound can be used to help diagnose a parenchymal or ductal laceration.[10]

9.6.4.9 OPERATIVE EVALUATION

Operative evaluation of the pancreas necessitates complete exposure of the organ. A central retroperitoneal haematoma must be thoroughly investigated, and intra-abdominal bile staining makes a complete evaluation essential to find the pancreatic or duodenal injury. In this case, a ductal injury must be assumed until excluded.

If the sphincter of Oddi and the distal biliary tract are intact, it is wise to attempt to preserve the head and neck of the pancreas. Major injuries to the body of the pancreas are usually treated by a distal pancreatectomy with splenectomy. If the injury is to the head of the pancreas, involving the duct and sphincter, a Whipple procedure must be contemplated. Increasingly, there is a move towards lesser procedures since the mortality of a Whipple procedure continues to be significant in the severely injured trauma patient. These injuries continue to be a major challenge for the trauma surgeon. It is essential to understand the manoeuvres necessary for gaining complete control of the duodenum and pancreas in order to completely explore and identify any injuries.

9.6.5 Pancreas Injury Scale

The organ injury scale developed by the American Association for the Surgery of Trauma (AAST)[11] has been accepted by most institutions that regularly deal with pancreatic trauma. See **Table 9.6.1** for the Pancreas Injury Scale.

9.6.6 Management

9.6.6.1 NON-OPERATIVE MANAGEMENT

In isolated blunt pancreatic injuries, exclusion of a major pancreatic duct injury with ERCP followed by expectant non-operative management (NOM) is gaining popularity. Recent reports utilizing early ERCP to identify and sometimes treat blunt pancreatic injuries by transpapillary stent insertion are showing promising results,[12,13] and can decrease the incidence of pancreatic-related complications and the failure rate

of NOM. A pancreatic duct stent appears useful for a proximal pancreatic fistula, but it may be complicated by a long-term stricture, whereas ductal stenting in the acute phase is potentially dangerous in that it may lead to a delay in necessary laparotomy and definitive repair of the pancreatic injury.[14] Because of the small size of the pancreatic duct distal to the ampulla, stenting is ordinarily not used in this location. Evidence suggests that endoscopic interventions are more successful in managing pancreatic fistulas and pseudocysts than in managing patients with main pancreatic duct stricture.[15]

NOM of low-grade (grades I and II) blunt pancreaticoduodenal injuries is safe despite occasional failures. A recent multicentre analysis strongly recommends this strategy for low-grade injuries.[16] Missed diagnoses continue to occur despite advances in CT scanning, but do not seem to cause an adverse outcome in most patients.[17] The vogue for conservative management of body and tail pancreatic duct injury has more recently been challenged with distal pancreatectomy, which is shown to have relatively low morbidity and mortality.

9.6.6.2 OPERATIVE MANAGEMENT

Many pancreatic injuries will only be confirmed following a CT scan, or at the time of surgery. The surgical approach is often for that of the presenting sign (e.g., peritonitis), and the pancreatic injury will be found at laparotomy. Commonly, there are associated injuries of the duodenum, bowel mesentery, and so on.

Table 9.6.1 Pancreas Injury Scale

Grade*	Type of Injury	Description of Injury
I	Haematoma	Minor contusion without duct injury
	Laceration	Superficial laceration without duct injury
II	Haematoma	Major contusion without duct injury or tissue loss
	Laceration	Major laceration without duct injury or tissue loss
III	Laceration	Distal transection or parenchymal injury with duct injury
IV	Laceration	Proximal** transection or parenchymal injury involving the ampulla
V	Laceration	Massive disruption of the pancreatic head

Note: See also Appendix B, 'Trauma Scores and Scoring Systems'.

* Advance one grade for multiple injuries up to grade III.
** The proximal pancreas is deemed to be that part of the pancreas to the *right* of the superior mesenteric artery and vein.

9.6.7 **Surgical Approach**

9.6.7.1 INCISION AND EXPLORATION (SEE ALSO SECTION 9.1: 'THE TRAUMA LAPAROTOMY')

Access to the pancreas in trauma is gained via a long midline incision.

Penetrating pancreatic trauma should be obvious. Once the retroperitoneum has been violated in penetrating trauma, it is imperative for the surgeon to do a thorough exploration of the central region.

Diagnosis of blunt pancreatic trauma is much more problematic. As the pancreas is a retroperitoneal organ, there may be no anterior peritoneal signs. The history can be helpful if information from the paramedics indicates that the vehicle's steering column was bent, or if the patient can give a history of epigastric trauma.

For complete evaluation of the gland, it is essential to see the pancreas from both the anterior and posterior aspects. To examine the anterior surface of the gland, it is necessary to divide the gastrocolic ligament and open the lesser sac. An extended Kocher manoeuvre is required so that the duodenum can be mobilized, and an adequate view gained of the pancreatic head, uncinate process, and posterior aspect. Injury to the tail requires mobilization of the spleen and left colon to allow medial reflection of the pancreas and access to the splenic vessels. Division of the ligament of Treitz and reflection of the fourth part of the duodenum and duodenojejunal flexure give access to the inferior aspect of the pancreas. Any parenchymal haematoma of the pancreas should be thoroughly explored, including irrigation of the haematoma, to exclude possible injury of the duct.

9.6.7.1.1 Access via the Lesser Sac

The stomach is then grasped and pulled inferiorly, allowing the operator to identify the lesser curvature and the pancreas through the lesser sac. Frequently, the coeliac artery and the body of the pancreas can be identified through this approach. The omentum is then grasped and drawn upwards. An opening is made in the omentum, and the operator's hand is passed into the lesser sac posterior to the stomach. This allows excellent exposure of the entire body and tail of the pancreas. Any injuries to the pancreas can be easily identified.

9.6.7.1.2 Duodenal Rotation (Kocher Manoeuvre)

If there is the possibility of an injury to the head of the pancreas, a Kocher manoeuvre is performed. The loose areola of tissue around the duodenum is bluntly dissected, and the entire second and third portions of the duodenum are identified and mobilized medially. This dissection is carried all the way medially to expose the inferior vena cava and a portion of the aorta. By reflecting the duodenum and pancreas towards the anterior midline, the posterior surface of the head of the pancreas can be completely inspected.

9.6.7.1.3 Right Medial Visceral Rotation

The inferior border of the proximal portion of the pancreas can be identified by performing a right medial visceral rotation. This is performed by taking down the ascending colon and then mobilizing the caecum, the terminal ileum, and the mesentery towards the midline. The entire ascending colon and caecum are then reflected superiorly towards the left upper quadrant of the abdomen. This gives excellent exposure of the entire vena cava, the aorta, and the third and fourth portions of the duodenum.

9.6.7.1.4 Left Medial Visceral Rotation

The descending colon on the left is mobilized, together with the spleen and the tail of the pancreas. These are rotated medially, allowing inspection of the tail and posterior and inferior aspects of the pancreas.

These manoeuvres allow for complete exposure of the first, second, third, and fourth portions of the duodenum along with the head, neck, body, and tail of the pancreas.

When pancreatic injury is suspected, extended exploration of the whole organ is imperative. Parenchymal lacerations that do not involve the pancreatic duct can be sutured when the tissue is not too soft and vulnerable. With or without the use of sutures, a worthwhile option in the treatment of such lacerations is fibrin sealing and collagen tamponade, and adequate drainage is essential.

9.6.7.2 PANCREATIC INJURY: SURGICAL DECISION-MAKING

9.6.7.2.1 Contusion and Parenchymal Injuries (AAST Grades I and II Injuries)

Relatively minor pancreatic lacerations and contusions comprise most injuries to the pancreas. If there is obvious disruption to the pancreatic duct, it should be ligated with distal pancreatic resection and, in the unstable trauma patient, with splenectomy.

9.6.7.2.2 Drainage Alone

Injuries to the tail and body of the pancreas that do not involve the duct can be drained, and with haemostasis this has become standard practice. Suction drainage should be used, as fewer intra-abdominal abscesses develop and there is less skin excoriation with a closed suction system.[18] A retrospective study of the Trauma Quality Improvement Program (TQIP) database, which included only patients with penetrating trauma of grades III and IV, concluded that resection is not associated with a significant decrease in mortality but is associated with a significant increase in length of stay (LOS). Drainage alone of the pancreatic bed may be a viable option, even for high-grade injuries.[19]

9.6.7.2.3 Laceration of the Distal Pancreas (AAST Grades II or III)

In most cases in which there is a major parenchymal injury of the pancreas to the left of the superior mesenteric vessels, a distal pancreatectomy is the procedure of choice, independent of the degree of ductal involvement. Spleen preservation is recommended in haemodynamically stable patients. After mobilization of the pancreas and ligation of the vessels, the pancreatic stump can be closed with sutures and the duct ligated separately, or it can be closed with a stapling device. A suction drain should be placed at the site of transection, as there is a high postoperative fistula rate. Suction drains are again preferable.

In the past decade, publications considering non-operative treatment of grade III pancreatic injuries have increased, showing that it can be safe. However, minimally invasive treatment modalities such as endoscopy and percutaneous drainage must be available in this situation, since most patients will develop pancreatic collections.

During laparotomy, indicators of pancreatic duct injury may be considered: direct visualization of the lesion, complete transection of the pancreas, laceration greater than half of the pancreas, centre perforation, and severe organ maceration.

> **Pitfall**
>
> Avoid the use of a linear guillotine stapler (GIA type), as the margin between the cut edge and the very small staples is unsafe. Rather, use a transverse anastomosis (TA) stapler, and leave 5 mm of tissue at the cut edge, outside of the staples.

Most authors agree that a pancreatectomy to the *left* of, and protecting, the superior mesenteric vessels usually leave enough pancreatic tissue and results in an acceptably low rate of insulin-dependent diabetes. Procedures associated with resection of greater than 80% of the pancreatic tissue are associated with a risk of adult-onset diabetes mellitus.

9.6.7.2.4 Splenic Salvage in Distal Pancreatectomy

Splenic salvage has been advocated where possible in *elective* distal pancreatectomy. However, this should be saved for the rare occasions when the patient is haemodynamically stable, and the injury is limited to the pancreas.

> **Pitfall**
>
> The technical problems of dissecting the pancreas free from the splenic vessels and ligating the numerous tributaries make the procedure contraindicated in an unstable patient with multiple associated injuries. When this operation is considered, the surgeon must clearly balance the extra time that it takes, and the problems associated with lengthy operations in injured patients, against the small risk of the development of overwhelming post-splenectomy infection (OPSI) postoperatively.

9.6.7.2.5 Ductal Injuries: Combined Injuries of the Head of the Pancreas and Duodenum (AAST Grades IV and V)

The injuries that vex the surgeon most, however, are those to the head of the gland, particularly those juxtaposed with or also involving the duodenum. Drainage of the head is a good alternative for grade IV injuries. Resection (Whipple procedure) is usually reserved for grade V patients who have destructive injuries or those in whom the blood supply to the duodenum and pancreatic head has been compromised. However, the Whipple procedure should be avoided in most situations due to high mortality. Damage control surgery (DCS) is usually a better choice, with preservation of all potentially viable tissue.

This is more so in austere, low-resource, and military environments.

Severe combined pancreaticoduodenal injuries account for less than 10% of injuries to these organs, and are commonly associated with multiple intra-abdominal injuries, particularly of the vena cava.[20] They are usually the result of penetrating trauma. The integrity of the distal common bile duct and ampulla on cholangiography, and the severity of the duodenal injury, will dictate the operative procedure. If the duct and ampulla are intact, simply repair with variations of drainage and pyloric exclusion. This includes extensive closed (suction) drainage around the injury site. Common duct drainage is not indicated.

9.6.7.2.6 Damage Control

Patients with severe pancreatic or pancreaticoduodenal injury (AAST grades IV and V) are not stable enough to undergo complex reconstruction at the time of initial laparotomy. Damage control, with the rapid arrest of haemorrhage and bacterial contamination and the placement of drains and packing, is preferable. It may be helpful to place a tube drain directly into the duct, both for drainage and to allow easier isolation of the duct at the subsequent operation. The damage control laparotomy is followed by a period of intensive care and continued aggressive resuscitation to correct physiological abnormalities and restore reserve before the definitive procedure.

9.6.7.2.7 Pyloric Exclusion

Pyloric exclusion has been widely reported for the management of severe combined pancreaticoduodenal injuries without major damage to the ampulla or the common bile duct. The rationale is to minimize exocrine pancreatic stimulation caused by gastric acid, and filling of the duodenum. The technique involves the temporary diversion of enteric flow away from the injured duodenum by closure of the pylorus and a distal gastro-jejunostomy. This is best achieved with access from the stomach through a gastrotomy and the use of a slowly absorbable suture. The alternative is a TA stapler across the pylorus. (*Note*: The GIA

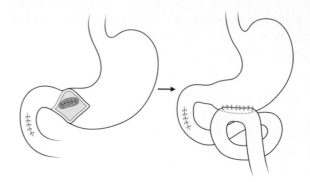

Figure 9.6.1 Pyloric exclusion and gastric bypass.

type of staple cannot be used due to its integral guillotine) (**Figure 9.6.1**).

Contrast studies have shown that the pylorus reopens within 2–3 weeks in 90%–95% of patients, allowing flow through the anatomical channel. The stomach is decompressed with a gastrojejunostomy.[21,22] Once the pylorus is open, the gastrojejunostomy usually closes spontaneously. There has been recent debate as to the need for the procedure, since even a nasogastric tube and use of proton pump inhibitors will be as effective.[20] Although the technique remains controversial, pyloric exclusion may be a useful option for grade III and IV combined pancreaticoduodenal injuries.

9.6.7.2.8 T-Tube Drainage

Some surgeons advocate closing the injury over a T-tube in combined injuries where the second part of the duodenum is involved. This ensures adequate drainage and allows the formation of a controlled fistula once the track has matured.

9.6.7.2.9 Pancreaticoduodenectomy (Whipple Procedure)

This is a major procedure to be practised in trauma only if no alternative is available,[22] and it will be required in less than 10% of combined injuries. Damage control with control of bleeding and of bowel contamination, and ligation of the common bile and pancreatic ducts, should be the rule. Indications for considering a pancreaticoduodenectomy are massive disruption of the pancreaticoduodenal complex, devascularization of the duodenum, and sometimes extensive duodenal injuries of the second part of the duodenum involving the ampulla or distal common bile duct.

The Whipple procedure (as first described for carcinoma of the ampulla)[23] is indicated only in the rare stable patient with this type of injury. The nature and severity of the injury and the co-existing damage to vessels are often accompanied by haemodynamic instability, and the surgeon must therefore control the initial damage and delay formal reconstruction until the patient has been stabilized. The results of this operation vary, and when patients with major retroperitoneal vascular injuries are included, mortality can approach 50%. More recently, in the largest series to date, for patients who underwent DCS or a staged Whipple procedure for complex pancreaticoduodenal trauma and the largest series with blunt trauma, in-hospital mortality was 13%.[24]

Damage control is an integral part of the approach to these devastating injuries. Krige et al. have reported their use of DCS in pancreatic trauma: in a series of predominately penetrating trauma and associated vascular injury, they reported a salvage rate of 45% using DCS.[25]

The role of pancreaticoduodenectomy in trauma was best summarized by Walt[26] in 1996:

Finally, to Whipple or not to Whipple, that is the question. In the massively destructive lesions involving the pancreas, duodenum and common bile duct, the decision to do a pancreaticoduodenectomy is unavoidable; and, in fact, much of the dissection may have been done by the wounding force. In a few patients, when the call is of necessity close, the overall physiologic status of the patient and the extent of damage become the determining factors in the decision. Though few in gross numbers, more patients are eventually salvaged by drainage, TPN [total parenteral nutrition] and meticulous overall care than by a desperate pancreaticoduodenectomy in a marginal patient.

9.6.8 Adjuncts

9.6.8.1 SOMATOSTATIN AND ITS ANALOGUES

Somatostatin and its analogue octreotide have been used to reduce pancreatic exocrine secretion in patients with acute pancreatitis. Despite meta-analysis, its role has not been clearly defined. Buchler[27] reported a slight but not significant reduction in the complication rate in patients with moderate to severe pancreatitis, but this was not verified by Imrie's group in Glasgow,[28] who found that somatostatin gave no benefit.

Somatostatin cannot be recommended in trauma on the current evidence, and a level 1 study is required.

9.6.8.2 NUTRITIONAL SUPPORT

Whether nutritional support is required should be considered at the definitive operation. Major injuries that precipitate prolonged gastric ileus and pancreatic complications may preclude gastric feeding. A feeding jejunostomy can be used but can lead to technical complications. A nasojejunal feeding catheter is a better and non-invasive alternative.

Elemental diets that are less stimulating to the pancreas are preferred. Total parenteral nutrition is far more expensive but may be used if enteral nutrition is not possible.

9.6.9 Pancreatic Injury in Children

The pancreas is injured in up to 10% of cases of blunt abdominal trauma in children, usually as a result of a handlebar injury. Whether these children with high-grade pancreatic injury should be operated upon or managed conservatively (the current vogue for the management of solid organ injuries in children) has been controversial. In most cases, a NOM approach is used, although considerable variability exists regarding NOM strategies[29]; however, there are increasing advocates of distal pancreatectomy in children, with body/tail transection providing an overall improved outcome. Splenic preservation is more important in children than adults, and a splenic-preserving distal pancreatectomy should be seriously considered in children. Where the expertise exists, this can be done as a laparoscopic procedure.

9.6.10 Complications

Pancreatic trauma is associated with up to 20% mortality. Early deaths result from the associated intra-abdominal vascular and other organ injuries, and later deaths from sepsis and the systemic inflammatory response syndrome (SIRS). Pancreatic injuries have postoperative complication rates of up to 40%, and the number rises with increasing severity of injury: with combined injuries and associated injuries, the complication rate approaches 62%.

Most complications are treatable or self-limiting, however, and could be avoided by an accurate assessment of whether the pancreatic duct was damaged. Pancreatic complications can be divided into those occurring early and those occurring late in the postoperative period.

9.6.10.1 EARLY COMPLICATIONS

9.6.10.1.1 Pancreatitis

Postoperative pancreatitis may develop in about 7% of patients. It may vary from a transient biochemical leak of amylase to a fulminant haemorrhagic pancreatitis. Fortunately, most cases run a benign course and respond to bowel rest and nutritional support.

9.6.10.1.2 Fistula

The development of a postoperative pancreatic fistula is the most common complication, increasing when the duct is involved, and the rate may be as high as 35%–40% in combined injuries. Most fistulas are minor (less than 200 mL of fluid per day), and self-limiting when there is adequate external drainage. However, high-output fistulas (> 7000 mL per day) may require surgical intervention for closure or prolonged periods of drainage with nutritional support. Management is directed locally at early adequate nutrition (preferably with distal enteral feeds through a feeding jejunostomy), adequate drainage, and transpapillary pancreatic stenting of confirmed ductal injuries.

9.6.10.1.3 Abscess Formation

Most abscesses are peripancreatic and associated with injuries to other organs, specifically the liver and intestine. A true pancreatic abscess is uncommon and usually results from inadequate debridement of necrotic tissue. For this reason, simple percutaneous drainage is generally not enough, and further debridement is required.

9.6.10.2 LATE COMPLICATIONS

9.6.10.2.1 Pseudocyst

Accurate diagnosis and surgical treatment of pancreatic injuries should result in a rate of pseudocyst formation of about 2%–3%. Accurate evaluation of the state of the duct will dictate management, and if the duct is intact, percutaneous drainage is likely to be successful. However, a pseudocyst together with a major ductal disruption will not be cured by percutaneous drainage, which will convert the pseudocyst into a chronic fistula. Current options include cystogastrostomy (open or endoscopic), endoscopic stenting of the duct, or resection.

9.6.10.2.2 Exocrine and Endocrine Deficiency

Pancreatic resection distal to the mesenteric vessels will usually leave enough tissue for adequate exocrine and endocrine function, as work has shown that a residual 10%–20% of pancreatic tissue is usually enough. Patients who have procedures that leave less functioning tissue will require exogenous endocrine and exocrine enzyme replacement.

Pearls and Pitfalls

- Any parenchymal haematoma of the pancreas should be thoroughly explored, including irrigation of the haematoma, to exclude possible injury of the duct.
- Suturing of parenchymal lesions (AAST grades I and II) to gain haemostasis simply leads to necrosis of the pancreatic tissue.
- Avoid the use of a linear guillotine stapler (GIA type), as the margin between the cut edge and the very small staples is unsafe. Rather, use a transverse anastomosis (TA) stapler, and keep all 5 mm of tissue at the cut edge, outside of the staples.
- The technical problems of dissecting the pancreas free from the splenic vessels and ligating the numerous tributaries make the procedure contraindicated in an unstable patient with multiple associated injuries. **Consider** splenectomy as well. When this operation is considered, the surgeon must clearly balance the extra time that it takes, and the problems associated with lengthy operations in injured patients, against the small risk of the development of overwhelming post-splenectomy infection (OPSI) postoperatively.

9.6.11 Summary of Evidence-Based Guidelines[20,30]

Table 9.6.2 gives a summary of the evidence-based guidelines for pancreatic trauma.

Table 9.6.2 Summary of EAST Evidence-Based Guidelines for Pancreatic Trauma

PICO Format	
P	**P**atient, **P**opulation, or **P**roblem
I	**I**ntervention, Prognostic factor, or Exposure
C	**C**omparison or Intervention (if appropriate)
O	**O**utcome you would like to measure or achieve

PICO	Recommendation
PICO Question 1	
For adults with grade I/II injury to the pancreas identified by CT scan (P), should operative intervention (I) or non-operative management (C) be performed?	**We conditionally recommend non-operative management for grade I/II pancreatic injuries diagnosed by CT scan.** Non-operative management appears to have low morbidity. If the pancreatic duct is not definitively intact, it seems reasonable to further evaluate the duct with additional tests, such as ERCP or MRCP, because this may change the grade of the injury and therefore the recommended treatment plan.
PICO Question 2	
For adults with grade III/IV injury to the pancreas identified by CT scan (P), should operative intervention (I) or non-operative management (C) be performed?	**We conditionally recommend operative management for grade III/IV pancreatic injuries diagnosed by CT scan.** Although there was no statistically significant difference between groups for any single outcome, our group feels that there is a cumulative trend towards increased morbidity after non-operative management. Treatment failures after non-operative management occur regularly, and treatment delays likely contribute to morbid complications and death.
PICO Question 3	
For adults undergoing an operation who are intraoperatively found to have a grade I/II pancreas injury (P), should resectional (I) or non-resectional management (C) be performed?	**We conditionally recommend non-resectional management for operative management of grade I/II pancreatic injuries.** Our pooled data analysis suggests that mortality from pancreas-related causes is generally low in this population and that there were significantly more intra-abdominal abscesses in the resection group.
PICO Question 4	
For adults undergoing an operation who are intraoperatively found to have a grade III/IV pancreas injury (P), should resectional (I) or non-resectional management (C) be performed?	**We conditionally recommend resection for operative management of grade III/IV pancreatic injuries.** Complications are frequent in both groups. In our pooled analysis, fistula development was associated with non-resection strategies. Pancreas-related mortality was higher in the non-resection group, but this finding was potentially confounded by incomplete mortality reporting and bias. Due to the very low quality of available data, this is a conditional recommendation.
PICO Question 5	
For adults with total destruction of the head of the pancreas (grade V) (P), should pancreaticoduodenectomy (I) or surgical treatment other than pancreaticoduodenectomy (C) be performed?	**No recommendation is given.** The literature on this topic is limited and dated. Surgical and resuscitation strategies have evolved significantly to include damage control procedures and early balanced resuscitations, making our ability to interpret the available literature limited. Grade V injury to the pancreas is extremely morbid, and the intraoperative and immediate postoperative rates of death are high.

(Continued)

Table 9.6.2 (*Continued*) Summary of EAST Evidence-Based Guidelines for Pancreatic Trauma

PICO Question 6	
For adults who have undergone an operation for pancreatic trauma (P), should routine octreotide prophylaxis (I) or no octreotide (C) be used?	**We conditionally recommend** against **the routine use of octreotide for postoperative prophylaxis related to traumatic pancreatic injuries to prevent fistula.** Data are limited, but pooled data show no difference in outcomes between groups. The subcommittee concluded that the less invasive (no medication) strategy would be preferable with no difference in outcomes.
PICO Question 7	
For adults undergoing distal pancreatectomy for trauma (P), should routine splenectomy (I) or splenic preservation (C) be performed?	**No recommendation is given.** Existing data do not support either treatment modality, although splenic preservation was only considered for stable patients. If either the stability of the patient or the surgeon's ability to safely preserve the spleen is in doubt, a distal pancreatectomy with splenectomy is a reasonable choice.

REFERENCES AND RECOMMENDED READING

References

1. Degiannis E, Glapa M, Loukogeorgakis SP, Smith MD. Management of pancreatic trauma. *Injury.* 2008;**39**:21–9.

2. Bradley EL III, Young PR Jr, Chang MC, Allen JE, Baker CC, Meredith W, et al. Diagnosis and initial management of blunt pancreatic trauma: guidelines from a multi-institutional review. *Ann Surg.* 1998;**227**:861–9.

3. Leppaniemi A, Haapiainen R, Kiviluoto T, Lempinen M. Pancreatic trauma: acute and late manifestations. *Br J Surg.* 1988;**75**:165–7.

4. Biffl W. Injury to the duodenum and pancreas. In Moore EE, Feliciano DV, Mattox KL, eds. *Trauma*, 8th ed. New York: McGraw-Hill Education, 2013:621–38.

5. Takishima T, Sugimoto K, Hirata M, Asari Y, Ohwada T, Katika A. Serum amylase level on admission in the diagnosis of blunt injury to the pancreas: its significance and limitations. *Ann Surg.* 1997 Jul;**226**:70–6.

6. Ahkrass R, Kim K, Brandt C. Computed tomography: an unreliable indicator of pancreatic trauma. *Am Surg.* 1996 Aug;**62**:647–51.

7. Thomson DA, Krige JE, Thomson SR, Bornman P. The role of endoscopic retrograde pancreatography in pancreatic trauma: A critical appraisal of 48 patients treated at a tertiary institution. *J Trauma Acute Care Surg.* 2014 Jun;**76(6)**:1362–6. doi:10.1097/TA.0000000000000227.

8. Bret PM, Reinhold C. Magnetic resonance cholangiopancreatography. *Endoscopy.* 1997 Aug;**29**:472–86.

9. Subramanian A, Dente CJ, Feliciano DV. The management of pancreatic trauma in the modern era. *Surg Clin N Am.* 2007 Dec;**87(6)**:1515–32, x. Review.

10. Hikida S, Sakamoto T, Higaki K, Hata H, Maeshiro K, Yamauchi K, et al. Intra-operative ultrasonography is useful for diagnosing pancreatic duct injury and adjacent tissue damage in a patient with penetrating pancreas trauma. *J Hepatobiliary Pancreat Surg.* 2004;**11**:272–5.

11. Moore EE, Cogbill TH, Malangoni MA, Jurkovich GJ, Shackford SR, Champion HR, et al. Organ injury scaling. II: pancreas, duodenum, small bowel, colon, and rectum. *J Trauma.* 1990;**30**:1427–9.

12. Kong Y, Zhang H, He X, Liu C, Piao L, Zhao G, et al. Endoscopic management for pancreatic injuries due to blunt abdominal trauma decreases failure of nonoperative management and incidence of pancreatic-related complications. *Injury.* 2014 Jan;**45(1)**:134–40. doi: 10.1016/j.injury.2013.07.017.

13. Wolf A, Bernhardt J, Patrzyk M, Heidecke CD. The value of endoscopic diagnosis and the treatment of pancreas injuries following blunt abdominal trauma. *Surg Endosc.* 2005 May;**19**:665–9.

14. Lin BC, Fang JF, Wong YC, Liu NJ. Blunt pancreatic trauma and pseudocyst: management of major pancreatic duct injury. *Injury.* 2007 May;**38**:588–93.

15. Biffl WL, Ball ChG, Moore EE, Lees J, Todd SR, Wydo S et al. Don't mess with the pancreas! A multicenter analysis of the management of low-grade pancreatic injuries. *J Trauma Acute Care Surg.* 2021; 91:820–8.

16. Velmahos GC, Tabbara M, Gross R, Willette P, Hirsch E, Burke P, et al. Blunt pancreatoduodenal injury: a

multicenter study of the research consortium of New England Centers for trauma (ReCONECT). *Arch Surg.* 2009 May;**144**: 13–9; discussion 419–20.

17. Fabian TC, Kudsk KA, Croce MA, Payne LW, Mangiante EC, Voeller GR, et al. Superiority of closed suction drainage for pancreatic trauma. A randomized prospective study. *Ann Surg.* 1990 Jun;**211**:724–8; discussion 728–30.

18. Mohseni S, Holzmacherc J, Sjolina G, Ahlb R, Saranic B. Outcomes after resection versus non-resection management of penetrating grade III and IV pancreatic injury: A trauma quality improvement (TQIP) databank analysis. *Injury.* 2018;**49**:27–32.

19. Coccolini F, Kobayashi L, Kluger Y, Moore EE, Ansaloni L, Biffl W et al. Duodeno-pancreatic and extrahepatic biliary tree trauma: WSES-AAST guidelines. *World J of Emerg Surg.* 2019;**14**:56 doi: 10.1186/s13017-019-0278-6.

20. DuBose JJ, Inaba K, Teixeira PG, Shiflett A, Putty B, Green DJ, et al. Pyloric exclusion in the treatment of severe duodenal injuries: results from the National Trauma Data Bank. *Am Surg.* 2008 Oct;**74**:925–29.

21. Seamon MJ, Pieri PG, Fisher CA, Gaughan J, Santora TA, Pathak AS, et al. A ten-year retrospective review: does pyloric exclusion improve clinical outcome after penetrating duodenal and combined pancreaticoduodenal injuries? *J Trauma.* 2007 Apr;**62**:829–33.

22. Whipple A. Observations on radical surgery for lesions of the pancreas. *Surg Gynecol Obstet.* 1946;**82**:623.

23. Thompson CM, Shalhub S, DeBoard ZM, Maier RV. Revisiting the pancreaticoduodenectomy for trauma: a single institution's experience. *J Trauma Acute Care Surg.* 2013 Aug;**75**:225–8. doi: 10.1097/TA.0b013e31829a0aaf.

24. Krige JE, Navsaria PH, Nicol AJ. Damage control laparotomy and delayed pancreatoduodenectomy for complex combined pancreatoduodenal and venous injuries. *Eur J Trauma Emerg Surg.* 2016 April; **42**:225–30. doi: 10.1007/s00068-015-0525-9.

25. Walt AJ. Pancreatic trauma. In Ivatury RR, Gayten CG eds. *The Textbook of Penetrating Trauma.* Baltimore Williams & Wilkins, 1996: 641–52.

26. Büchler M, Friess H, Klempa I, Hermanek P, Sulkowski U, Becker H, et al. Role of octreotide in the prevention of postoperative complications following pancreatic resection. *Am J Surg.* 1992 Jan;**163**: 125–30; discussion 130–1.

27. McKay C, Baxter J, Imrie C. A randomized, controlled trial of octreotide in the management of patients with acute pancreatitis. *Int J Pancreatol.* 1997 Feb;**21**:13–9.

28. Naik-Mathuria BJ, Rosenfeld EH, Gosain A, Burd R, Falcone Jr. RA, Takkar R, et al. al. Proposed clinical pathway for non-operative management of high-grade pediatric pancreatic injuries based on a multicenter analysis: A Pediatric Trauma Society collaborative. *J Trauma Acute Care Surg.* 2017 Oct;**83(4)**:589–96. doi: 10.1097/TA.0000000000001576.

29. Ho VP, Patel NJ, Bokhari F, Madbak FG, Hambley JE, Yon JR et al. Management of adult pancreatic injuries: A practice management guideline from the Eastern Association for the Surgery of Trauma. *J Trauma Acute Care Surg.* 2017 Jan;**82(1)**:185–99. doi: 10.1097/TA.0000000000001300.

30. Biffl WL, Moore EE, Croce M, Davis JW, Coimbra R, Karmy-Jones R, et al. Western Trauma Association critical decisions in trauma: management of pancreatic injuries. *J Trauma Acute Care Surg.* 2013;**75(6)**.

Recommended Reading

Injury to the duodenum and pancreas. In Moore EE, Feliciano DV, Mattox KL, eds. *Trauma*, 9th ed. New York: McGraw-Hill Education, 2021: 621–38

Phillips B, Turco L, McDonald D, Mause E, Walters RW. A subgroup analysis of penetrating injuries to the pancreas: 777 patients from the National Trauma Data Bank, 2010–2014. *J Surg Res.* 2018 May;**225**:131–41. doi: 10.1016/j.jss.2018.01.014.

9.7 Spleen

9.7.1 Overview

'The spleen is the most commonly injured organ in blunt abdominal trauma'.[1] Most injuries can be successfully managed non-operatively, although this is dependent on the grade of injury (anatomy) and the haemodynamic effects on the patient (physiology). Other considerations include associated injuries, comorbidities (including anticoagulation), and age.

The goal of non-operative management (NOM) is spleen preservation. This approach has evolved in the setting of blood component volume resuscitation, improved cross-sectional imaging allowing more accurate assessment of the anatomy of the injury, the increased availability of embolization, and a better understanding of the importance of splenic function. Despite the widespread use of NOM, open splenectomy remains a life-saving trauma intervention for many patients. Regardless of the resources available, for the shocked patient, operative intervention with splenectomy remains the treatment of choice.

9.7.2 Anatomy

The spleen is the largest single mass of lymph tissue and is situated within the layers of the dorsal mesogastrium. The 3–7 splenic segments, each with their own blood supply, are separated by avascular planes. The splenic artery, a branch of the coeliac axis, provides the principal blood supply to the spleen. The artery gives rise to a superior polar artery, from which the short gastric arteries arise. The splenic artery then gives rise to superior and inferior terminal branches that enter the splenic hilum. The artery and the splenic vein are embedded in the superior border of the pancreas. With a blood flow of approximately 170 mL/min/100 g, injury to this organ can result in significant blood loss.

Three splenic suspensory ligaments maintain the intimate association between the spleen and the diaphragm (lienophrenic ligament), left kidney (lienorenal ligament), and splenic flexure of the colon (lienocolic ligament). The gastrosplenic ligament contains the short gastric arteries. These attachments place the spleen at risk of avulsion during rapid deceleration. The spleen is also relatively delicate and can be damaged by impact from the overlying ribs. The splenic capsule varies in thickness, being thicker in children than in older adults. This probably contributes to a higher success rate of NOM in the former group.

9.7.3 Diagnosis

The diagnosis of probable splenic injury is based on clinical and radiological assessment. In the case of haemorrhagic shock in conjunction with a positive focussed assessment with sonography for trauma (FAST), the surgeon will need to make the decision to take the patient to the operating room based on the probable likelihood of solid organ injury. For such patients, attempting to confirm the diagnosis with CT scan or attempting to avoid an operation with embolization may prove fatal.

9.7.3.1 CLINICAL

The patient may complain of left upper quadrant pain or referred pain to the left shoulder, and there may be local tenderness. Signs of hypovolaemia (tachypnoea, tachycardia, or hypotension) might be present.

Consideration of the pattern of injury will also alert the surgeon to the possibility of splenic injury. Clinical evidence of rib fractures in the lower left chest from a direct blow, or a penetrating injury that traverses the space between the left 9th to 11th ribs posteriorly, places the spleen at risk.

9.7.3.2 ULTRASOUND

Extended focussed abdominal sonography for trauma (eFAST) has become an important tool in the assessment of circulation in the haemodynamically compromised patient, as part of the primary survey. The finding of free intra-abdominal fluid, particularly if it is most obvious around the spleen and in the left paracolic gutter, indicates a possible splenic injury.

9.7.3.3 COMPUTED TOMOGRAPHY (CT) SCAN

Dual-phase CT scanning can provide an accurate diagnosis of vascular and parenchymal damage in splenic trauma and is the preferred modality to confirm the grade of injury.

Provided the patient is not haemodynamically compromised and has responded to blood volume resuscitation, an arterial phase scan which includes the splenic artery followed by a (delayed) portal–venous phase will identify parenchymal lesions and any evidence of vascular injury (blood pooling, contrast blush, pseudoaneurysm [PSA], or arteriovenous fistula).

9.7.4 Splenic Injury Scale[2]

The Organ Injury Scale (OIS) of the American Association for the Surgery of Trauma (AAST) is based on the most accurate assessment of injury, whether it is by radiological study (CT scan), laparotomy, laparoscopy, or autopsy evaluation (**Table 9.7.1**). The 2018 update of the AAST OIS introduced contrast-enhanced CT imaging and takes into consideration evidence of vascular injury. This is relevant because CT evidence of a contrast blush (active extravasation) is an important

Table 9.7.1 Splenic Injury Scale: 2018 Revision[2]

AAST Grade*	AIS Severity	Imaging Criteria (CT Findings)	Operative Goals	Pathologic Criteria
I	2	**Haematoma** Subcapsular haematoma < 10% surface area **Laceration** Parenchymal laceration < 1 cm depth	**Haematoma** Subcapsular haematoma < 10% surface area **Laceration** Parenchymal laceration < 1 cm depth Capsular tear	**Haematoma** Subcapsular haematoma < 10% surface area **Laceration** Parenchymal laceration < 1 cm depth Capsular tear
II	2	**Haematoma** Subcapsular haematoma 10%–50% surface area Intraparenchymal haematoma < 5 cm in **Laceration** Laceration 1–3 cm	**Haematoma** Subcapsular haematoma 10%–50% surface area Intraparenchymal haematoma < 5 cm in diameter **Laceration** 1–3 cm	**Haematoma** Subcapsular haematoma 10%–50% surface area Intraparenchymal haematoma < 5 cm in diameter **Laceration** Laceration 1–3 cm depth
III	3	**Haematoma** Subcapsular haematoma > 50% surface area Ruptured subcapsular or intraparenchymal haematoma > 5 cm **Laceration** Parenchymal laceration > 3 cm depth Any injury in the presence of a liver vascular injury or active bleeding contained within liver parenchyma	**Haematoma** Subcapsular haematoma > 50% surface area Ruptured subcapsular or intraparenchymal haematoma > 5 cm **Laceration** Laceration > 3 cm in depth	**Haematoma** Subcapsular haematoma > 50% surface area Ruptured subcapsular or intraparenchymal haematoma > 5 cm **Laceration** Parenchymal laceration > 3 cm depth
IV	4	**Laceration** Parenchymal laceration involving segmental or hilar vessels producing > 25% devascularization **Disruption** Any injury in the presence of a splenic vascular injury, or active bleeding confined within the splenic capsule	**Laceration** Parenchymal laceration involving segmental or hilar vessels producing > 25% devascularization	**Laceration** Parenchymal laceration involving segmental or hilar vessels producing > 25% devascularization
V	5	**Vascular injury** Any injury in the presence of splenic vascular injury with active bleeding extending beyond the spleen into the peritoneum **Disruption** Shattered spleen	**Vascular injury** Hilar vascular injury which devascularizes the spleen **Disruption** Shattered spleen	**Vascular injury** Hilar vascular injury which devascularizes the spleen **Disruption** Shattered spleen

Note: Vascular injury is defined as a pseudoaneurysm or arteriovenous fistula, and it appears as a focal collection of vascular contrast that decreases in attenuation with delayed imaging. Active bleeding from a vascular injury presents as vascular contrast, focal or diffuse, that increases in size or attenuation in delayed phase. Vascular thrombosis can lead to organ infarction.

*Grade based on highest grade assessment made on imaging, at operation, or on pathologic specimen. More than one grade of splenic injury may be present and should be classified by the higher grade of injury. Advance one grade for multiple injuries up to a grade III.

predictor of failure of NOM. Evidence of vascular injury (PSA, arteriovenous fistula, or blush) signifies at least a grade IV injury and is an indication to consider embolization if available.

9.7.5 Management

9.7.5.1 NON-OPERATIVE MANAGEMENT (NOM)[3,4]

The goal of NOM is spleen preservation. This approach was initially established in the paediatric population and is now well described with a splenic preservation rate of more than 90%. Similarly, most adult patients with blunt splenic injury are also successfully managed non-operatively. This has come about via the implementation of blood component resuscitation for haemorrhagic shock limiting the development of coagulopathy, as well as improved access to cross-sectional imaging which facilitates accurate grading. The use of embolization as an adjunct to NOM has improved the success rates for high-grade injuries (AAST grade IV and V).[4,5]

The advantages of NOM over operative management include preservation of the immunological function of the spleen and avoidance of overwhelming post-splenectomy infection (OPSI), the avoidance of complications of laparotomy and non-therapeutic laparotomies, lower rates of blood transfusion, lower costs associated with hospitalization, and lower rates of morbidity and mortality.[6]

NOM of splenic injury includes the monitoring and tracking of vital signs, serial physical examination, and monitoring of serum haemoglobin and haematocrit. It does not include strict bed rest and may include embolization. Safe NOM requires haemodynamic stability, the absence of peritonism or other indication for laparotomy, accurate assessment of grade of injury via CT scan, and admission into a hospital with timely access to personnel, operating room capabilities, and blood products.

The success of NOM is dependent on the selection of appropriate patients. After resuscitation and completion of the initial assessment, haemodynamically stable patients should undergo CT scan. Patients with AAST grade I, II, or III splenic injuries, who have no associated intra-abdominal injuries requiring surgical intervention, are obvious candidates for NOM. Patients with higher-grade splenic injuries (AAST grade IV and V) can also be successfully treated non-operatively. They should be monitored closely to detect any signs that indicate ongoing bleeding and therefore a need for intervention. Ideally, this should be in a high-dependency or intensive

care unit. Patients who are sedated and intubated with traumatic brain or other injuries should have continuous blood pressure monitoring. There is no evidence that bed rest or restricted activity is beneficial. Moreover, there is little evidence to support the use of serial CT scans, without clinical indications, to monitor progress.

Embolization, if available, is a useful adjunct to NOM, and is the treatment of choice to facilitate NOM of high-grade injuries. Early embolization is associated with improved salvage rates, as demonstrated in a number of prospective studies.[7]

The indications for embolization include identification of vascular injury on CT angiography (PSA, arteriovenous fistula) or active extravasation (either intraparenchymal or intraperitoneal), AAST grade IV or V injury, or evidence of ongoing bleeding with a significant drop in haemoglobin level and tachycardia. It should be noted that current World Society of Emergency Surgery (WSES) guidelines do not recommend routine embolization of AAST grade III injuries.[7]

Failure of NOM, defined as the need for surgical intervention, is associated with increasing grade of injury, moderate (250–500 mL) or high-volume (> 500 mL) haemoperitoneum, high Injury Severity Score (ISS), age over 55 years (especially when combined with a high ISS), comorbidities, and the presence of PSA or arteriovenous fistula. However, it is the identification of a contrast blush on CT scan that has been identified as one of the more reliable predictors of failure of NOM.

The risk of delayed re-bleeding of the spleen after NOM is acceptably low, reportedly in the range of 1%–8%. Whilst re-bleed is considered more likely if a high-grade injury has been managed non-operatively, prophylactic embolization of the splenic artery in adults with grade IV and V injuries has been reported to result in a NOM success rate of 96% (**Table 9.7.2**).

9.7.5.2 OPERATIVE MANAGEMENT

As was highlighted earlier, splenectomy is the treatment of choice for patients with haemorrhagic shock not responding to resuscitation and with free fluid on eFAST, and in patients with a high-grade injury and obvious need for a laparotomy for any reason. In most situations, these patients will be too shocked to be safely put through the CT scanner, leaving the surgeon to confirm the probable solid organ injury at laparotomy. Although splenic preservation is desirable, most patients who require an operation due to splenic bleeding will have a splenectomy performed.

Table 9.7.2 Evidence-Based Guidelines for Selective Non-Operative Management of Splenic Injury[3]

Level of Evidence	Recommendation
I	Patients who have diffuse peritonitis or who are haemodynamically unstable after blunt abdominal trauma should be taken urgently for laparotomy.
II	1. A routine laparotomy is not indicated in the haemodynamically stable patient without peritonitis presenting with an isolated splenic injury. 2. The severity of splenic injury (as suggested by CT grade or degree of haemoperitoneum), neurologic status, age > 55, and/or the presence of associated injuries are not contraindications to a trial of non-operative management in a haemodynamically stable patient. 3. In the haemodynamically normal blunt abdominal trauma patient without peritonitis, an abdominal CT scan with intravenous contrast should be performed to identify and assess the severity of injury to the spleen. Angiography should be considered for patients with American Association for the Surgery of Trauma (AAST) grade of greater than III injuries, the presence of a contrast blush, moderate haemoperitoneum, or evidence of ongoing splenic bleeding. Non-operative management of splenic injuries should only be considered in an environment that provides capabilities for monitoring, serial clinical evaluations, and an operating room available for urgent laparotomy.
III	1. After blunt splenic injury, clinical factors such as a persistent systemic inflammatory response, increasing/persistent abdominal pain, or an otherwise unexplained drop in haemoglobin should dictate the frequency of and need for follow-up imaging for a patient with blunt splenic injury. 2. Contrast blush on CT scan alone is not an absolute indication for an operation or angiographic intervention. Factors such as patient age, grade of injury, and the presence of hypotension need to be considered in the clinical management of these patients. 3. Angiography may be used either as an adjunct to non-operative management for patients who are thought to be at high risk for delayed bleeding or as an investigative tool to identify vascular abnormalities such as pseudoaneurysms that pose a risk for delayed haemorrhage. Pharmacologic prophylaxis to prevent venous thromboembolism can be used for patients with isolated blunt splenic injuries without increasing the failure rate of non-operative management, although the optimal timing of safe initiation has not been determined.
Unanswered questions	1. Frequency of haemoglobin measurements 2. Frequency of abdominal examinations 3. Intensity and duration of monitoring 4. Is there a transfusion trigger after which operative or angiographic intervention should be considered? 5. Time to reinitiating oral intake 6. The duration and intensity of restricted activity (both in-hospital and after discharge) 7. Optimum length of stay for both the intensive care unit (ICU) and hospital 8. Necessity of repeated imaging 9. Timing of initiating chemical deep venous thrombosis (DVT) prophylaxis after a splenic injury 10. Should patients with severe injuries and/or embolized injuries receive post-splenectomy vaccines? 11. Is there an immunologic deficiency after splenic embolization?

9.7.6 **Surgical Approach**

Whilst little has changed with the surgical technique of splenectomy over the years, the frequency of this operation has decreased significantly, due to the increased successful use of the NOM approach. Access to the spleen in trauma is best performed via a long midline incision, from the xiphisternum to the infra-umbilical midline. When indicated, the spleen is mobilized under direct vision. In paediatric patients, a midline incision should also be used, rather than a subcostal incision, since there is better access to the entire abdominal cavity if there is injury to other intra-abdominal structures.

The spleen is best approached by a surgeon standing on the patient's right-hand side. The table can also be rotated slightly to the right. The spleen is mobilized under direct vision. Great care and gentle handling are necessary to avoid pulling on the spleen, avulsing the capsule, and making a minor injury worse by stripping the capsule off the lower pole.

Medial traction by the operator's non-dominant hand will give access to the lienophrenic, lienorenal, and lieno-colic ligaments.

- The spleen is gently pulled upwards and medially, and the lienorenal and lienocolic ligaments are divided.
- The spleen is then gently pulled downwards, and the lienophrenic ligaments are divided with scissors, close to the spleen, between the spleen and the diaphragm.
- The short gastric vessels between the greater curvature of the stomach and the spleen must be divided between ligatures. These vessels must be divided **away** from the greater curvature, as there is a danger of avascular necrosis of the stomach if they are divided too close to the stomach itself.
- The spleen is pulled forward, and several packs can be placed in the splenic bed to hold it forward so that it can be inspected.
- The hilum can be controlled with the surgeon's left hand, giving the anaesthetic staff an opportunity to catch up with blood volume resuscitation.

In the presence of competing major injuries that require urgent intervention (e.g., severe traumatic brain injury requiring craniotomy), ongoing haemodynamic compromise, or if the spleen has sustained damage at the hilum, a routine splenectomy should be performed. In the stable patient and in the absence of other life-threatening injuries, splenic preservation could be considered.

9.7.6.1 SPLEEN NOT ACTIVELY BLEEDING

If not actively bleeding, the spleen can be left alone.

9.7.6.2 SPLENIC SURFACE BLEED ONLY

These bleeds will usually stop with a combination of manual compression, packing, diathermy, argon beam, and fibrin adhesives in combination with other haemostatic agents.

9.7.6.3 MINOR LACERATIONS

These may be sutured using absorbable sutures, with or without Teflon pledgets. Suturing is time-consuming and mostly not helpful in trauma patients. The superficial lacerations are best treated with fibrin adhesive and collagen tamponade. These measures are best taken at the beginning of the operation, and the spleen packed; upon completion of the operation, the pack can be removed without displacing the collagen fleece.

9.7.6.4 MESH SPLENORRHAPHY AND PARTIAL SPLENECTOMY

Mesh splenorrhaphy is rarely deployed and even more rarely successful. If the lacerations involve only one pole or one half of the organ, the respective vessels could be ligated.

Prior to resection, the spleen should be mobilized. Stapler resection makes organ conservation possible in many cases, and it represents a valuable alternative to sutured partial splenectomy or splenorrhaphy. Its greatest advantages are simplicity of use, the practicality of the instrument itself, and the reduction in time and blood transfusion.

Whilst splenorrhapy and partial splenectomy are rarely used nowadays, patients who have proceeded to theatre due to lack of access to timely embolization should be considered for spleen preservation surgery, but only **if physiology allows**.

9.7.6.5 SPLENECTOMY

In the presence of other major injuries, with haemodynamic instability, if the spleen has sustained damage at the hilum, or if the patient has proceeded to theatre because of failure of NOM, a routine splenectomy should be carried out.

Following careful mobilization of the spleen, access to the splenic pedicle can be anterior or posterior. Care must be taken to avoid injuring the tail of the pancreas, which lies very close to the hilum of the spleen. The splenic pedicle may be secured with suture ties or vascular cutting-staples.

9.7.6.6 DRAINAGE

The splenic bed is *not* routinely drained after splenectomy. If the tail of the pancreas has been damaged, a closed suction drain should be placed in the area affected.

TIPS AND TRICKS

The following ctricks will make the operation easier in most cases:

- Alexis™ wound retractor (or equivalent)
- LigaSure™, particularly good for controlling the short gastric arteries
- Automatic cutting–stapling devices
- A stool to stand on
- A good headlight
- A fixed body wall retractor (or a strong assistant)
- Cell saver

9.7.7 Perioperative Considerations

9.7.7.1 HAEMOSTATIC RESUSCITATION

Modern resuscitative techniques involving early identification and correction of coagulopathy and the use of massive transfusion protocols have contributed to the increased success of NOM, even in high-grade splenic injury.

9.7.7.2 REPEAT IMAGING

Whilst repeat contrast-enhanced CT scan may identify latent vascular injury, only 4% of routine repeat scans lead to a change in clinical management.[12] Current WSES guidelines advise that repeat CT scanning should only be performed if there is a clinical change[8] (e.g., a sudden increase in left upper quadrant pain, or clinical signs of bleeding). Patients with a grade IV or V injury without definite vascular injury may be considered for a repeat CT at 48 to 72 hours to exclude the development of PSA. Currently, though, this is not strongly supported by the literature, as outlined in a systematic review published in 2020.[8]

9.7.7.3 MOBILIZATION

Early mobilization and discharge, especially after grade I or II injury, have become common practice. Failure of NOM is not associated with the day of mobilization, with strict bed rest now considered unnecessary.

9.7.7.4 RETURN TO NORMAL ACTIVITIES

Eighty percent of grade I–II injuries will appear completely healed on ultrasound by day 50, and 80% of grade III–V injuries within 75 days.[8] The WSES guidelines recommend restricting activity (including contact and non-contact sports) for 4 to 6 weeks for grade I and II injuries, and for 2 to 4 months for grade III–V injuries.[9,10]

9.7.7.5 VENOUS THROMBOEMBOLISM (VTE) PROPHYLAXIS

VTE is a significant cause of morbidity and mortality in patients who survive the first 24 hours after major injury. All patients with splenic injury should have mechanical prophylaxis in the form of graduated compression stockings and/or sequential pneumatic compression devices. Splenic injury is not a contraindication to chemoprophylaxis, and low-molecular-weight heparin (LMWH) should be commenced early, ideally within 48 hours.[10]

9.7.8 Outcomes

The success rate of selective NOM is > 90%, increasing to 100% in some series with embolization.[11] NOM failure rates of 4%–15% have been published recently. This is increased in the presence of PSA and arteriovenous fistula, and increases to 67%–82% in the presence of an active contrast blush on CT scan.

For the majority of patients who require splenectomy, the clinical signs are evident, and approximately 60% proceed to theatre within 2 hours. For those patients who have failed NOM, 95% will proceed to splenectomy within 72 hours, and 1.5% within 3 to 5 days. The risk of delayed rupture for all grades is estimated to be between 0.27% and 1.4% over 6 months.[11,12]

Mortality after NOM (including with embolization) is <1%. This increases to 3.6% after splenectomy, and up to 5%–15% after delayed rupture. This highlights the need to prevent delayed rupture, including the use of early splenectomy when indicated.

See **Table 9.7.3** for post-splenectomy vaccination guidelines.

Table 9.7.3 Post-Splenectomy Vaccination Guidelines

Evidence	Recommendation
Level 1	• None
Level 2	• Non-elective splenectomy patients should be vaccinated at least 14 days post-splenectomy or at time of discharge from the hospital. • Asplenic patients should be revaccinated at the appropriate time interval for each vaccine.

Level 3	• Asplenic or immunocompromised patients (with an intact but non-functional spleen) should be vaccinated as soon as the diagnosis is made.
	• When adult vaccination is indicated, the following **five** vaccinations should be administered:
	  ○ Pneumococcal vaccine naïve: Conjugate pneumococcal vaccine (PCV13) followed by polyvalent pneumococcal vaccine (PPSV23) > 8 weeks later
	  ○ Previous PPSV23 vaccination: PCV13 > 1 year after PPSV23
	  ○ MenACWY (Menactra®), two doses, given at least 2 months apart
	  ○ MenB-FHbp (three-dose series) at 0, 2, and 6 months **or** MenB-04C (two-dose series) at least one month apart
	  ○ *Haemophilus influenzae* type B vaccine (HibTITER)
	• Paediatric vaccination should be performed according to the recommended paediatric dosage and vaccine types, with special consideration made for children less than 2 years of age.

Vaccine	Dose	Route	Revaccination
13-valent pneumococcal (PCV13, Prevnar 13)	0.5 mL	IM	None
23-valent pneumococcal (PPSV23, Pneumovax®)	0.5 mL	IM or SC	Once at 5 years
Meningococcal / Diphtheria conjugate (MENACWY)	0.5 mL	IM	At 2 months and every 5 years
Serogroup B Meningococcal (MENB-FHbp)	0.5 mL	IM	At 2 months and 6 months
Serogroup B Meningococcal (MENB-4C)	0.5 mL	IM	Once at > 1 month
Haemophilus influenzae type B conjugate	0.5 mL	IM	None

9.7.9 **Vaccination and Prevention of OPSI**[14]

If the spleen is removed or devascularized, resulting in functional asplenia, the loss of function places the individual at high risk of infection with the risk of OPSI by organisms such as *Streptococcus pneumoniae*, *Haemophilus influenzae* type B, and *Neisseria meningitidis*. The incidence is estimated at 0.05%–2% of such patients, with a mortality reportedly as high as 50%.

National guidelines recommend vaccination against pneumococcus, meningococcus, and *Haemophilus influenzae* type B after the seventh postoperative day. Antibiotics are recommended for a minimum of 3 years. Vaccination is also recommended after embolization, to protect against severe infection during a period of likely hyposplenism. Antibiotics are not required in embolized patients.

For patients who have had angioembolization, without removal of the spleen, vaccination is **not** recommended.

Patients should be informed of the lifelong defect in their immune system and be encouraged to keep their pneumococcus and influenza immunizations current. These patients are also more susceptible to malaria than the rest of the population.

REFERENCES AND RECOMMENDED READING

REFERENCES

1. Schneider AB Gallaher J, Raff L, Purcell LN, Reid T, Charles A. Splenic preservation after isolated splenic blunt trauma: the angioembolization paradox *Surgery*. 2021 Aug;**170(2)**:628–33. doi: 10.1016/j.surg.2021.01.007. Epub 2021 Feb 19.

2. Kozar RA, Crandall M, Shanmuganathan K, Zarzaur B, Coburn M, Cribari C, et al. Organ injury scaling

2018 update: Spleen, liver and kidney. *J Trauma Acute Care Surgery.* 2018 Dec;**85(6)**:1119–22. doi: 10.1097/TA.0000000000002058.

3. Stassen, NA, Bhullar I, Cheng JD, Crandall ML, Friese RS, Guillamondegui OD, et al. Selective nonoperative management of blunt splenic injury: an Eastern Association for the Surgery of Trauma practice management guideline *J Trauma.* 2012 Nov;**73(5 Suppl 4)**:S294–300. doi: 10.1097/TA.0b013e3182702afc. Available from www.east.org (accessed September 2023).

4. Skattum J, Naess PA, Eken T, Gaarder C. Refining the role of splenic angiographic embolization in high-grade splenic injuries. *J Trauma Acute Care Surg.* 2013;**74(1)**:100–3; discussion 103–4.

5. Gaarder C, Dormagen JB, Baptist J, Torsten E, Skaga NO, Klow, NE, et al. Nonoperative Management of Splenic Injuries: Improved Results with Angioembolization. *J Trauma.* 2006 July;**61(1)**:192–8. doi 10.1097/01.ta.0000223466.62589.d96.

6. Requarth JA, D'Agostino RB Jr, Miller PR. Nonoperative management of adult blunt splenic injury with and without splenic artery embolotherapy: a meta-analysis. *J Trauma.* 2011 Oct;**71(4)**:898–903; discussion 903. doi: 10.1097/TA.0b013e318227ea50.

7. Raikhlin A, Baerlocher MO, Asch O, Myers A. Imaging and transcatheter arterial embolization for traumatic splenic injuries: review of the literature. *Can J Surg.* 2008;**51**:464–72.

8. Amico F, Anning R, Bendinelli C, Balogh ZJ, Participants of the 2019 World Society of Emergency Surgery (WSES) Nijmegen splenic injury collaboration group. Grade III blunt splenic injury without contrast extravasation – World Society of Emergency Surgery Nijmegen consensus practice. *World J Emerg Surg.* 2020 Aug 3;**15(1)**:46. doi: 10.1186/s13017-020-00319-y.

9. Savage SE, Zarzaur BL, Magnotti LJ, Weinberg JA, Maish GO, Bee TK, et al. *J Trauma.* 2008 Apr;**64(4)**:1085–92. doi: 10.1097/TA.0b013e31816920f1.

10. Rowell SE, Biffl WL, Brasel K, Moore EE, Albrecht RA, DeMoya M, et al. Western Trauma Association Critical Decisions in Trauma: Management of adult blunt splenic trauma-2016 updates. *J Trauma Acute Care Surg.* 2017;**82(4)**:787–93. doi: 10.1097/TA.0000000000001323.

11. Coccolini F, Giulia Montori G, Catena F, Kluger Y, Biffl W, Moore EE, et al. Splenic Trauma: WSES classification and guidelines for adult and paediatric patients. *World J Emerg Surg.* 2017 Aug 18;**12**:40. doi: 10.1186/s13017-017-0151-4.

12. Zarzaur BL, Kozar R, Myers JG, Claridge JA, Scalea TM, Neideen TA, et al. The splenic injury outcomes trial: an American Association for the Surgery of Trauma multi-institutional study. *J Trauma Acute Care Surg.* 2015 Sept;**79(3)**:335–42. doi: 10.1097/TA.0000000000000782.

13. Zarzaur BL, Rozycki GS. An update on nonoperative management of the spleen in adults. *Trauma Surg Acute Care Open.* 2017 Jun 9;**2(1)**:e000075. doi: 10.1136/tsaco-2017-000075. eCollection 2017.

14. Freeman JJ, Yorkgitis BK, Haines K, Koganti D, Patel N, Maine R, et al. Vaccination after spleen embolization: a practice management guideline from the Eastern Association for the Surgery of Trauma. *Injury.* 2022 Nov;**53(11)**:3569–74. doi: 10.1016/j.injury.2022.08.006. Epub 2022 Aug 4.

9.8 The Urogenital System

9.8.1 **Overview**

Urogenital trauma refers to injuries to the kidneys, ureters, bladder, and urethra, the female reproductive organs in the pregnant and non-pregnant state, and the penis, scrotum, and testes.

Death from penetrating bladder trauma was mentioned in Homer's *Iliad*, as well as by Hippocrates and Galen, whilst Evans and Fowler in 1905 demonstrated that the mortality from penetrating intraperitoneal bladder injuries could be reduced from 100% to 28% with laparotomy and bladder repair. Ambroise Paré observed death following a gunshot wound of the kidney, with haematuria and sepsis, and it was only in 1884 that nephrectomy became the recommended treatment for renal injury.

9.8.2 **Renal Injuries**

Injury to the kidney is seen in up to 10% of patients with blunt or penetrating abdominal injuries; however, most cases involve blunt rather than penetrating injury. Serious renal injuries are frequently associated with injuries to other organs, with multiorgan involvement in 80% of patients with penetrating trauma and 75% of those with blunt trauma.

Haematuria, defined as more than five red blood cells per high-power field, is present in over 95% of patients who sustain renal trauma; however, the absence of haematuria does not preclude significant renal injury.

9.8.2.1 DIAGNOSIS

The first investigation is to look for gross haematuria, followed by urinalysis to check for microscopic haematuria.

Pitfall

Haematuria is the hallmark of urological injury, but up to 30% of patients with severe renal trauma will have no haematuria whatsoever. Whilst most patients with significant abdominal trauma may have microscopic haematuria, often in the absence of relevant renal injury, a high index of suspicion is then needed, based on the mechanism of injury and the presence of abdominal and pelvic injury.

The patient's haemodynamic status will determine the subsequent steps, for blunt and penetrating trauma.

9.8.2.1.1 Unstable Patient

The management of unstable patients is immediate surgery.

9.8.2.1.2 Stable Patient

Computed tomography (CT) has replaced intravenous urography as the primary modality for the assessment of suspected renal injuries. The investigation of choice is the multiphase, double- or triple-contrast CT scan, but this can misgrade the renal injury. More commonly, however, it does allow the grading of renal injuries, and forms the basis for non-operative treatment, possibly up to and including non-vascular grade IV injuries and blunt renal artery thrombosis.

CT is requested when there is gross haematuria or suspicion of trajectory likely to involve the kidneys. Renal injury findings are sometimes picked up during routine abdominal CT for abdominal trauma. It has been shown that the size of the haematoma can be related to the grade of renal injury, which is a useful correlation in suboptimal studies and where older machines are used.

Contrast-enhanced ultrasound can also allow the visualization of active intrarenal bleeding, but this study may not be readily available in most centres. Duplex Doppler ultrasound can allow visualization of arteriovenous (AV) fistulas and active intrarenal bleeds.

9.8.2.2 RENAL INJURY SCALE[1]

Table 9.8.1 outlines the renal injury scale (2018 revision).

9.8.2.3 MANAGEMENT

See the Western Trauma Association (WTA) algorithm on management of renal injury found on CT scan (**Figure 9.8.1**).[2]

See the American Urology Association guidelines, updated as Urotrauma 2020 (**Table 9.8.2**).[3]

Up to half of renal stab injuries and up to one-third of gunshot injuries in one series can be treated non-operatively, provided excellent diagnostic methods can visualize the injuries.

In principle, management can be guided by the severity of the injury, and many patients can be treated non-operatively.[5,6]

9.8.2.3.1 Unstable Patient

At laparotomy, it will become apparent whether the kidneys are the source of the shock. Should a large retroperitoneal haematoma be present in the region of the kidney, then the kidney should be managed according to the WTA algorithm (see **Figure 9.8.2**).

This haematoma would most likely be centred around the hilum or be very tense, thus indicating the high likelihood of the kidney being the source of bleeding. A lateral approach through Gerota's fascia will allow easy control of the renal hilum to inspect the source of bleeding. A kidney can only be left unexplored if the haematoma is small, lateral, and non-expanding and the cause of hypotension is found somewhere else.

Packing of the retroperitoneum can be applied under these haemodynamic circumstances **only after** the significant source of bleeding from the kidney has been

Table 9.8.1 Renal Injury Scale, 2018 Revision

AAST Grade*	AIS Severity	Imaging Criteria (CT Findings)	Operative Goals	Pathologic Criteria
I	2	**Haematoma** Subcapsular haematoma and/or parenchymal contusion without laceration **Laceration** None	**Haematoma** Nonexpanding subcapsular haematoma and/or parenchymal contusion without laceration **Laceration** None	**Haematoma** Subcapsular haematoma and/or parenchymal contusion without parenchymal laceration **Laceration** None
II	2	**Haematoma** Perirenal haematoma confined to Gerota's fascia **Laceration** *Renal parenchymal laceration*: < 1 cm depth without urinary extravasation	**Haematoma** Subcapsular haematoma 10%–50% surface area Intraparenchymal haematoma < 5 cm in diameter **Laceration** *Renal parenchymal laceration*: < 1 cm depth without urinary extravasation	**Haematoma** Subcapsular haematoma 10%–50% surface area Intraparenchymal haematoma < 5 cm in diameter **Laceration** *Renal parenchymal laceration*: < 1 cm depth without urinary extravasation
III	3	**Laceration** *Renal parenchymal laceration*: > 1 cm depth without collecting system rupture or urinary extravasation **Vascular** Any injury in the presence of a kidney vascular injury or active bleeding contained within Gerota's fascia	**Laceration** *Renal parenchymal laceration*: > 1 cm depth without collecting system rupture or urinary extravasation	**Laceration** Renal parenchymal laceration: > 1 cm depth without collecting system rupture or urinary extravasation
IV	4	**Laceration** Parenchymal laceration extending into urinary collecting system with urinary extravasation **Disruption** Renal pelvis laceration and/or complete ureteropelvic disruption Segmental renal vein or artery injury Active bleeding beyond Gerota's fascia into the retroperitoneum or peritoneum Segmental or complete kidney infarction(s) due to vessel thrombosis without active bleeding	**Laceration** Parenchymal laceration extending into urinary collecting system with urinary extravasation **Disruption** Renal pelvis laceration and/or complete ureteropelvic disruption Segmental renal vein or artery injury Active bleeding beyond Gerota's fascia into the retroperitoneum or peritoneum Segmental or complete kidney infarction(s) due to vessel thrombosis without active bleeding	**Laceration** Parenchymal laceration extending into urinary collecting system **Disruption** Renal pelvis laceration and/or complete ureteropelvic disruption Segmental renal vein or artery injury Active bleeding beyond Gerota's fascia into the retroperitoneum or peritoneum Segmental or complete kidney infarction(s) due to vessel thrombosis without active bleeding

(Continued)

Table 9.8.1 (*Continued*) Renal Injury Scale, 2018 Revision

AAST Grade*	AIS Severity	Imaging Criteria (CT Findings)	Operative Goals	Pathologic Criteria
V	5	**Vascular injury** Main renal artery or vein laceration or avulsion of the hilum Devascularized kidney with active bleeding **Disruption** Shattered kidney with loss of identifiable parenchymal anatomy	**Vascular injury** Main renal artery or vein laceration or avulsion of the hilum Devascularized kidney with active bleeding **Disruption** Shattered kidney with loss of identifiable parenchymal anatomy	**Vascular injury** Main renal artery or vein laceration or avulsion of the hilum Devascularized kidney with active bleeding **Disruption** Shattered kidney with loss of identifiable parenchymal anatomy

Note: *Vascular injury* is defined as a pseudoaneurysm or arteriovenous fistula, and appears as a focal collection of vascular contrast that decreases in attenuation with delayed imaging. Active bleeding from a vascular injury presents as vascular contrast, focal or diffuse, that increases in size or attenuation in the delayed phase. Vascular thrombosis can lead to organ infarction.

*Grade based on highest grade assessment made on imaging, at operation or on pathologic specimen. More than one grade of kidney injury may be present and should be classified by the higher grade of injury. Advance one grade for bilateral injuries up to grade III.

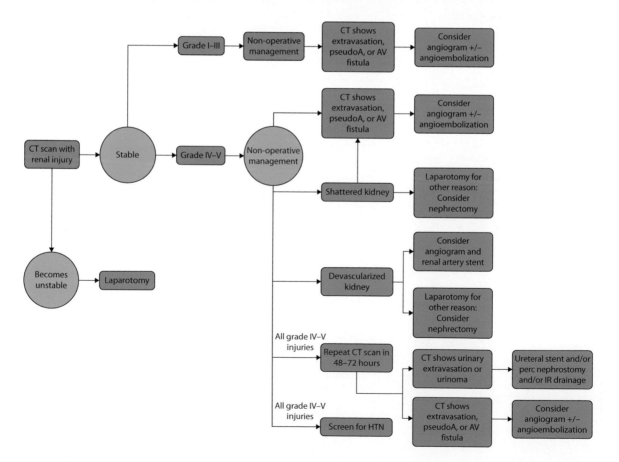

Figure 9.8.1 Western Trauma Association (WTA) algorithm for renal injury found on CT scan. *Abbreviations*: CT, computed tomography; HTN, hypertension.

Table 9.8.2 American Urological Association Guidelines[4]

Renal Trauma Guidelines

1. Clinicians should perform diagnostic imaging with intravenous (IV) contrast-enhanced computed tomography (CT) in stable blunt trauma patients with gross haematuria or microscopic haematuria and systolic blood pressure < 90 mmHg. (Standard; Evidence Strength: Grade B)

2. Clinicians should perform diagnostic imaging with IV contrast-enhanced CT in stable trauma patients with mechanism of injury or physical exam findings concerning for renal injury (e.g., rapid deceleration, significant blow to flank, rib fracture, significant flank ecchymosis, or penetrating injury of abdomen, flank, or lower chest). (Recommendation; Evidence Strength: Grade C)

3. Clinicians should perform IV contrast-enhanced abdominal/pelvic CT with immediate and delayed images when there is suspicion of renal injury. (Clinical Principle)

4. In haemodynamically stable patients with renal injury, clinicians should use non-invasive management strategies. (Standard; Evidence Strength: Grade B)

5a. In haemodynamically unstable patients with no or transient response to resuscitation, the surgical team must perform immediate intervention (surgery or angioembolization in selected situations). (Standard; Evidence Strength: Grade B)

5b. For haemodynamically unstable patients with radiographic findings of large perirenal haematoma (> 4 cm) and/or vascular contrast extravasation in the setting of deep or complex renal laceration (AAST Grade 3-5), surgeons should perform immediate intervention (angioembolization or surgery). (Recommendation; Evidence Strength: Grade C)

6. Clinicians may initially observe patients with renal parenchymal injury and urinary extravasation. (Clinical Principle)

7. Clinicians should perform follow-up CT imaging for renal trauma patients having either (a) deep lacerations (AAST Grade IV–V) or (b) clinical signs of complications (e.g., fever, worsening flank pain, ongoing blood loss, or abdominal distention). (Recommendation; Evidence Strength: Grade C)

8a. Clinicians should perform urinary drainage in the presence of complications such as enlarging urinoma, fever, increasing pain, ileus, fistula, or infection. (Recommendation; Evidence Strength: Grade C)

8b. Drainage should be achieved via ureteral stent and may be augmented by percutaneous urinoma drain, percutaneous nephrostomy, or both. (Expert Opinion)

Ureteral Trauma Guidelines

9a. Clinicians should perform IV contrast-enhanced abdominal/pelvic CT with delayed imaging (urogram) for stable trauma patients with suspected ureteral injuries. (Recommendation; Evidence Strength: Grade C)

9b. Clinicians should directly inspect the ureters during laparotomy in patients with suspected ureteral injury who have not had preoperative imaging. (Clinical Principle)

10a. Surgeons should repair traumatic ureteral lacerations at the time of laparotomy in stable patients. (Recommendation; Evidence Strength: Grade C)

10b. Surgeons may manage ureteral injuries in unstable patients with temporary urinary drainage followed by delayed definitive management. (Clinical Principle)

10c. Surgeons should manage traumatic ureteral contusions at the time of laparotomy with ureteral stenting or resection and primary repair, depending on ureteral viability and clinical scenario. (Expert Opinion)

11a. Surgeons should attempt ureteral stent placement in patients with incomplete ureteral injuries diagnosed postoperatively or in a delayed setting. (Recommendation; Evidence Strength: Grade C)

11b. Surgeons should perform percutaneous nephrostomy with delayed repair as needed in patients when stent placement is unsuccessful or not possible. (Recommendation; Evidence Strength: Grade C)

11c. Clinicians should initially manage patients with ureterovaginal fistula using stent placement when possible. In the event of stent failure, clinicians may pursue additional surgical intervention. (Recommendation; Evidence Strength: Grade C)

12a. Surgeons should repair ureteral injuries located proximal to the iliac vessels with primary repair over a ureteral stent, when possible. (Recommendation; Evidence Strength: Grade C)

(Continued)

Table 9.8.2 (*Continued*) American Urological Association Guidelines

12b. Surgeons should repair ureteral injuries located distal to the iliac vessels with ureteral reimplantation or primary repair over a ureteral stent, when possible. (Recommendation; Evidence Strength: Grade C)

13a. Surgeons should manage endoscopic ureteral injuries with a ureteral stent and/or percutaneous nephrostomy tube, when possible. (Recommendation; Evidence Strength: Grade C)

13b. Surgeons may manage endoscopic ureteral injuries with open repair when endoscopic or percutaneous procedures are not possible or fail to adequately divert the urine. (Expert Opinion)

Bladder Trauma Guidelines

14a. Clinicians must perform retrograde cystography (plain film or CT) in stable patients with gross haematuria and pelvic fracture. (Standard; Evidence Strength: Grade B)

14b. Clinicians should perform retrograde cystography in stable patients with gross haematuria and a mechanism concerning for bladder injury, or in those with pelvic ring fractures and clinical indicators of bladder rupture. (Recommendation; Evidence Strength: Grade C)

15. Surgeons must perform surgical repair of intraperitoneal bladder rupture in the setting of blunt or penetrating external trauma. (Standard; Evidence Strength: Grade B)

16. Clinicians should perform catheter drainage as treatment for patients with uncomplicated extraperitoneal bladder injuries. (Recommendation; Evidence Strength: Grade C)

17. Surgeons should perform surgical repair in patients with complicated extraperitoneal bladder injury. (Recommendation; Evidence Strength: Grade C)

18. Clinicians should perform urethral catheter drainage without suprapubic (SP) cystostomy in patients following surgical repair of bladder injuries. (Standard; Evidence Strength: Grade B)

Genital Trauma Guidelines

19. Clinicians should perform retrograde urethrography in patients with blood at the urethral meatus after pelvic trauma. (Recommendation; Evidence Strength: Grade C)

20a. Clinicians should establish prompt urinary drainage in patients with pelvic fracture–associated urethral injury. (Recommendation; Evidence Strength: Grade C)

20b. Clinicians should perform percutaneous or open suprapubic tube placement as preferred initial management for most pelvic fracture urethral injury (PFUI) cases. (Recommendation; Evidence Strength: Grade C)

21. Surgeons may place suprapubic tubes (SPTs) in patients undergoing open reduction internal fixation (ORIF) for pelvic fracture. (Expert Opinion)

22. Clinicians may perform primary realignment (PR) in haemodynamically stable patients with pelvic fracture–associated urethral injury. (Option; Evidence Strength: Grade C)

Clinicians should not perform prolonged attempts at endoscopic realignment in patients with pelvic fracture–associated urethral injury. (Clinical Principle)

23. Clinicians should monitor patients for complications (e.g., stricture formation, erectile dysfunction, and incontinence) for at least one year following urethral injury. (Recommendation; Evidence Strength: Grade C)

24. Surgeons should perform prompt surgical repair in patients with uncomplicated penetrating trauma of the anterior urethra. (Expert Opinion)

25. Clinicians should establish prompt urinary drainage in patients with straddle injury to the anterior urethra. (Recommendation; Evidence Strength: Grade C)

Bladder Trauma Guidelines

26. Clinicians must suspect penile fracture when a patient presents with penile ecchymosis, swelling, cracking, or snapping sound during intercourse or manipulation and immediate detumescence. (Standard; Evidence Strength: Grade B)

27. Surgeons should perform prompt surgical exploration and repair in patients with acute signs and symptoms of penile fracture. (Standard; Evidence Strength: Grade B)

28. Clinicians may perform ultrasound in patients with equivocal signs and symptoms of penile fracture. (Expert Opinion)

(Continued)

Table 9.8.2 (*Continued*) American Urological Association Guidelines

29. Clinicians must perform evaluation for concomitant urethral injury in patients with penile fracture or penetrating trauma who present with blood at the urethral meatus, gross haematuria, or inability to void. (Standard; Evidence

30a. For blunt scrotal injuries, clinicians should perform scrotal ultrasonography for most patients having findings suggestive of testicular rupture. (Recommendation; Evidence Strength: Grade C)

30b. For most penetrating scrotal injuries, clinicians should perform prompt surgical exploration with repair or orchiectomy (when non-salvageable), given the high rate of testicular injury and the limited sensitivity of ultrasound in this setting. (Recommendation; Evidence Strength: Grade C)

30c. Surgeons should perform scrotal exploration and debridement with tunical closure (when possible) or orchiectomy (when non-salvageable) in patients with suspected testicular rupture. (Standard; Evidence Strength: Grade B)

31. Surgeons should perform exploration and limited debridement of non-viable tissue in patients with extensive genital skin loss or injury from infection, shearing injuries, or burns (thermal, chemical, or electrical). (Standard; Evidence Strength: Grade B)

32. Surgeons should perform prompt penile replantation in patients with traumatic penile amputation, with the amputated appendage wrapped in saline-soaked gauze, in a plastic bag, and placed on ice during transport. (Clinical Principle)

33. Clinicians should initiate ancillary psychological, interpersonal, and/or reproductive counselling and therapy for patients with genital trauma when loss of sexual, urinary, and/or reproductive function is anticipated. (Expert Opinion)

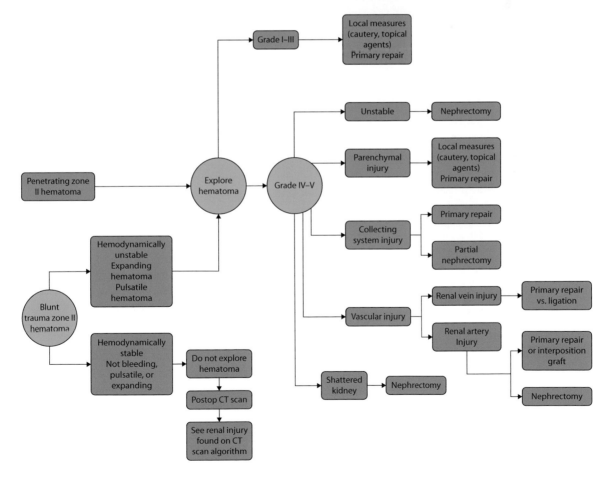

Figure 9.8.2 WTA algorithm for the management of zone II haematoma and renal injury discovered at laparotomy. *Abbreviation*: CT, computed tomography.

excluded (i.e. to control oozing from the surface of the kidney or fascia).

Pitfall

Logistics in unstable patients in theatre are not favourable for an on-table angiogram.

A 'single-shot' intravenous urogram can be performed in the emergency room (the patient is too unstable for a formal CT scan) by injecting 2 mL/Kg radiographic contrast medium, followed by a single plain X-ray film of the abdomen, taken 10 minutes after the contrast was injected. The impact of this study on actual surgical management has become controversial over the years.

9.8.2.3.2 Stable Patient

In recent years, it has been recognized that many renal injuries can be managed without operation, and angio-embolization is a worthwhile option if the skills are readily available.

Liberal use of contrast-enhanced CT angiography scans has made conservative management much more straightforward. Even when the patient requires a laparotomy, automatic exploration of Gerota's fascia in lateral haematomas can be avoided. This has been practised in penetrating trauma as well.

Continued clinical evaluation in the ward or intensive care unit should include assessment for haematuria. Any development of microscopic haematuria, or failure to clear haematuria, should prompt a follow-up contrast CT scan. AV fistula formation can then be detected in the injured kidney, and appropriate angioembolization carried out.

9.8.2.3.3 Grades 1 and 2

These comprise most renal injuries and can usually be treated non-operatively.

9.8.2.3.4 Grade 3

These comprise major lacerations through the cortex extending to the medulla or collecting system with or without urinary extravasation. Drainage may be necessary.

9.8.2.3.5 Grade 4

These are 'catastrophic' injuries and include multiple renal lacerations and vascular injuries involving the renal pedicle. These injuries often require surgery and may need nephrectomy. The most significant vascular injury following blunt trauma is thrombosis of the main renal artery, caused by deceleration with intimal tear and propagation of thrombus in the renal artery.

*Partial nephrectomy should **not** be contemplated in the patient with competing injuries, or potential or actual haemodynamic instability.*

9.8.2.3.6 Grade 5

Pelvi-ureteric junction injuries are a rare consequence of blunt trauma, and are caused by sudden deceleration, which creates tension on the renal pedicle. The diagnosis may be delayed because haematuria is absent in one-third of patients. Pelvi-ureteric junction injuries are classified into avulsion (complete transection) and laceration (incomplete tear). Nephrectomy is usually required.

9.8.2.4 SURGICAL APPROACH

Access should be by midline laparotomy, even if an isolated renal injury is suspected, since the likelihood of other injuries is always present.

The kidneys are usually explored after dealing with intra-abdominal emergencies unless they are the source of ongoing bleeding. Ideally, control of the renal pedicle should be obtained before opening Gerota's fascia. The lateral approach can still allow for quick control of the hilum after slightly manipulating the affected kidney. Remember: the renal artery is shorter and the renal vein longer on the left kidney, and vice versa on the opposite side.

Some advocate a direct approach to suspected peripheral penetrating injuries as being faster and equally safe. A left medial visceral rotation on the left, including division of Gerota's fascia and medial rotation of the left kidney, or an extended Kocher manoeuvre on the right can also afford good control of the aorta, inferior vena cava (IVC), and renal vessels if required.

The right renal artery can be found by dissecting posteriorly between the aorta and the IVC (**Figure 9.8.3**). Dissection lateral to the IVC may lead to inadvertent isolation of a segmental branch of the right renal artery. The vessels are then controlled by loops to allow rapid occlusion should bleeding occur on opening Gerota's fascia. The right renal vein is easily controllable after reflection of the right colon and duodenum, and must be mobilized to expose the artery. It always should be

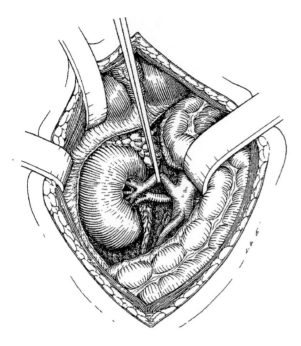

Figure 9.8.3 Access to the right kidney.

repaired, if possible, because of the lack of collateral venous drainage.

The peritoneum over the aorta is opened, and the anterior wall of the aorta followed up to the left renal vein. After exposing the retroperitoneum from the right

or the left, the left renal artery is identified by dissecting upwards on the lateral aspect of the aorta above the inferior mesenteric vein. The left renal vein crosses the aorta just below the level of the origin of the renal arteries (**Figures 9.8.4** and **9.8.5**).

Access to the left renal artery may also be improved by one of two manoeuvres:

- Ligation of the adrenal, gonadal, and lumbar tributaries of the left renal vein will enhance the mobilization of the vein to expose the renal artery.
- Ligation of the distal renal vein at the IVC can improve exposure of the origin of the renal artery. The collateral drainage via the lumbar gonadal and adrenal vessels will be sufficient to deal with the venous drainage on the left (**Figure 9.8.6**).

After control of the renal pedicle has been obtained, Gerota's fascia can be opened or debrided as necessary. Care must be taken not to strip the renal capsule from the underlying parenchyma, as this may bleed profusely. The mobilized kidney now can be examined, debrided, trimmed, and sutured with drainage (**Figure 9.8.7**).

The kidney tolerates a single ischaemic event much better than repeated ischaemic times. However, the maximum warm ischaemic time that the kidney will tolerate is less than 1 hour, although this can be prolonged by ice packing.

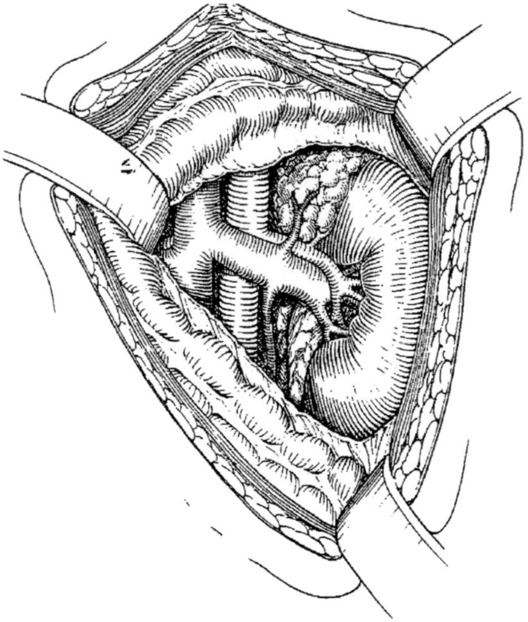

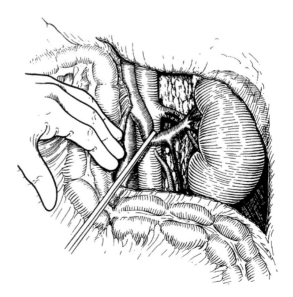

Figure 9.8.4 Access to the left kidney.

Figure 9.8.5 Access to the left renal vessels.

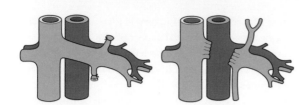

Figure 9.8.6 Division of the left renal vein.

With complete vascular isolation for up to 30 minutes, Gerota's fascia is then opened, and the injured kidney debrided by sharp dissection, and sutured or partially amputated. The renal pelvis collecting system should be closed with a running absorbable suture to provide a watertight seal. Nephrectomy will be required in less than 10% of stable patients.

Cover can then be effected using the renal capsule, omentum, meshes, and so on, replacing the kidney within Gerota's fascia, and draining the area with a suction drain until it is draining minimally, and urine collections have been excluded.

Nephrostomy tubes or ureteric stents can be used either immediately or later in cases of major renal trauma with extravasation.

9.8.2.5 ADJUNCTS

- *Pledgets*: The kidney does not hold sutures well. Care should be taken to ensure that the suture is not over-tightened, as it will cut through. The use of pledgets, though not essential, may be helpful.
- *Sealants*: Urine leakage is common. Tissue sealants can be practical additional means of sealing the suture line.
- *Drains*: Whenever a nephrectomy or a repair is performed, the high incidence of fluid (urine or blood) mandates the use of a suction drain.

9.8.2.6 POSTOPERATIVE CARE

Urinomas, whether sterile or infected; perinephric abscesses; and delayed bleeding are the most common complications of conservative management. They are often amenable to imaging and percutaneous, transureteric, or angiographic management. Even when the kidney appears to be shattered into several pieces, drainage of the surrounding urinomas seems to encourage healing and help avoid sepsis.

Hypertension secondary to scarring and the renin–angiotensin response (Page kidney) is a rare late complication.[7]

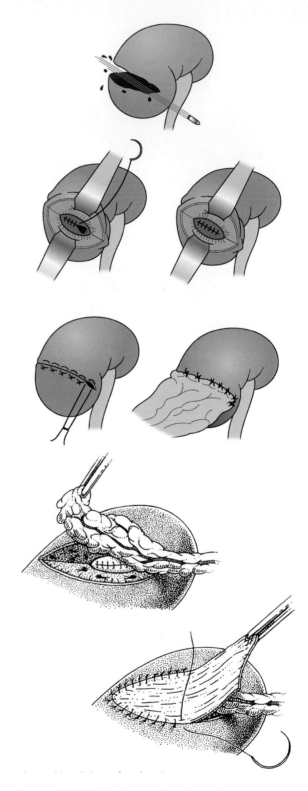

Figure 9.8.7 Techniques of renal repair.

9.8.3 **Ureteric Injuries**

Significant ureteric injuries are often missed or not picked up until late, after the onset of complications or deterioration in renal function.

9.8.3.1 DIAGNOSIS

Patients with ureteric injury present without even microscopic haematuria in up to 50% of cases, and the injuries are mostly associated with penetrating trauma, although ureteric avulsion and rupture can happen in blunt trauma, especially in the paediatric population. Ureteric injuries may even be missed by high-dose IVP, and a high index of suspicion is essential. Intraoperative recognition may be facilitated by the intravenous or intraureteral injection of indigo carmine or methylene blue.

9.8.3.2 SURGICAL APPROACH

The procedures described for access to the retroperitoneal great vessels also allow perfect exposure to both ureters. Ureteric injuries are rare, usually due to penetrating trauma, so that local exploration and mobilization of part of the ascending or descending colon alone may be sufficient, depending on the site of injury. Minimal dissection of the periureteric tissues should take place, except at the precise level of injury, in order to preserve the delicate blood supply. Ureteric injuries close to the kidney are accessed by left or right medial visceral rotation, as described above. Ureteric injuries near the bladder may be accessed by opening the peritoneal layer in the region and mobilizing the bladder.

9.8.3.2.1 Unstable Patients

Unstable patients require immediate surgery and exploration of the ureter after life-threatening injuries have been dealt with, ideally preceded by one-shot on-table IVP.

If the patient requires an abbreviated laparotomy, the ureteric injury can be safely left alone, stented, or ligated until the patient returns to the operating theatre for definitive procedures; indeed, successful repair has frequently been effected after delayed or missed presentation. Percutaneous nephrostomy can be used as a post-operative adjunct for the ligated ureter.

In unstable patients with associated colonic injuries, especially those requiring colectomy, even nephrectomy can be justified.

9.8.3.2.2 Stable Patients

Stable patients with fresh injuries between the pelvi-ureteric junction and the pelvic brim are treated by end uretero-ureterostomy with spatulation and interrupted suturing over a double-J stent (**Figure 9.8.8**).

The stent can be safely left *in situ* for 4–6 weeks. It has been suggested that stents can be omitted in injuries requiring minimal debridement, such as stab wounds, but not in gunshot wounds, where stenting results in significantly fewer leaks. Injuries to the pelvi-ureteric junction and its vicinity are treated in the same fashion, but a tube nephrostomy should be added.

Injuries around the pelvic brim are best treated by uretero-neocystostomy, with an anti-reflux reimplantation. More advanced repair methods include the retrocolic transuretero-ureterostomy, and the creation of a Boari flap with attached uretero-neocystostomy.

In the case of loss of long segments where anastomosis to the contralateral ureter is not possible, an end-ureter-ostomy could be brought out, or nephrectomy done in rare cases of serious associated injuries in the area.

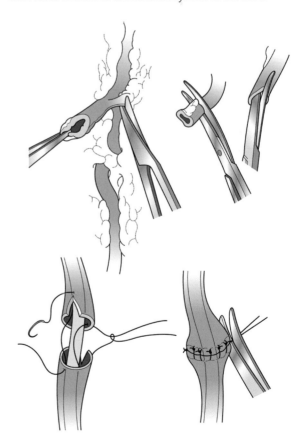

Figure 9.8.8 Technique of ureteric repair.

After surgery, the bladder is drained transurethrally, or ideally suprapubically, and closed suction drains can be placed retroperitoneally in proximity to the repaired ureter; these can be expected to drain for several days.

9.8.3.3 COMPLICATIONS

Complications comprise stricture with hydronephrosis, leakage from the anastomosis, and infected urinomas, especially in late diagnosis, most of which are amenable to percutaneous management.

9.8.4 Bladder Injuries

Bladder injuries are mainly due to blunt trauma and are found in about 8% of pelvic fractures. Penetrating trauma is due to gunshot, stabs, impalement, or iatrogenic injuries, the latter mostly in relation to orthopaedic pelvic fixation.

9.8.4.1 DIAGNOSIS

Signs and symptoms vary from inability to void and frank haematuria, to vague abdominal or suprapubic tenderness without haematuria in a small percentage of cases.

Intraperitoneal injuries may be associated with a higher serum creatinine and urea, and low sodium, but this biochemical derangement takes some time to develop. Elevated serum creatinine levels are due to absorption of urine through the peritoneum.

Ultrasound and CT scanning can be of use to demonstrate free fluid in the abdomen, the presence of clots in the bladder, and a change in bladder filling and shape (with sonar probe compression). A CT cystogram can be done as part of an abdominal CT study and can differentiate between intra- and extraperitoneal bladder injuries.

Retrograde cystography is the method of choice in the emergency room, as it is very accurate if a large enough volume of contrast (about 7 mL/kg) is instilled, and at least two separate projections (anteroposterior and lateral views) are obtained. Post-micturition films are essential. A minimum of 350 mL dilute contrast medium should be instilled.

Contrast extravasation will delineate loops of bowel and the peritoneal contours in intraperitoneal ruptures, whilst it will track along the pelvic bones, scrotum, obturator areas, and so on in extraperitoneal ruptures.

9.8.4.2 MANAGEMENT

Urgent operative treatment is indicated in all intraperitoneal, and some types of extraperitoneal, injuries, whilst others require delayed surgery. Most penetrating injuries require immediate surgery.

Urethral or suprapubic catheter drainage with a large-bore catheter, for up to 2 weeks, will allow most extraperitoneal injuries from blunt trauma to heal; surgery will be needed only if a cystogram at that stage shows ongoing leakage. Contraindications to non-operative management are bladder neck injury, the presence of bony fragments through the bladder wall, infected urine, and associated female genital injuries.

Extraperitoneal bladder repair during a laparotomy for other trauma is often easily accomplished, but it may be dangerous if it requires opening into a tamponaded pelvic haematoma, and it is inappropriate in the context of damage control.

9.8.4.3 SURGICAL APPROACH

Bladders can be repaired easily and with few complications with absorbable sutures.

All repairs should be carried out through an intraperitoneal approach, from within the lumen of the bladder, after performing an adequate longitudinal incision on the anterior surface in order to avoid entering lateral pelvic haematomas. In cases of gunshot wound, *both* wounds to the bladder must be sought and identified. In some situations, it will be necessary to open the bladder widely, explore, and repair from within. Single-layer mass suturing is indicated in extraperitoneal ruptures, but for intraperitoneal ruptures closure should be in separate layers.

Percutaneous suprapubic catheterization can be very difficult if the bladder is detached from the posterior urethra and is not very full because of shock and partial emptying into the pelvic cavity. The recommended technique is to place a long intravenous catheter, such as a single-lumen central line, into the partially empty bladder under ultrasound guidance, inflate the bladder with warm saline until very distended, and then insert the suprapubic catheter under ultrasound guidance.

The presence and patency of both ureteric orifices must be confirmed in all cases. If suturing in the vicinity, these should be cannulated with a size 5 feeding tube or ureteric catheter.

A large-bore transurethral or suprapubic catheter, or both, can be used, the latter being fed extraperitoneally into the bladder, and a drain left in the Retzius space. A cystogram will be done in most cases after 10 days to 2 weeks, followed by removal of the suprapubic catheter.

9.8.5 Urethral Injuries

Urethral injuries can have the most disastrous consequences of all genitourinary trauma, such as incontinence, long-lasting impotence, and strictures. They should be addressed as early as possible.

9.8.5.1 DIAGNOSIS

The mechanism of injury, a pelvic fracture, and blood at the meatus must alert the surgeon to the possibility of a urethral rupture, mainly of the posterior urethra from blunt trauma.

Rectal examination is mandatory before urethral catheter insertion, and a high-riding prostate will suggest that the urethra is disrupted. Rupture of the female urethra is, fortunately, very uncommon.

Once rupture is suspected, two completely different approaches are practised and acceptable.

- Retrograde urethrography is performed by placing a small Foley catheter in the fossa navicularis, with the patient in the oblique position.
- The preferable approach, however, is not to intervene with an emergency procedure at all. This is particularly important if a pelvic haematoma is present, due to the risk of effectively causing a compound injury. It is preferable to place a suprapubic catheter (it will be necessary to allow the bladder to fill until it is palpable prior to the insertion of the suprapubic catheter). A cystogram and, if necessary, cystoscopy can then be done under controlled circumstances at a later stage.

9.8.5.2 MANAGEMENT

9.8.5.2.1 Suprapubic Cystostomy

The mainstay of immediate treatment is the placement of a suprapubic catheter for urinary drainage. This can be done as an isolated open procedure, as an open procedure during a laparotomy, or using a percutaneous method. The isolated open method requires a lower midline laparotomy incision, and an intraperitoneal approach to the bladder to avoid entering a pelvic haematoma. Suprapubic placement during a laparotomy done for other reasons follows the same principles.

Percutaneous placement is done using specifically designed trochar and catheter kits.

The procedure requires a full bladder, as identified clinically or on ultrasound. If this is not the case, and the patient is not in a condition to produce a lot of urine, a small intravenous catheter can be placed under ultrasonic guidance using the Seldinger technique, and the bladder can then be distended with saline until a standard percutaneous method can be used.

9.8.5.3 RUPTURED URETHRA

Urethral injuries are most often associated with pelvic fractures, especially anterior arch fractures with displacement. Although blood at the urethral meatus, gross haematuria, and displacement of the prostate are signs of urethral disruption, their absence does not exclude urethral injury.

The male urethra is divided into two portions:

- The *posterior urethra* is made up of the *prostatic urethra* and the *membranous urethra*, which courses between the prostatic apex and the perineal membrane. The membranous urethra is prone to injury from pelvic fracture because the puboprostatic ligaments fix the apex of the prostate gland to the bony pelvis, and shearing forces are applied to the urethra when the pelvis is disrupted.
- The *anterior urethra* is distal to that point. It is susceptible to blunt force injuries along its path in the perineum (such as from direct blows or fall-astride injuries).

The conventional treatment for urethral injury is to divert the urinary stream with a suprapubic catheter and refer to a specialist centre for delayed reconstruction of the urethral injury. Early endoscopic realignment (within 1 week of injury) using a combined transurethral and percutaneous transvesical approach is advocated by some experts.

Anterior urethral trauma may present late, with symptoms of urethral stricture.

9.8.5.3.1 Urethral Repair

Immediate surgical intervention is recommended for the following conditions:

- All penetrating injuries of the posterior urethra, and most of the anterior urethra.
- Posterior urethral injuries associated with rectal injuries and bladder neck injuries.
- Where there is wide separation of the ends of the urethra.
- Penile fracture.

Accurate approximation and end-to-end anastomosis are recommended for injuries to the anterior urethra, whilst for membranous urethra injuries, realignment and stenting over a Foley catheter for 3 or 4 weeks may be sufficient. This can be achieved by an open lower-midline laparotomy and passage of Foley catheters from above and below, with ultimate passage into the bladder, or via flexible cystoscopy and manipulation.

Patients managed with a suprapubic catheter alone should have their definitive urethral repair after about 3 months from the injury.

Primary realignment may have better results than delayed repair, but delayed primary repair (on days 8–10) is recommended when there is a large haematoma.

9.8.6 Injury to the Scrotum

9.8.6.1 DIAGNOSIS

Ultrasound of the scrotum is indicated in evaluation of blunt trauma to the testicle, and can differentiate between torsion, disruption, and haematoma.

9.8.6.2 MANAGEMENT

The blood supply to the scrotum is so good that penetrating trauma usually can be treated by debridement and suturing.

If the tunica vaginalis of the testis is disrupted, the extruding seminiferous tubules should be trimmed off and the capsule closed as soon as possible, in order to minimize host reaction against the testis.

Loss of scrotal skin with exposed testicle, a well-described occurrence after burns and other trauma, often can be remedied by the creation of pouches in the proximal thigh skin and subsequent approximation, with little effect on the testicles.

9.8.7 Gynaecological Injury and Sexual Assault

Any evidence of gynaecological injury requires external and internal examination using a speculum, and exclusion of associated urethral and anorectal injuries. If rape is suspected or reported, the official sexual assault evidence collection kit should be used, and detailed clinical notes should be made.

The patient must be counselled, and informed consent must, where possible, be obtained for all examinations.

Reporting of all cases of sexual assault should be carried out by the treating physician, in order to minimize underreporting by the already traumatized patient.

9.8.7.1 MANAGEMENT

Lacerations of the external genitalia and vagina can be sutured under local or general anaesthesia, and a vaginal pack left in for 24 hours to minimize the swelling.

Intrapelvic organs are dealt with at laparotomy by suturing, hysterectomy, or oophorectomy. Oxytocin is used to minimize uterine bleeding and colostomy to avoid soiling.

Additional supportive care for the psychological effects of sexual assault should be made available.

9.8.7.2 GUIDELINE

Antiretroviral treatment is more effective if instituted within 3 hours of injury, and sexually transmitted disease and pregnancy prophylaxis should be given according to standard protocols. Baseline blood tests required include human immunodeficiency virus (HIV) status, hepatitis B, full blood count, and liver and renal function; follow-up arrangements must be made to monitor medication and HIV status.

9.8.8 Injury of the Pregnant Uterus

Aggressive resuscitation of the mother and the foetus must be carried out in keeping with Advanced Trauma Life Support® recommendations. Midline laparotomy always should be used when surgery is necessary, but simple intrauterine death is best managed by induced labour at a later stage (see also Section 14.3).

REFERENCES AND RECOMMENDED READING

References

1. Kozar RA, Crandall M, Shanmuganathan K, Zarzaur BL, Coburn M, Cribari C, et al. Organ injury scaling 2018 update: spleen, liver, and kidney. *J Trauma Acute Care Surg.* 2018 Dec;85(6):1119–22. doi: 10.1097/TA.0000000000002058.

2. Brown CVR, Alam HB, Brasel K, Hauser CJ, de Moya M, Martin M, et al. Western Trauma Association critical decisions in trauma: management of renal trauma. *J Trauma Acute Care Surg*. 2018;85(5):1021–5. doi: 10.1097/TA.0000000000001960.

3. Morey AF, Brandes S, Dugi 3rd DD, Armstrong JH, Breyer BN, Broghammer JA, et al. Urotrauma: AUA guideline. *Urology*. 2014 Aug;**192(2)**:327–35. doi: 10.1016/j.juro.2014.05.004. Epub 2014 May 20.

4. American Urological Association Education and Research 2014. Updated 2020: www.auanet.org (accessed online September 2023).

5. Armenakas NA, Duckett CP, McAninch JW. Indications for non-operative management of renal stab wounds. *J Urol*. 1999 March;**161(3)**:768–71.

6. Velmahos GC, Demetriades D, Cornwell EE 3rd, Belzberg H, Murray J, Asensio J, et al. Selective management of renal gunshot wounds. *Br J Surg*. 1998 Aug;**85(8)**:1121–4.

7. Montgomery RC, Richardson JD, Harty JI. Posttraumatic renovascular hypertension after occult renal injury. *J Trauma*. 1998 Jul;**45(1)**:106–10.

Recommended Reading

RENAL INJURIES

Kim FJ, Da Silva RD. Genitourinary trauma. In Feliciano DV, Mattox KL, Moore EE eds. *Trauma*, 9th Edn. McGraw Hill Education, New York. 2021:729–826.

Santucci R. 2015 William Hunter Harridge lecture: how did we go from operating on nearly all injured kidneys to operating on almost none of them? *Am J Surg*. 2016;**211(3)**:501e505.

Ureteric injuries

Armenakas NA. Current methods of diagnosis and management of ureteral injuries. *World J Urol*. 1999 April;**17**:78–83.

Velmahos GC, Degiannis E, Wells M, Souter I. Penetrating ureteral injuries: the impact of associated injuries on management. *Am Surg*. 1996 June;**62(6)**:461–8.

Bladder

Haas CA, Brown SL, Spirnak JP. Limitations of routine spiral computerized tomography in the evaluation of bladder trauma. *J Urol*. 1999 July;**162(1)**:50–2.

Volpe MA, Pachter EM, Scalea TM, Macchia RJ, Mydlo JH. Is there a difference in outcome when treating traumatic intraperitoneal bladder rupture with or without a suprapubic tube? *J Urol*. 1999 April;**161(4)**:1103–5.

Scrotum

Chang AJ, Brandes SB. Advances in diagnosis and management of genital injuries. *Urol Clin North Am*. 2013 Aug;**40(3)**:427–38. doi: 10.1016/j.ucl.2013.04.013. Epub 2013 May 29. Review

Cline KJ, Mata JA, Venable DD, Eastham JA. Penetrating trauma to the male external genitalia. *J Trauma*. 1998 Mar;**44(3)**:492–4.

Munter DW, Faleski EJ. Blunt scrotal trauma: emergency department evaluation and management. *Am J Emerg Med*. 1989 Mar;**7(2)**:227–34.

The Pelvis 10

Pelvic fractures may be due to low- or high-energy trauma, and they consist of pelvic ring fractures, and acetabular fractures mainly due to blunt trauma. The likelihood of associated injuries in high-energy trauma is 65%, usually involving the abdominal and pelvic viscera. In the haemodynamically unstable patient with severe pelvic fracture, there is a 90% risk of associated injury, a 50% risk of extra-pelvic bleeding, and a 30% risk of intra-abdominal bleeding.

The magnitude of pelvic bleeding as one of the 'hidden bleeding sources' is still underestimated or missed completely.

Identification of a pelvic injury as a bleeding source is a mandatory step in the primary survey of the Advanced Trauma Life Support® (ATLS). Early extended focussed assessment with sonography for trauma (eFAST) and pelvic X-ray will guide the initial decision-making. The identification of an unstable pelvic ring fracture and the stabilization and/or compression of the pelvis by an external compression device ('reduce the pelvic volume') are potentially life-saving procedures that must be done in the emergency room (ER). Severe pelvic injuries require a multidisciplinary team involving trauma-trained surgeons, anaesthesiologists, interventional radiologists, and orthopaedic surgeons. If adequate orthopaedic experience is unavailable, consideration should be given towards early transfer of this patient to a more skilled institution as soon as the patient's condition allows.

Formal treatment protocols for pelvic injuries have been shown to decrease mortality and should be developed in every hospital treating pelvic injuries.

10.1 ANATOMY

The surgical anatomy of the pelvis is the key to understanding pelvic injuries:

- The pelvic inlet is a circular structure that is immensely strong, but routinely gives way *at more than one point* should enough force be applied to it. Therefore, isolated fractures of the anterior or posterior pelvic ring are uncommon – look for the disruption of the opposite side of the pelvic ring as well.
- The forces required to fracture the pelvic ring do not respect the surrounding organ systems.
- The pelvic cavity is divided into the true and the false pelvis; *true pelvis* refers to the space enclosed by the pelvic girdle below the pelvic brim and is located between the pelvic inlet and the pelvic floor.
- External iliac vessels are in the false pelvis and may rarely cause major haemorrhage from iliac wing and acetabular fractures. Most major pelvic bleeding originates in the true pelvis from the internal iliac vessels. Eighty-five percent of bleeding is venous in origin.
- The pelvis has a rich collateral blood supply, especially across the sacrum and posterior part of the ileum. The cancellous bone of the pelvis also has an excellent blood supply. More than 85% of pelvic haemorrhage is venous in origin, mainly from fracture sites. However, in the haemodynamically unstable patient with severe pelvic injury, arterial bleeding is frequent (> 50%). Important for the treatment is that the surgeon must deal with fractures, arterial bleeding, and venous bleeding.
- Post-mortem examination has shown that the pelvic peritoneum that 'should' tamponade pelvic haematomas can accommodate more than 3000 mL. However, in cases of severe pelvic fractures, where the retroperitoneal compartment is disrupted and the external bony barrier is not stable, haematoma may extend upwards towards the mediastinum ('chimney effect') or downwards into the medial thigh in case of rupture of the pelvic floor.
- All iliac vessels, the sciatic nerve roots including the lumbosacral nerve, and the ureters cross the sacroiliac (SI) joint; disruption of this joint may cause severe haemorrhage, and sometimes causes arterial and

venous obstruction of the iliac vessels as well as nerve palsy. Fortunately, injuries to the ureters are rare.

- The pelvic organs (bladder, rectum, and female reproductive organs) as well as abdominal organs (parts of the colon and small bowel in the false pelvis) are prone to shear and compression forces acting on the pelvis during the impact of injury.
- Apart from blunt compression injury, the bladder can also rupture due to fracture penetration.
- The pelvis also features the acetabulum, a major structure in weight transfer to the leg. Failure to appreciate injury or inappropriate treatment will lead to severe disability.

10.2 CLASSIFICATION

The two most-used classification systems are mainly based on the direction and location of applied force (Young and Burgess), or fracture pattern allowing judgement on the stability of the pelvic ring (Tile). The different classification systems are all based on grade of fracture stability, and close correlation with risk of bleeding has been shown. However, no fracture pattern can exclude significant haemorrhage. In practice, no major differences have been shown between the two systems.[1]

10.2.1 Tile's Classification[2]

Tile's classification is one of the most used and classifies fractures into three main types (from A1 to C3). Pelvic ring fractures can be classified into three types, using the Tile classification, based on their severity. See **Figures 10.1** and **10.2**.

10.2.1.1 TYPE A: COMPLETELY STABLE

Posterior pelvic integrity is intact. Rarely related to massive bleeding (however, severe wing fracture dislocation may cause bleeding in rare cases). This involves isolated fracture of the iliac wing or pubic rami, mostly caused by direct compression (**Figure 10.1**). These are stable fractures, to be treated conservatively.

10.2.1.2 TYPE B: VERTICALLY STABLE BUT ROTATIONALLY UNSTABLE

B-type fractures are subdivided into externally (B1) and internally (B2) rotated fractures. Sometimes, one side with internal rotation and the other side with external rotation may present at the same time – this is B3.

Type B1: This is the most common type of fracture, also known as an 'open book' fracture. There is horizontal (external rotational) instability due to an anterior lesion (disruption of the symphysis and/or fracture of the superior and inferior pubic rami) combined with a posterior disruption of the anterior *or* posterior ligaments of the SI joint. The impact on the sacrum itself is small. It can result in bleeding in an enlarged pelvic cavity. Injury of the lower urogenital tract, rectum, and vagina and severe soft tissue damage due to the rotation are frequently seen in these cases. Internal or external stabilization is required.

Type B2: Less common, this is a lateral compression-type injury, which results in an intrinsically stable fracture of the pelvic ring, with an impression of the posterior complex in the sacral bone and mostly damage at the pubic arch. Perforation of the bladder can be caused by the anterior fracture, as can hypovolaemic shock due to severe disruption of the soft tissues of the pelvic diaphragm; organ injury to the lower urogenital tract and rectum can be seen in these cases.

Type B3: This is a combined B1 and B2 injury.

10.2.1.3 TYPE C: WHOLLY UNSTABLE IN ROTATIONAL AND VERTICAL PLANES

There is complete horizontal and vertical instability, due to anterior and posterior fractures and/or disruptions (complete SI disruption or displaced vertical sacral fracture). A fall from height, as well as anteroposterior shearing forces in a dashboard impact in a motor vehicle crash, results in this type of fracture (disruption of symphysis pubis or fractures of rami combined with complete SI joint disruption or displaced vertical sacral/medial wing fracture). A C-type fracture may involve one hemipelvis (C1 or C2) or both hemipelves (C3) and is the result of extensive mechanical force; it has the highest risk of major artery bleeding due to shearing dislocation in the posterior pelvic ring. A C-type fracture is most often the 'killing fracture'. Major dislocations put pelvic organs (bladder, urethra, rectum, vagina, and sciatic and femoral nerves) at high risk of related injuries. Extreme acceleration and deceleration forces also increase the risk of intra-abdominal and abdominal retroperitoneal shearing injuries (to the bowel, mesentery, and kidney arteries).

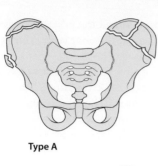

Type A

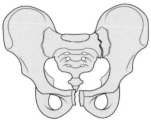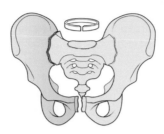

Type B1 Fracture ("unilateral open-book"). Rotationally unstable fracture (external rotation)

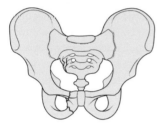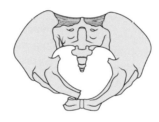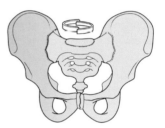

Type B2 Fracture (lateral compression). Rotationally unstable fracture (internal rotation)

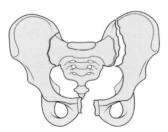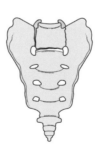

Type C

Type C 'Jumper's fracture'
Anterior pelvic ring may be intact, but posteriorly the
(spinal integrity to pelvis is completely disrupted
spinopelvic dissociation).

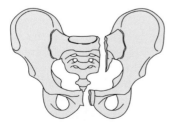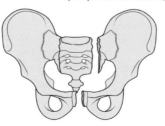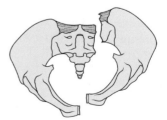

Figure 10.1 Tile's classification of fractures of the pelvis.

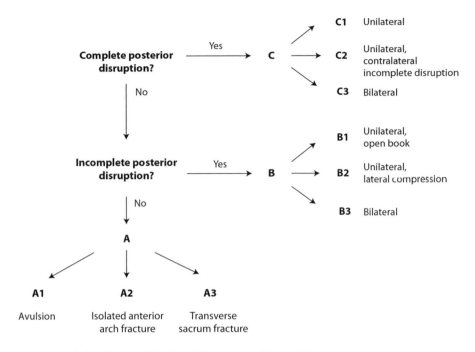

Figure 10.2 Summary of the Tile classification of fractures of the pelvis.

10.2.1.4 **A JUMPER'S FRACTURE**

A *jumper's fracture* is a special type of C-type pelvic ring fracture. The posterior integrity of the pelvic ring, as well as the integrity of the lumbar spine to the pelvis, is completely gone (also known as *spinopelvic dissociation*). The phenomenal appearance to this injury is that there often is no disruption to the anterior pelvic ring, which makes it difficult to identify from plain X-rays. Jumper's fracture is due to landing on feet when falling from height. The pelvis stops moving down when the feet contact the ground, but the rest of the body doesn't, resulting in spine and medial parts of the sacrum (just below the lowest lumbar spine) being fractured and 'pushed' down into the pelvis (**Figure 10.1**). This injury may have bleeding and often affects sciatic and sacral nerves, resulting in cauda equina syndrome. Computed tomography (CT) is required for an accurate diagnosis.

10.2.1.5 **ACETABULAR FRACTURES**

Acetabular fractures do not involve the integrity of the posterior pelvic ring. However, some acetabular fractures may be easy to mistake and mix with pelvic ring injury, especially the ones involving major fracture of the medial iliac wing in close vicinity of the SI joint.

Acetabular fracture-related major bleeding is rare and seldom involves the major internal iliac vessels. However, severe dislocation in acetabular fracture may also involve external iliac vessels, resulting in bleeding or blunt arterial distension injury with thrombosis.

10.2.1.6 **FRACTURE COMBINATIONS**

In some cases, there are combined pelvic fractures, involving both the pelvic ring and the acetabulum. There is no classification for these combined fractures, and both pelvic ring and acetabulum fractures are classified on an individual basis. Clinically, the most dislocated component results in the most likely source of bleeding.

10.2.2 **Young and Burgess Classification[3]**

This system is based primarily on the direction of the force causing the injury: anterior posterior compression (APC) types II and III, lateral compression (LC) type III, and vertical shear (VS) fractures are characterized by major ligamentous disruption. VS fractures include the isolated vertical force vectors, and combined mechanism (CM) fractures include pelvic ring disruptions that do not fall into any single category. See **Figures 10.3** and **10.4**.

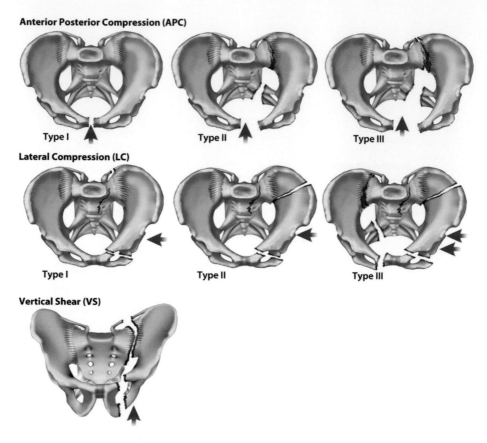

Figure 10.3 Young and Burgess's classification of fractures of the pelvis.

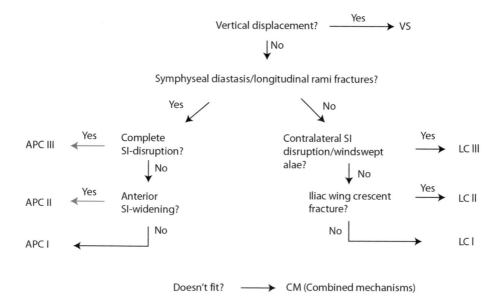

Figure 10.4 Summary of the Young and Burgess classification of fractures of the pelvis. *Abbreviations*: APC, Anterior posterior compression; LC, lateral compression; VS, vertical shear.

10.2.2.1 ANTEROPOSTERIOR COMPRESSION (APC) (TYPES 1, 2, AND 3)

- *APC-1*: Stable injury pattern with 'sprain' of the pubic symphysis (< 2.5 cm diastasis); no injury to the posterior elements.
- *APC-2*: Rotationally unstable injury pattern with complete disruption of pubic symphysis (> 2.5 cm diastasis) and disruption of the anterior SI ligament.
- *APC-3*: Rotationally and vertically unstable injury pattern with complete disruption of pubic symphysis (> 2.5 cm diastasis) and complete disruption of the anterior and posterior SI ligaments.

10.2.2.2 LATERAL COMPRESSION (LC) (TYPES 1, 2, AND 3)

- *LC-1*: Stable injury pattern with transverse pubic rami fractures and stable impaction fractures of the ipsilateral sacrum. Minimal or no internal rotation deformity.
- *LC-2*: Rotationally unstable injury pattern with transverse pubic rami fractures, unstable posterior fracture/dislocation of the ipsilateral SI joint, and internal malrotation of the injured hemipelvis. The 'classic' LC-2 pattern is reflected by a trans-iliosacral ('crescent') fracture dislocation.
- *LC-3*: Rotationally and vertically unstable injury pattern with ipsilateral and contralateral injury to the posterior elements ('windswept pelvis').

10.2.2.3 VERTICAL SHEAR (VS)

The VS injury pattern consists of a complete disruption of the pubic symphysis (with or without associated pubic rami fractures) and a complete disruption of the SI joint (with or without associated fractures of the iliac wing and sacrum). The injured hemipelvis is externally rotated and vertically translated, resulting in a combined rotational and translation instability.

10.2.2.4 COMBINED MECHANISM (CM)

This is any combination of any of the above, combined with haemodynamic instability.

10.3 CLINICAL EXAMINATION AND DIAGNOSIS

Pelvic fractures should be easily identified if ATLS guidelines are followed (i.e. clinical palpation of the pelvic brim from the SI joint to the pubic symphysis, and a routine chest X-ray and pelvic X-ray for any blunt injury in a patient unable to walk). In the absence of X-ray facilities, a clinical examination can be performed with gentle bimanual palpation of the brim of the pelvis from the SI joints to the pubic symphysis. Difference of height of the superior anterior iliac spine can be found in C-type injuries. Any palpable defect or boggy swelling is indicative of a pelvic disruption. In the absence of these signs, gentle bimanual lateral and antero-posterior compression (not distraction!) of the pelvis can be performed. Any instability felt indicates the presence of major pelvic instability, associated with life-threatening blood loss, requiring appropriate measures. The absence of clinical instability does not, however, preclude an unstable pelvic fracture. One-third of such trauma victims with pelvic ring fractures sustain circulatory instability on arrival. eFAST is needed to exclude intra-abdominal bleeding in these patients. Pelvic fracture–related intra-abdominal bladder rupture results in free fluid in the abdominal cavity. However, ultrasound does not have the sensitivity to tell the difference between blood and urine.

Inspection of the skin may reveal lacerations in the groin, perineum, or sacral area, indicating an open pelvic fracture, the result of gross deformation. Evidence of perineal injury or haematuria mandates radiological evaluation of the urinary tract from below upwards (retrograde urethrogram, followed by cystogram or CT cystogram, followed by an excretory urogram as appropriate) when the physiology allows. Inspection of the urethral meatus may reveal a drop of blood, indicating urethral rupture. There seems to be little evidence to support the fear of converting partial urethral rupture into a complete rupture by gently trying to insert a Foley catheter. Urological tract imaging is mandated if you cannot pass a catheter easily with the return of clear urine. Blood at the meatus, or a high-riding prostate, should have raised the alert, and the most highly skilled person available should be utilized to insert an in-dwelling catheter with great care. Inability to pass the catheter easily mandates a cystourethrogram to define the suspected urethral injury. If there is resistance, the patient should have a suprapubic catheter inserted.

Inspection of the anus may reveal lacerations of the sphincter mechanism. Diligent rectal examination (and, in females, a vaginal examination) may reveal blood in the rectum and/or discontinuity of the rectal wall, indicating a rectal laceration, and similarly in the vagina. In male patients, the prostate is palpated; a high-riding prostate indicates a complete urethral avulsion. A full neurological examination is performed of the perineal area, sphincter mechanism, and femoral and sciatic nerves.

The CT scanner is the diagnostic modality of choice in the haemodynamically stable patient, and CT angiography as a routine is particularly helpful.

10.4 RESUSCITATION

The priorities for resuscitating patients with pelvic fractures are no different from the standard. These injuries produce a real threat to the circulation, and management is geared towards controlling this. Management is based on haemodynamic status. Because of the capacity of the pelvis to continue to bleed, these patients require urgent control of haemorrhage. Most contemporary treatment protocols rely on pelvic stabilization and interventional radiology, alone or in combination. Other (damage control) options (including resuscitative endovascular balloon occlusion of the aorta [REBOA]) may be needed for the unstable exsanguinating patient and when angiography is unavailable.

Since pelvic bleeding is commonly associated with traumatic coagulopathy, early blood and coagulation factor substitution is mandatory. Viscohaemostatic assays (VHAs) should be routine in such patients. Volume resuscitation should be based on blood and blood products to prevent further dilutive coagulopathy.

10.4.1 Haemodynamically Normal Patients

There is usually an isolated injury, possibly requiring external or internal (open) reduction and fixation to limit future instability and disability. The management is not critically urgent and can be done either as immediate surgery in cases of isolated injury or in a delayed fashion within the first week after trauma.

10.4.2 Haemodynamically Stable Patients (Transient Responders)

Patients responding to initial volume resuscitation need external stabilization of the pelvic ring. Several principal methods exist for external stabilization of the pelvic ring:

- External compression by circumferential wrap with standard hospital draw sheets or special devices, such as the SAM® Sling (SAM Medical, Tualatin, OR, USA) or Arrow Traumatic Pelvic Orthotic Device

(T-POD™) Pelvic Stabilization Device (Teleflex, Morrisville, NC, USA). Such devices are applied in the ER or, in some trauma systems, in a preclinical setting.
- External fixators which can be applied over the iliac crest or in the supra-acetabular region of the iliac bone. The latter may be technically more difficult to apply; however, it gives significantly more stability to the pelvic ring (**Figure 10.5**).
- Standard external fixation with an AO external fixator frame.
- The pelvic C-clamp, applied close to the level of the SI joint, is effective in providing pelvic compression. The application may be more difficult and cannot be performed in cases with dorsal iliac bone fractures. A pelvic X-ray needs to be done before application of a C-clamp to exclude an *os ilium* fracture at the insertion site of the clamp.

Pitfalls

- Do not place the compression device too low or too high over the abdomen itself. It is important to centre the compression **at the level of the greater trochanters and internally rotate the legs before applying the compression**. This will optimize the vector of compression force to the acetabulum area to the middle of the pelvis and compress both the anterior and posterior parts of the pelvic ring.
- They are easy to place; however, they give less stability to the bony pelvis than an external fixator or a C-clamp. In addition, access to the abdomen or the femoral vessels is limited. Also, intensive care unit (ICU) nursing is hampered by such devices. Therefore, the surgeon should consider replacing the sheet or T-Pod in the operating room (OR) with, for example, an external fixator.

If patients continue to bleed after external fixation in the OR, additional bleeding control needs to be done by either interventional angiography or pelvic packing, as described in Section 10.4.3.

10.4.3 Haemodynamically Unstable Patients (Non-Responders)

A severely disrupted pelvic fracture may present as the classical non-responder to any volume or blood restoration.

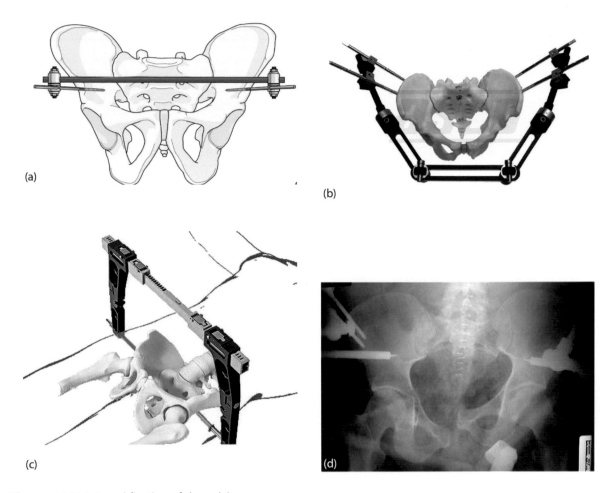

Figure 10.5 External fixation of the pelvis.

These patients tend to exsanguinate rapidly, and immediate measures are required to control bleeding.

> *If the bleeding is considered possibly to be arterial in nature, especially with a blush on a CT scan, there may be indication for REBOA as a temporizing action until angioembolization can be achieved. (See Chapter 15.3.)*

- The goal of the treatment is to decrease pelvic bleeding by temporary means and to find possible adjacent bleeding sites.
- Applying a pelvic binder or sheet, as described above, is the first step. In C-type fractures, the C-clamp may be beneficial if available and can be applied quickly.

> *A quickly and correctly applied pelvic binder is better than spending too much time on a C-clamp.*[4]

- Pelvic X-rays will help in working with the binder. It gives the idea of dislocation and needed reduction (compression) forces applied with the binder.
- Angioembolization and REBOA require access to the groin (common femoral artery). A pelvic binder will block this access initially, but it may be repositioned. An unstable pelvic ring must not be left without stabilization during the procedure.
- Depending on the available resources, extra-peritoneal pelvic (EPP) packing or interventional angioembolization is the next choice for bleeding control. Pelvic angioembolization is only a choice if there is no other urgent need for surgical interventions and it is available within a short delay. The full-scale resuscitation needs to be possible throughout the embolization process; therefore,

remote or small angiography suites are not suitable for these patients.

- If the patient has undergone CT which reveals an arterial blush, the most effective management is angioembolization.
- Angioembolization should *precede* the pelvic packing if the haemodynamics are not improving. Every hour of delay counts in angioembolization.[5] Pelvic packing has little effect on major arterial bleeding but will reduce the pelvic volume and have a tamponing effect on venous bleeding. Since 80%–90% of the bleeding is venous, in almost all cases with arterial bleeding there is concomitant venous bleeding.
- Angioembolization and pelvic packing are considered as complementary procedures.

Persistent bleeding after packing may require angioembolization, and vice versa.

- In haemodynamically crushing patients ('patients *in extremis*'), the clamping of the thoracic aorta can temporarily support the haemodynamics, decrease the arterial pelvic bleeding, and buy time for both establishing and catching up with the fluid resuscitation.
- REBOA can be used for proximal bleeding control (Zone 3 at the level of bifurcation) or as both resuscitative support and bleeding control (Zone 1 at the level of the thoracic aorta).
- REBOA may serve as a bridge to definitive haemostatic treatment after severe pelvic trauma.

Pitfall

REBOA, as well as clamping of the thoracic aorta, will **only** control arterial bleeding, and may *not* stop the bleeding but only buy time. It does not control venous bleeding. Venous bleeding is best controlled with a pelvic binder.

10.5 EXTERNAL FIXATION

Traditional external fixation cannot provide complete stability or compression. A force applied to a segment of a circle cannot stabilize defects outside of that segment; it can only do so in one dimension and will aggravate disruption outside of the segment across which it is applied. Generally, external fixators are best suited for APC and LC fractures, and pelvic C-clamps are best suited for VS types. Points of fixation include the following.

10.5.1 Iliac-Crest Route

This can be carried out without fluoroscopic imaging and is the method of choice for ER external fixation; it is technically less demanding and faster for acute application but is associated with a higher failure rate.

10.5.2 Supra-Acetabular Route

This requires more accurate pin placement under fluoroscopic guidance, a C-arm, and a radio-transparent orthopaedic table. Its main benefits are a higher resistance to failure, since it is attached through a much stronger part of the bone, and normally only one pin is required.

10.5.3 Pelvic C-Clamp

Pelvic C-clamps are applied close to the maximum diameter of the pelvis at the level of the SI joint and should be more effective in providing pelvic compression. Their application may be more difficult, and not carried out in all trauma centres.

10.6 LAPAROTOMY

If the patient is exsanguinating or requires surgery for other injuries, or angiography is delayed or unavailable, it is prudent to perform a laparotomy to treat or exclude intra-abdominal bleeding. In such a case, the peritoneal incision should be limited at its lower end to a few centimetres below the umbilicus, if feasible. If the major source of bleeding is the pelvis, consider extraperitoneal packing of the pelvis with intact peritoneum in the presence of a large or expanding pelvic haematoma, which should preferably be performed *first* (i.e., before the laparotomy). Packing of the pelvis will be most effective against a stabilized pelvic ring (external fixation). If pelvic bleeding persists, direct exploration with suturing or ligature of lacerations of major blood vessels may be required.

In the unstable patient, other sources of intra-abdominal bleeding must be excluded. Consider damage control surgery (DCS) (see Chapter 6).

- Temporary closure of the abdominal wall is preferable, using a negative-pressure (sandwich) technique.

- Angiography should be performed after DCS for control of any remaining pelvic bleeding by embolization of the bleeding vessels. EPP packing should be considered.

In the stabler patient, if bleeding persists, explore the pelvis and tamponade the area, with suturing or ligature of lacerations of the major blood vessels, repair of anatomical structures (bladder and rectum) where possible, and cystostomy and/or colostomy with rectal washout as required. If it is required and possible at this stage, undertake internal fixation of the pelvic ring in case of non-complex fracture types such as a symphyseolysis. All complex types of fractures should be taken care of by external fixation.

After the initial haemorrhage has been controlled, general DCS principles apply to EPP, and the patient is returned to the OR for definitive surgery when physiology has been restored (36–48 hours).

Pitfall

A caveat of pack removal is that the longer the packs are left in, the greater the risk of pelvic sepsis. Definitive internal fixation of the pelvis is ideally performed early, but timing will obviously depend on the physiology.

Formal treatment protocols for pelvic injuries
have been shown to decrease mortality and should be
developed in every hospital treating pelvic injuries.

Pitfall

Requirements for blood average 15 units for open pelvic fractures. To avoid dilutional coagulopathy, protocols for massive transfusion should be instituted. Volume replacement is ultimately only an adjunct to the treatment of haemorrhagic shock – stopping the bleeding. VHA is invaluable in monitoring and correcting any coagulopathies that may arise.

10.7 EXTRAPERITONEAL PELVIC (EPP) PACKING

A total of 80%–90% of pelvic bleeding is venous, arising from the multiple venous plexuses around the pelvis. This bleeding is not controllable by arterial embolization.

The properly performed EPP packing with a stabilized pelvic ring will be able to control venous and some arterial bleeding. In the most effective packing technique, the packing is done in the true pelvis.

Extraperitoneal packing was first described in 1985 by Pohleman,[6] and the technique was further described by Ertel in 2001[7] and Smith in 2005.[8] The original technique was more aggressive, but the current technique stops below or medial to the external iliac vessels at the pelvic brim.

World Society of Emergency Surgery (WSES) guidelines[9] recommend pelvic packing as the first choice (although with a low level of recommendation), whilst the EAST guideline (currently being updated) suggests that angioembolization is a treatment of choice for the bleeding pelvis (see **Table 10.1**).[10,11] Comparative studies will not contribute further evidence to this debate. Therefore, the availability of the necessary resources in the local trauma system will influence the surgeon's decision in this context.

If the source of the bleeding is in doubt, or FAST or diagnostic peritoneal lavage (DPL) results are positive, it is wise to perform an exploratory laparotomy to treat or rule out intra-abdominal bleeding. In the presence of a large or expanding pelvic haematoma, EPP packing should be performed by grabbing the edges of the peritoneum and entering the preperitoneal space from the midline (**Figure 10.6**).

If other sources of bleeding have been ruled out, the EPP packing can be done without entering the abdomen via a lower midline suprapubic incision.

10.7.1 Technique of Extraperitoneal Packing[12,13]

- The patient is positioned supine, and, if necessary, to provide a firm surface to pack against, an anterior external fixator with bilateral single supra-acetabular pins and external fixator, or a C-clamp, is applied.
- A 5 cm midline suprapubic incision is made, and the fascia anterior to the rectus muscle is exposed.
- The fascia is divided in the midline until the symphysis can be palpated directly (the pre-peritoneal plane has been reached), protecting against urinary bladder damage. From the symphysis, the pelvic brim is followed laterally and posterior to the SI joint (first bony irregularity felt), first on the side of major bleeding (most often, the side of SI joint disruption).

Table 10.1 Eastern Association for the Surgery of Trauma (EAST) Practice Guideline: Management of Pelvic Injury

Level of Evidence	Question and Recommendations
	Which Patients with Hemodynamically Unstable Pelvic Fractures Warrant Early External Mechanical Stabilization?
III	1. The use of a pelvic orthotic device (POD) does not seem to limit blood loss in patients with pelvic haemorrhage. 2. The use of a POD effectively reduces fracture displacement and decreases pelvic volume. Level III recommendation.
	Which Patients Require Emergency Angiography?
I	1. Patients with pelvic fractures and haemodynamic instability or signs of ongoing bleeding after nonpelvic sources of blood loss have been ruled out should be considered for pelvic angiography/embolization. 2. Patients with evidence of arterial intravenous contrast extravasation (ICE) in the pelvis by CT may require pelvic angiography and embolization regardless of haemodynamic status.
II	1. Patients with pelvic fractures who have undergone pelvic angiography with or without embolization, who have signs of ongoing bleeding after nonpelvic sources of blood loss have been ruled out, should be considered for repeat pelvic angiography and possible embolization. 2. Patients older than 60 years with major pelvic fracture (open book, butterfly segment, or vertical shear) should be considered for pelvic angiography without regard for haemodynamic status.
III	1. Although fracture pattern or type does not predict arterial injury or need for angiography, anterior fractures are more highly associated with anterior vascular injuries, whereas posterior fractures are more highly associated with posterior vascular injuries. 2. Pelvic angiography with bilateral embolization seems to be safe with few major complications. Gluteal muscle ischaemia/necrosis has been reported in patients with haemodynamic instability and prolonged immobilization or primary trauma to the gluteal region as the possible cause, rather than a direct complication, of angioembolization. 3. Sexual function in males does not seem to be impaired after bilateral internal iliac arterial embolization.
	What Is the Best Test to Exclude Intra-abdominal Bleeding?
I	1. Focussed assessment with sonography for trauma (FAST) is not sensitive enough to exclude intraperitoneal bleeding in the presence of pelvic fracture. 2. FAST has adequate specificity in patients with unstable vital signs and pelvis fracture to recommend laparotomy to control haemorrhage. Level I recommendation.
II	1. Diagnostic peritoneal tap (DPT)/diagnostic peritoneal lavage (DPL) is the best test to exclude intra-abdominal bleeding in the haemodynamically unstable patient. 2. In the haemodynamically stable patient with a pelvic fracture, CT of the abdomen and pelvis with intravenous contrast is recommended to evaluate for intra-abdominal bleeding regardless of FAST results.
	Are There Radiologic Findings Which Predict Haemorrhage?
II	1. Fracture pattern on pelvic X-ray does not single-handedly predict mortality, haemorrhage, or the need for angiography. 2. Presence/location of hematoma does not predict or exclude the need for angiography and possible embolization. 3. CT of the pelvis is an excellent screening tool to exclude pelvic haemorrhage. 4. Absence of contrast extravasation on CT does not always exclude active haemorrhage. 5. Pelvic haematoma > 500 cm³ in size has an increased incidence of arterial injury and need for angiography.
III	1. Isolated acetabular fractures are as likely to require angiography as pelvic rim fractures. 2. If a retrograde urethrocystogram is required, it should be performed after CT with intravenous contrast.

(Continued)

Table 10.1 (*Continued*) Eastern Association for the Surgery of Trauma (EAST) Practice Guideline: Management of Pelvic Injury

Level of Evidence	Question and Recommendations
	What Is the Role of Non-Invasive Temporary Pelvic Binder (TBP) External Fixation Devices?
III	1. TPBs effectively reduce unstable pelvic fractures as well as definitive stabilization, and decrease pelvic volume. 2. TPBs may limit pelvic haemorrhage but do not seem to affect mortality. Level III recommendation. 3. TPBs work as well as, or better than, emergent EPF in controlling haemorrhage.
	Which Patients Warrant Retroperitoneal (Preperitoneal) Packing?
III	1. Retroperitoneal pelvic packing is effective in controlling haemorrhage when used as a salvage technique after angiographic embolization. 2. Retroperitoneal pelvic packing is effective in controlling haemorrhage when used as part of a multidisciplinary clinical pathway including a POD or C-clamp.

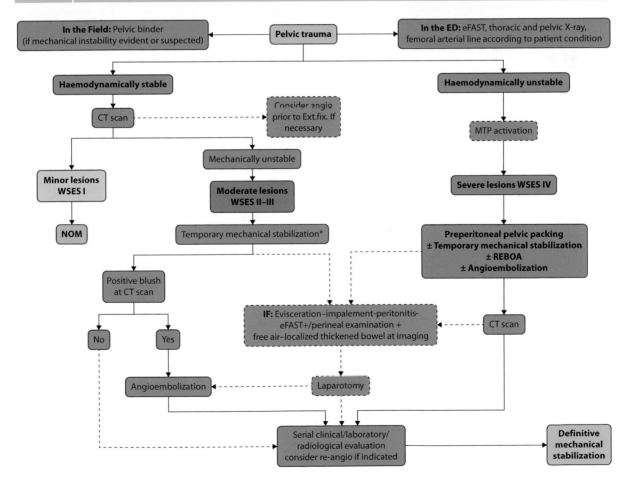

Figure 10.6 World Society of Emergency Surgery (WSES) guidelines for management of a pelvic fracture. *Abbreviations*: Angio, angiography; CT, computed tomography; ED, emergency department; eFAST, extended focussed assessment with sonography for trauma; MTP, massive transfusion protocol; NOM, non-operative management; REBOA, resuscitative endovascular balloon occlusion of the aorta.

- The bladder and rectum are then held to the opposite side, whilst the plane is opened bluntly down to the pelvic floor, avoiding injury to vascular and nerve structures in the area.
- The space is then packed with vascular or abdominal swabs, starting posteriorly and distal to the tip of the sacrum, and building the packs cranially and anteriorly.
- The procedure is then repeated on the opposite side.
- Packing a pelvis efficiently implies also addressing arterial bleeding. This requires applying force whilst packing. In an unbroken pelvis with an intact pelvic floor, one should be able to accommodate three large abdominal swabs on each side. In severe pelvic fractures, efficient packing might require much more (more than 10 packs not being unusual). The number of packs needed is defined by the available space and the appropriate force applied.
- Closure is by using standard DCS techniques including negative-pressure dressings.

As in the abdomen, the packs should be removed after 24–48 hours.

10.8 ASSOCIATED INJURIES

Associated injuries can only be managed once the patient is haemodynamically stable. In case of associated bleeding, the sequence of bleeding control interventions on the pelvis and other bleeding sites depends on the individual choice of the surgeon. Normally, the assumed most prominent bleeding is targeted first. Procedures for damage control may be the only available option.

10.8.1 Head Injuries

These are the most commonly associated major injuries. It is worthwhile remembering that 'C' precedes 'D' during resuscitation and management: the CT scan and neurosurgical procedures must wait for haemodynamic stability, and haemodynamic stability may be achieved only after DCS.

10.8.2 Intra-abdominal Injuries

These are frequently masked by pelvic pain. Retroperitoneal haematomas may break through into the peritoneal cavity,

causing a false-positive result on eFAST or DPL. In the presence of a pelvic fracture, CT scanning is the diagnostic modality of choice in the stable patient. In all other patients, diagnostic ultrasound is preferred. If open DPL is performed, the entry point should be above the umbilicus to avoid entering extraperitoneal haematomas tracking up the anterior abdominal wall. A low threshold should be maintained for laparotomy because of associated intraperitoneal injury.

10.8.3 Bladder and Urethral Injuries

Bladder injuries are the most common accompanying injury of pelvic fractures. It is important to distinguish between extraperitoneal and intraperitoneal bladder injuries. Whilst intraperitoneal bladder injuries demand primary surgical repair, extraperitoneal bladder injuries can be handled non-surgically (by suprapubic catheter). (See Section 9.8 on urological trauma.)

10.8.4 Urethral Injuries

Urethral injuries should be managed conservatively. Primary urethral repair by cystoperineal traction sutures results in minimal disability in the hands of experts when performed immediately in stable patients. For the majority, suprapubic cystostomy (preferably under ultrasonic guidance) and delayed urethral repair are required. If the patient needs to be taken to the operating theatre for extraperitoneal packing, it is usually very simple to railroad a catheter transurethrally into the damaged area and then pass it under vision into the bladder. (See Section 9.8 on urological trauma.)

Endo-urological techniques with two cystoscopes can also allow early (2–7 days) primary realignment, which is accompanied by a significant decrease in stricture formation and need for further extensive surgery. Suprapubic cystostomy and delayed urethral repair may be needed if the patient is unstable but does not require surgery for other reasons. Septic complications with urethral injuries in the presence of pelvic fractures requiring fixation do not seem to be of concern.[14]

10.8.5 Anorectal Injuries[15]

Injuries of the anus and rectum are managed according to the degree of damage to the sphincters and anorectal mucosa. Injuries superficial to these require only debridement and dressings. Deep injuries require diversion colostomy and drainage.

Pitfalls

- Presacral drainage is *not* required and may disrupt the nervous plexuses.
- There is doubt about the benefit of prograde mechanical cleansing (washout) of the rectum due to the risk of pelvic infection introduced by washing faeces into the pelvic cavity.

Sphincter repair is best left for the experts, but repeated debridement and early approximation of mucosa to skin should limit infection and scarring.

10.8.6 Vaginal Injuries

All vaginal injuries should be explored under a general anaesthetic. Vaginal lacerations should be managed as follows:

- High lesions should be repaired and closed.
- Lower lesions should be packed and addressed after the patient is stable.

10.9 OPEN PELVIC FRACTURES

Complex pelvic fractures with open pelvic injury can be the most difficult of all injuries to treat. Initially, they can cause devastating haemorrhage and may later be associated with overwhelming pelvic sepsis and distant multiple organ failure.

10.9.1 Diagnosis

For those patients who present with compound pelvic fractures and are haemodynamically stable, diagnostic studies such as plain films of the pelvis, three-dimensional CT scans, and CT angiography should be rapidly carried out. The injuries to the rectum and vagina must be assessed.

10.9.2 Surgery

All patients with open (compound) pelvic fractures should be taken to the OR as soon as the necessary diagnostic studies have been carried out. Control of pelvic bleeding can be temporarily achieved by packing the open wound and then making the decision of whether to obtain a pelvic arteriogram (which will be positive in 15% of cases), or to move rapidly to external fixation of the anterior pelvis and consideration for posterior stabilization as well. These decisions are made on an individual basis, considering the patient's status, the injury pattern, and the surgeon's experience in dealing with these complex injuries, and then carrying out the further diagnostics, keeping in mind that there is also a high risk of internal pelvic bleeding and other associated pelvic-area injuries.

Based on the location of the injury, colostomy may be required in order to prevent contamination of the wound in the post-injury period. In general, all injuries involving the perineum and perianal area should have a diverting colostomy. However, in the damage control situation, contamination must be controlled (if necessary, by temporary occlusion), but establishment of a colostomy should be postponed until the patient's physiology has returned to normal.

10.10 SUMMARY

A haemodynamically normal patient can be safely transferred for stabilization of unstable fractures within hours after injury and following control of the associated damage.

- Associated injuries should only be managed once the patient is haemodynamically stable.
- Procedures for damage control may be the only available option for the unstable patient.
- External stabilization of the pelvic ring is the basis of all initial management.
- Correction of coagulopathy, and blood restoration using a massive transfusion protocol, is the second step and a prerequisite for the creation of a stable clot in the retroperitoneum.
- If necessary, further bleeding control can be achieved by either angioembolization or extraperitoneal packing.
- Extraperitoneal packing should be performed prior to opening the abdomen, where possible.
- Packing controls both venous and some arterial bleeding, whilst angioembolization only addresses arterial bleeders.

ANAESTHESIOLOGICAL CONSIDERATIONS

- Thirty per cent mortality if the patient arrives at the hospital in severe shock.
- Pelvis can hold 4 to 6 L of blood before a tamponade effect occurs.
- 30%–49% of patients require greater than 10 units of blood.
- Large-bore intravenous catheters in the upper part of the body.
- High risk of trauma-induced coagulopathy.
- Inadvertent entry into the retroperitoneal haematoma can cause uncontrollable bleeding.
- In pregnancy, engorgement of the pelvic vasculature increases the risk of retroperitoneal haemorrhage after lower abdominal or pelvic trauma.
- Assessment of volume status may be confusing, especially in younger patients.
- Haematocrit levels, central venous pressure readings, and arterial blood pressures can be unreliable.
- A base deficit with metabolic acidosis as obtained via arterial blood gas can be a better indicator of shock severity.
- The patient who survives to haemorrhage and coagulopathy will face the risk of pulmonary emboli.
- Early thromboprophylaxis and point-of-care viscoelastic monitoring.

REFERENCES AND RECOMMENDED READING

References

1. Osterhoff G, Scheyerer MJ, Fritz Y, Bouaicha S, Wanner GA, Simmen HP, et al. Comparing the predictive value of the pelvic ring injury classification systems by Tile and by Young and Burgess. *Injury.* 2014 Apr;**45(4)**:742–7. doi: 10.1016/j.injury.2013.12.003.
2. Tile M. Acute pelvic fractures: causation and classification. *J Am Acad Orthop Surg.* 1996 May;**4(3)**:143–51. doi: 10.5435/00124635-199605000-00004.
3. Young JW, Burgess AR, Brumback RJ, Poka A. Pelvic fractures: value of plain radiography in early assessment and management. *Radiology.* 1986 Aug;**160(2)**:445–51 doi: 10.1148/radiology.160.2.3726125.
4. Bakhshayesh P, Boutefnouchet T, Tötterman A. Effectiveness of non-invasive external pelvic compression: a systematic review of the literature. *Scand J Trauma Resusc Emerg Med.* 2016 May;**24**:73. doi: 10.1186/s13049-016-0259-7.
5. Matsushima K, Piccinini A, Schellenberg M, Cheng V, Heindel P, Strumwasser A, et al. Effect of door-to-angio-embolization time on mortality in pelvic fracture: every hour of delay counts. *J Trauma Acute Care Surg.* 2018 Nov;**85(5)**:685–92. doi: 10.1097/TA.0000000000001803.
6. Pohleman T, Gänsslen A, Bosch U, Tscherne H. The technique of packing for control of haemorrhage in complex pelvic fractures. *Tech Orthop.* 1995;**9**:267–70.
7. Ertel W, Keel M, Eid K, Platz A, Trentz O. Control of severe haemorrhage using C-clamp and pelvic packing in multiply injured patients with pelvic ring disruption. *J Orthop Trauma.* 2001 Sep-Oct;**15(7)**:468–74. doi: 10.1097/00005131-200109000-00002.
8. Smith WR, Moore EE, Osborn P, Agudelo JF, Morgan SJ, Parekh AA, et al. Retroperitoneal packing as a resuscitation technique for haemodynamically unstable patients with pelvic fractures: report of two representative cases and a description of technique. *J Trauma.* 2005 Dec;**59**:1510–14. doi: 10.1097/01.ta.0000197330.81352.94.
9. Coccolini F, Stahel PF, Montori G, Biffl W, Horer TM, Catena F, et al. Pelvic trauma: WSES classification and guidelines. *World J Emerg Surg.* 2017 Jan;**12(5)**. doi: 10.1186/s13017-017-0117-6. eCollection 2017. Review.
10. Costantini TW, Coimbra R, Holcomb JB, Podbielski JM, Catalano R, Blackburn A et al. Current management of hemorrhage from severe pelvic fractures: results of an American Association for the Surgery of Trauma multi-institutional trial. AAST Pelvic Fracture Study Group. *J Trauma Acute Care Surg.* 2017 Jun;**82(6)**:1030–8. doi: 10.1097/TA.0000000000001465.
11. Cullinane DC, Schiller HJ, Zielinski MD, Bilaniuk JW, Collier BR, Como J, et al. Eastern Association for the Surgery of Trauma practice management guidelines for hemorrhage in pelvic fracture–update and systematic review. *J Trauma.* 2011 Dec;**71(6)**:1850–68. doi: 10.1097/TA.0b013e31823dca9a.
12. Filiberto DM, Fox AD. Preperitoneal pelvic packing: technique and outcomes. *Int J Surg.* 2016. Sep;**33(Pt B)**:222–4. doi: 10.1016/j.ijsu.2016.05.072. Epub 2016 Jul 1.

13. Burlew CC. Preperitoneal pelvic packing: a 2018 EAST Master Class Video Presentation. *J Trauma Acute Care Surg*. 2018 July;**85(1)**:224–8. doi: 10.1097/TA.0000000000001881.

14. Johnsen NV, Vanni AJ, Voelzke BB. Risk of infectious complications in pelvic fracture urethral injury patients managed with internal fixation and suprapubic catheter placement. *J Trauma Acute Care Surg*. 2018 Sep;**85(3)**:536–40. doi: 10.1097/TA.0000000000002012.

15. Fry RD. Anorectal trauma and foreign bodies. *Surg Clin N Am*. 1994 Dec;**74(6)**:1491–505.

Recommended Reading

HAEMORRHAGE

Petersen DJ. Pelvic hematoma and hemodynamic instability in the absence of fracture; 2018. *J Trauma Acute Care Surgery*. 2018 Jul;**85(1)**:218–9. doi: 10.1097/TA.0000000000001900

REBOA

Napolitano LM. Resuscitative endovascular balloon occlusion of the aorta: indications, outcomes, and training. *Crit Care Clin*. 2017 Jan;**33(1)**:55–70. doi: 10.1016/j.ccc.2016.08.011. Review.

Pieper A, Thony F, Brun J, Rodière M, Boussat B, Arvieux C, et al. Resuscitative endovascular balloon occlusion of the aorta for pelvic blunt trauma and life-threatening hemorrhage: A 20-year experience in a Level I trauma center. *J Trauma Acute Care Surg*. 2018 Mar;**84(3)**:49–453. doi: 10.1097/TA.0000000000001794.

Moore LJ, Martin CD, Harvin JA, Wade CE, Holcomb JB. Resuscitative endovascular balloon occlusion of the aorta (REBOA) for control of non-compressible truncal hemorrhage in the abdomen and pelvis. *Am J Surg*. 2016 Dec;**212(6)**:1222–30. doi: 10.1016/j.amjsurg.2016.09.027.

Extremity Trauma **11**

11.1 OVERVIEW

Extremity injuries often look dramatic, and they occur in 85% of patients who sustain blunt trauma. But this should not distract the clinician's attention away from major sources of bleeding in the non-compressible compartments. Musculoskeletal injuries of the axial skeleton and long bones can, however, be associated with major blood loss and life-threatening situations. Seemingly minor extremity trauma can lead to serious long-term functional deficit and loss of productivity. Musculoskeletal injuries are the most frequent reasons why blunt trauma patients have operative interventions. However, in some circumstances, the relevance of such injuries assumes major importance.

Fractures of the bony skeleton may occur in isolation or as part of multiple injuries. Catastrophic external bleeding, mostly in military settings or in penetrating injury in civilian settings due to gunshot wounds (GSWs) and explosive devices, will lead directly to hypovolaemic shock. In the [C]-A-B-C (circulation, airway, and breathing control) concept, circulation control ('[C]') will be applied by a combat application tourniquet (CAT) in the pre-hospital setting, even before airway control.

Multiple fractures, especially femoral shaft fractures, contribute to hypovolaemia as well. The possibility must be borne in mind when there are multiple long bone fractures associated with vascular damage, and non-visible but ongoing bleeding is occurring. Where this is the case, and direct control of the bleeding is not possible, a timely and appropriately applied tourniquet may buy time to stabilize the patient and treat other life-threatening injuries.

11.2 MANAGEMENT OF SEVERE INJURY TO THE EXTREMITY

The primary survey and resuscitation must take priority.

11.2.1 Life-Saving

- Notice ongoing external bleeding, and control it (direct pressure, pressure bandage, or tourniquet).
- Exclude or detect other bleeding sources.

11.2.2 Limb-Saving

- Assess limb injuries, making careful note of distal perfusion.
- Involve the orthopaedic, vascular, and plastic surgeons early.
- Perform fasciotomy.
- Restore impaired circulation.
- Cover open wounds with a sterile dressing and give tetanus toxoid and antibiotic prophylaxis.
- Debride non-viable tissue.
- Restore skeletal stability.
- Achieve temporary wound closure.
- Commence rehabilitation.

DOI: 10.1201/9781003258124-14

CORRECT APPLICATION OF A TOURNIQUET

1. Identify the area of bleeding.
2. Apply tourniquet 10 cm above the area of bleeding.
3. If not able to apply 10 cm above the area of bleeding, apply tourniquet 'high and tight', meaning as proximal to the root of the extremity as possible.
4. Tighten Velcro as much as possible.
5. Turn windlass to achieve bleeding control.
6. If not sufficient control, a secondary tourniquet must be applied *proximally* to the initially placed tourniquet.
7. Note the time of application (*Note*: White tag on the CAT).

Pitfall

It is important to remember that a fracture is not a separate entity from the soft tissue damage that accompanies it – it is simply an extension of the energy transferred to the soft tissue. Injury that involves bone, and the principles of management, are the same.

A fracture is a soft tissue injury in which broken bone is present. (Unknown)

During the past two decades, a better understanding of the individual injuries, and technical advances in diagnostic evaluation and surgery (allowing revascularization of the extremity, stabilization of the complex fracture, and reconstruction of the soft tissues), medicine, and rehabilitation, have led to an increased frequency of attempts at limb salvage. In some of these patients, however, limb salvage may have subsequent deleterious results, being associated with a high morbidity and a poor prognosis and often requiring late amputation (27%–70%) despite initial success. In these, early or primary amputation might even be beneficial. Especially in elderly, significant comorbidity (diabetes, pre-existent limb ischaemia, smoking) should be included in decision-making as well.

Amputation is not an expression of failure. Sometimes it is the best way for the patient to resume regular activity.

The management of the mangled limb remains a vexing problem; it should be multidisciplinary and involve the combined skills of the orthopaedic, vascular, plastic, and reconstructive surgeons, as well as the rehabilitation specialist. Poorly coordinated management often results in more complications, increased duration of treatment, and a less favourable outcome for the patient. Ultimately, the decision to amputate or repair is often a difficult one, and best shared with a senior colleague. The cost of

rehabilitation is often less – and the time shorter – if a primary amputation is performed, than if lengthy and repeated operations are undertaken, and persistent painful debility or an insensate or flail limb is still the outcome. A successful limb salvage is defined by the overall function and satisfaction of the patient.

11.3 MANAGEMENT OF VASCULAR INJURY OF THE EXTREMITY

Vascular injuries are present in 25%–35% of all penetrating trauma to the extremities. Whilst physical exam is reliable, ankle pressure indices (API), computed tomography (CT) angiography, and duplex ultrasound are all useful adjuncts. Except for inconsequential intimal injuries and distal artery injuries, most extremity vascular injuries should be repaired.

Extremity arterial injury after penetrating trauma is common in military conflict or civilian trauma centres. Most peripheral arterial injuries occur in the femoral and popliteal vessels of the lower extremity. Loss of distal pulse, and unilateral cool or pale extremities, are the most significant hard signs of vascular impairment. It can be confirmed by Doppler ultrasound and supported by lack of signal on pulse oximetry. In severe hypovolaemic shock (systolic blood pressure [SBP] < 60 mmHg), however, it is not always easy to evaluate vascular impairment in the acute phase. After primary survey and resuscitation, the extremity should be assessed again. Other soft signs of vascular injury include an expanding or pulsating haematoma, a false aneurysm, continuous murmurs of arteriovenous fistulas, progressive swelling of an extremity, and unexplained ischaemia or dysfunction. A significant percentage of these patients have no physical findings suggesting vascular trauma; thus, routine further investigation has been advocated.

The most common cause of peripheral vascular injury is penetrating trauma, which includes a spectrum from simple puncture wounds to wounds resulting from high-energy missiles.

Normal pulses do not rule out vascular injuries.

Ten per cent of significant and major vascular injuries have no physical findings. Penetrating trauma also includes iatrogenic injuries such as those following percutaneous catheterization of the peripheral arteries for diagnostic procedures, access for monitoring, or REBOA. When a needle or catheter dislodges an arteriosclerotic plaque or elevates the intima, a vessel may thrombose, leading to acute ischaemia in a limb. The key, therefore, is to maintain a high index of suspicion based on the mechanism of injury and the proximity of vascular structures.

Recently, duplex scanning of blood vessels has been shown to be a useful adjunct in determining if an arteriogram is indicated. A positive duplex scan is valuable, but a negative one does not exclude vascular injury. A positive duplex scan, or an ankle–brachial index of less than 0.9 in a distal pulse, is a mandatory indication for arteriogram and possible operation.

The gold standard for confirming a suspected vascular injury remains the CT arteriogram.[1] However, CT arteriography should not be performed in the patient who is unstable needing emergency laparotomy or thoracotomy, nor when the injury is obvious, or the limb ischaemic. The arteriogram should be delayed until after resuscitation and treatment of the life-threatening emergency. On-table operating room angiography is considered in these circumstances.

If doubt exists, an angiogram should be obtained.

Blunt trauma also may cause peripheral vascular injuries, with shear injuries as the most common cause. Contusions or crushing injuries may produce transmural or partial disruption of arteries, resulting in elevation of the intima and the formation of intramural haematomas. Blunt trauma such as posterior dislocation of the knee may cause total disruption of a major vessel. Blunt trauma may also indirectly contribute to vascular occlusion by creating large haematomas in proximity to the vessel. These haematomas may lead to arterial spasm, distortion, or compartment syndromes that interfere with arterial flow.

In principle, it is wise to fix the bony skeleton before embarking on definitive vascular repair. However, this can be catastrophic if ischaemia is present. **Shunting takes priority**. The following protocol should be used (in the order listed):

- Initial assessment for ischaemia
- Exploration of the vessels
- Fasciotomy if required and in case of any doubt
- Temporary stenting (shunting) of the vein and artery
- Surgical stabilization of the skeleton
- Definitive repair of the vascular damage

Damage control of the extremity injury should take place in the same fashion as in the abdomen. The wound should not be closed.

There are five options open to the surgeon when vascular damage is encountered: vessels may be repaired, replaced (grafted), ligated (and bypassed), stented, or shunted.

11.3.1 Shunts

Intraluminal shunts may be manufactured out of intravenous tubing, nasogastric tubing, biliary T-tubes, or even chest drain tubing, depending on the size of the vessel to be shunted. Commercially made shunts (as used routinely in carotid surgery) are on the market, and others are now being made specifically for trauma. Essentially, the shunt is secured proximally and distally into the injured vessel – there is *no* need for heparinization – and this allows time for other damage control procedures to take precedence whilst maintaining perfusion of the limb. When possible, both artery and vein should be shunted if both are damaged. If not possible, the vein should be tied off. Whilst shunts may be left in place during prolonged periods of resuscitation, they should be removed as soon as clinically feasible to limit shunt-related complications.[2]

Some injury complexes should raise a specific suspicion of vascular damage, for example a supracondylar fracture of the humerus, and posterior dislocation and high-energy impact periarticular fractures of the knee. The presence of palpable pulses does not exclude arterial injury, and a difference of 10% in the measured Doppler pressure compared with the opposite uninjured limb (i.e. API < 0.9) mandates urgent CT or conventional angiography. This is not hard to do, and the technique is well described elsewhere. An absent pulse mandates exploration if the level of injury is known, and angiography if it is not.

Repairs, particularly graft replacements of injured vessels, should only be attempted by those competent to do them, and only in limbs where the viability of the soft tissues is not in doubt (i.e. after fasciotomy). Ligation may be done as a measure of desperation in the exsanguinating patient, and limb survival is often surprising. However, the availability of temporary intravascular shunts should limit the need for arterial ligation as a damage control manoeuvre. If ligation is deemed necessary, claudication pain may be dealt with later. Extra-anatomical bypass has no place in the setting of damage control and trauma surgery. Endovascular stenting is becoming rapidly a procedure of choice in some areas (e.g., traumatic aortic rupture) but requires facilities and expertise that may not always be available. Long-term patency rates of extremity stenting are unknown at this point.

The Eastern Association for the Surgery of Trauma (EAST) first published guidelines for evaluation and treatment of such trauma in 2002. Since that time, there have been advancements in the management of penetrating lower extremity arterial trauma. The current guidelines are in **Table 11.1**.[3]

Table 11.1 Eastern Association for the Surgery of Trauma (EAST) Guidelines for the Management of Lower Extremity Arterial Injury

Level of Evidence	Recommendation
I	1. Computed tomographic angiography (CTA) may be used as a primary diagnostic study for evaluation of penetrating lower extremity vascular injury when imaging is required.
II	1. Patients with hard signs of arterial injury (pulse deficit, pulsatile bleeding, bruit, thrill, expanding haematoma) should be surgically explored. There is no need for arteriogram in this setting unless the patient has an associated skeletal or shotgun injury. Restoration of perfusion to an extremity with an arterial injury should be performed in less than 6 hours to maximize limb salvage. 2. Patients (without hard signs of vascular injury) who have abnormal physical examination findings and/or ankle brachial index (ABI) of < 0.9 should have further evaluation to rule out vascular injury 3. Patients with normal physical examination findings and an ABI > 0.9 may be discharged (in the absence of other injuries requiring admission).
III	1. In cases of haemorrhage from penetrating lower extremity trauma in which manual compression is unsuccessful, tourniquets may be used as a temporary adjunct for haemorrhage control until definitive repair. 2. The use of temporary intravascular shunts may be indicated to restore arterial flow in combined vascular–orthopaedic injuries (Gustilo IIIC fractures) to facilitate limb perfusion during orthopaedic sterilization. 3. Temporary intravascular shunts may be indicated in damage control situations to facilitate limb perfusion when the physiological status of the patient, or operative capabilities, prevent definitive repair. 4. There are no data to support the routine use of endovascular therapies following infra-inguinal trauma. 5. Embolization of profunda branches tibial vessels is acceptable, and there are no data to support preferential use of coils or n-butyl-2-cyanoacrylate glue. 6. The role of non-invasive Doppler pressure monitoring with duplex ultrasonography to confirm or exclude arterial injury is not well defined. There may be a role for these studies in patients with soft signs of vascular injury or with proximity injuries. 7. Non-operative observation of asymptomatic non-occlusive arterial injuries is acceptable. 8. Repair of occult and asymptomatic non-occlusive arterial injuries managed non-operatively, and subsequently requiring repair, can be done without significant increase in morbidity. 9. Simple arterial repairs fare better than grafts. If complete repair is required, vein graft seems to be the best choice. Polytetrafluoroethylene (PTFE), however, is also an acceptable conduit. 10. PTFE may be used in a contaminated field. Effort should be made to obtain soft tissue coverage. 11. Tibial vessels may be navigated if there is no documented flow distally. 12. Early four-compartment lower legs fasciotomy should be applied liberally when there is an associated injury, or when there has been prolonged ischaemia. If not performed, compartment pressures should be closely monitored. 13. Arteriography for proximity is indicated only in patients with shotgun injuries. 14. Completion arteriogram should be performed after arterial repair.
Unanswered questions	None

11.3.2 Chemical Vascular Injuries

The frequency of chemical injury to blood vessels has increased secondary to iatrogenic injury and the intra-arterial injection of illicit drugs. These agents may cause intense vasospasm or direct damage to the vessel wall, often associated with intense pain and distal ischaemia.

Chemical vascular injuries may be treated with intra-arterial or intravenous administration of 10,000 units heparin to prevent distal thrombosis. Reserpine (0.5 mg) also has been recommended, although its only effect experimentally has been to protect against the release of catecholamines from the vessel walls. Other vasodilators and thrombolytic enzymes have been tried, with variable results. A reliable combination is 5000 units heparin in 500 mL Hartmann's solution (Ringer's lactate), to which is added 80 mg papaverine to combat arterial spasm. This is administered in boluses of 20–30 mL intra-arterially every 30 minutes, or intravenously at the rate of 1100 units heparin per hour.

11.4 CRUSH SYNDROME

Severely compressed limbs and large volume of muscle will all have an element of crush syndrome associated with them unless one is dealing with a traumatic amputation by a sharp instrument such as a chainsaw or machete. As such, a watch must be kept for the development of a compartment syndrome and/or myoglobinuria.

11.5 MANAGEMENT OF OPEN FRACTURES

Sepsis is a constant threat to the healing of open fractures. Risk factors for infection are:

- Severity of injury (especially injury to the soft tissue envelope of a limb)
- Type of contamination
- Delay from injury to surgical care (> 6 hours)
- Failure to use timely prophylactic antibiotics
- Inappropriate wound debridement
- Lack of coverage of bony structures
- Inappropriate wound closure (including primary wound closure) in contaminated and contused wounds

11.5.1 Severity of Injury (Gustilo Classification)[4]

Table 11.2 The Gustilo Classification of Open Fracture Injury[4]

Fracture Grade	Description
Grade I	• Wound is less than 1 cm with minimal soft tissue injury. • Wound bed is clean. • Bone injury is simple with minimal comminution.
Grade II	• Wound is greater than 1 cm with moderate soft tissue injury. • Wound bed is moderately contaminated. • Fracture contains moderate comminution from direct trauma.
Grade III	• Following fracture, automatically results in classification as type III: • Segmental fracture with displacement. • Fracture with diaphyseal segmental loss. • Fracture with associated vascular injury requiring repair. • Farmyard injuries or highly contaminated wounds. • High-velocity gunshot wound. • Fracture caused by crushing force from a fast-moving vehicle.
Grade IIIA	• Wound is greater than 10 cm with crushed tissue and contamination. • Soft tissue coverage of bone is usually possible. • Wound sepsis rate is ±4%.
Grade IIIB	• Wound is greater than 10 cm with crushed tissue and contamination; there is periosteal stripping and bone exposure, usually associated with contamination. • Soft tissue injury is extensive – cover is inadequate and requires a regional or free flap. • Wound sepsis rate is ±52%.
Grade IIIC	• A fracture in which there is a major vascular injury requiring repair for limb salvage; major soft tissue injury is not necessarily significant. • Wound sepsis rate is ±42%. • Fractures can be classified using the Mangled Extremity Severity Score. • In some cases, it will be necessary to consider below-knee amputation.

11.5.2 **Sepsis and Antibiotics**

Sepsis is a constant threat to healing, and the main risk factors include the severity of the injury, the delay from injury to surgical care, failure or delays in use of prophylactic antibiotics, and inappropriate wound closure.

The early use of prophylactic antibiotics is important, but it must be recognized that antibiotics are an adjunct to appropriate wound care. The introduction of the Thomas splint and improved understanding of the need for surgical wound care are credited with reducing the mortality rate for open fractures of the femur from 80% to 16% during the First World War.[5] During the Spanish Civil War, Truetta reported a septic mortality rate of 0.6% in 1069 open fractures with a policy of aggressive wound excision and debridement, reduction of the fracture, stabilization with plaster, and leaving the traumatic wound open.[6]

Secondary soft tissue management with coverage of the bone by reconstructive surgery, including free flaps, has the best results if completed within the first week.

Recent consensus guidelines (by EAST) recommend that antibiotics be discontinued 24 hours after wound closure for grade I and II fractures. For grade III wounds, the antibiotics should be continued for only 72 hours after the time of injury, or for not more than 24 hours after soft tissue coverage of the wound is achieved, whichever occurs first. Agents effective against *Staphylococcus aureus* appear to be adequate in fractures classified by Gustilo classification as grade I and II fractures; however, the addition of broader Gram-negative coverage may be beneficial for grade III injuries.[7]

11.5.3 **Venous Thromboembolism**

Deep venous thrombosis prophylaxis remains an integral part of management of patients with severe limb injury. Ideally, both mechanical and chemical prophylaxis should be used.[8]

11.5.4 **Timing of Skeletal Fixation in Polytrauma Patients**

Most comparative studies have shown a reduction in the risk of post-traumatic respiratory compromise after early, definitive fixation of fractures (within 48 hours) both for isolated injuries and for multisystem trauma. The maintenance of patient homeostasis is the most important factor during surgery. Provided this is respected, early surgery is safe. There is also evidence of reduction in mortality, duration of mechanical ventilation, thromboembolic events, and cost in favour of early

fixation. There is no evidence that early fixation alters the outcome in those with concomitant head injury.

EAST guidelines make the following recommendation: In trauma patients with open or closed femur fractures, we suggest early (<24 hours) open reduction and internal fracture fixation. This recommendation is conditional, and the strength of the evidence is low. Early stabilization of femur fractures shows a trend (statistically insignificant) toward lower risk of infection, mortality, and VTE. Therefore, the panel concludes that the desirable effects of early femur fracture stabilization probably outweigh the undesirable effects in most patients. Conditional recommendation (low quality of evidence).[9]

The acute stabilization by early external fixation as part of damage control orthopaedics may obviate some of the risks. In cases where damage control surgery is indicated, a phased approach by temporary fixation in the acute phase is followed by definitive reconstruction as a secondary procedure. Long bone fractures like femur, tibia, and humerus can be stabilized with a simple unilateral frame. Periarticular fracture can be treated initially with a bridging external fixation. Localization of pin placement is dictated by anatomy of relevant structures such as the radial nerve in case of a humeral shaft external fixation. The definitive care by internal fixation should be considered as well.

Pin placement should be as far as possible from the definitive approach.

11.5.4.1 RESPIRATORY INSUFFICIENCY[10]

Episodes of respiratory insufficiency often occur after orthopaedic injury. Extremity injury may occur as part of a multisystem insult, with associated head, chest, and other injuries. Hypoxia, hypotension, and tissue injury provide an initial 'hit' to prime the patient's inflammatory response; operative treatment of fractures constitutes a modifiable secondary insult. In addition, post-traumatic fat embolism has been implicated in the respiratory compromise that appears after orthopaedic injury, especially following intramedullary nailing.

11.5.4.2 HEAD INJURY

In approximately 5% of long bone fractures of the leg, the patient is physiologically unstable due to haemodynamic instability, raised intracranial pressure, or other problems. Temporary methods of fixation are attractive in this setting. Although some studies have suggested that early nailing of a femoral fracture may be harmful in patients with a concomitant head injury, there is no compelling evidence that early long bone stabilization in mildly, moderately, or severely brain-injured patients enhances or worsens the outcome.[11] However, time-consuming procedures should be avoided, and early transfer to an intensive care unit (ICU) environment with a staged approach to the orthopaedic trauma should be considered.

11.6 LIFE-THREATENING LIMB TRAUMA: LIFE VERSUS LIMB

Certain skeletal injuries by their nature indicate significant forces sustained by the body and should prompt the treating surgeon to look for other associated injuries. Other limb injuries, presenting with crush injury with extensive soft tissue damage, concomitant vascular or nerve injury, and major bony disruption, pose other threats to either life or limb, and it is on these that this topic concentrates.

Despite huge advances in the management of these injuries, and the resultant decrease in amputation rates associated with them, there remains a small group of patients who present with 'mangled limbs', produced by mechanisms of high-energy transfer or crush in which there is vascular disruption in combination with severe open comminuted fractures and moderate loss of soft tissue. These injuries most frequently affect healthy individuals during their prime years of gainful employment and can result in varying degrees of long-term functional and emotional disability.

There are many ways to classify major limb injuries and their complications, and these scoring systems can be found towards the end of this chapter.

The salvage of severe lower extremity fractures can be extremely challenging. Even if the surgical team is successful in preserving the limb, the functional result may be unsatisfactory because of residual effects of injuries to muscle and nerve, bone loss, and the presence of chronic infection. Failed efforts at limb salvage consume resources and are associated with increased patient mortality and high hospital costs.

Many lower extremity injury severity scoring systems have been developed to assist the surgical team with the initial decision to amputate or salvage a limb.[12] Prospective studies have, however, sounded a note of caution about relying exclusively on a scoring system to make these important decisions.

11.6.1 Scoring Systems

11.6.1.1 MANGLED EXTREMITY SYNDROME INDEX (MESI)

Gregory et al.[13] proposed a Mangled Extremity Syndrome Index (MESI) (**Table 11.3**). The injury was categorized according to the integument, nerve, vessel, and bone

Table 11.3 Mangled Extremity Syndrome Index

Criterion	Score
Injury Severity Score	
< 25	1
25–50	2
> 50	3
Integument Injury	
Guillotine	1
Crush/Burn	2
Avulsion/Degloving	3
Nerve Injury	
Contusion	1
Transection	2
Avulsion	3
Vascular injury	
Vein transected	1
Artery transected	1
Artery thrombosed	2
Artery avulsed	3
Bone injury	
Simple	1
Segmental	2
Segmental comminuted	3
Bone loss < 6 cm	4
Articular	5
Articular with bone loss > 6 cm	6
Delay in time to operation	1 point per hour > 6 hours
Age (Years)	
< 40	0
40–50	1
50–60	2
> 60	3
Pre-existing disease	1
Shock	2

Score < 20: Functional limb salvage can be expected. Score > 20: Limb salvage is improbable.

injury. A point system quantified injury severity, delay in revascularization, ischaemia, age of the patient, pre-existing disease, and whether the patient was in shock.

11.6.1.2 PREDICTIVE SALVAGE INDEX SYSTEM

Howe et al.[14] proposed a predictive index incorporating the level of the arterial injury, degree of bony injury, degree of muscle injury, and interval for warm ischaemia time (**Table 11.4**). Variables such as additional injuries and the presence of shock were not felt to be predictive of amputation. Of the patients, 43% underwent amputation, with infrapopliteal injuries being associated with the highest amputation rate (80%).

Table 11.4 Predicted Salvage Index System

Criterion	Score
Level of Arterial Injury	
Suprapopliteal	1
Popliteal	2
Infrapopliteal	3
Degree of Bone Injury	
Mild	1
Moderate	2
Severe	3
Degree of Muscle Injury	
Mild	1
Moderate	2
Severe	3
Interval from Injury to Operating Room (Hours)	
< 6	0
6–12	2
> 12	4

Salvage: Score < 7. Amputation: Score > 8.

11.6.1.3 MANGLED EXTREMITY SEVERITY SCORE (MESS)

Johansen et al.[15] described the MESS (**Table 11.5**), which characterizes the skeletal and soft tissue injury, warm ischaemia time, presence of shock, and age of the patient, as a means of solving the dilemma of which patients need amputation. A MESS value greater than 7 predicted amputation.

Table 11.5 Mangled Extremity Severity Score (MESS)

Factor	Score
Skeletal/Soft Tissue Injury	
Low energy (stab, fracture, civilian gunshot wound)	1
Medium energy (open or multiple fracture)	2
High energy (shotgun or military gunshot wound)	3
Very high energy (above plus gross contamination)	4
Limb Ischaemia	
Pulse reduced or absent but perfusion normal	1*
Pulseless, diminished capillary refill	2*
Patient is cool, paralysed, insensate, numb	3*
Shock	
Systolic blood pressure always > 90 mmHg	0
Systolic blood pressure transiently < 90 mmHg	1
Systolic blood pressure persistently < 90 mmHg	2
Age (Years)	
< 30	0
30–50	1
> 50	2

* Double the value if the duration of ischaemia is over 6 hours. Score > 7 predicted amputation.

In a further paper, 25 years on, the authors suggested that whilst a MESS > 7 predicted amputation *at that time*, advances in care have meant that this number must be re-evaluated.[16]

11.6.1.4 NISSSA SCORING SYSTEM

McNamara et al.[17] and others have retrospectively evaluated the MESS. Attempts have been made to address criticisms of the MESS by including nerve injury in the scoring systems and by separating the soft tissue and skeletal injury components of the MESS. The result is the NISSSA (**n**erve injury, **i**schaemia, **s**oft tissue injury/contamination, **s**keletal injury, **s**hock/blood pressure, **a**ge) scoring system (**Table 11.6**), which is considered more sensitive and more specific than the MESS.

Table 11.6 NISSSA (Nerve Injury, Ischaemia, Soft Tissue Injury/Contamination, Skeletal Injury, Shock/Blood Pressure, Age) Scoring System

Factor	Score
Nerve Injury	
Sensate	0
Loss of dorsal	1
Partial plantar	2
Complete plantar	3
Ischaemia	
None	0
Mild	1*
Moderate	2*
Severe	3*
Soft Tissue Injury/Contamination	
Low	0
Medium	1
High	2
Severe	3
Skeletal Injury	
Low energy	0
Medium energy	1
High energy	2
Very high energy	3
Shock/Blood Pressure	
Normotensive	0
Transient hypotension	1
Persistent hypotension	2
Age (Years)	
< 30	0
30–50	1
> 50	2

* Double the value if the duration of ischaemia exceeds 6 hours.
Score > 11 predicted amputation.

Pitfall

Scoring systems clearly have their limitations when the resuscitating surgeon is faced with an unstable polytrauma patient. Thus, these scoring systems are not universally accepted. They have shortcomings with respect to reproducibility, prognostic value, and treatment planning in this context. These factors can lead to inappropriate attempts at limb salvage when associated life- and limb-threatening injuries might be overlooked if attention is focused mainly on salvage of the mangled limb, or to an amputation when salvage may have been possible. Whilst experience with these scoring systems is generally limited, they may provide some objective parameters on which clinicians can base difficult decisions regarding salvage of life or limb. Any recommendations derived from them must be judged in terms of available technology, expertise, patient desire, and commitment to the treatment course.

In summary, the decision of whether to amputate primarily or to embark on limb salvage and continue with planned repetitive surgeries is complex, and is based on:

- Life-saving?
- Technically possible?
- Function expected?
- Patient's specific situation, preferences, and compliance.

Prolonged salvage attempts that are unlikely to be successful should be avoided, especially in patients with insensate limbs and predictable functional failures. Scoring systems should be used only as a guide for decision-making. The relative importance of each of the associated trauma parameters (apart from prolonged warm ischaemia time or risking the life of a patient with severe, multiple-organ trauma) is still of questionable predictive value. A good understanding of the potential complications facilitates the decision-making process in limb salvage versus amputation.

11.7 COMPARTMENT SYNDROME[18–20]

Compartment syndrome may occur after extremity injury, with or without vascular trauma. Increasing pressure within the closed fascial space of a limb compromises the blood supply of muscle. Early clinical diagnosis and treatment are important to prevent significant morbidity.

The classical 5Ps (pain, paraesthesia, paralysis, pallor, and pulselessness) are described as classical signs, but they are unreliable and above all late parameters.

Rather, the clinician should rely on the '5Ps of pain':

- Pain out of proportion to the injury
- Pain at rest
- Pain in passive and active movement
- Pain on palpation
- Pain increasing rapidly

In comatose or paralysed and sedated patients, one cannot monitor clinical signs at all! In this type of trauma patient, the threshold to perform fasciotomy must be even lower.

Compartment syndrome occurs relatively commonly, following trauma or ischaemia to an extremity, with or without vascular injury. It is important to emphasize that reperfusion following vascular repair plays a major role. As such, the classical clinical findings may be absent prior to vascular repair. Once the diagnosis of compartment syndrome is made, urgent fasciotomy is indicated. This applies to both upper and lower limbs.

The measurement of intra-compartment pressure[21] using proprietary devices like the Stryker® (Stryker, Kalamazoo, MI, USA) is invaluable when doubt exists about the diagnosis. This can be particularly helpful in cases not accessible for physical examination such as the unconscious patient and those in intensive care, sedated and ventilated. It is important that measurements be taken on both lower legs at the same place (e.g., in the tibialis anterior muscle 2 cm below and lateral to the tibial tubercle) for comparison.

Pitfall

A pulse still may be palpable, or recordable on the Doppler, even though a compartment syndrome exists.

A novel non-invasive approach to intra-compartmental pressure measurement is pressure-related ultrasound.[22]

The lower leg is the most common site, but in crush injuries and high-energy impact, it can also occur in the leg above the knee and the upper extremity, especially the forearm.

11.8 FASCIOTOMY

> *Should there be doubt over whether the compartment syndrome is significant, a fasciotomy should be performed.*

Fasciotomy must be performed *before* arterial exploration when an obvious arterial injury exists, or when there is a suspicion of high intra-compartmental pressures.

It is important to note that fasciotomy is different from escharotomy. The latter is performed in a patient with circumferential full-thickness burns; it involves splitting of the tight, contracted, charred-skin envelope and does not involve dividing the fascia of the muscle compartments. Escharotomy can be done by non-surgeons at the bedside under sedation, whilst fasciotomy requires intimate knowledge of anatomy and should be done by surgeons, in theatre, under general anaesthesia and controlled conditions.

The indications for fasciotomy can be divided into three scenarios:

1. Therapeutic
2. Prophylactic
3. Diagnostic

1. *Therapeutic fasciotomy*: This is done for a patient with an established compartment syndrome. The causes, signs, and operative technique are described elsewhere in this chapter.
2. *Prophylactic fasciotomy*: When a patient has had an ischaemic limb (e.g., stab wound of the brachial artery, absent pulses, and cold limb) for several hours, but the limb is still clearly viable (see below for signs of non-viability), the limb may be safely revascularized. However, after several hours of ischaemia, revascularization will almost certainly be followed by reperfusion syndrome of the arm, which will result in significant swelling. If a 'prophylactic' fasciotomy is not done at the same time, the patient will almost inevitably develop compartment syndrome within a

few hours postoperatively and will need to be brought back to theatre for a therapeutic fasciotomy. The technique for prophylactic fasciotomy is as for therapeutic.

3. *Diagnostic fasciotomy*: When a patient has had an ischaemic limb for several hours (e.g., gunshot wound of superficial femoral artery, absent pulses, and cold limb), it is critical to assess whether the limb is viable before revascularization is done. Revascularizing a dead limb (especially a leg) will result in overwhelming reperfusion syndrome and may be rapidly deadly. In general, an ischaemic limb can be revascularized up to 6 hours, but this is not a hard-and-fast rule. The viability of the limb depends on several factors, including the presence of collateral supply and the metabolic rate within the limb (i.e., a patient who has been running prior to getting shot may have less time before the leg becomes non-viable).

Signs of ischaemia include a cold, pale, painful limb, followed by loss of sensation and loss of motor function and, at a late stage, rigidity (e.g., a rigid ankle joint). Once rigidity sets in, viability is questionable. Once 'fixed skin staining' occurs (dark skin patches), the limb is clearly non-viable and must be amputated.

When presented with questionable viability, it is important to start with a 'diagnostic' fasciotomy before making a decision regarding revascularization. The technique is as for therapeutic fasciotomy, but in this case the procedure is done to inspect the musculature. Viable muscles are bright in colour and contract when stimulated with a diathermy, whilst dead muscles appear pale, are often swollen, and there is no sign of contraction on electrical stimulation.

Usually the anterior and peroneal compartment muscles are more sensitive to ischaemia, and they may become non-viable whilst the posterior compartment muscles are still viable. In this case, one may still proceed to revascularize the leg, and observe the leg postoperatively. The anterior and peroneal muscles may necrose, at which time they may be debrided, and the wound subsequently closed, or skin grafted. The patient will require a lifelong splint to prevent foot-drop. However, if diagnostic fasciotomy reveals more than two non-viable compartments, revascularization is not advisable.

Note that a diagnostic fasciotomy, if followed by revascularization, has also acted as a 'prophylactic' fasciotomy.

11.8.1 Lower Leg Fasciotomy

It is critically important that the fasciotomy is comprehensive and adequate, releasing all four lower limb compartments (**Figure 11.1**).

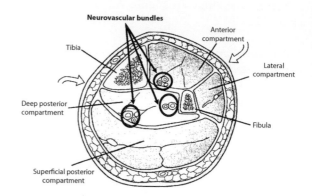

Figure 11.1 Cross section of lower leg, showing compartments.

Several techniques have been described for the lower leg:

- Two-incision, four-compartment fasciotomies
- One-incision fasciotomy
- Fibulectomy
- Subcutaneous fasciotomy

Pitfall

In trauma, there is **no place** for single-incision fasciotomy, subcutaneous fasciotomy, or fibulectomy.

Two-incision, four-compartment fasciotomies only.

11.8.1.1 TWO-INCISION, FOUR-COMPARTMENT FASCIOTOMY[23]

The skin must be opened widely to allow a good view of the underlying fascia. It is critical that the fascia is split over its entire length, and this can only be done under direct vision. Care must be taken not to damage the saphenous veins, which may constitute the major system of venous return in such an injured leg.

Two long incisions are made:

Lateral incision

- The lateral incision starts anterolaterally over the fibula, 2–3 cm below the head.
- Retract skin.
- Start by making a transverse incision at mid-point across the septum (**Figure 11.2**). The horizontal part of the 'H' is to identify the septum and can be placed anywhere on the lateral side.
- Cut the fascia on either side of the septum using curved scissors.

malleolus posterior to the medial border of the tibia.

- The subcutaneous tissue is pushed away by blunt dissection, and the superficial and deep posterior compartments are opened separately.

Pitfall

Care must be taken not to damage the saphenous veins medially, which may constitute the major system of venous return in such an injured leg.

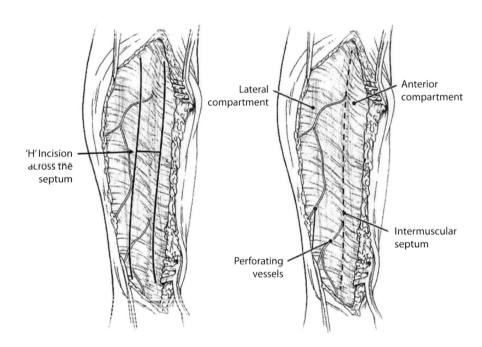

Figure 11.2 Technique of 'H' incision over lateral and anterior compartments.

Pitfall

On the lateral side, the common peroneal nerve, running down the entire lateral side as far as 2 cm above the lateral malleolus, should be identified and preserved.

Medial incision

- A long posteromedial incision is made 2 cm medial to, and below, the tibial tuberosity, running down the entire lower leg, 2–3 cm behind the posterior border of the tibia, as far as 2 cm above the medial

11.8.1.2 SINGLE-INCISION FASCIOTOMY

This is a longer procedure, and it is more difficult to do adequate decompression for major trauma.

It should never be practised in the trauma situation.

11.8.1.3 FIBULECTOMY

This is a difficult procedure, leading to extensive blood oozing, and may well result in damage to the peroneal artery.

It should never be practised in the trauma situation.

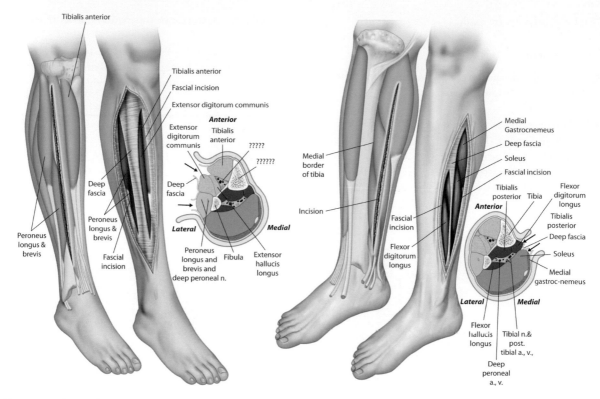

Figure 11.3 Fasciotomy.

11.8.1.4 SUBCUTANEOUS FASCIOTOMY

It should never be practised in the trauma situation.

11.8.2 **Upper Leg**[24]

In the upper leg, compartments of quadriceps (ventral), hamstrings (dorsal), and adductors (medial) should be opened. Be aware that ongoing arterial bleeding from the injury can occur from branches of the profunda branches of the femoral artery, and selective angio-embolization may be needed, or, if not applicable, ligation of the profundal femoral artery.

11.8.3 **Upper and Lower Arm**[25,26]

In the upper arm, the biceps (ventral) and triceps compartment (dorsal) can be at risk.

In the lower arm, the dorsal compartment of the extensors can be opened by direct approach. Ventral fasciotomy of the flexors should be completed with release of the carpal tunnel distally and division of the *lacertus fibrosis* in the elbow region proximally (**Figure 11.3**).

Incisions of the dorsal and volar compartments of the forearm (Figure 11.4):

- A 'lazy S' incision is made from the elbow epicondyle through the palm and carpal tunnel distally.
- Although uncommonly affected, a second dorsal incision can be made over the mobile wad posteriorly from the lateral epicondyle to the wrist.

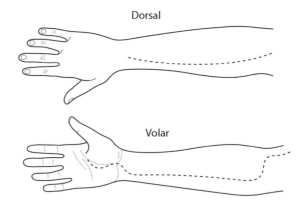

Figure 11.4 Fasciotomy incisions for the forearm.

11.9 COMPLICATIONS OF MAJOR LIMB INJURY

Table 11.7 outlines fracture complications.

Table 11.7 Complications of Fractures

Skin and soft tissue	Skin and tissue loss, wound infection, coverage failure
Bone and fracture site	Compartment syndrome with necrosis of muscle/nerve injury Deep infection – acute or chronic Bone loss, delayed union, malunion/loss of alignment, non-union fixation problems – failure of hardware Peri-implant fracture
Nerve	Direct injury or ischaemic damage Chronic regional pain syndrome
Vascular	Arterial occlusion, venous insufficiency Deep vein thrombosis, compartment syndrome due to reperfusion
Joint motion	Associated joint surface fracture Contracture, late arthritis
Secondary	Ototoxicity, nephrotoxicity, myonecrosis from antibiotics Secondary spread of infection, sepsis/multiple organ failure/death
Psychosocial	Depression, loss of self-worth Economic hardship, questionable employment status, marital problems
Functional	Chronic pain Disability – muscle strength/endurance Decrease in activities of daily function Loss of ability to return to work, inability to participate in recreational activities
Cosmesis	Scars, bulky flaps

In a review of 53 mangled lower extremities, Bondurant et al. compared primary with delayed amputation in terms of morbidity and cost.[27] Patients undergoing delayed ablation had longer periods of hospitalization (22.3 vs. 53.4 days) and more surgical procedures (1.6 vs. 6.9) at greater cost ($28,964 vs. $53,462). Six patients with delayed amputation developed sepsis from the injured lower extremity and died, and, whilst no patient with a primary amputation developed sepsis or died, their quality of life was very poor.

The decision to amputate primarily is difficult. At the initial examination, the extent of the eventual loss of soft tissue can never be fully appreciated, distal perfusion is also difficult to assess (many patients are shocked), and the neurological evaluation is often unreliable (as a result of associated head injury or ischaemia and soft tissue disruption). Any thoughts of limb salvage should always maintain the priority of life over limb, thus minimizing systemic complications and missed injuries. To facilitate this early decision-making, several guidelines have been devised providing management of injuries which might eventually require amputation.[28]

11.10 SUMMARY

It seems preferable to perform early, definitive long bone stabilization in polytrauma patients. Recent consensus guidelines suggest that, for patients with dominant head or chest injuries, the timing of long bone stabilization should be individualized according to the patient's clinical condition. Damage control orthopaedics has a real place in limb salvage.[28]

REFERENCES AND RECOMMENDED READING

References

1. Seamon MJ, Smoger D, Torres DM, Pathak AS, Gaughan JP, Santora TA, et al. A prospective validation of a current practice: the detection of extremity vascular injury with CT angiography. *J Trauma*. 2009 Aug;**67(2)**:238–43; discussion 243–4. doi: 10.1097/TA.0b013e3181a51bf9.

2. Mathew S, Smith BP, Cannon JW, Reilly PM, Schwab CW, Seamon MJ. Temporary arterial shunts in damage control: experience and outcomes. *J Trauma Acute Care Surg*. 2017 Mar;**82(3)**:512–7. doi: 10.1097/TA.0000000000001334.

3. Fox N, Rajani RR, Bokhari F, Chie WC, Kerwin, A, Seamon MJ, et al. Evaluation, and management of penetrating lower extremity arterial trauma: an Eastern Association for the Surgery of Trauma practice management guideline. *J Trauma Acute Care Surg*. 2012;**73(5) Supplement 4**:S315–20. doi: 10.1097/TA.0b013e31827018e.

4. Gustilo RB, Mendoza RM, Williams DN. Problems in the management of type III (severe) open fractures: a new classification of type III open fractures. *J Trauma*. 1984 Aug;**24**:742–6. doi: 10.1097/00005373-198408000-00009.

5. Gustilo RB, Anderson JT. Prevention of infection in the treatment of one thousand and twenty-five open fractures of long bones: retrospective and prospective analyses. *J Bone Joint Surg Am*. 1976 Jun;**58(4)**:453–8.

6. Truetta J. War surgery of extremities: treatment of war wounds and fractures. *Br Med J*. 1942;**1**:616.

7. Hoff WS, Bonadies JA, Cachecho R, Dorlac WC. EAST Practice Management Guidelines Work Group: update to Practice Management Guidelines for prophylactic antibiotic use in open fractures. *J Trauma*. 2011 Mar;**70(3)**:751–4. doi: 10.1097/TA.0b013e31820930e5. 10.1097/TA.0b013e31820930e5. Available from www.east.org (accessed online September 2023).

8. Rogers FB, Cipolle MD, Velmahos G, Rozycki G. Practice management guidelines for the prevention of venous thromboembolism in trauma patients: the EAST practice management guidelines work group. *J Trauma*. 2002 July;**53(1)**:142–64. doi: 10.1097/00005373-200207000-00032. Available from www.east.org (accessed online September 2023).

9. Gandhi RR, Overton T, Haut ER, Lau B, Vallier H, Rohs T, et al. Optimal timing of femur fracture stabilization in polytrauma patients: a practice management guideline from the Eastern Association for the Surgery of Trauma. *J Trauma Acute Care Surg*. 2014 Nov;**77(5)**:787–795. doi: 10.1097/TA.0000000000000434. (accessed online September 2023)

10. Robinson CM. Current concepts of respiratory insufficiency syndromes after fracture. *J Bone Joint Surg Br*. 2001 Aug;**83(6)**:781–91. doi: 10.1302/0301-620x.83b6.12440.

11. Scalea TM, Scott JD, Brumback RJ, Burgess AR, Mitchell KA, Kufera JA, et al. Early fracture fixation may be 'just fine' after head injury: no difference in central nervous system outcomes. *J Trauma*. 1999 May;**46(5)**:839–46. doi: 10.1097/00005373-199905000-00012.

12. Bosse MJ, MacKenzie EJ, Kellam JF, Burgess AR, Webb LX, Swiontkowski MF, et al. A prospective evaluation of the clinical utility of the lower-extremity injury-severity scores. *J Bone Joint Surg*. 2001;**83A**:3–14. doi: 10.2106/00004623-200101000-00002.

13. Gregory RT, Gould RJ, Peclet M, Wagner JS, Gilbert DA, Wheeler JR, et al. The Mangled Extremity Syndrome (MES): a severity grading system for multisystem injuries of the extremities. *J Trauma*. 1985 Dec;**25(12)**:1147–50.

14. Howe HR Jr, Poole GV Jr, Hansen KJ, Clark T, Plonk GW, Koman LA, et al. Salvage of lower extremities following combined orthopedic and vascular trauma: a predictive salvage index. *Am Surg*. 1987 Apr;**53(4)**:205–28.

15. Johansen K, Daines M, Howey T, Helfet D, Hansen ST Jr. Objective Criteria accurately predict amputation following lower extremity trauma. *J Trauma*. 1990 May;**30(5)**:568–72; discussion 572–3. doi: 10.1097/00005373-199005000-00007.

16. Johansen K, Hansen ST Jr. MESS (Mangled Extremity Severity Score) 25 years on: time for a reboot? *J Trauma Acute Care Surg*. 2015 Sep;**79(3)**:495–6. doi: 10.1097/TA.0000000000000767.

17. McNamara MG, Heckman JD, Corley FG. Severe open fractures of the lower extremity: a retrospective evaluation of the Mangled Extremity Severity Score (MESS). *J Orthop Trauma*. 1994;**8(2)**:81–7. doi: 10.1097/00005131-199404000-00001.

18. Perron AD, Brady WJ, Keats TE. Orthopedic pitfalls in the ED: acute compartment syndrome. *Am J Emerg Med*. 2001 Sept;**19(5)**:413–16. Review. doi: 10.1053/ajem.2001.20038.

19. Tiwari A, Haq AI, Myint F, Hamilton G. Acute compartment syndromes. *Br J Surg*. 2002 Apr;**89(4)**:397–412. doi: 10.1046/j.0007-1323.2002.02063.x.

20. Schmidt AH. Acute compartment syndrome. *Orthop Clin North Am*. 2016 Jul;**47(3)**:517–25. doi: 10.1016/j.ocl.2016.02.001. Review.

21. Hammerberg EM, Whitesides TE Jr, Seiler JG 3rd. The reliability of measurement of tissue pressure in compartment syndrome. *J Orthop Trauma*. 2012 Sept;**26(9)**:e166; author reply e166. doi: 10.1097/BOT.0b013e3182673a3f.

22. Sellei RM, Wollnitz J, Reinhardt N, de la Fuente M, Radermacher K, Weber C, Kobbe P, Hildebrand F. Non-invasive measurement of muscle compartment elasticity in lower limbs to determine acute compartment syndrome: clinical results with pressure related ultrasound. *Injury*. 2020 Feb;**51(2)**:301–6. doi: 10.1016/j.injury.2019.11.027. Epub 2019 Nov 21.

23. Mubarak SJ, Owen CA. Double incision fasciotomy of the leg for decompression in compartment syndromes. *J Trauma*. 1977 Mar;**59(2A)**:184–7.

24. Ojike NI, Roberts CS, Giannoudis PV. Compartment syndrome of the thigh: a systematic review. *Injury*. 2010 Feb;**41(2)**:133–6. doi: 10.1016/j.injury.2009.03.016. Epub 2009 Jun 24.

25. Kalyani BS, Fisher BE, Roberts CS, Giannoudis PV. Compartment syndrome of the forearm: a systematic review. *J Hand Surg Am*. 2011 Mar;**36(3)**:535–43. doi: 10.1016/j.jhsa.2010.12.007.

26. Kistler JM, Ilyas AM, Thoder JJ. Forearm compartment syndrome: evaluation and management. *Hand Clin.* 2018 Feb;**34(1)**:53–60. doi: 10.1016/j.hcl.2017.09.006. Review.

27. Bondurant FJ, Cotler HB, Buckle R, Miller-Crotchett P, Browner BD. The medical and economic impact of severely injured lower extremities. *J Trauma.* 1988;**28**:1270–3. doi: 10.1097/00005373-198808000-00023.

28. Scalea TM, DuBose J, Moore EE, West M, Moore FA, McIntyre R, et al. Western Trauma Association critical decisions in trauma: management of the mangled extremity. *J Trauma Acute Care Surg.* 2012 Jan;**72(1)**:86–93. doi: 10.1097/TA.0b013e318241ed70.

Recommended Reading

Harris AM, Althausen PL, Kellam J, Bosse MJ, Castillo R. Complications following limb-threatening lower extremity trauma. *J Orthop Trauma.* 2009 Jan;**23(1)**:1–6. doi: 10.1097/BOT.0b013e31818e43dd.

Helgeson MD, Potter BK, Burns TC, Hayda RA, Gajewski DA. Risk factors for and results of late or delayed amputation following combat-related extremity injuries. *Orthopedics.* 2010 Sep 7;**33(9)**:669. doi: 10.3928/01477447-20100722-02.

Head Trauma 12

12.1 INTRODUCTION

Traumatic brain injury (TBI) is a leading cause of death and disability worldwide. Approximately 69 million individuals are estimated to suffer TBI from all causes each year.[1]

The incidence of TBI is increasing in low- and middle-income countries (LMICs) because of increased transport-related injuries, and young men are particularly affected. Ninety per cent of TBI related deaths occur in these countries.[2] The elderly cohort is also increasing in most countries due to low-impact falls. On average, 39% of patients with severe TBI die from their injury, and 60% have an unfavourable outcome. Trauma patients with co-existing TBI have a higher mean length of stay in hospital, higher hospital cost, and increased percentage of disability compared with trauma victims without TBI.[3]

The mortality and morbidity of TBI are attributed to the **primary brain injury** which includes diffuse axonal injury and intracranial haematomas and the **secondary brain injury** due initially to hypoxia, hypotension, and cerebral ischaemia. Early evacuation of intracranial haematomas and the correction of secondary physiological derangements save lives and improve outcome.

Damage control resuscitation aims to rapidly restore normal ventilation and oxygenation, correct hypovolaemia and hypotension, reverse hypothermia, and correct coagulopathy. *Hypotensive resuscitation* may be used for penetrating trauma, but the systolic blood pressure (SBP) should be kept above 90 mmHg to maintain cerebral perfusion. Prompt imaging by computed tomography (CT) whenever possible facilitates the treating team's immediate decisions.

12.2 INJURY PATTERNS AND CLASSIFICATION

TBIs are classified according to severity, mechanism of injury, and pathology.

DOI: 10.1201/9781003258124-15

12.2.1 Severity

The *severity of TBI* is assessed clinically with the Glasgow Coma Scale (GCS), which evaluates the neurological status of the patient (see Appendix B.2). It is essential to realize that the GCS is not a single number, and each of its three components have clinical value. Additional clinical signs and symptoms, such as focal neurological deficits, abnormal pupillary light reflexes, pupil inequality (anisocoria), and seizures, contribute to the classification of TBI severity.

- *Mild TBI*: Brief loss of consciousness for a few seconds or minutes, post-traumatic amnesia (PTA) for less than an hour, normal brain-imaging results, and GCS score 13–15.
- *Moderate TBI*: Loss of consciousness for less than 24 hours, PTA for 1–24 hours, abnormal brain-imaging findings, and GCS score of 9–12.
- *Severe TBI*: Loss of consciousness or coma for more than 24 hours, PTA for more than 24 hours, abnormal brain-imaging findings, and GCS score of 3–8.

12.2.2 Pathological Classification of TBI

- *Focal brain injuries*: Impact forces acting directly on the head create a wide range of focal lesions including contusion, brain laceration, epidural or subdural haematoma, and subarachnoid or intracerebral haemorrhage. Contrecoup injury occurs when the brain impacts the opposite side of the skull to the impact. Fast acquisition of brain imaging promotes early diagnosis and prompt intervention that may critically affect patient outcome. However, most patients with TBI do not have a lesion suitable for neurosurgical intervention.
- *Diffuse brain injuries*: Sudden head movement, usually rapid deceleration often seen in motor vehicle

accidents, results in *diffuse axonal injury* (DAI). The CT scan shows diffuse cerebral oedema, multiple petechial haemorrhages, loss of grey-white differentiation, loss of basal cisterns, and subarachnoid spaces and small ('slit') ventricles. DAI is frequently devastating for the patient and leads to extensive damage to the white matter and a variety of profound neurological deficits.[4]

The pathologies of TBI are frequently present in various combinations, further complicating patient management and outcome prediction.

Both the severity and type of TBI are directly associated with the **mechanism** of injury and the forces applied to the brain.

12.2.2.1 BLUNT HEAD TRAUMA

Blunt head trauma carries a high risk for secondary brain damage, represents the main cohort of patients suffering from severe post-injury morbidity, and is the main diagnostic target for a trauma team. The most frequent causes of blunt head injury are motor vehicle collisions, falls, and assaults, which result in scalp lacerations, scalp haematomas, and skull fractures.

Fractures of the skull vault are classified as closed or open (compound), linear, comminuted, or depressed. Skull base fractures may result in periorbital haematomas and cerebrospinal fluid (CSF) leaks from the nose or ears. The significance of skull fractures should not be underestimated. All open depressed skull fractures should be surgically treated, especially if the underlying dura is damaged. A closed depressed fracture may or may not require surgery.

12.2.2.2 PENETRATING HEAD TRAUMA

Penetrating injuries are caused mainly by bullets from firearms, and less commonly by knife or machete wounds and bomb blast fragments. A bullet causes a spreading shock wave in the brain, causing collateral brain damage in addition to the primary track of the projectile. The projectile may ricochet internally off the skull or perforate the skull and scalp in its path. Patients with penetrating cerebral injury require emergency craniotomy if there is a significant mass effect from a haematoma or projectile fragments. However, removal of bone or projectile fragments should not be pursued at the expense of damaging normal brain tissue. Patients presenting with

a GCS of 5 or less after resuscitation, and CT findings of bilateral brain injury, have a particularly poor prognosis, and conservative treatment may be indicated.

12.2.2.3 BLUNT CEREBROVASCULAR INJURY (BCVI)

BCVIs are rare yet potentially devastating injuries affecting 1% to 3% of blunt trauma patients.[3] Over the past three decades, significant advances have been made in our understanding of the mechanisms and pathophysiology underlying these injuries. The development of screening criteria (**Table 12.1**)[4] and an injury

Table 12.1 Denver Screening Criteria for Blunt Cerebrovascular Injury
Signs and Symptoms of BCVI
Potential arterial haemorrhage from neck / Nose / Mouth
Cervical bruit in a patient < 50 years of age
Expending cervical haematoma
Focal neurological defect: Hemiparesis, vertebrobasilar symptoms, Horner's syndrome
Neurological deficit inconsistent with head CT
Stroke on CT or MRI
Risk Factors for BCVI
High-energy transfer mechanism
Displaced mid-face fracture: Le Fort II or Le Fort III
Mandible fracture
Complex skull fracture / Basilar skull fracture / Occipital condyle fracture
Severe TBI with GCS < 6/15
Cervical spine fracture, subluxation, or ligamentous injury at any level
Near hanging with anoxic brain injury
Clothesline-type injury or seatbelt abrasion with significant pain, swelling, or altered mental status
TBI with thoracic injury
Scalp degloving
Thoracic vascular injury
Blunt cardiac rupture
Upper rib fractures
GCS, Glasgow Coma Scale MRI, magnetic resonance imaging TIA, transient ischaemic attack

Table 12.2 Denver Grading System for Blunt Cerebrovascular Injury

Grade	Description
I	Luminal irregularity or dissection with < 25% luminal narrowing
II	Dissection or intramural haematoma with > 25% narrowing, intraluminal thrombosis, or raised intimal flap
III	Pseudoaneurysm
IV	Occlusion
V	Transection with free extravasation

Table 12.3 The PICO Format

P	Patient, Population, or Problem	How would I describe the patient group?
I	Intervention, Prognostic factor, or Exposure	Which main intervention, prognostic factor, or exposure is considered?
C	Comparison or Intervention (if appropriate)	What is the main alternative to compare with the intervention?
O	Outcome you would like to measure or achieve	What can be accomplished, measured, improved, or affected?

grading scale (**Table 12.2**)[5] has been central to our ability to detect, accurately describe, prognosticate, and treat BCVIs.

Early diagnosis and treatment are critical to minimize the morbidity and mortality associated. One of the most feared complications is a stroke, which may occur in up to 20% of patients, most commonly in the early (< 72 hours) post-injury period. Early initiation of antithrombotic therapy (ATT) has been demonstrated to decrease the risk for stroke, stroke-related morbidity and mortality, and overall mortality in patients with BCVIs.

Since the original Eastern Association for the Surgery of Trauma (EAST) practice management guideline (PMG) was published, new data and controversy have emerged regarding various aspects in the diagnosis and management of BCVIs. The following PMG addresses several issues related to the use of screening protocols, screening of cervical spine injuries, the role of ATT, and endovascular stents in patients with BCVIs. See **Tables 12.3** and **12.4**.[6]

In summary, the EAST PMG is as follows:
- In adult patients with blunt polytrauma, it is recommended that a screening protocol to detect BCVI be used.
- In adult patients with high-risk cervical spine injuries, it is recommended that CT angiography (CTA) be performed to detect BCVI.
- In adult patients with low-risk cervical spine injuries, it is recommended that screening CTA be performed to detect BCVI.
- In adult patients with BCVI, it is recommended that ATT be used to prevent both stroke and mortality.
- In adult patients with Grade II and Grade III BCVIs, it is recommended **against** the use of routine endovascular stenting as an adjunct to ATT to decrease the risk of stroke.

12.3 PHYSIOLOGICAL PARAMETERS IN TBI

In addition to clinical assessment, three types of brain monitoring are used in patients with severe TBI: intracranial pressure (ICP), cerebral perfusion pressure (CPP), and advanced cerebral monitoring including brain oxygen (PbrO$_2$). Multimodality monitoring is not always available, and decisions on management are made on a clinical basis with the additional CT brain result if available. The application of TBI guidelines may therefore not be applicable in resource-poor environments.

12.3.1 Mean Arterial Pressure (MAP)

MAP is defined as the average arterial pressure during a single cardiac cycle and is an indicator of the haemodynamic status in an injured patient. It is represented mathematically by the formula:

$$\frac{SAP + 2DAP}{3}$$

where *SAP* is systolic pressure, and *DAP* is diastolic pressure.

12.3.2 Intracranial Pressure

ICP is the pressure inside the skull and is affected by variations in CSF volume, brain water, cerebral blood volume, and venous return of the brain. The normal ICP range is 7–15 mmHg. Values persistently over 20 mmHg

Table 12.4 Eastern Association for the Surgery of Trauma (EAST) Practice Management Guideline for Blunt Cerebrovascular Injury

PICO	Recommendation
PICO Question 1	
In adult patients with blunt polytrauma (P), should a screening protocol (I) versus no screening protocol (C) be used to detect BCVI (O)?	We recommend using a screening protocol for the detection of BCVI in adult patients with blunt polytrauma. **Strong recommendation**
PICO Question 2A	
In adult patients with high-risk cervical spine injuries (P), should a screening computed tomography angiography (CTA) (I) versus no screening CTA (C) be performed to detect BCVI (O)?	On the basis of these considerations, we recommend screening CTA in patients with high-risk cervical spine injuries to detect BCVI. **Strong recommendation**
PICO Question 2B	
In adult patients with low-risk cervical spine injuries (P), should a screening CTA (I) versus no screening CTA (C) be performed to detect BCVI (O)?	On the basis of these considerations, we conditionally recommend BCVI screening in patients with low-risk cervical spine injuries to detect BCVI. **Conditional (intermediate) recommendation**
PICO Question 3	
In adult patients diagnosed with BCVI (P), should ATT (I) versus no ATT (C) be administered to decrease the incidence of stroke (O1) or mortality (O2)?	**On the basis of the available literature, we recommend the use of ATT to decrease the incidence of both stroke and mortality in patients with BCVI.** This should be done as early and safely as possible following confirmation of the diagnosis, and consideration should be given towards a multidisciplinary discussion of the optimal ATT among patients with concomitant injuries in whom therapy may exacerbate or worsen bleeding. Data support the use of ATT in patients diagnosed with BCVI, but there is no evidence to support a particular treatment. The use of various medications should be individualized.
PICO Question 4	
In adult patients with Grade II or III BCVIs (P), should routine endovascular stenting (as an adjunct to ATT) (I) versus ATT alone (C) be performed to reduce the risk of stroke (O1) or mortality (O2)?	Given the rarity of the injury and the lack of well-controlled prospective clinical trials, the level of evidence on which to base **recommendations is low to very low.** Currently, routine endovascular stent placement in the acute setting cannot be supported, but there may be individual cases (e.g., persistent or enlarging pseudoaneurysm) in which it would be considered appropriate and potentially beneficial to a patient.

are abnormal and may indicate the presence of an intracranial mass lesion such as a haematoma, or cerebral oedema that requires surgical intervention.

12.3.3 Cerebral Perfusion Pressure

CPP is the net pressure gradient that drives cerebral blood flow (CBF) to the brain. It can be calculated by the formula: MAP − ICP.

The normal CPP range is 60–70 mmHg in adults in the supine position.

12.3.4 Cerebral Blood Flow

CBF represents the blood supply to the brain at any given time. Normal values are around 50–55 mL/min/100 g of brain tissue, which corresponds to 15% of the cardiac output in the adult. It is autoregulated tightly according to the brain's metabolic demands, the blood pressure, and the arterial blood CO_2 pressure ($PaCO_2$) and arterial oxygen pressure (PaO_2) values, and it shows significant derangement in severe TBI.

12.4 PATHOPHYSIOLOGY OF TBI[7]

The initial stages of cerebral injury are characterized by two main elements: direct tissue damage and impaired regulation of CBF and metabolism. This 'ischaemia-like' pattern leads to accumulation of lactic acid due to anaerobic glycolysis, increased membrane permeability, and consecutive oedema formation. On a cellular level, an excessive release of neurotransmitters takes place, along with an increase of free radicals and fatty acids, occurring from membrane degradation of cellular and vascular structures. These events lead to programmed cell death (apoptosis).

12.5 MANAGEMENT OF TBI

Current evidence-based *Guidelines for the Management of Traumatic Brain Injury (TBI)* are published by the Brain Trauma Foundation.[8,9]

Current evidence-based *Guidelines for the Management of Paediatric Severe Traumatic Brain Injury (TBI)* are published by the Brain Trauma Foundation.[10]

Time to treatment should be minimized to minimize secondary brain injury. Advanced Trauma Life Support (ATLS®) principles are applied. An abbreviated neurological examination provides important baseline information. Maintenance of blood pressure and oxygenation is fundamental.

- Maintain SBP at ≥ 100 mmHg for patients 50 to 69 years old or at ≥ 110 mmHg for patients 15 to 49 or > 70 years old. This may decrease mortality and improve outcomes (level III evidence).
- Following restoration of blood volume, pressor support with noradrenaline may be required if the CPP is not maintained.
- Keep arterial blood oxygen saturation (SaO_2) > 95%.
- Keep PaO_2 > 80 mmHg (> 10.5 kPa).

Autoregulation: The normal brain maintains a constant CBF over a wide range of blood pressure. However, autoregulation is frequently deranged in severe TBI, and the brain becomes more vulnerable to hypotension. Other systemic brain insults which aggravate secondary brain injury are:

- Anaemia (Hb < 10 g/dL)
- Hyponatraemia (serum sodium < 142 mmol/L)
- Hyperglycaemia (blood sugar > 10 mmol/L)
- Hypoglycaemia (blood sugar < 4.6 mmol/L)
- Fever (temperature > 36.5 °C)

Many intensive care units have developed basic care protocols for the management of severe TBI patients. An imaging and clinical examination (ICE) protocol has also been developed for managing severe TBI without ICP monitoring.[11] This has been applied in resource-poor countries but has not yet been compared to the protocols which include ICP and CPP monitoring.

12.6 CPP THRESHOLD

An adequate CPP is achieved by optimizing blood pressure and minimizing ICP.[9] This will ensure the delivery of adequate blood flow and oxygenation to the brain. The CPP to aim for is 60 to 70 mmHg. A CPP of 60 mmHg is adequate provided the MAP is greater than 70 mmHg. A level below 60 mmHg may result in cerebral ischaemia and should be avoided (level IIB evidence).

CPPs maintained at > 70 mmHg should be avoided because the patient may develop fluid overload, pulmonary oedema, and respiratory failure (level III evidence).

To maintain adequate CPP (> 70 mmHg), blood pressure must be kept high and ICP low.

12.7 ICP MONITORING

Management of patients with severe TBI using information from ICP monitoring is recommended to reduce in-hospital and 2-week post-injury mortality (level IIB evidence).[9] Treating ICP > 22 mmHg is recommended because values above this level are associated with increased mortality (level IIB evidence).[9] A combination of ICP values and brain CT findings should be used to determine the need for treatment (level III evidence).[6] ICP monitoring is frequently not available in LMICs.

12.7.1 ICP Monitoring Devices

Measurement of ICP currently requires a burr hole or direct placement at craniotomy.

- *Intraventricular catheter*: This is the most accurate, cost-effective, and reliable ICP monitoring method. A hole is drilled through the skull, and the catheter is inserted through the brain into the lateral ventricle. When the ICP is high, catheter placement can be challenging, because the ventricles are compressed and may be shifted from their normal position.
- *Intraparenchymal catheter*: The calibration of these catheters may drift over several days, and re-calibration may not be available. Some of the newer catheters can measure brain oxygen tension ($PBrO_2$) and temperature in addition to ICP.
- *Subarachnoid, subdural, and epidural catheters*: These are unreliable.

12.7.1.1 CSF DRAINAGE

An external ventricular drain (EVD) can be used to drain CSF and assist with ICP reduction. An EVD system zeroed at the midbrain with continuous drainage of CSF may be considered to lower ICP burden more effectively than intermittent use (level III evidence).[9] Use of CSF drainage to lower ICP in patients with an initial GCS < 6 during the first 12 hours after injury may be considered (level III evidence).[9]

12.7.2 ICP Management: Do's and Don't's

12.7.2.1 HYPERVENTILATION

Hyperventilation lowers $PaCO_2$, which causes cerebral vasoconstriction. This will reduce brain swelling and lower ICP; however, severe hyperventilation causes excessive vasoconstriction, and the local alkalosis that results will further interfere with oxygen delivery, resulting in cerebral ischaemia.

Prolonged prophylactic hyperventilation with $PaCO^2$ of ≤ 35 mmHg (< 3 kPa) is not recommended.

Hyperventilation is recommended as a temporizing measure for the reduction of elevated ICP, but hyperventilation should be avoided during the first 24 hours after injury when CBF often is reduced critically. If hyperventilation is used, jugular vein oxygen saturation (SjO_2) or $PbrO_2$ measurements are recommended to monitor oxygen delivery (level IIB evidence).[9]

12.7.2.2 OSMOTHERAPY (MANNITOL AND HYPERTONIC SALINE)

Although hyperosmolar therapy may lower ICP, the Brain Trauma Foundation Guidelines found insufficient evidence about effects on clinical outcomes to support a specific recommendation, or to support the use of any specific hyperosmolar agent, for patients with severe TBI.[9] Mannitol or hypertonic saline used prior to ICP monitoring should be restricted to patients with signs of trans-tentorial herniation (coning) or progressive neurologic deterioration not attributable to extracranial causes. Mannitol is effective for control of raised ICP at doses of 0.25 to 1 g/kg body weight over 15 minutes. Arterial hypotension (SBP < 90 mmHg) should be avoided. Repeated mannitol may lose its effect and aggravate cerebral oedema. A serum osmolality > 320 mOsm/kg and a serum sodium > 155 mmol/L should be avoided. Mannitol is the drug of choice for improving ICP, but bears a high risk of hypovolaemia, arterial hypotension, and hypernatraemia, as well as recently identified nephrotoxicity. Hypertonic saline could reduce ICP without causing significant hypovolaemia.

12.7.2.3 BARBITURATES AND PROPOFOL

High-dose barbiturate administration may be used to control elevated ICP refractory to maximum standard medical and surgical treatment. Haemodynamic stability is essential before and during barbiturate therapy.

Although propofol is recommended for the control of ICP, it is not recommended for improvement in mortality or 6-month outcomes. Caution is required, as high-dose propofol can produce significant morbidity (level IIB evidence).[9]

12.7.2.4 STEROIDS

The use of steroids is *not* recommended for improving outcome or reducing ICP. In patients with moderate or severe TBI, high-dose methylprednisolone is associated with increased mortality and is contraindicated (level I evidence).[9]

12.8 IMAGING

Skull X-rays are of limited use, unless a CT scan is not available, or a penetrating injury has occurred.

CT scan is the investigation of choice for TBI. All patients with moderate or severe TBI should have a head CT scan. Deteriorating neurological status, amnesia, and focal neurological signs are additional criteria. According to the New Orleans criteria,[12] mild TBI patients with a GCS of 15 and normal neurological examination after blunt trauma should undergo CT if one of the following is present:

* Headache
* Vomiting
* Age over 60 years
* Drug or alcohol intoxication
* Short-term memory deficit
* Seizures

For haemodynamically unstable patients requiring immediate non-cranial surgery, the imaging is postponed.

Pitfall

There is an association between cerebral injury and carotid vascular injury.

It is recommended that, whenever possible in blunt head injury, a CT angiogram of the neck for assessment of the carotid and vertebral arteries be performed at the time of the initial CT scan.

12.9 INDICATIONS FOR SURGERY

Surgery aims to facilitate the insertion of an ICP monitor, CSF drainage, the evacuation of a significant space-occupying lesion, and bony decompression. Decision-making is primarily based on clinical assessment (drop in GCS, pupillary abnormality, focal neurological deficit) and CT scan findings. Surgery to reduce ICP is only meaningful and safe if systemic haemodynamics and oxygenation are stable. Not all intracranial haematomas require removal; only those causing or having the potential to cause significantly raised ICP warrant surgery (e.g., a large epidural haematoma should be evacuated quickly). A thin-layer acute subdural haematoma or traumatic subarachnoid haemorrhage may not need surgery.

Indications to perform emergency surgical treatment in the remote or rural setting are:

* Inability to perform head CT on a neurologically deteriorating patient
* Transfer to the nearest neurosurgical unit is more than 2 hours away
* A sizeable intracranial haematoma

The remote general surgeon should contact the regional neurosurgeon for support and advice.

12.9.1 Burr Holes and Emergency Craniotomy

Rapidly expanding intracranial haematoma is a surgical emergency. These surgical interventions can be performed by a non-neurosurgeon and avert progressive brain injury and death.

12.9.1.1 EMERGENCY BURR HOLE CRANIOTOMY[13]

Clear indications exist for performing a burr hole: GCS ≤ 8 with imaging evidence of an epidural haematoma causing midline shift and unequal pupils. In the absence of a head CT, a very high clinical suspicion (e.g., a palpable fracture, with an ipsilateral fixed dilated pupil, and deteriorating neurologic status) is the only exception for performing an emergency craniotomy without imaging. Otherwise, without imaging and/or with a GCS above 8, the craniotomy is contraindicated.

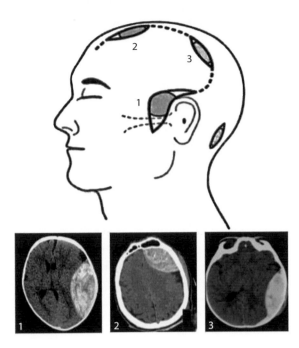

Figure 12.1 Diagram demonstrating position of standard burr holes, and frequent locations of epidural haematomas that are decompressed: (1) temporal (above the zygomatic arch), (2) frontal (over the coronal suture, approximately 10 cm cephalad and in line with the mid-pupillary line), and (3) parietal (over the parietal eminence).

Burr hole drilling sites are shown in **Figure 12.1**, relative to haematoma positions. The basic steps in burr hole technique are:

- Confirm the correct side and position of the haematoma.
- Shave the scalp.
- Infiltrate the scalp with local anaesthetic (e.g., 0.5% bupivacaine [Marcaine®] and 1/200,000 adrenaline).
- Make a 3 cm incision straight down to the bone.
- Push the periosteum with a knife/swab and insert the self-retaining retractor.
- If you are using the Hudson brace for 'manual' burr holes, start drilling perpendicularly to the skull and simultaneously apply saline wash.
- Stop when you feel a difference in tissue resistance.
- The perforator creates a conical opening, and the burr converts this into a cylindrical opening.
- If the haematoma is epidural, a dark blood clot will be identified and can be aspirated. If it is subdural, open the dura with a sharp knife.

- If no blood comes out, review location and side *without further delaying patient transfer.*
- If fresh blood continues to ooze from the wound, do **not** try to tamponade.

The instrument usually used is the Hudson brace (**Figure 12.2**).

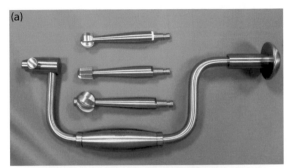

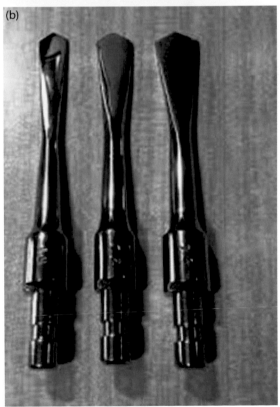

Figure 12.2 Hand-driven burr hole craniotomy: (a) Hudson brace with a set of burrs and (b) the 'V'-shaped perforators below.

12.9.1.2 EMERGENCY CRANIOTOMY[14]

This is a more complex surgical procedure that requires a non-neurosurgeon to have some training and familiarity. The scalp is raised as a myocutaneous flap, and the burr holes are placed and then joined using the Gigli saw if a craniotome is unavailable. The frontotemporal craniotomy is the commonest type used in trauma (**Figure 12.3**).

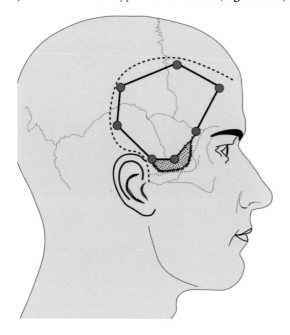

Figure 12.3 Diagram shows a frontotemporal craniotomy for evacuation of an intracranial haematoma. Note the line of the scalp incision, the position of the burr holes, and the removal of bone down to the floor of the middle cranial fossa.

Depressed fractures should be elevated when the depth of the depression meets or exceeds the thickness of the adjacent skull table to alleviate compression of the underlying cortex. A burr hole is placed at the edge of the fracture in order to place an elevator beneath an impacted depressed fracture. Loose bone fragments and debris are removed, haemostasis is obtained, and the dura underlying the fracture is repaired. Avoid elevating depressed fractures overlying the major venous sinuses.

12.9.1.2.1 Penetrating Cranial Injury

Patients with penetrating cerebral injury require emergency craniotomy or craniectomy to wash out and debride the wound and to evacuate haematomas. Marked cerebral swelling frequently develops around the projectile track, and a decompressive craniectomy is required to adequately decompress the brain. Removal of deep bone or projectile fragments should not be pursued at the expense of damaging normal brain tissue. Patients presenting with a GCS score of ≤ 5 after resuscitation, or CT findings of bilateral brain injury, have a poor prognosis, and non-operative treatment may be indicated.

12.9.1.2.2 Decompressive Craniectomy

Removal of large segments of skull helps to control ICP. The commonest is the unilateral craniectomy or frontal-temporal-parietal flap; it is frequently used by neurosurgeons as a primary procedure in LMICs in the absence of ICP monitoring to evacuate acute haematomas and decompress swollen brain. The technique has been described by Quinn et al.[10] The bifrontal-temporal craniectomy is used mainly for bilateral diffuse swelling. In advanced countries, the craniectomy is used for acute subdural haematoma evacuation or as a secondary or salvage operation for intractable intracranial hypertension. Removal of the skull commits the patient to a second operation to replace the flap (cranioplasty).

12.10 ADJUNCTS TO CARE

12.10.1 Infection Prophylaxis[15]

- Closed fractures of the base of the skull with nasal CSF or otorrhea should **not** receive antibiotic prophylaxis.

> *The incidence of infection does not change; the incidence of antibiotic resistance is increased.*

- Open (compound) fractures of the skull should be treated in the same way as other compound fractures.
- Intravenous (IV) antibiotics are administered for a trauma craniotomy at the induction of anaesthesia (cephalosporin, amoxicillin, or flucloxacillin).
- Broad-spectrum antibiotic prophylaxis is recommended for penetrating craniocerebral injuries (cephalosporin, amoxicillin/clavulanate).[15]

12.10.2 Seizure Prophylaxis

Seizure activity in the early post-traumatic period following TBI may cause secondary damage as a result of increased metabolic demands, raised ICP, and excess neurotransmitter release.

Anticonvulsants are indicated for patients who have had a seizure after TBI. The treatment regimen is also shown to decrease the incidence of early post-traumatic seizures (PTSs) (within 7 days of injury) and is continued for 6 months to 1 year. Early seizures are not associated with a worse outcome.

Prophylactic use of phenytoin or valproate is not recommended for preventing late post-traumatic seizures.

Phenytoin (20 mg/kg loading dose and then 4–5 mg/kg at night) is recommended to decrease the incidence of early PTSs (within 7 days of injury for a 7-day duration only), when the overall benefit is thought to outweigh the complications associated with such treatment. However, early PTSs have not been associated with worse outcomes. There is insufficient evidence to recommend levetiracetam compared with phenytoin regarding efficacy in preventing early PTSs and toxicity (level IIA evidence).[6]

12.10.3 Nutrition

Patients should be fed as soon as possible (via a naso- or orogastric tube) to attain basal caloric replacement; at the latest, feeding by day 5–7 post injury is recommended to decrease mortality (level IIA evidence).[6]

12.10.4 Deep Vein Thrombosis (DVT) Prophylaxis

Low-molecular-weight heparin (LMWH) or low-dose unfractioned heparin may be used in combination with mechanical prophylaxis (pneumatic calf compression stockings) until the patient is ambulant. However, there is a theoretical risk for expansion of intracranial haemorrhage.

In addition to compression stockings, pharmacologic prophylaxis may be considered if the brain injury is stable, and the benefit is considered to outweigh the risk of increased intracranial haemorrhage. There is insufficient evidence to support recommendations regarding the preferred agent, dose, or timing of pharmacologic prophylaxis for DVT (level III evidence).[9]

LMWH is usually commenced 48 hours after craniotomy if the patient is stable and the postoperative scan is satisfactory.

12.10.5 Steroids

The use of steroids is **not recommended** for improving outcome or reducing ICP. In patients with moderate or severe TBI, high-dose methylprednisolone is associated with an increased mortality and is contraindicated (level I evidence).[6]

12.11 PAEDIATRIC CONSIDERATIONS

The approach for the paediatric TBI patient is like that followed in the adults.[10] Preservation of SBP > 90 mmHg is critical. Young children and babies are more susceptible to hypovolaemia and anaemia from blood loss compared with adults.

12.12 PEARLS AND PITFALLS

- Always follow the ATLS principles (avoid D before completing ABC).
- Do not attribute a deterioration in level of consciousness (D) to alcohol or drug abuse (E)!
- Keep in mind the C-spine protection in the presence of significant TBI.
- Control major bleeding from a scalp wound (especially in children).
- Closely monitor TBI patients to detect early clinical deterioration in neurological status, despite an early normal CT scan.
- GCS should not be used solely as a single number. It is calculated from three different parameters, each of which has its own significance. The trend is important.
- Hypotensive resuscitation applies in combined TBI and systemic penetrating injury.
- ICP elevation is caused by various intracranial pathologies. Management of intracranial hypertension with conservative measures should not divert attention from identifying the specific cause, and its management including exploratory burr holes if CT is not available.
- Progressive bleeding within the cranial cavity causes death. Death is due to elevation of ICP, brain shift, and herniation of brain that compresses and damages the brain stem.
- Proceed to emergency burr hole or craniotomy when indicated to avoid further harm to the patient. Preferably contact a neurosurgeon to discuss the case.

12.13 SUMMARY

Traumatic brain injuries are a major cause of mortality and morbidity. Primary treatment in TBI focusses on prevention of secondary brain injury, mainly through preservation of normovolaemia and adequate tissue oxygenation. Emergency burr holes or craniotomy may be required when there is delay reaching a neurosurgeon and the patient is deteriorating or likely to deteriorate further. Temporizing measures before surgery may include hyperventilation and hyperosmolar agents such as mannitol or hypertonic saline.

ANAESTHESIOLOGICAL CONSIDERATIONS

- Rapid sequence intubation with meticulous efforts to preserve cerebral perfusion will form part of the damage control resuscitation of the patient with severe TBI.
- Coughing or straining, which increases ICP, should be carefully avoided.
- Time is of the essence; only strictly needed procedures are allowed to delay CT scan for diagnosis and potential neurosurgical treatment.
- Take care of the neck during intubation and surgery. Consider manual inline stabilization of the cervical spine.
- An early arterial line will form part of standard monitoring in severe brain injury, without delaying surgery.
- In the situation of an emergent need for craniotomy if arterial access is proving difficult, avoid delay and proceed with surgery. Ultrasound guidance and the use of Seldinger arterial cannulation techniques may improve the speed and reliability of arterial access in the trauma patient.
- Monitor end-tidal CO_2, and avoid hyperventilation (unless there is evidence of brain herniation, when this may be used as a temporizing measure). Blood gases will help guide ventilation; the arterial–end-tidal CO_2 difference should be accounted for when titrating ventilation.
- Elevate the head end of the operating table 10–15 degrees if blood pressure is maintained.
- Maintain adequate intravenous fluids; correct hypothermia; maintain glycaemic control; insert a nasogastric tube if the anterior skull base has been cleared of fractures (otherwise, insert an orogastric tube); be aware of blood loss, and replace as required; and replace clotting factors and platelets as indicated. *Note*: Severe brain injury may be associated with severe coagulopathy.
- Avoid hypotonic solutions and human albumin.
- For the TBI patient, the aim is to reduce the secondary brain injury by improving the balance between oxygen demand and delivery.
- Hypertonic saline can be used to treat raised ICP.
- Oxygen delivery to the brain cells is improved by securing the airway; assuring proper ventilation and oxygenation; restoring adequate circulation, oxygen carrying capacity, and perfusion pressure; and aiming for reducing cerebral oedema by facilitating venous drainage (head up) and adequate serum sodium levels. Oxygen demand is reduced by adequate sedation using anaesthetics that can reduce the $CMRO_2$ (cerebral metabolic rate of oxygen).
  - Prevention of secondary brain injury is the aim.
- In combined injuries (no single TBI), compromises of the above-mentioned aims often must be done. Preservation of cerebral perfusion and oxygenation must be given high priority.
  - Maintain mean arterial pressure (MAP), normocapnia, and normoglycaemia. Avoid hypothermia.
- Be aware of fluid balance and blood loss, and replace as required; replace clotting factors and platelets indicated.
- Rapid sequence intubation with care of cervical spine, avoidance of increased intracranial pressure (ICP) (coughing/straining), maintenance of MAP (hence, cerebral perfusion pressure), and avoidance of obstruction of cerebral venous drainage (tube ties, neck position, etc.).
  - Monitor end-tidal CO_2, and ventilate to normocapnia (confirm with blood gas when possible).
- Ketamine and propofol are safe in TBI patients and can be used in the acute setting until haemodynamics is under control. Thereafter, propofol is mostly used for short-term anaesthesia/sedation maintenance.
  - Insert a nasogastric tube if the anterior skull base has been cleared of fractures (otherwise, insert an orogastric tube).

REFERENCES AND RECOMMENDED READING

References

1. Dewan MC, Rattani A, Gupta S, Baticulon RE, Hung YC, Punchak M, et al. Estimating the global incidence of traumatic brain injury. *J Neurosurg.* 2018 Apr;**1**:1–18. doi: 10.3171/2017.10.JNS17352.

2. Rosenfeld JV, Maas AI, Bragge P, Morganti-Kossmann MC, Manley GT, Gruen RL. Early management of severe traumatic brain injury. *Lancet.* 2012;**380(9847)**:1088–98. doi: 10.1016/S0140-6736(12)60864-2.

3. Centers for Disease Control (CDC). Traumatic brain injury and concussion. Get the facts. 2017. Available from: https://www.cdc.gov/traumaticbraininjury/get_the_facts. html (accessed online September 2023)

4. Geddes AE, Burlew CC, Wagenaar AE, Biffl WL, Johnson JL, Pieracci FM, et al. Expanded screening criteria for blunt cerebrovascular injury: a bigger impact than anticipated. *Am J Surg.* 2016;**212(6)**:1167–74. doi: 10.1016/j.amjsurg.2016.09.016. Epub 2016 Sep 29.

5. Biffl WL, Moore FF, Offner PJ, Broga KE, Franciose RJ, Burch JM. Blunt carotid arterial injuries: implications of a new grading scale. *J Trauma.* 1999;**47(5)**:845–53 doi: 10.1097/00005373-199911000-00004.

6. Kim DY, Biffl W, Bokhari F, Brakenridge S, Chao E, Claridge JA, et al. Evaluation and management of blunt cerebrovascular injury. An EAST practice management guideline. *J Trauma Acute Care Surg.* 2020 Jun;**88(6)**:875–87. doi: 10.1097/TA.0000000000002668.

7. McGinn MJ, Povlishock JT. Pathophysiology of traumatic brain injury. *Neurosurg Clin N Am.* 2016 Oct;**27(4)**:397–407. doi: 10.1016/j.nec.2016.06.002.

8. Carney N, Totten AM, O'Reilly C, Ullman JS, Hawryluk GW, Bell MJ, et al. Guidelines for the management of severe traumatic brain injury, Fourth Edition. *Neurosurgery.* 2017 Jan 1;**80(1)**:6–15. doi: 10.1227/NEU.0000000000001432.

9. *Guidelines for the Management of Severe Traumatic Brain Injury.* 4th Edn. The Brain Trauma Foundation. 2016. Available from https://braintrauma.org/coma/guidelines/ guidelines-for-the-management-of-severe-tbi-4th-ed (accessed online September 2023)

10. *Guidelines for the Management of Pediatric Severe Traumatic Brain Injury (TBI).* 3rd Edn. The Brain Trauma Foundation. 2019. Available from https://braintrauma.org/ coma/guidelines/pediatric (accessed September 2023)

11. Chesnut RM, Temkin N, Dikmen S, Rondina C, Videtta W, Petroni G, et al. A Method of managing severe traumatic brain injury in the absence of intracranial pressure monitoring: the imaging and clinical examination protocol. *J Neurotrauma.* 2018 Jan 1;**35(1)**:54–63. doi: 10.1089/neu.2016.4472.

12. Bouida W, Marghli S, Souissi S, Ksibi H, Methammem M, Haguiga H, et al. Prediction value of the Canadian CT head rule and the New Orleans criteria for positive head CT scan and acute neurosurgical procedures in minor head trauma: a multicenter external validation study. *Ann Emerg Med.* 2013 May;**61(5)**:521–7.

13. Wilson MH, Wise D, Davies G, Lockey D. Emergency burr holes: "How to do it". *Scand J Trauma Resusc Emerg Med.* 2012 Apr 2;**20**:24. doi: 10.1186/1757-7241-20-24.

14. Quinn TM, Taylor JJ, Magarik JA, Vought E, Kindy MS, Ellegala DB. Decompressive craniectomy: technical note. *Acta Neurologica Scandinavica.* 2011 Apr;**123(4)**:239–44. doi: 10.1111/j.1600-0404.2010.01397.x.

15. Bayston R, de Louvois J, Brown EM, Johnston RA, Lees P, Pople IK. Use of antibiotics in penetrating craniocerebral injuries. "Infection in Neurosurgery" Working Party of British Society for Antimicrobial Chemotherapy. *Lancet.* 2000 May 20;**355(9217)**:1813–7.

Recommended Reading

Maas AI, Dearden M, Teasdale GM, Braakman R, Cohadon F, Iannotti F, et al. EBIC-guidelines for management of severe head injury in adults. European Brain Injury Consortium. *Acta Neurochir (Wien).* 1997;**139(4)**:286–94. doi: 10.1007/BF01808823.

Rosenfeld JV. *Practical Management of Head and Neck Injury.* Elsevier, Churchill Livingstone. 2012. ISBN 978-0-7295-3956-2.

Rosenfeld JV, Bell RS, Armonda R. Current concepts in penetrating and blast injury to the central nervous system. *World J Surg.* 2015;**39(6)**:1352–62. doi: 10.1007/s00268-014-2874-7.

Alam HB, Vercruysse G, Martin M, Brown CVR, Brasel K, Moore EE, Sava J, Ciesla D, Inaba K; Western Trauma Association Critical Decisions in Trauma Committee. Western Trauma Association critical decisions in trauma: Management of intracranial hypertension in patients with severe traumatic brain injuries. *J Trauma Acute Care Surg.* 2020 Feb;**88(2)**:345–51. doi: 10.1097/TA.0000000000002555.

Burns **13**

13.1 OVERVIEW

Globally, burns are a serious public health problem. There are over 300,000 deaths each year from fires alone, with more deaths from scalds, electrical burns, and other forms of burns. Fire-related deaths alone rank among the 15 leading causes of death among children and young adults aged 5–29 years. Over 95% of fatal fire-related burns occur in low- and middle-income countries. South-East Asia alone accounts for just over one-half of the total number of fire-related deaths worldwide, and females in this region have the highest fire-related burn mortality rates globally.[1]

High-income countries have made considerable progress in lowering rates of burn-related death and disability, through combinations of proven prevention strategies and improvements in the care of burn victims. Most of these advances in prevention and care have been incompletely applied in low- and middle-income countries.

Burns are common, often disfiguring, disruptive to families and work, financially burdensome, and **painful**. The concept of near-total early wound excision cannot be overstated for large burns, and the clock starts ticking for the wound and the patient from the moment of injury. Delay to resuscitation and operation is harmful! Major burns cause massive tissue destruction and result in activation of a cytokine-mediated inflammatory response that leads to dramatic pathophysiologic effects at sites local to and distant from the burn.

13.2 BURNS PATHOPHYSIOLOGY

The early (ebb) phase (24–48 hours) of a major burn injury is characterized by decreased cardiac output, and decreased blood flow to all organs. The decreased cardiac output is due to loss of intravascular volume, direct myocardial depression, and increased pulmonary and systemic vascular resistance (PVR and SVR, respectively) and haemoconcentration, and can lead to metabolic acidosis and venous desaturation ($\downarrow SVO_2$). Decreased urine flow results from decreased glomerular filtration, and elevated aldosterone and antidiuretic hormone (ADH) levels. Oxygenation and ventilation problems may occur due to inhalation injury and the systemic effects of burns, including adult respiratory distress syndrome (ARDS), but also when there are circumferential chest burns requiring escharotomy. Compartment syndrome ensues if there is a circumferential burn which does not undergo escharotomy to release the constriction.

Compartment syndrome can also occur in the abdomen, extremities, or orbits without local or circumferential burns. Mental status can be altered because of psychological stress, hypoxia, hypotension, inhaled toxins, and administered drugs (**Figure 13.1**).

At 48–72 hours, the hypermetabolic-hyperdynamic (flow) phase starts, characterized by increased oxygen consumption, carbon dioxide production, and cardiac output, with enhanced blood flow to all organs including skin, kidney (glomerular filtration rate [GFR]), and liver, and decreased SVR. Increased venous oxygen saturation ($\uparrow SVO_2$) is related to peripheral arteriovenous shunting. The markedly decreased SVR mimics sepsis. Lungs and airways may continue to be affected because of inhalation injury and ARDS, and pulmonary oedema can occur due to redistribution of resuscitation fluids and resultant hypervolaemia. The altered mental status may be related to continued systemic inflammatory response syndrome (SIRS) and continued drug therapy. Release of catabolic hormones and insulin resistance lead to muscle protein catabolism and hyperglycaemia.

DOI: 10.1201/9781003258124-16

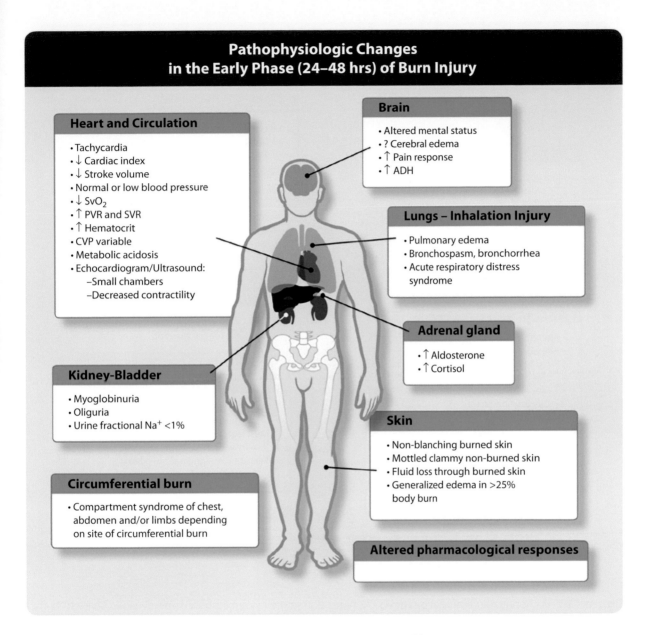

**Pathophysiologic Changes
in the Early Phase (24–48 hrs) of Burn Injury**

Heart and Circulation

- Tachycardia
- ↓ Cardiac index
- ↓ Stroke volume
- Normal or low blood pressure
- ↓ SvO$_2$
- ↑ PVR and SVR
- ↑ Hematocrit
- CVP variable
- Metabolic acidosis
- Echocardiogram/Ultrasound:
  – Small chambers
  – Decreased contractility

Brain

- Altered mental status
- ? Cerebral edema
- ↑ Pain response
- ↑ ADH

Lungs – Inhalation Injury

- Pulmonary edema
- Bronchospasm, bronchorrhea
- Acute respiratory distress syndrome

Adrenal gland

- ↑ Aldosterone
- ↑ Cortisol

Kidney-Bladder

- Myoglobinuria
- Oliguria
- Urine fractional Na$^+$ <1%

Skin

- Non-blanching burned skin
- Mottled clammy non-burned skin
- Fluid loss through burned skin
- Generalized edema in >25% body burn

Circumferential burn

- Compartment syndrome of chest, abdomen and/or limbs depending on site of circumferential burn

Altered pharmacological responses

Figure 13.1 Pathophysiologic changes in the early phase (24–48 hours) of burn injury.

13.3 **ANATOMY**

Apart from simple erythema (sunburn), all other burns constitute an open wound of greater or lesser severity. To create a dramatic analogy, a burn is like an evisceration with exposed bowel. In the case of the burn, it is the dermis (**Figure 13.1**) that is exposed to a lesser or greater extent, resulting in significant losses of fluid from the body, along with loss of the bacterial barrier, leaving the path open for infection as well as loss of heat by convection and conduction (**Figures 13.2** and **13.3**).

In physiological terms, there is a significant loss of protein, primarily albumin; electrolytes; and

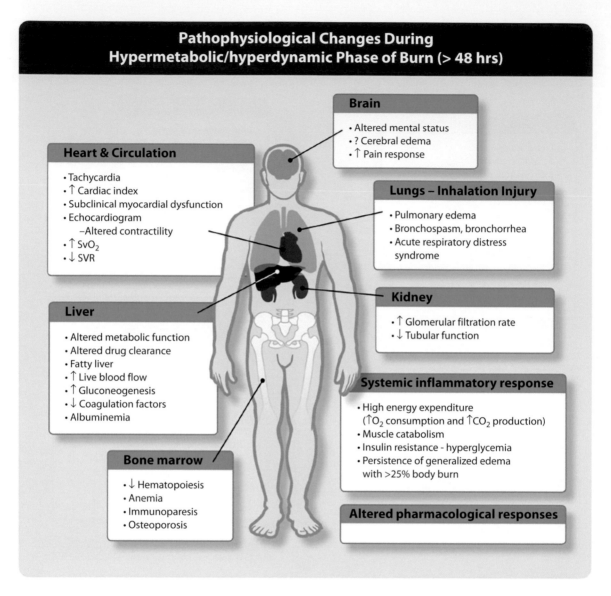

Figure 13.2 Pathophysiological changes at 48–72 hours during the hypermetabolic/hyperdynamic phase of burn.

haemoconcentration, along with a massive increase in energy requirements to heal the wound.

The burn wound is divided into three areas (**Figure 13.4**):

- The zone of coagulation
- The zone of stasis
- The zone of hyperaemia

Inadequate resuscitation or the inappropriate use of ice or iced water to cool the burn may lead to deepening the burn due to vasoconstriction in the zone of stasis, extending the zone of coagulation.

13.4 SPECIAL TYPES OF BURN

13.4.1 Chemical Burns

First aid should be extended for chemical burns to 30 minutes of washing. Alkali goes deep as it dissolves fat, but acid can 'tan' the skin and be surprisingly

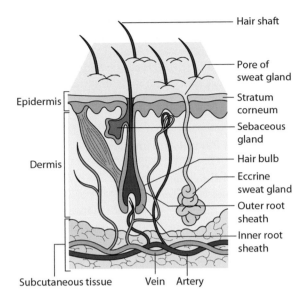

Figure 13.3 Layers and structures of the skin.

shallow, although diagnosis of depth for these chemicals is just plain difficult. Time, however, does tell.

Hydrofluoric acid will continue to injure until the fluorine is chelated. Extreme pain is the hallmark as nerves are irritated. Neuropathic pain is common for months afterwards. After washing the area, the next step is to introduce cations to the injury front. Ca++ and Mg++ are used. Techniques include:

- Calcium added to gel and applied topically.
- Calcium gluconate solution added to dimethyl sulphoxide (DMSO), especially useful for soaking fingertips.

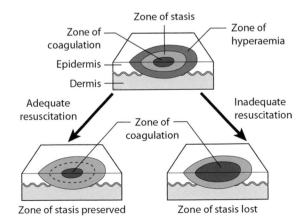

Figure 13.4 Zones of a burn.

- Intra-arterial infusion of calcium.
- Bier's block with calcium gluconate.
- Hypocalcaemia can result from small areas burned with concentrations > 10%. The amount of calcium that may need to be intravenously infused is staggering. Beware!

13.4.2 **Electrical Injury**

Electrical burns are always more extensive than the surface wound indicates. This is especially so for high-voltage (> 1000 volts) injuries. Low-voltage domestic current injury is often seen on the fingers and thumb. The wound frequently extends down to joints, so the operator should be ready to create flap coverage at the time of excision.

Cardiac arrhythmias can result. Loss of consciousness is a prime indicator of this. A 12-lead electrocardiogram (ECG), a rhythm strip, and cardiac-specific troponin levels are the minimum investigations. If normal and no loss of consciousness, no further cardiac-specific investigation or management is needed. Otherwise, cardiac monitoring, echocardiography, and cardiology input are indicated.

High-voltage electrical injuries are associated with devastating injuries, both burn and musculoskeletal. Posterior dislocation of the shoulder; compression fractures of the spine; trauma from being thrown – to the ribs, chest, and long bones; and head trauma should be sought and excluded. The nature of the injury is different to other burn aetiology including low-voltage burns. The body is a volume conductor; therefore, narrower-diameter areas accumulate heat. The current runs up the periosteum, nerves, and vessels whilst affecting muscle cells also. Electroporation of cell walls particularly injures myocytes, with cell necrosis increasing over 5 days; if the muscle looks abnormal at first, it is destined to die! Early release with full-length fasciotomy of the compartments should be performed and re-looks planned. There will always be more to do. In the upper limb, carpal tunnel and Guyon's canal releases should be incorporated in the extensile incisions. Remember that deep muscles, such as the pronator quadratus and rotator cuff, will be most affected.

Early excision of obviously dead tissue combined with fasciotomy are performed immediately, with planned take-backs at regular intervals for further debridement.

13.5 DEPTH OF THE BURN

Burns have been traditionally divided into first, second, and third degree, but the terms 'partial thickness' (superficial and deep) and 'full thickness' are more informative and will be used here. There is also a group of 'indeterminate' thickness burns, which represent a separate challenge.

13.5.1 Superficial Burn (Erythema)

'Sunburn' is painful, dry, and not blistered, and it will fade on its own within 7 days. It requires no debridement and is not counted in the calculation of percentage of total burn surface area (TBSA). Simple oral analgesics and anti-inflammatory agents are usually all that is needed.

13.5.2 Superficial Partial Thickness

These involve the entire epidermis down to the basement membrane and no more than the upper third of the dermis. Rapid re-epithelialization occurs in 1–2 weeks. Because of the large number of remaining epidermal cells and the good blood supply, there is a very small zone of injury or stasis beneath the burn eschar (**Figure 13.5**).

A superficial partial-thickness (SPT) burn is wet, often blistered, intensely painful, and red or white (including in coloured races); it blanches on pressure and will generally heal without split-skin grafting (SSG), usually within 10–14 days. The hairs remain attached when they are pulled. The skin still feels elastic and supple. These burns are often caused by hot water and steam. They do not scar.

13.5.3 Deep Partial Thickness

Destruction of the epidermis occurs down to the basement membrane plus the middle third of the dermis. Re-epithelialization is much slower (2–4 weeks) due to fewer remaining epidermal cells and a lesser blood supply. More collagen deposition will occur, especially if the wound has not been excised and grafted within 3 weeks. The depth of the wound has a significant risk of conversion to full thickness, particularly if infection supervenes. The zone of stasis is much larger than in an SPT injury because of the lower blood flow and greater initial injury to the remaining epidermal cells (**Figure 13.6**).

A deep partial-thickness (DPT) burn is often a mixture of wet and dry. The drier it is, the deeper. Sensation is variable but is still present to touch, although often less painful. The skin texture is thicker and more rubbery. Red patches do not blanche on pressure but exhibit 'fixed skin staining' due to capillary stasis. The hairs will come out readily when pulled. If not excised, these burns take 4–6 weeks to heal and scar badly. The function of a re-epithelialized DPT burn is poor due to the fragility of the epidermis and the rigidity of the scar-laden dermis.

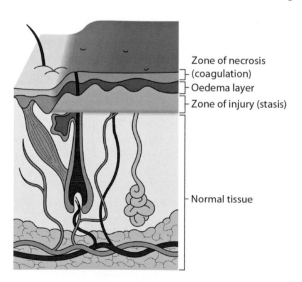

Figure 13.5 Superficial partial-thickness burn.

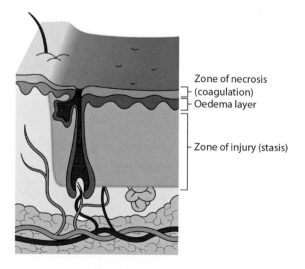

Figure 13.6 Deep partial-thickness burn.

13.5.4 'Indeterminate' Partial-Thickness Burns

Indeterminate burns are usually a mixture of SPT and DPT burns and may exhibit the clinical features of both. The history may help in deciding which is the predominant element and enable management decision-making.

13.5.5 Full Thickness

Full-thickness burns involve the entire epidermis and at least two-thirds of the dermis, leaving very few dermal and epidermal cells to regenerate. Spontaneous healing is very slow, over 4 weeks. Sharp debridement is needed to remove the eschar. Scarring is usually severe if the wound is not skin-grafted, and there is a high risk of infection.

Full-thickness burns are thick, dry, insensate, leathery, and usually black or yellow. Thrombosis is often visible in the surface vessels. The hairs have been burned off. Escharotomies and fasciotomies may be indicated for circumferential full-thickness burns. If left, these burns will contract, become infected, and scar badly. They require early excision (ideally within the first 24–48 hours) and grafting. All electrical burns are full thickness, as are many flame and chemical burns.

13.6 **TOTAL BODY SURFACE AREA BURNED (TBSA)**

For the purposes of calculating the TBSA as a percentage of the entire body surface area, only SPT and DPT burns, along with full-thickness burns, are included in the calculation. Erythema – simple 'sunburn' – alone is ignored.

All units involved in the management of burns should have a clearly established protocol, and this should include the use of a burns resuscitation chart that also shows TBSA affected, in diagrammatic form (traditionally, the 'rule of nines' in the adult, and the Lund and Browder chart in the child; **Figure 13.7**). The patient's

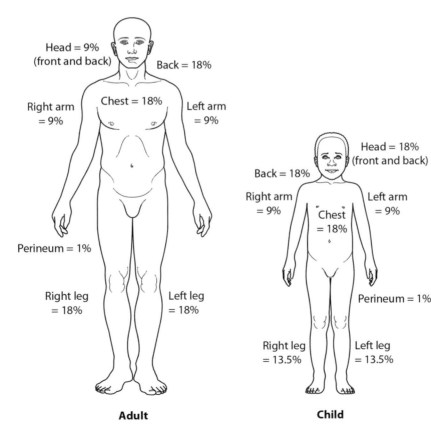

Figure 13.7 Body surface area.

palm, *including the fingers*, represents approximately 1% TBSA and is useful when calculating patchy burns.

It must be emphasized that TBSA calculation is only a starting point for working out a plan of management. Subsequent management is dictated by the patient's response – not by calculated numbers!

13.7 MANAGEMENT

13.7.1 Safe Retrieval

As with all trauma, this will follow the usual Advanced Trauma Life Support (ATLS®) protocols of 'airway, breathing, circulation, disability, and exposure – the ABCDEs.

However, it may, in addition, include removing the casualty from the source of burning *without concomitant risk to the rescuer*. This may mean that electrical power supplies must be switched off, chemical and fuel spillages contained, and fires extinguished to allow rescuers access to the casualty. Burning clothing must be removed, and caustic substances washed off as much as possible, but little time should be spent at the scene.

Do not forget that a burned patient is still a trauma patient and may well have suffered other major injuries in addition to the burn.

13.7.2 First Aid

Do: Cool the burn with *lukewarm* running water. If a tap is not available, use a bucket and jug. Continue for 10 minutes; this provides analgesia and limits burn size. Remember to monitor body temperature. In intubated patients, this process should not exceed 30 minutes.

Don't: Use ice or iced water as these may extend the depth of burn. Do not let the patient get cold; removing burning clothing and leaving the patient exposed to the elements will very quickly result in hypothermia.

The principle is to cool the burn but to keep the patient warm.

Any burn produces inflammation and associated swelling and capillary leakage. The greater the TBSA affected, the greater the inflammatory response, so that any burn of over 20% TBSA will produce a total-body systemic reaction with resultant SIRS. This is unavoidable and should be anticipated.

13.7.3 Initial Management

13.7.3.1 AIRWAY

A rapid assessment of the circumstances of the burn may well alert the medical team to the potential for an airway burn. Fires in an enclosed space (such as house fires) with combustible material and a prolonged extrication time will clearly represent a significant risk.

The inability to make a high-pitched sound ('eeee'), redness, blisters, or smoke inside the teeth means the upper airway has been injured. Endoscopy or laryngoscopy, with liberal application of local anaesthesia, can help judge the severity of injury and guide the need for intubation.

Aspiration of caustic substances may produce a chemical pneumonitis, and steam inhalation from boiling water may cause significant airway injury. When obvious signs of airway injury exist, including stridor, obvious airway burns, redness and swelling of the uvula and pharynx, and wheezing breath sounds or respiratory distress, not only should supplemental oxygen be administered, but early intubation should be accomplished before swelling closes the upper airway.

When in doubt, INTUBATE.

It is easier to subsequently extubate a stable patient who has been intubated early, than to try a late intubation on a patient whose airway is swollen, distorted, and burnt.

Pitfall

Use the biggest tube possible, as narrow tubes become clogged with thick, sooty secretions, and **do not cut the tube short**. The amount of swelling is startling!

13.7.3.2 INHALATIONAL TOXICITY

Carbon monoxide intoxication most often presents with coma or obtundation, rarely the oft-described cherry-red appearance, and is best diagnosed with carboxyhaemoglobin (COHb) levels on blood gas analysis. Treatment is high-dose oxygen.

Remember that the peak level of carbon monoxide is present at the scene, and not at first measurement in the hospital.

Pitfall

Do **not** rely on a pulse oximeter (which measures oxygen saturation). COHb preferentially saturates haemoglobin compared to oxygen, and the oximeter will read close to 100% ('cherry-red colour'), even though the oxygen on the haemoglobin has been displaced. Monitor with COHb levels and serum lactate for tissue hypoxia.

Any carbon monoxide level of over 10% is regarded as toxic, and 100% oxygen should be given until the carbon monoxide level has fallen to below 5%.

Cyanide (often a result of combustible plastics and synthetic materials) is another poisoning agent that should be excluded, and antidotes given if identified.

13.7.3.3 ANALGESIA

Partial-thickness burns are intensely painful and usually require repeated doses of intravenous opiates, titrated against the pain. Analgesia must always be given, even if the child or adult cannot communicate with you. However, the deeper the burn gets, the fewer nerve endings survive, to the point where full-thickness burns are insensate. Providing early, adequate pain relief will reduce stress to the patient and attending medical staff alike, and should be a priority in management after airway control.

13.7.3.4 INTRAVENOUS ACCESS

Intravenous access, preferably central access, should be initiated (if necessary, through the burn itself), and at the same time, blood samples taken for full blood count, electrolytes, blood type and screen, and glucose. If possible, arterial blood gases with an assessment of COHb should be obtained, and a note made of the fraction of inspired oxygen (FiO_2), so that the degree of pulmonary shunting can be calculated. This may be helpful if subsequent ventilation is required.

In patients with a greater than 50% burn, it is likely that a consumption coagulopathy may develop; therefore, a thromboelastogram should be performed, or a conventional coagulation screen.

Pitfalls

- When possible, central lines should be used in larger burns, as with oedema, other lines may not remain in the vein. The lines should be sutured in place, as dressings will not hold them.

- Central lines are best placed above the diaphragm initially, as abdominal pressure can rise so severely that fluid will not flow. The earlier fluid resuscitation is commenced, the lower the mortality and morbidity from acute kidney injury, wound progression, and early and late infection of wound and lung.

13.7.3.5 EMERGENCY MANAGEMENT OF THE BURN WOUND

Coverage of the burn wound in the emergency setting is best accomplished with large quantities of 'clingfilm,' which has been shown to be sterile and is available in industrial quantities. Clingfilm reduces pain by covering exposed nerve endings, and contains and reduces fluid losses, whilst still allowing proper inspection of the burn wound. The old practice of 'mummifying' the patient in swathes of gauze and crepe bandages (with or without the addition of underlying silver creams) is unhelpful, painful for the patient, messy, time-consuming, inefficient for nursing staff, and obstructive to the clinician.

13.7.3.6 FLUID RESUSCITATION

All burns over 20% constitute 'major burns.' All of these will require intravenous fluid replacement, a urinary catheter to monitor output, a nasogastric tube for early feeding, and at least high-care nursing. Lesser percentage burns may be treated by aggressive oral rehydration, but particularly in infants it is better to err on the side of caution, and some units still routinely resuscitate those under 12 years, who have a greater than 10% TBSA burn, with intravenous fluids.

Pitfalls

- All fluid replacement formulae are only *guidelines* to resuscitation. Adequacy of resuscitation is based on urine output rather than slavishly following a formula such as the Parkland formula for fluid requirements.
- Fluid losses start at the time of burn, and fluid replacement is calculated *from the time of burn*, and not from the time of admission to hospital.

The modified Parkland formula is traditionally used to work out requirements for the first 24 hours but has been replaced by the American Burns Association Consensus Formula.2

This is an algorithm for the safe resuscitation of both children and adults. It segregates burns based on *predicted* fluid needs in an attempt to avoid overzealous crystalloid resuscitation and by adjusting the fluid rate in accordance with hourly urine output.

American Burn Association Consensus Formula

- 2–4 mL/kg/Percent (%) burn in the first 24 hours.
  - Give half in the first 8 hours *post burn*.
  - Give half in the next 16 hours *post burn*.
- Modify this as follows:
  - Adults   2 mL/kg/Percent (%) burn in the first 24 hours.
  - Children 3 mL/kg/Percent (%) burn in the first 24 hours.
  - Electrical 4 mL/kg/Percent (%) burn in the first 24 hours.
- **Modify according to urine output:**
  - Adults   Adjust fluid rate for a urine output of 0.5 mL/hour.
  - Children Adjust fluid rate for a urine output of 1 mL/hour. **If the child is < 30 kg, add maintenance fluids that include dextrose or dextrose saline** *in addition to the Consensus Formula.*

Pitfalls

- If too much fluid is given, capillary leakage will increase, producing 'fluid creep' and increasing oedema as the fluid shifts into the 'third space', increasing the likelihood of SIRS and ARDS.[3] The exception would be if there were myoglobinuria, as in electrical burns, where an output of over 1.0 mL/kg/hour would be required for an adult.
- If the patient is hypotensive on admission, it is wrong to attribute signs of shock to the burn until all other sources of shock have been ruled out. Burn shock does not usually develop in the first 24 hours post burn.
- *Antibiotics are not indicated for early burns* within 72 hours of injury, as the burn is still essentially sterile.

13.7.3.7 ASSOCIATED INJURIES

It is easy to focus on the burn alone and miss any associated injuries. A careful history will give clues to not only the type and depth of the burn, but also the possibility of the associated injuries. A full examination is essential once analgesia is adequate, intravenous lines (which may have to transgress a burned area of skin) are running, oxygen is being administered, and the burn has been covered.

Any other injuries found during examination of the patient must be dealt with according to clinical need. Injuries that are bleeding take priority, and the normal principles of resuscitation, including damage control, apply. Most orthopaedic injuries may be deferred for definitive treatment until the resuscitation phase of the burn injury is over. This is usually within the first 48 hours. However, if the patient requires early tangential excision and SSG, and the patient's physiology is not compromised, it may be appropriate to attend to orthopaedic conditions at the same time.

The clinician must be alert to the possibility of deliberate abuse, especially in children, where the nature and distribution of the burn are inconsistent with the story given by the parent or caregiver. The pattern of burn and an unacceptably late presentation may further give clues to a deliberate, 'punishment' burn. When suspicion exists, it is important to document the burn injury meticulously, with photographs if possible. Other signs of abuse should be looked for, and social services contacted if appropriate.

13.7.4 Escharotomy and Fasciotomy

In any trauma resuscitation, the purpose is to combat shock, defined as tissue hypoxia inadequate to the needs of that tissue's survival. Burns are no different, but they present with some special challenges, particularly when the airway is compromised, or when circumferential full-thickness burns with a thick, unyielding eschar produce a tourniquet effect. This can occur around the chest, neck, or limbs, producing a slow asphyxiation or critical limb ischaemia. Recognition of the need for escharotomy is vital and needs to be acted upon, usually within the emergency department or, if immediately available, the operating room. An escharotomy is indicated for relief of pressure in a limb or torso to allow vascular supply or ventilation. Circumferential deep limb burns with a large overall burn area requiring large-volume fluid resuscitation comprise the commonest scenario. The eschar does not expand to accommodate, and so fluid accumulates, and pressure rises. This process takes some time to reach a crescendo – some 6–8 hours. In an awake patient, the same symptoms and signs as a tight plaster cast are complained of:

- Increasing, unbearable, deep aching pain
- Loss of active muscle movement

- Extreme pain with forced stretching of muscle groups
- Cool digits
- Slowed capillary refill
- Loss of digital Doppler signal

The feel of a limb that needs escharotomy can be likened to squeezing an apple – no give. It is common for limbs to be firm, but if there is 'give', escharotomy is not (yet) indicated. If pulses are lost and there is still 'give' to palpation, first check another limb and the blood pressure. Hypovolaemia may be the cause.

An escharotomy (skin) is not necessarily
a fasciotomy (fascia).

The technique is simple. A warmed operating room is preferable, though not required, for performance of an escharotomy; but good lighting, instruments to achieve haemostasis, and preferably an assistant are. In an awake patient, local anaesthetic injected proximally and into areas of a partial-thickness burn makes the procedure quite possible. A full-thickness burn is insensate. A scalpel, artery forceps, sutures, and ligatures should be at hand; diathermy is a good alternative in the ventilated patient.

Incisions are made in the axial planes. The upper limb wishes to be in a pronated position when oedematous, so it must be forced into full supination; otherwise, the incisions can easily cross flexure creases, leading to division of longitudinal structures and contracture. An antimicrobial cream is applied to the wounds, and a non-stick absorbent dressing loosely bandaged.

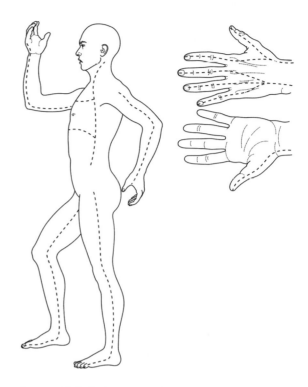

Figure 13.8 Escharotomy sites.

Pitfall

If the procedure has been delayed, efflux of metabolites will cause hypotension and hyperkalaemia. Be prepared!

Linear incisions are made to allow the escharotomy wounds to gape apart, relieving the tension. The escharotomy wounds must be extensive enough to reach normal tissue. Although a scalpel is usually adequate to achieve this, diathermy may be necessary.

Figure 13.8 shows the main incision lines for the release of eschar causing constriction. Escharotomy should be a largely painless procedure, as it is only transgressing devitalized tissue, except at its limits where it may encroach upon living tissues which will be normally sensate, or even hypersensate. This not only will alert the clinician to stop but also ensures that constriction rings of dead eschar are not left at the limits of the escharotomy.

Pitfall

Despite escharotomy release, some tissues – especially in limbs – may remain ischaemic, particularly where there has been an electrical burn, which is always full thickness and frequently produces significant myonecrosis. In these cases, it may be necessary to extend the escharotomy into a fasciotomy to release the compartment syndrome. Fasciotomy is usually accompanied by profuse bleeding if the tissue within is still viable, and it is wise to be prepared for this.

13.7.5 **Definitive Management**

13.7.5.1 **'CLOSING' THE BURN WOUND**

Burns are not static wounds: they are 'pathology-in-evolution'. The longer the burn remains uncovered by either the patient's own skin or an effective biological alternative, the longer it remains a significant breach of the skin's antibacterial barrier and a significant source of heat and fluid loss to the body, analogous to bowel evisceration.

From about 72 hours post burn, surface bacteria migrate into the remaining deep dermis and below, rendering topical antiseptics and antibiotics ineffective, and increasing the chances of systemic septicaemia. For these reasons, there has been a move towards early excision of the wound and SSG where necessary. Clearly, not all burns require grafting. Hot water and scalds from steam will often heal on their own within 10 days, despite their dramatic initial appearances. It is wise to wait for this time before deciding to operate. The SSG rate for these burns has been almost halved by such an approach. However, *all* burns should undergo an initial cleaning and debridement under anaesthesia as soon as possible after admission, preferably within the first 48 hours. The reasons for this are fourfold:

- This cleans the wound thoroughly and enables an appropriate choice of dressing, as clingfilm is difficult to secure for more than 48 hours.
- It allows a proper inspection of the burn and removal of blisters, because it is not unusual for the area of the burn to be underestimated in the emergency room, and a 9% burn may turn out to be 16%, putting it into the 'major burn' category, with all its attendant requirements.
- It is often (wrongly) assumed that blistered burns are always SPT burns. Blistered skin should be removed, unless it is slack, so that the clinician can be sure there is no deeper burn beneath. It is safer to excise the blister and assess the depth of the burn beneath, as it may turn out to be DPT or even full thickness.
- If it is seen that excision and SSG are required, this may be accomplished at the same surgical procedure.

13.7.5.2 TECHNIQUE OF EXCISION AND SPLIT-SKIN GRAFTING (SSG)

Both of these techniques can be accomplished by using either the Humby knife (or a modification of it) or an electric dermatome. The 'set' of the blade (depth of cut) will need to be greater for excision than for the harvesting of skin for SSG.

13.7.5.3 TUMESCENT TECHNIQUE

Blood loss can be significant in both procedures but may be minimized by using tourniquets for the limbs, or the 'tumescent technique' on the torso, if skin availability is problematic.

- The technique uses 2 mL 1:1000 adrenaline (epinephrine) + 40 mL 0.5% plain bupivacaine added to 1000 mL of warm normal saline.
- Take a 19-gauge 3.5-inch spinal needle, and attach a giving set to the bag, which is placed in a pressurized

infusion device or spring-loaded self-filling syringe, and the injection given subdermally.

- The raised skin should feel cold (and look white in Caucasian races).
- Once the skin has been harvested or the burn excised, adrenaline-soaked abdominal packs (5 mg in 1000 mL normal saline) can be applied to the wound bed, with a significant reduction in blood loss.

SSGs are secured by skin clips, tissue glue, or sutures, depending on the site, and then covered with several layers of paraffin gauze to prevent movement, followed by dry gauze and bandaging. Vacuum dressing has become a ready alternative.

If infection has been a problem, activated nanocrystalline silver (e.g., Acticoat®, Smith and Nephew, London, UK) may be applied and secured in place with water-soaked gauze and bandages. The dressing will remain bacterially active for up to 4 days and may also have anti-inflammatory properties.

The choice of site for harvesting skin depends on the site that is burned (e.g., back or eyelids), and what skin is available:

- Neck skin is good for eyelids.
- Inner arm skin is good for the face.
- Wherever possible, match the colour, texture, and hair growth.
- When skin substitutes are not an option, re-harvesting donor sites is usually possible within 10–14 days.
- Scalp skin is thicker, is usually of good quality, and regenerates faster. When all else fails, it will provide an extra source.

13.7.5.4 WOUND COVERAGE

Local burn wound care aims to protect the wound surface, maintain a moist environment, promote burn wound healing, and limit burn wound progression whilst minimizing discomfort for the patient. If needed, topical antimicrobials are used in conjunction with appropriate basic wound care.

Local treatment of burn wounds includes cleansing and debridement and routine burn wound dressing changes, typically incorporating topical antimicrobial agents; however, there is no consensus on which agent or dressing is optimal for burn wound coverage to prevent or control infection or to enhance wound healing (**Table 13.1**).[4]

Wound coverage can be a dilemma. In the first instance, for burns > 30% TBSA, a temporary cover with Biobrane®

Table 13.1 Topical Antimicrobial Agents Used for Burns

Antimicrobial Agents	Clinical Indications	Effectiveness	Contraindications	Adverse Effects
Silver sulphadiazine (1% cream) with or without cerium	• Small, medium, and large surface area burns	• Decreases colonization of wounds • Alleviates pain • Broad spectrum • No evidence to support improved wound healing or reduction in bacterial wound infections	• Burns near eyes • Pregnancy • Breastfeeding • Newborns < 2 months • Allergic to sulphonamides • Signs of re-epithelialization	• Skin hypersensitivity • Neutropenia (usually transient) • Leukopenia (usually transient) • Methemoglobinemia
Silver-containing dressings (e.g., Acticoat and Aquacel Ag)	• Small, medium, and large surface area burns	• Stronger antimicrobial activity, longer duration of action than silver sulphadiazine, some evidence for reduced wound infection rates	• Burns near eyes • Pregnancy • Allergic to silver	• Systemic silver uptake • Temporary staining of the skin
Bacitracin ointment 500 units/gram	• Small surface area burns • Face • Ears • Perineum • Graft sites • Alternative, if allergic to sulphonamides	• Ease of application and of removal • Painless • Frequent dressing changes	• Bacterial resistance • Signs of re-epithelialization	• Yeast colonization • Skin hypersensitivity
Combination antibiotic ointment (e.g., bacitracin, neomycin, and polymyxin B)	• Small surface area burns • Face • Ears • Perineum • Graft sites • Alternative if allergic to sulphonamides	• Ease of application and of removal • Painless • Frequent dressing changes	• Bacterial resistance • Allergic reaction • Signs of re-epithelialization	• Yeast colonization • Skin hypersensitivity • Ototoxicity and nephrotoxicity with neomycin-containing ointments (e.g., Neosporin)
Mupirocin ointment/ Cream 2%	• Small, medium surface area burns • Face • Ears • Nose • Perineum • Alternative if allergic to sulphonamides	• Gram-positive coverage includes methicillin-resistant *Staphylococcus aureus* (MRSA) • Ease of application and of removal • Painless • Frequent dressing changes	• Bacterial resistance • Allergic reaction • Signs of re-epithelialization	• Yeast colonization • Skin hypersensitivity

(Continued)

Table 13.1 (*Continued*) Topical Antimicrobial Agents Used for Burns

Antimicrobial Agents	Clinical Indications	Effectiveness	Contraindications	Adverse Effects
Mafenide (8.5% cream, 5% solution)	• Ears • Nose • Dense bacterial proliferation	• Excellent eschar penetration • Penetrates cartilage • Gram-negative coverage includes *Pseudomonas*	• Burns > 40% total body surface area • Allergic to sulphonamides	• Metabolic acidosis (inhibits carbonic anhydrase) • Painful • Inhibits epithelial regeneration
Chlorhexidine	• Only superficial burns	• Does not interfere with re-epithelialization • Can be used with silver sulphadiazine • Generally used as a cleansing agent	• Deep burns • Caution in neonates – rare association with cutaneous burns	• Skin hypersensitivity
Povidone-iodine	• Small, medium surface area burns	• Only when no other agent is available	• Children under 2 years • Pregnancy • Breastfeeding • Thyroid disorders • Signs of re-epithelialization	• Cytotoxicity (toxic to fibroblasts, reduces cell proliferation) • Painful • Skin hypersensitivities • Chemical burn • Iodine toxicity • Renal failure • Acidosis • Anaphylaxis
Acetic acid	• Antiseptic, topical agent often used in a diluted form as an adjunct in the setting of *Pseudomonas aeruginosa*	• Gram-negative bacteria including *P. aeruginosa*	• Superficial burns have been described from misuse	• High concentrations inhibit epithelialization, inhibit PMNs and fibroblasts

Note: Topical antimicrobial agents may increase risk of host fungal infections. Nystatin ointment or powder may be useful in combination with topical antimicrobials to decrease fungal colonization.

(Mylan, Canonsburg, PA, USA) – a bilaminate biosynthetic skin substitute composed of nylon mesh, coated with porcine collagen peptides bonded to a silicone membrane – serves to seal the excised wound and, in the case of a debrided partial-thickness burn, may well be its final coverage with the wound healing.[5] For excised full-thickness burns, Biobrane has a short life span if applied to fat but longer on fascia. It does need to be replaced by more permanent wound coverage before it goes 'sour', which is characterized by loss of adherence, then fluid accumulation, which then turns to pus in a few days. However, it is expensive, and therefore not accessible to many centres.

Prontosan Gel® may be used as temporary cover.

Versajet II (Smith and Nephew) debridement is frequently used for mid-dermal burns prior to application of Biobrane and for multiple applications with children.[6] It is a hydrodissector that works in some way like a pressure washer combined with suction. It is excellent for preservation of live dermis, and as such, early facial excision and unmeshed allograft have obviated the need for autografting in all but the worst facial burns.

Smaller deep burns are autografted at this stage, with the meshed-versus-unmeshed debate being beyond the scope of this chapter. Less or no mesh expansion gives better cosmesis, especially in people with any skin colour; more frequent seroma/haematoma formation; and less area coverage.

Permanent wound coverage for a large or massive burn usually becomes a patchwork quilt of different applications. Dermal replacement template, widely expanded (1:4) meshed autograft or using a Meek (Humeca, Woodstock, GA, USA) technique with narrow meshed allograft overlay (torso) or unmeshed autograft (face/hands). Originally designed by Cicero Meek, from the University of South Carolina, in 1963, the Meek technique involves using a Meek–Wall microdermatome producing widely expanded postage stamp autografts, in which pre-folded gauzes are used to gain a regular distribution of the autografts. The gauze pleats are pulled out on all the four sides to provide uniform expansion of the islands of grafts. When faced with large surface area burns and limited donor sites, the Meek technique is a satisfactory method to cover large wounds.[7]

- The Meek method provides true expansion up to 9:1.
- Small graft remnants can be utilized.
- Grafting of full-thickness burns up to 70%–75% TBSA becomes possible with one harvest of the donor sites.
- The reliability of graft take is equal or better.
- Epithelialization is achieved within 3–4 weeks, depending on the expansion ratio.

13.7.5.5 BURN WOUND EXCISION AND CLOSURE

The larger the burn, the more quickly it should be removed. In massive burns, operation should proceed as soon as the patient has regained normothermia, passing urine appropriately and coagulation corrected. Blood loss is much decreased if excision takes place within the first 24 hours.

General issues that need to be attended to before commencing a large wound excision include:

- A clear, pre-determined operative plan that encompasses the initial and subsequent procedures, including donor site usage: what is going where, mesh expansion ratio, along with which coverage is temporary and which permanent.
- Large and secure venous access.
- An operating room warmed so that the air surrounding the patient is at least 32° C and preferably much warmer than that (latent heat of evaporation from the moist wound will come from the atmosphere rather than the patient).
- Regular 'checking in' with the anaesthetic team.
- Multiple surgical teams operating simultaneously.
- Frequent use of thromboelastography (TEG)/rotary thromboelastometry (RoTEM).
- Availability of blood and blood products in large quantities.
- Pre-set 'bail-out' endpoints and methods.
- Cold, electrolyte-rich drinks for the operating room staff!

Small burns can be dealt with in a routine operating room set-up as long as the patient is being kept warm.

The following protocol is an example:

- Appropriate antibiotic prophylaxis is used routinely.
- Hair is clipped.
- The wounds are washed with warmed antiseptic solution (aqueous chlorhexidine).
- Normal saline with 1 ampoule of 1:1000 adrenaline is injected subdermally with a 19-gauge needle and Pitkin self-loading syringe. Do not go deeply, as subcutaneous vessels can be severed with loss of the accompanying fat lobule and graft loss.
- Tourniquets are used on limbs with appropriate padding and timekeeping. If the area for tourniquet application is burned, excision of the wound after injection occurs first.
- Excision is affected by either sequential, tangential excision using a hand or powered dermatome or with diathermy in massive and very deep burns. Living dermis is white, and live fat is glistening yellow.

- It is important to finish one small area at a time before moving on, as any bleeding will obscure the detail by staining. Further unnecessary tissue removal may follow.
- Wounds are covered with 1:200,000 adrenaline-soaked dressings, with limbs being wrapped in aqueous chlorhexidine-soaked sponges/lap pads and bandaged.
- Let the tourniquet down!

13.7.6 Assessing and Managing Airway Burns

13.7.6.1 UPPER AIRWAY

Suspicion is the watchword, with early intervention before the opportunity to protect the airway by intubation has been lost. Listening to the respiration is vital, and dyspnoea with hoarse, coarse breathing or stridor should prompt immediate action.

Upper airway burns to the larynx and trachea may be suspected by the history (e.g., a steam valve blew into the face) or by inspection of the mouth, tongue, and oropharynx, which may be red, infected, and swollen. These burns usually require intubation but generally resolve within 36 hours. It is important to remember that the burn is 'pathology-in-evolution' and that the early signs will get worse in the next 24 hours.

13.7.6.2 LOWER AIRWAY

The deep, 'alveolar' burn is much more difficult to detect or predict. The rate of onset is slower, and it may only manifest itself 3–5 days after the burn. Some indication that a lower airway burn is present may come from the history of prolonged smoke exposure and raised COHb levels. Blood gases should be taken whenever possible, and the ventilation–perfusion shunt worked out by plotting the FiO_2 against the PaO_2 (partial pressure of oxygen in arterial blood).

The intubated patient with suspected inhalational injury should have a bronchoscopy performed to assess the degree of injury graded by the Abbreviated Injury Score (AIS 1–4) Increasing AIS is correlated to a higher need of resuscitative fluids in the first 24 hours post-injury. Patients with AIS 3–4 on initial bronchoscopy should have the procedure repeated after 24–48 hours. The optimal management, if possible, is early extubation, thus enabling the patient to clear their own airway. If using inhalation therapy, anticholinergics should be avoided, as these dry the airway and reduce the mobilization of foreign airway particles.

Heparin 10,000 IU 6 hourly nebulization (with or without N-acetyl-cysteine) has been shown in randomized controlled trials (RCTs) to be an effective liberator of inspissated muco-necrotic debris. Additional fluid therapy may be required with pulmonary burns.

13.7.7 Tracheostomy

Early tracheostomy should be considered, especially if the area of the burn includes the neck. It is quite acceptable to place a tracheostomy through the site of a burn. Once the oedema has occurred, placement of a tracheostomy is far more difficult and hazardous. The tracheostomy should be well secured, as if it is displaced, replacement may prove very difficult.

Pitfall

Remember that with neck oedema secondary to the burn, the tracheal tube may be pulled out. Use an adjustable, or long, tracheostomy tube, and do not rely just on fixation to the skin anteriorly.

13.8 SPECIAL AREAS

The face, hands, perineum, and feet are special areas that need special attention to obtain a good outcome.

13.8.1 Face

Biobrane is very useful for SPT burns of the face. It needs to be held in place firmly with compression for 48 hours to 'bond'. This may be accomplished by crepe bandaging, which is then removed after 2 days. Biobrane reduces pain and may be left in place until it begins to separate by itself after about 10 days, leaving new epithelium that does not need to be grafted. Unmeshed allograft is also used for deep partial-thickness facial burns after Versajet debridement in much the same way.

13.8.2 Hands

Function is the priority for burned hands. Wrapping up in boxing glove–type dressings will rapidly result in stiff, contracted hands, so whenever possible leave the hands exposed or with minimal dressings. The practice of smothering burned hands in silver sulphadiazine cream and then placing them in plastic bags is not recommended. Superficial partial-thickness burns can be covered with copious amounts of mupirocin ointment to combat staphylococcal and streptococcal infection, keep the burn supple, and allow the occupational therapist the freedom to work without restriction. Deeper burns to the hand may be covered with a biosynthetic dressing such as Biobrane.

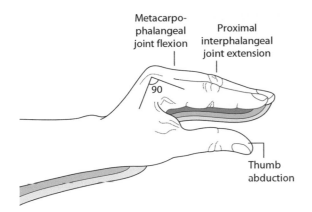

Figure 13.9 Functional position of the hand.

If escharotomy is needed, it is important to try to preserve the 'pinch grip' between finger and thumb. For this reason, the incisions should be on the ulnar side of the thumb, and the radial side of the fingers. It may be necessary to splint the hand at night to prevent contracture. This must be done in the 'intrinsic-plus' or 'position of function', with the wrist slightly dorsiflexed, the meta carpophalangeal joints at a right angle, and the fingers in full extension (**Figure 13.9**).

The splint is best applied from the palmar surface and wrapped gently around the edges of the index and little fingers to stop them falling off the splint platform. It is important to place paraffin gauze between the fingers on the splint to prevent adherence to each other, with the potential for later syndactyly.

13.8.3 **Perineum**

Early catheterization is recommended, as is nursing by exposure as much as possible. Nappies/diapers coated with silver sulphdiazine cream are comfortable and practical, for both adults and children. Chlorhexidine gluconate and nystatin can be added to the mix. A temporary colostomy for faecal diversion should be considered.

13.8.4 **Feet**

Apart from preventing syndactyly, as mentioned previously, the importance of burns to the feet is the ability to be able to weight-bear, and to prevent foot-drop during the recovery period. Splints will be needed to maintain the ankle joint at a right angle.

Weight-bearing on a SSG will rapidly result in destruction of the graft. If a full-thickness burn of the sole of the foot is present, it may take the skills of a reconstructive plastic surgeon to embark on lengthy cross-leg flap procedures to obtain adequate coverage that will withstand body weight. In resource-constrained countries, a below-knee amputation may seem a drastic measure, but frequently returns the patient to work and their family quicker.

13.9 **ADJUNCTS IN BURN CARE**

13.9.1 **Nutrition in the Burned Patient[8]**

A dietitian is an essential member of the burns team. All patients with a major burn (> 20% TBSA) should have a nasogastric tube or fine-bore feeding tube for early enteral nutrition. This should ideally be started within 18 hours of the burn. Not only does this help in the early replacement, but it also protects against gut bacterial translocation and systemic sepsis. The best way to determine calorie requirement is by indirect calorimetry performed on a regular basis whilst in a post-absorptive state. Oxygen consumption and carbon dioxide production are measured, and a formula produces resting energy expenditure, thereby enabling nutritional supplementation to be accurately delivered to the individual as they progress through the post-burn state.

Estimating the nutritional needs of burn patients is essential to the healing process.[9] There is no single formula that can accurately determine how many calories a patient needs, so it is important to monitor a patient's nutritional condition closely. Using a metabolic cart is the most accurate way to determine needs and tailor the nutrition to the recovery phase.

Protein requirements generally increase more than energy requirements and appear to be related to the amount of lean body mass. The body loses protein through the burn, and this will be reflected in a significant drop in serum albumin level over the first week, which will take at least a month to recover despite assiduous nutritional care. However, most increased protein requirements come from muscle breakdown for use in extra energy production. Providing an increased intake of protein does not stop this obligatory breakdown; it simply provides the materials needed to replace lost tissue.

Carbohydrates provide the majority of calorie intake under most conditions, including the stress of burns. Providing adequate calories from carbohydrates spares incoming protein from being used for fuel. The body breaks down carbohydrates into glucose that the body then uses for energy.

Fat is needed to meet essential fatty acid requirements and provide needed calories. Common recommendations include giving 30% of calories as fat, although this can be higher if needed (40%) in the recovery phase. Excess fat intake has been implicated in decreased immune function, and intake levels should be monitored carefully. Vitamins and trace elements are also necessary.

13.9.1.1 PAEDIATRIC BURN NUTRITION

Providing adequate calories and nutrients is a difficult task when treating burn injuries. This task becomes even more difficult when the patient is a child.

13.9.2 Ulcer Prophylaxis[10]

(See also Chapter 17 on critical care.)

Good, early (within 24 hours) enteral nutrition may in addition protect against the development of stress ulceration.

In the presence of good nutritional policies, sucralfate should be used for prophylaxis. H_2 receptor-blockers and protein pump inhibitors should be reserved for therapy, and **not** used for prophylaxis, especially in the ventilated patient in whom nosocomial and *Candida* ventilator-associated pneumonia (VAP) is a major risk factor.

13.9.3 Venous Thromboembolism Prophylaxis[11]

(See also Section 17.15.2.)

Patients with major burns are at high risk of venous thromboembolism. Venous thromboembolic prophylaxis is often forgotten. Sequential compression devices can be placed over burns and grafts with impunity, and fractionated heparin is needed in startlingly high doses. Anti-factor Xa levels can be used to titrate the dose to achieve 0.2–0.4 U/mL.[12]

A range of 30–80 mg every 12 hours is required.

13.9.4 Vitamin C

Vitamin C infusion carries level II and III evidence as support, although it is not universally accepted.[13]

- Consider a continuous ascorbic acid (vitamin C) infusion (66 mg/kg/hour for 24 hours) in burn patients sustaining injury ≥ 30% TBSA.
- Infusion should be begun within 6 hours of burn injury.
- The fluid volume associated with the ascorbic acid infusion should be included in the total volume of fluid resuscitation calculated according to the Parkland formula.
- Total fluid volume infused, with rate adjusted to maintain a urine output in adults of 50–100 mL/hour.
- Point-of-care glucose testing becomes inaccurate during and after vitamin C infusion, and therefore serum glucose levels are required.

13.9.5 Anabolic Steroids[14]

Use of oxandrolone, an anabolic steroid, is also well supported by evidence. Decreased time to donor-site healing, decreased weight and nitrogen loss, and additional gain in lean body mass are all significant. A dose of 0.1 mg/kg/day in divided doses has been established.

13.9.6 Antibiotics

Antibiotic prophylaxis is **not** routinely used for burns; however, the great difficulty with burns patients is differentiating inflammation from infection. There is no substitute for good wound care, hand-washing, and infection control measures, including good microbiological surveillance, and when treatment is deemed appropriate it should be, when possible, goal directed and of short duration. Tissue excised during tangential excision should be sent for culture, and, when skin-grafting, cultures (sometimes obtained by local punch biopsy) should again be sent. The risk of fungal infection is high in these patients, and this should be taken into consideration with those patients who are not responding to broad therapy antibiotic treatment.

13.9.7 **Other Adjuncts**

- Bowel management is mundane but germane. Evacuation of hard stool, instillation of aperients such as sorbitol 30 mL every 8 hours until a liquid stool is forthcoming, followed by insertion of a faecal management system have made everyone's life easier and decrease the amount of faecal wound contamination considerably.
- Preventing pressure on burned ears is a constant battle but imperative, as cosmetic defects result from pressure necrosis. Foam covered with plastic with a central cut-out when side-rolled helps.
- Tube security is problematic when facial burns are present. The tie will cause pressure and an unsightly line of scar in partial-thickness wounds.
- Propranolol, a non-selective beta blocker, binds to beta receptors on skeletal, muscle, and fat cells and decreases proteolysis and lipolysis. This treatment is particularly efficacious in the young and is dosed to an endpoint of a decrease in heart rate of 25% below resting. Four times daily administration is often needed for children, as the burn response leads to a much-shortened half-life.

13.10 **PALLIATIVE CARE FOR BURNS**[15,16]

Burns in LMICs, and even in high-income countries, that are extensive or with mass-casualty burn incidents may require triaging of the patients who have a very low chance of survival. Patients should be allowed to have an airway secured but may not necessarily be ventilated, and just enough fluid is administered to allow sufficient analgesia infusions to be provided. They should be catheterized and the family allowed to be present, along with social and spiritual support. The 'lethal-dose 50' is a useful cutoff and will vary per location. Keep in mind that inhalation injury per se increases the risk of death by around 15%. Two recent review papers give some practical advice on how to manage the palliation process.

13.11 **SUMMARY**

Burns are a huge problem worldwide, with the majority occurring in countries that are ill-equipped to deal with them as resources are few, transport is lacking, and cultural influences militate against early referral to modern facilities. Education is the cornerstone of prevention, and up to 95% of burns in developing countries are preventable.

Burn care remains a 'team effort', and no amount of highly skilled grafting in the operating room will be rewarded by a happy and functional outcome if the feeding, nursing, intensive care, physiotherapy, or occupational therapy is lacking.

REFERENCES

1. Vos T, Abajobir AA, Abate KH, Abbafati C, Abbas KM, Abd-Allah F, et al. Global, regional, and national incidence, prevalence, and years lived with disability for 328 diseases and injuries for 195 countries, 1990–2016: a systematic analysis for the Global Burden of Disease Study. 2016. *The Lancet*. 2017;390(10100):1211–1259.
2. Gibran NS, Wiechman S, Meyer W, et al. Summary of the 2012 ABA Burn Quality Consensus Conference. *J Burn Care Res*. 2013;34(4):361–385.
3. Rogers AD, Karpelowsky J, Millar AJW, Argent A, Rode H. Fluid creep in major paediatric burns. *Eur J Pediatr Surg*. 2010,**20**.133–138.
4. Topical agents and dressings for local wound care: https://www.uptodate.com/contents/topical-agents-and-dressings-for-local-burn-wound-care?sectionName=Dressings&search=parklandformula&topicRef=350&anchor=H2088109107&source=see_link#H2088109107. (accessed September 2023)
5. Tan H, Wasiak J, Paul E, Cleland H: Effective use of Biobrane® as a temporary wound dressing prior to definitive slit-skin graft in the treatment of severe: A retrospective analysis. *Burns*. 41(5):969–976. doi: 10.1016/j.burns.2014.07.015. (accessed September 2023).
6. Smith and Nephew Versajet. Details available from: http://www.smith-nephew.com/key-products/advanced-wound-management/versajet/. (accessed online January 2019)
7. Heidekrueger, P.I., Broer, P.N., Ninkovic, M. (2017). The Meek Technique in the Treatment of Burns. In: Shiffman, M., Low, M. (eds.). *Burns, Infections and Wound Management. Recent Clinical Techniques, Results, and Research in Wounds*, vol 2. Springer, Cham. https://doi.org/10.1007/15695_2017_29
8. Jacobs DO, Kudsk KA, Oswanski MF, Sacks GS, Sinclair KE. Practice management guidelines for nutritional support of the trauma patient. In *Eastern Association for the Surgery of Trauma. Practice Management Guidelines*. Available from www.east.org (accessed January 2019).
9. Burn nutrition calculator. Available from: https://surgicalcriticalcare.net/burn_nutrition.html (accessed online September 2023))

10. Stress Ulcer Prophylaxis. A Surgicalcriticalcare.net Guideline. 2023. https://surgicalcriticalcare.net/Guidelines/Stress%20Ulcer%20Prophylaxis%202023.pdf. (accessed September 2023).

11. Venous thromboembolism prophylaxis in surgery and trauma patients. SurgicalCriticalCare.net. 2023. https://surgicalcriticalcare.net/Guidelines/DVT%20prophy-laxis%202023.pdf. (accessed September 2023).

12. Lin H, Faraklas I, Cochran A, Saffle J. Enoxaparin and anti-factor Xa levels in acute burn patients. *J Burn Care Res.* 2011; 31(1):1–5.

13. Nakajima M, Kojiro M, Aso S, Matsui H, Fushimi K, Kaita Y, et al. Effect of high-dose vitamin C therapy on severe burn patients: a nationwide cohort study. *Crit Care.* 2019;23:407. doi: 10.1186/s13054-019-2693-1

14. Li H, Guo Y, Yang Z, Roy M, Guo Q. The efficacy and safety of oxandrolone treatment for patients with severe burns: A systematic review and meta-analysis. *Burns.* 2016;42(4):717–727.

15. Den Hollander D, Albertyn R, Ambler J. Palliation, end-of-life care and burns; concepts, decision-making and communication – A narrative review. *African Journal of Emergency Medicine.* 2020;**10(2)**:95–98, https://doi.org/10.1016/j.afjem.2020.01.003.

16. Den Hollander D, Albertyn R, Ambler J. Palliation, end-of-life care and burns; practical issues, spiritual care, and care of the family – A narrative review II, *African Journal of Emergency Medicine.* 2020;**10(4)**:256–260. https://doi.org/10.1016/j.afjem.2020.07.011.

RECOMMENDED READING

Greenwood JE. Development of patient pathways for the surgical management of burn injury. *A NZ J Surg.* 2006;**76**: 805–11.

Herndon D, Ed. *Total Burn Care.* 3rd Edition. 2007. Saunders Elsevier. Philadelphia PA.

Orgill DP. Excision and skin grafting of thermal burns. *N Engl J Med.* 2009 Feb 26;**360**(**9**):893–901. doi: 10.1056/NEJMct0804451.

Tenenhaus M, Rennekampff H-O. Topical agents and dressings for local burn wound care. https://www.uptodate.com/contents/topical-agents-and-dressings-for-local-burn-wound-care?sectionName=Dressings&search=parklandformula&topicRef=350&anchor=H2088109107&source=see_link#H2088109107.

Vercruysse GA, Alam HB, Martin MMJ, Brasel K, Moore EE, Brown CV, et al. Western Trauma Association critical decisions in trauma: Preferred triage and initial management of the burned patient. *J Trauma Acute Care Surg.* 2019 Nov; 87(5): 1239–1243. doi: 10.1097/TA.0000000000002348

Special Patient Situations **14**

14.1 PAEDIATRIC TRAUMA

14.1.1 Introduction

Unintentional injury is the most common cause of death in children throughout the world. In most countries, blunt trauma, often caused by falls or traffic-related accidents, constitute more than 90% of injuries. However, gunshots are now the leading cause of death of children under 12 years of age in the United States.[1,2]

Many will be treated in a hospital with limited expertise in paediatric trauma care. Paediatric anatomy and physiology have potential clinical implications, and the need for referral should be considered as soon as the patient will tolerate safe transfer to an appropriate facility.

The provider caring for a traumatically injured paediatric patient must be aware of key differences, such as management of the paediatric airway, the risk for hypothermia, and pliable rib cage and significant pulmonary contusion in the absence of rib fractures. Some critical points in adult management have significantly contributed to paediatric trauma management, including balanced resuscitation strategies, early use of blood products, prophylaxis of venous thromboembolism, and, more recently, use of whole blood instead of component therapy. Similarly, some paediatric trauma strategies have changed the way adult patients are managed including non-operative management of solid organ injury.

14.1.2 Injury Patterns

Certain injury patterns of paediatric trauma are well recognized:[1,2]

- Lap belt complex
  - Pancreatic contusion or transection from epigastric blow
  - *Duodenal injury*: Typically, haematoma

- Chance fracture of the lumbar spine
- Horizontal contusion of the anterior abdominal wall
- It is important to note that such injuries could be minimized by proper use of appropriate child restraints in vehicles. These include four-point harnesses for babies and booster seats for older children.
- Liver and spleen injury
- Pedestrian–vehicle crash (PVC) complex
- Forward-facing infant complex (small children should not be placed in a seat with an active airbag as the force of the airbag may cause serious damage to the small child)
- Flexion fracture of the cervical spine (which occurs most commonly in the upper cervical vertebrae)
- Flexion fracture of the cervical spine
- *The common bicycle scenarios*:
  - Handlebar in the epigastrium, and splenic, liver, duodenal, or pancreatic injury
  - The fall astride with urethral or perineal injury
- *Non-accidental injury (NAI)*: Injury patterns suggestive of NAI are very well known. The most vulnerable group with the highest mortality rates is infants. The presence of a severe head injury in an infant without a clear history of a fall from a significant height or a vehicle collision should always arouse suspicion. Other suspicious injuries include a femur fracture or multiple rib fractures in a child who is not yet able to walk, or multiple fractures/bruises of different ages.

Pitfall

Child abuse is far more common than appreciated. A high index of suspicion should be applied to all trauma cases. Unless there is hypervigilance, a child may be treated and sent back to the abusive environment that brought him or her to hospital.

DOI: 10.1201/9781003258124-17

14.1.3 Pre-Hospital

Pre-hospital interventions should be limited to basic life support with airway and ventilatory support, securing haemostasis of external bleeding, and basic attempts to secure vascular access. Extensive unsuccessful roadside resuscitative procedures are a common cause of morbidity and mortality. The younger the child and the more unstable his or her condition, the greater the tendency should be to 'scoop and run' to the nearest **appropriate** facility.

If a haemodynamically unstable child is treated at an interim facility prior to transfer for definitive care, care should be taken to avoid unnecessary imaging without immediate therapeutic consequence, particularly computed tomography (CT) scanning, to avoid delay in reaching definitive care.

Pitfall

Avoid increasing radiation exposure by doing unnecessary X-rays, or X-rays that may need to be repeated by the receiving facility.

14.1.4 Resuscitation Room

14.1.4.1 AIRWAY

The indications for airway control are identical to those in the adult patient. The routine administration of oxygen and the stepwise system of management according to severity of airway compromise are the cardinal features of paediatric airway management. Orotracheal intubation without force, done by an experienced anaesthesiologist, will minimize the post-extubation stridor that can result from a traumatic intubation. A surgical airway is seldom necessary. If it is required, a tracheostomy should be performed.

In a trauma setting, a cricothyroidotomy is the appropriate surgical airway in older children. As noted in the current (10th) edition of Advanced Trauma Life Support (ATLS®), a surgical airway is rarely indicated in infants or small children. It can be performed in older children who have a palpable cricoid membrane, typically children older than 12 years of age. Potential complications include creation of a false passage, haemorrhage, and laryngeal and tracheal trauma with subsequent stenosis and vocal cord paralysis.

Pitfalls

- Ensure that appropriate supplies, suction, medication, and endotracheal tube sizes are **next to you** prior to attempts at intubation.
- The anterior airway in children is critical to intubation. Proper positioning with a shoulder roll whilst still maintaining cervical spine stabilization is essential and can ensure appropriate visualization of the airway.
- Surgical airways can be performed in older children who have a palpable cricoid membrane, typically children older than 12 years of age.
- The danger of tube dislodgement is commonly due to failure to secure the tube adequately, or the endotracheal tube may be too small. Re-assess placement frequently and after each time the patient is moved.
- Secure the very small endotracheal tube with soft adhesive tape, rather than the standard 'trachy tape' which may kink the small, soft tube.
- The airway of the obligate nasal breather (the neonate or infant) must not be compromised with a nasogastric tube.

The cervical spine (C-spine) in children can be cleared by a combination of the National Emergency X-Radiography Utilization Study (NEXUS) low-risk criteria and the Canadian C-Spine Rule. Caution is advised for nonverbal and/or unconscious children.[3] In these children, plain radiographs should be performed. If these images are inadequate or show hints suggesting bony injury, a CT of the C-spine should be considered. Magnetic resonance imaging (MRI) is used to evaluate ligamentous integrity and to evaluate the spinal cord in cases of suspected contusion.

There are numerous scoring systems that guide the clinician as to whether to do a CT brain in the child with a mild TBI (traumatic brain injury). The most validated of these is the Pediatric Emergency Care Applied Research Network (PECARN) guidelines, and these have been adopted by ATLS.[4]

If the child is getting a CT brain, one can include the first three cervical vertebrae. Many C-spine injuries in children occur at this location, and it avoids radiation across the thyroid which may be associated with thyroid cancer later in life. The rest of the C-spine can be imaged by plain film, as mentioned above. Plain films in children have better yields than in adults.

There is much debate about the ability to rule out C-spine injury in the obtunded child who cannot be examined. Children are at higher risk of ligamentous injury, which may not be detected by a normal CT view. As such, some units would routinely do an MRI, whereas others would maintain spine motion restriction until the child wakes up and can be assessed clinically.

14.1.4.2 BREATHING

Hypoventilation is a prominent cause of hypoxia in the injured child. Because the child depends primarily on diaphragmatic breathing, one must be particularly cautious of conditions that impair diaphragmatic movement (tension pneumothoraces, diaphragmatic rupture, and severe gastric dilatation) and treat expeditiously. Always apply an end-tidal CO_2 monitor.

Clinically relevant haemothorax or pneumothorax should be addressed with tube thoracostomy. The compliant paediatric chest wall predisposes children to underlying pulmonary contusion, often *without* rib fractures.

14.1.4.3 CIRCULATION

Frequent assessment of circulatory status is important. Children have effective compensatory mechanisms for compensating for blood loss, depending predominantly on an adequate heart rate. Tachycardia, peripheral vasoconstriction, and signs of inadequate central nervous system perfusion predominate. Hypotension is a late sign of blood loss, reflecting a class IV shock with greater than 40% blood volume loss.[5] It is for this reason that it is generally not recommended to target hypotensive resuscitation as is recommended in adults.

The practitioner must recognize and treat shock aggressively. The primary management of bleeding is surgical haemostasis. Rapid vascular access is obtained, tailored to the severity of the child's shock and the practitioner's experience: a peripheral line is considered adequate for initial resuscitation. If a peripheral line cannot be obtained, an intraosseous line should be the fallback option and is well tolerated in children with a low complication rate. Central lines are reserved for the larger child and the more experienced physician. Although most children respond rapidly to crystalloid resuscitation, early use of blood products in a child with hypovolaemic shock and ongoing bleeding is indicated.

Tip

Limit crystalloid administration in bleeding patients to a single bolus of 20 mL/kg, then switch to blood if necessary. Adhere to a balanced transfusion ratio, aiming for 1:1:1 fresh frozen plasma (FFP), packed red blood cells (pRBCs), and platelets (PLTs). Initiate a massive transfusion protocol if > 40 mL/kg product administration is anticipated. If initiating massive transfusion, administer tranexamic acid (TXA) (1 g or 15 mg/kg dosing within 3 hours of injury, followed by continuous IV infusion at 2 mg/kg/h for >8 h or until bleeding stops).[6]

Resuscitative endovascular balloon occlusion of the aorta (REBOA) can be considered in the adolescent as a bridge to definitive care or embolization in unstable patients with pelvic fractures or catastrophic intra-abdominal bleeding. A femoral artery diameter of at least 6 mm is required to accommodate the French gauge (FG) 7 sheath, and the balloon should be slowly and cautiously inflated to the point of occlusion to avoid vascular injury to the smaller-calibre aorta. FG 4 units are becoming available (Cobra-OS®, Frontline Medical Technologies, London, ONT, Canada).[7]

Do not delay the transfer of the unstable child to the operating room – establish good access, and the anaesthesiologist can resuscitate whilst the surgeon stops the bleeding. **Never** transfer a haemodynamically unstable patient to the CT scanner. Hypothermia during resuscitation and transfer must be avoided. The urinary output is an invaluable aid to determine the adequacy of resuscitation after the initial phase.

The Western Trauma Association (WTA) algorithm for paediatric emergency resuscitative thoracotomy (ERT) is shown in **Figures 14.1** and **14.2**.

14.1.4.4 DISABILITY

Make a quick neurological assessment including the Glasgow Coma Scale (GCS) score, pupils, and movements of all extremities. The GCS of an infant or toddler is a modified scale to be more appropriate to their developmental stage (see **Table 14.1**).

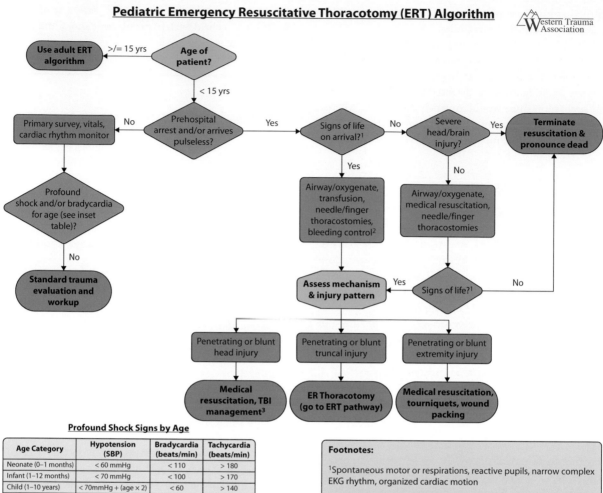

Figure 14.1 Western Trauma Association (WTA) algorithm for paediatric resuscitative thoracotomy.

14.1.4.5 CARDIAC ARREST

In children, cardiac arrest usually is not caused by ventricular fibrillation, and is often heralded by bradycardia, pulseless electrical activity, or asystole. The primary objective of resuscitation should be to correct the underlying cause (such as tension pneumothorax, hypovolaemia, hypothermia, or hypoxia). If return of spontaneous circulation is not achieved, resuscitative thoracotomy is indicated; however, the success rate in patients with cardiac arrest after blunt trauma is low.

14.1.5 Specific Organ Injury

14.1.5.1 HEAD INJURY

Head injury remains the leading cause of traumatic death in children. The medical and surgical management of paediatric TBI aims to minimize secondary brain injury and is based on the results of serial neurologic examination, radiographic evaluation, and, in severe TBI, invasive monitoring.

Diffuse brain injury occurs commonly in children. Surgery is recommended for mass lesions, neurologic

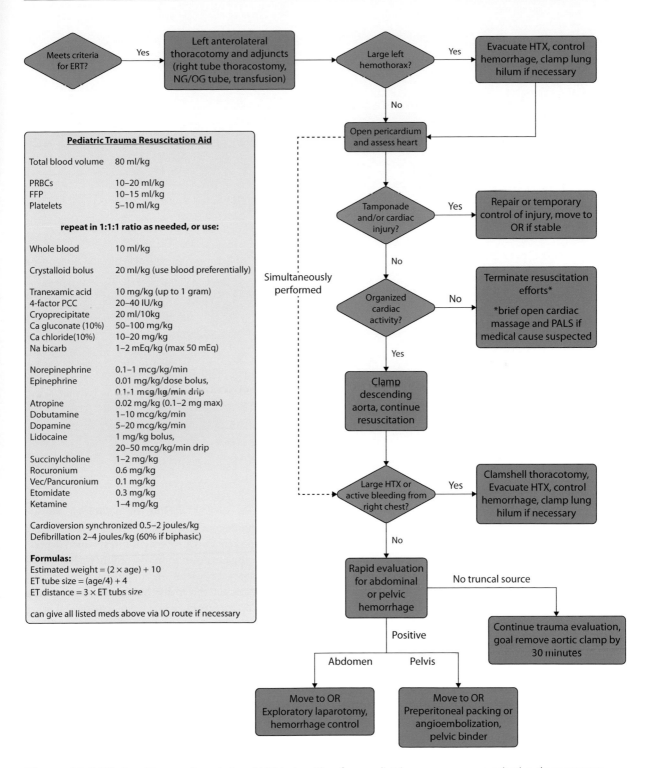

Figure 14.2 Western Trauma Association (WTA) algorithm for paediatric emergency resuscitative thoracotomy (RT) sequence.

Table 14.1 Paediatric Glasgow Coma Scale (PGCS)

	> 1 Year			< 1 Year	Score
Eye opening	Spontaneously			Spontaneously	4
	To verbal command			To shout	3
	To pain			To pain	2
	No response			No response	1
Motor response	Obeys			Spontaneous	6
	Localizes pain			Localizes pain	5
	Flexion-withdrawal			Flexion-withdrawal	4
	Flexion abnormal (decorticate rigidity)			Flexion abnormal (decorticate rigidity)	3
	Extension (decerebrate rigidity)			Extension (decerebrate rigidity)	2
	No response			No response	1
Verbal response	> 5 Years	2–5 years		0–23 months	
	Orientated	Appropriate words / phrases		Smiles / Coos appropriately	5
	Disorientated / Confused	Inappropriate words		Cries but is consolable	4
	Inappropriate words	Persistent cries and screams		Persistent inappropriate crying and screaming	3
	Incomprehensible sounds	Grunts		Grunts, agitated, restless	2
	No response	No response		No response	1
Total paediatric Glasgow Coma Scale (3–15/15)					

deterioration, and/or clinical evidence of herniation. Specific clinical markers of deterioration or herniation include pupillary dilation, bradycardia with uncal and trans-tentorial herniation, hemiplegia with uncal and subfalcine herniation, and stereotyped responses to painful stimuli with brainstem compromise. Any new neurologic deficit or sign of herniation should be considered a neurologic emergency that warrants re-evaluation for further medical or surgical intervention.

In general, children have a lower incidence of intracranial mass lesions requiring surgical drainage after blunt injury compared with adults. Signs of sudden neurologic deterioration must prompt urgent neurosurgical evaluation and CT scan that supersede all other priorities except the management of the airway and the treatment of hypovolaemic shock.[8]

CT is the most accurate imaging modality to evaluate paediatric patients with a suspected head injury. Repeat CT head is indicated in mild TBI patients in association with a decline in neurologic status. Electroencephalogram (EEG) and MRI are appropriate adjuncts in patients with persistent unexplained depression of neurologic examination discordant with CT findings. Laboratory evaluation in the initial management of TBI focusses on the identification of coagulopathy that can exacerbate intracranial haemorrhage and other metabolic derangements associated with worsened outcomes (hyponatraemia and hyperglycaemia).

Blunt cerebrovascular injury (BCVI) in children is relatively rare but occurs more commonly than previously recognized and, when accompanied by vessel occlusion and infarction, can be catastrophic. BCVI screening in children is an area of active research, as utilization of the adult screening criteria can result in over-exposure to radiation.[9] Skull base fracture had the strongest association with BCVI, and additional significant associations included C-spine and mandible fractures. Patients with a vehicular mechanism of injury and a low GCS (≤ 8) should be considered for cranio-cervical CT angiography.

Pitfall

Over-diagnosing 'raised intracranial pressure' on the CT head of a child. Remember that normally a child's brain fills the cranium more than in an adult, and relative 'attenuation' of sulci can be normal.

The risk of radiation and subsequent mutagenesis and cancer in children comprise an important factor to consider. **One should always employ the ALARA principle ('As Low As Reasonably Achievable')** when imaging children. CT scan is associated with the highest radiation dose, and its necessity must carefully be considered before its utilization. An ultrasound of the abdomen may be technically easier due to less abdominal wall tissue, but the fluid volume required to be 'positive' is far less, and often missed. If CT scan is going to be used as a modality, consider reducing the phases (e.g., 'Is a delayed phase really required?') and the dosing schedule.

A resource is available online to guide these techniques: www.imagegently.org[10]

Therapeutic hypothermia has not been shown to be of benefit in paediatric TBI. The Cool Kids study was one of the largest to look at this and was terminated early due to futility.[11]

14.1.5.2 THORACIC INJURY

Young children have a more flexible thoracic cage than adults. Rib fractures in children are uncommon and indicate major injury. Rib fractures in a child < 3 years old without major mechanism are highly suspicious for NAI. Pulmonary contusion is the most common injury to the chest and is commonly seen in the absence of rib fractures. Contusions are typically delayed in appearance on chest X-ray. If pathological findings (of pulmonary contusion) are visible on the admission chest X-ray, then the contusion is severe, and hypoxia should be expected to worsen over the next 1–2 days. Aortic injury is rare in children due to the elasticity of the aorta.

In the unstable child, performing extended focussed assessment with sonography for trauma (eFAST) can provide important information in assessing the causes of shock (e.g., cardiac tamponade, tension pneumothorax, etc.), with no radiation and with little to no delay in treatment.[12]

Pitfall

Intercostal drains require a specific technique of insertion. Because of the thin chest wall of a child, there will not be enough tissue to create an air seal around the tube, nor enough tissue to close the defect properly when removing the tube. As a result, always make the incision approximately 1½–2 rib spaces below the intercostal space you intend to use and tunnel the chest tube over the ribs and into the intercostal space.

14.1.5.3 ABDOMINAL INJURY[13]

Abdominal injuries must be suspected after high-energy trauma. The upper abdominal organs have little protection from the rib cage and musculature. Not surprisingly, the spleen and the liver are the most frequently injured intra-abdominal organs in children. Most children with abdominal injuries from blunt trauma can be safely treated non-operatively. For the trauma surgeon, the challenge is to identify expeditiously those patients who require surgical intervention. Patients with haemoperitoneum and haemodynamic instability not responding to resuscitation, those with clear signs of peritonitis or bowel injury as evidenced by free intraperitoneal air, or those with penetrating abdominal trauma should be explored urgently. Diaphragmatic rupture and intraperitoneal bladder rupture are other early indications for surgery.

Hollow viscus injuries are relatively rare, and symptoms can be vague in the early stage after trauma. Repeated examination remains essential in the early diagnosis of these injuries. Free fluid in the absence of solid organ injury on a CT scan in a patient with an appropriate injury mechanism (e.g., lap belt injury) is highly indicative of an intestinal lesion. A lap belt sign should almost mandate a CT scan of the abdomen due to its high association with abdominal injuries. Associated chance fractures of lumbar spine are frequently related to these injuries.

Duodenal injuries are uncommon, with diagnosis often being delayed and associated with serious complications. In the absence of significant trauma, a duodenal injury in a child under 2 years should arouse suspicions of child abuse.

Pancreatic injuries are rare, and diagnosis often is delayed. Contusions can be treated non-operatively. The management of the patient with the CT appearance of transection through the body of the gland (AAST grade II injuries) is controversial. Conservative treatment appears to give results that are equivalent to distal pancreatectomy with preservation of pancreatic function.[14]

14.1.5.4 GENITOURINARY INJURY

The hallmark of genitourinary tract injury is haematuria. However, the degree of haematuria does not correlate with injury severity, and the absence of blood in the urine does not exclude significant urological injury. The kidneys are most involved. Less than 5% of children with renal injuries will need operative treatment. A CT scan of the abdomen is highly sensitive and specific, although it does not reliably exclude bladder rupture unless dedicated cystography views with bladder distension are obtained. Genital trauma in children should always have sexual abuse ruled out as a cause.

14.1.5.5 PELVIC INJURY

Pelvic fractures in children are typically due to mechanisms that exert significant force on the pelvic ring, such as a pedestrian struck by a motor vehicle. The ATLS primary and secondary surveys are stressed even more to ensure that there is no missed injury, as up to half of all pelvic fractures in children have an associated musculoskeletal, head, or visceral injury. In addition, the pelvis can hold a significant volume of blood, and children can exsanguinate due to a missed or untreated pelvic injury. Placement of a pelvic binder as described in this volume can be a life-saving measure and tamponade the haemorrhage associated with pelvic injuries. Identification of the pelvic injury radiographically can assist with appropriate reduction and treatment modalities.

14.1.5.6 SPINE INJURY

Ligamentous laxity in paediatric spines may lead to significant movement of the vertebrae without any fracture of the vertebrae. Spinal cord damage may occur during the movement but will not be indicated on X-ray or CT scan due to the lack of fractures or subluxation. Such injury (known as SCIWORA, or spinal cord injury without radiologic abnormality) is more common in children. Pseudo-subluxation may also occur in the upper cervical vertebrae for the same reason.

14.1.5.7 SUSPECTED NON-ACCIDENTAL INJURY (NAI)

Successful management of the abused child requires recognition at the level of treating providers as well as institutional support and resources for the provision of the appropriate medical, social, and psychological support. It is critical for physicians to feel the moral responsibility of being mandatory reporters of such injuries in abused children as well as being willing to discharge the often-onerous legal duties that such cases usually entail. In the ideal circumstances, physicians do not have to accuse any party of deliberate injury to the child but merely raise the alarm on its possibility so that the case can be satisfactorily investigated.

History that is suggestive of abuse includes:

- History does not match the mechanism required for the injury.
- Differing or changing history from the same person or different people.
- Multiple medical visits at different hospitals.
- Delay in seeking medical care.

Some specific injury patterns unique to abuse include:

- Burns to the buttocks and feet. This is from a forced immersion into hot water. (See **Figure 14.3**.)
- Subdural haematoma in a child too young to walk and fall onto head. This is a classic feature of the 'shaken baby syndrome'. Features of this syndrome also include retinal haemorrhages, and a fundoscopy should be carried out in suspected cases.
- 'Bucket handle' fractures of the epiphysis from man-handling a child. (See **Figure 14.4**.)

14.1.6 Analgesia

For children, an age-appropriate pain scale should be taken and be repeated. For each age group, there are observational, behavioural, and self-reporting pain scales available ranging from neonatal to 12-year-olds. A

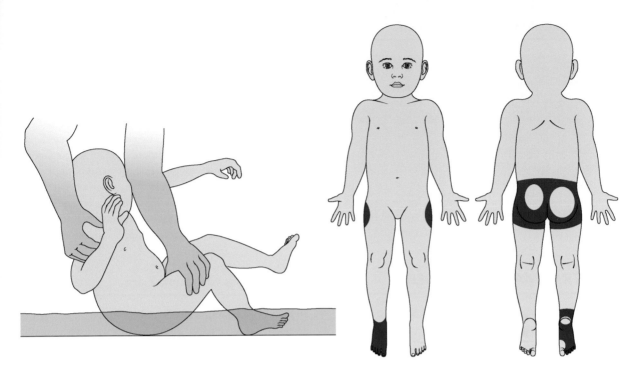

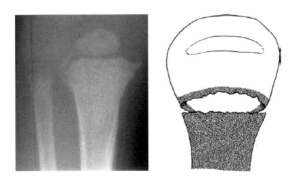

Figure 14.3 Areas at risk for non-accidental burns.

very prevalent fear of providing children with appropriate analgesia needs to be overcome.

Dosage of any paediatric drug is generally based on weight. Weight may be known by a caregiver, but more often in an emergency, it must be estimated. Length-based weight prediction devices are available in many forms, the most widely known being the Breslow tape.

A rough guide to estimating an average habitus child's weight is:

(Age × 2) + 8. In the older child, it should be (Age × 2) + 9.

Figure 14.4 Bucket handle fractures of the epiphysis.

Opiates are appropriate for acute pain and should be offered to the paediatric trauma patient to reduce pain and anxiety.

> ***Adequate titrated doses of morphine are***
> ***0.1 mg/kg 4 hourly or when required.***

Such an approach will facilitate resuscitation and assessment and does not mask important clinical signs. Careful monitoring of respiratory and haemodynamic status, and level of consciousness, is essential. Ketamine remains a useful alternative or second agent, can be given via several routes (including intranasal), and carries less respiratory side effects. Animal studies have shown neurodevelopmental delay in children equivalent to less than 3 years old; however, this has subsequently been shown only with repeated doses or prolonged infusions. Adverse effects of ketamine are better tolerated in a child than in an adult. Methoxyflurane has the advantages that it can be administered by inhalation and is becoming more popular for use in children refusing IV access. It is important to ensure that opioid analgesia is used in a judicious manner at discharge, with a limit on the number of tablets provided for home use and a focus on multimodal treatment. Generous opioid-based home analgesia regimens have been recently associated with high rates of development of dependency and adverse effects.[15]

14.1.7 Anaesthesiology in Children

Table 14.2 Anaesthesiology Considerations in Paediatric Trauma

- The danger of tube dislodgement, commonly due to failure to secure the tube adequately, or tube migration with head positioning may occur (especially into the right main bronchus), or the endotracheal tube may be too small (less of a problem when using cuffed tubes).
- The airway of the obligate nasal breather (the neonate or infant) must not be compromised with a nasogastric tube.

14.2 TRAUMA IN THE ELDERLY

14.2.1 Definition of 'Older' and Susceptibility to Trauma

Population ageing is a global phenomenon.[16] In 2020, there were 1 billion people worldwide aged 60 years and over (outnumbering children age under 5): approximately 13% of the total global population. By 2050, all regions (Africa aside) will have nearly a quarter of their populations aged above 60 years. Twenty-five per cent of Europe's present population is already aged 60 years and over. The number of persons aged 80 years and over will triple from 137 million in 2017 to 425 million in 2050. More older persons will mean more 'older trauma'.

Who is an 'older patient'? It depends. In 2001, the World Health Organisation's (WHO) Africa Minimum Data Set Project collaborators adopted the age of 50 years as 'old' in sub-Saharan Africa.[17] Accepted practice in the UK is that any patient over 75 years is classified as 'older'. But it is wise to be pragmatic and make a judgement based on the perceived interplay of chronological, local geographic, socio-economic, and biological factors. In current trauma scoring systems, the break-point for an age-linked increased risk of complication and mortality ranges from 45 to 55 years of age. In the United States, the 12.5% of the population over the age of 65 accounts for almost one-third of all deaths from injury. The UK Trauma Audit Research Network records a linear increase in post-trauma mortality with age.[18] Although age is a major factor in trauma, it is not the most important. The severity of the injury, pre-existing comorbidities, and medications play major parts in the increased morbidity and mortality of this population.[19] Older

people seem to both be more susceptible to trauma and experience higher mortality rates and complications.[20]

The presence of age-related comorbidities, in particular osteoporosis as well as cardiovascular, cerebrovascular, and renal impairments,[21] and concurrent multiple medications (polypharmacy) interact and summate to become potential and significant determinants of adverse outcome.

Certain medications (e.g., zopiclone and benzodiazepines) are prescribed more commonly and for longer among the older generations, yet by impairing reactions, these medications render them more susceptible to road traffic crashes and head injury.[22] In the United States, falls are the leading cause of fatalities in the construction industry: older workers have a higher rate of fatal falls than younger workers.

14.2.2 Access to Trauma Care

Despite pre-hospital trauma triage criteria, older trauma patients are less likely to be transported to a major trauma service. They thus have poorer outcomes than younger trauma patients and attract greater costs and lengths of stay which may increase with age and injury severity. Yet outcomes for older trauma patients who are afforded active intervention may be substantially better than preconceptions might suggest, with concomitant cost and time savings.[23] Awareness of these issues is essential in management of the elderly trauma patient.

14.2.3 Physiology

The older person's response to bodily insult, whether disease or trauma, may be atypical or even masked, in part due to the ageing process, and in part due to existing comorbidity and medication. Ageing is a risk factor for microvascular dysfunction and hyperpermeability. Apart from age-related remodelling of the vascular wall, endothelial barrier integrity and function in the periphery and at the blood–brain barrier decline with age. General physiological, cellular, and molecular changes occur in the vascular system as a product of ageing. Ageing leads to barrier dysfunction and vascular hyperpermeability[23] in the periphery and the blood–brain barrier; and age-related increases occur in oxidative stress, inflammatory markers, and apoptotic signalling. Oxidative stress can have a negative impact in all forms of major surgery including trauma surgery; this is particularly marked in an ageing population.[24] Careful and open-minded assessment is essential in management where, because of the interplay of the above factors, the older trauma patient may not only present with vague and misleading signs, but also end up precipitously *in extremis*.

The following potential age-related changes should be borne in mind.

14.2.3.1 RESPIRATORY SYSTEM

- Decreased lung elasticity; decreased pulmonary compliance
- Alveolar collapse and loss of surface area available for gas exchange
- Atrophy of bronchial epithelium, leading to a decrease in clearance of particulate foreign matter
- Chronic bacterial colonization of the upper airway

14.2.3.2 CARDIOVASCULAR SYSTEM

- Diminished pump function; lower cardiac output
- Inability to mount an appropriate response to both intrinsic and extrinsic catecholamines
- Reduced flow to vital organs
- Commonly prescribed medications may blunt normal physiological responses

14.2.3.3 NERVOUS SYSTEM

- Progressive brain atrophy
- Decline in cerebral and cognitive functions
- Hearing and visual impairment
- Proprioceptive impairment
- Gait impairment; loss of muscle bulk/strength
- Blunted baroreceptor function (predisposes to postural hypotension)
- Decreased cerebral blood flow (exacerbated by atherosclerosis)

14.2.3.4 RENAL

- Decline in renal mass
- Normal serum creatinine no longer implies normal renal function
- Increased vulnerability to nephrotoxic agents (e.g., non-steroidal anti-inflammatory drugs [NSAIDs] and angiotensin-converting enzyme [ACE] inhibitors)

14.2.3.5 MUSCULOSKELETAL

- Osteoporotic fractures with minimal energy transfer
- Diminution of vertebral body height
- Decrease in muscle mass

14.2.3.5.1 Multiple Rib Fractures

Rib fractures occur in 10% of trauma patients and are associated with lung contusions, haemopneumothorax, and cardiac injuries; they are also common in the elderly. Complications of multiple rib fractures, including increased pneumonia rates, ventilator dependence, intensive care unit (ICU) and hospital length of stay (LOS), and mortality, in adults aged ≥ 65 years were compared to younger patients with similar injury severity. Mortality risk increases by 19% and nosocomial infection risk increases by 29% with each additional rib fracture. Due to continuous chest wall motion during respiration, ribs require significantly longer to heal than fractures that can be immobilized; disability prevalence approaches 40% 6 months after injury. Due to the impact of rib fractures on outcomes in older adults, Eastern Association for the Surgery of Trauma (EAST) practice management guidelines (PMGs) for this population were developed.[25] Specifically, selection criteria for ICU admission, the use of locoregional anaesthesia, and non-invasive positive-pressure ventilation (NIPPV) are not well defined. Similarly, the utility of incentive spirometry (IS) and both single as well as multimodal pain medications is unclear in older adults. Recovery of patients from chest wall injury is prolonged, with low-severity injuries leading to chronic pain syndromes and high-severity injuries impacting quality of life and functional independence.

The EAST guidelines are helpful in managing such injuries.[25]

Non-Surgical Management and Analgesia Strategies for Older Adults with Multiple Rib Fractures: A Systematic Review, Meta-Analysis, and Practice Management Guideline (See **Table 8.4**).

14.2.3.6 INFLUENCE OF COMORBID CONDITIONS[19]

In addition to the physiological changes listed above, the onset of age-related disorders may predispose to an impaired response to injury. These can include any chronic degenerative disease, and especially disease in any major organ or bodily system (e.g., metabolic disorder or obesity), which might occur in isolation or in any combination.

14.2.4 Multiple Medications: Polypharmacy

A clear correlation exists between the number of medications taken and the likelihood of drug-induced complications. As ageing advances, the rates of drug metabolism diminish. Drug accumulations with associated unwanted interactions become more likely. In turn, a misleading clinical picture may emerge which may mask vital changes in signs.

Polypharmacy has a multitude of effects on the cardiovascular system in this patient population in which beta-blockade, calcium-channel blockers, and cardiac glycosides are common medications which lead to negative inotropic, dromotropic, and chronotropic effects. Under normal circumstances, this is the desired effect of the medication; however, with an acute insult, these medications prevent the host from mounting a normal physiologic response to compensate and maintain homeostasis.

14.2.5 Analgesia

Just as a younger patient would be afforded, the older person needs appropriate and adequate analgesia in any given trauma context. In fact, a major risk factor for hospital-acquired delirium in the elderly is undertreatment of pain. This allows for an improvement in physiological variables such as neuroendocrine stress responses and pulmonary function.[19] This, in turn, renders the older patient potentially more suitable for a major surgical procedure and consequently for rapider recovery.

Suggested guiding principles include:

- Be mindful of the patient's physical state and co-existing medications and utilize the most appropriate category of analgesic.
- Opioids should not be avoided unless specifically contraindicated.
- Start analgesia with a lower dose (70% of that for a healthy adult) and titrate as required.
- Consider a multimodal approach to pain treatment to reduce total dosages.
- An analgesic regimen which augments an effective afferent block (regional analgesia) may be effective and medication sparing.

14.2.6 Anticoagulants

Patients on anticoagulants found to have a significant intracranial haemorrhage require aggressive management. Reversal of the anticoagulant must be achieved rapidly.

The new oral anticoagulants such as dabigatran (Pradaxa®), apixaban (Eliquis®), and rivaroxaban (Xarelto®) are indicated for a variety of clinical conditions that affect the elderly. These include treatment of venous thromboembolism, stroke prophylaxis in non-valvular atrial fibrillation, and acute coronary syndrome. The new oral anticoagulants have a different mechanism of action than warfarin (Coumadin), acting to inhibit Xa and Thrombin IIa in the coagulation cascade. Only dabigatran has a direct reversal agent, idarucizumab (Praxbind®, Boehringer Ingelheim). Several other targeted antidote reversal agents are in development.

Reversal of anticoagulation caused by warfarin historically relied on the use of vitamin K and fresh frozen plasma (FFP). Recent literature suggests relying on prothrombin complex concentrates. Vitamin K and FFP therapy often requires 30–60 min to thaw the FFP. Furthermore, large volumes of FFP in the range of 30 cc/kg (4–12 units) are often required for adequate reversal. The time to infuse the necessary volume of FFP can complicate care. Treatment with vitamin K and prothrombin complex concentrates avoids these limitations.

Reversal of the anticoagulation caused by warfarin or new oral anticoagulants should be based on current institution-specific guidelines that are under constant revision.

14.2.7 Decision to Operate

Mortality data and survival curves for major abdominal surgery in the octogenarian population indicate it is safer than previously thought. These data enable risk stratification and prediction of outcomes.

Although wound healing is slower than in comparable younger patients, the result is qualitatively similar[12,14].

14.2.8 Outcome

Mortality rates are higher for comparable injuries compared with younger patients. The following guidelines have been recommended.

In summary, the surgeon should:

- Accept the potential for a decreased physiological reserve.
- Suspect comorbid disease.
- Suspect multiple medications and polypharmacy.
- Suspect atypical manifestations of any given situation with masked signs.
- Look for subtle signs of organ dysfunction by aggressive monitoring (e.g., renal function).

- Assume that any alteration in mental status is associated with brain injury, and only accept age-related deterioration after exclusion of injury.
- Be aware of poorer outcomes and sudden physiological deterioration.
- Be aware of the distinction between aggressive care and futile care.

14.2.9 Anaesthetic Considerations in the Elderly[27]

Table 14.3 Anaesthesiology Considerations in the Elderly

- Elderly trauma patients must be diagnosed and treated aggressively owing to their limited reserve capacities. 'Halfway is no way' for the elderly. This principle should be followed until/unless treatment is seen as futile.
- Age-related physiological changes may slow drug onset and exacerbate adverse physiological effects. Patience and careful monitoring are required to avoid the undesirable consequences of overdose. Doses of anaesthetics typically need to be reduced, in some cases dramatically, and a longer time for onset of effects can be expected.
- Whilst endotracheal intubation is easily performed in most trauma patients, this becomes more complicated in the elderly (especially with limited neck and jaw movement).
- Consider non-invasive ventilation (NIV) or high-flow nasal oxygen early, if no contraindication, to support the patient, thus avoiding endotracheal intubation.
- If an epidural or other regional anaesthesia techniques are indicated, these should be performed as soon as possible, other contraindications (such as anticoagulants) allowing (night shift work, do not delay until the next day).
- Be aware of a markedly increased susceptibility to pressure sores and skin injury in the unconscious elderly trauma patient.
- Be cautious in the use of anticoagulants and platelet inhibitors which might exacerbate traumatic bleeding, thus requiring this effect to be 'counteracted'. On the other hand, excessive bleeding is a possible signal of underlying problems which might not benefit from uncritical procoagulant therapy.

Source: Ref. 26.

14.3 TRAUMA IN PREGNANCY[34]

Trauma in pregnancy is the leading non-obstetric cause for maternal mortality.[35] In addition, trauma can cause placental abruption, which is a leading cause for foetal death, even after minor trauma.[36]

Trauma in pregnancy remains a challenge with the need for multidisciplinary management and the fact that, when the pregnancy is at a viable stage (usually around 22–26 weeks), one is dealing with *two* patients. Engage gynaecology early in the process. The ABCDE basics apply in the same way as in the non-pregnant patient, but there are anatomic and physiological changes that require consideration.

The management goals include rapid maternal assessment and resuscitation which enable identification and treatment of maternal life-threatening injuries, preventing hypoxia, hypotension, acidosis, and hypothermia. Awareness of anatomical and physiological changes that occur during pregnancy allows for interventions in the pregnant trauma patient that maintain utero-placental perfusion and foetal oxygenation, thereby ensuring both maternal and foetal care are optimized. These include mucosal congestion and laryngeal oedema (difficult to intubate), increased oxygen consumption and plasma volume (reduced oxygen carrying capacity and increased risk of hypoxia), delayed gastric emptying and gastric reflux (risk of aspiration), gravid uterus (aortocaval compression resulting in hypotension), and increased pelvic circulation (risk of large-volume occult haemorrhage – intrauterine, retroperitoneal, or from pelvic fractures).

In the pregnant patient, prioritisation of maternal care is the safest and fastest means of ensuring foetal survival.

Pitfall

The risk of hypotension from the enlarged uterus occluding the inferior cava is a common but avoidable pitfall.

In the pregnant patient, always check for vaginal haemorrhage.

Caesarean section delivery is indicated for foetal distress after resuscitation of a stable mother. Signs of foetal distress include bradycardia, cardiac pauses, sudden decelerations, lack of foetal movement on ultrasound, and the presence of foetal parts extruded through the vagina. If the pregnant trauma patient is unstable, standard trauma resuscitation, triage, and intervention are indicated. A Caesarean section can be performed at the time of a trauma laparotomy or via a midline vertical lower abdominal incision.

With the advent of REBOA, a Caesarean section should be considered for any occlusive vascular instrument placement, like resuscitative thoracotomy with aortic cross-clamping, as this abruptly deprives the foetus of circulation.

Finally, a perimortem delivery is indicated when there is clear indication of the impending death of the mother and there is still viability of the foetus.

In the pregnant patient, always check for vaginal haemorrhage.

Pitfall

The risk of hypotension from the enlarged uterus occluding the inferior cava is common but avoidable pitfall.

Radiographic studies indicated for maternal evaluation, including abdominal CT, should not be deferred or delayed due to concerns regarding foetal exposure to radiation.[37]

14.3.1 Evaluation

- Early maternal resuscitation, ultrasound evaluation of the foetal heart, and the use of cardiotocography are recommended in the evaluation of these patients.
- Suppression of premature labour may be required.
- Administration of RhoGAM® anti-D antibody (Kedrion Biopharma, Melville, NY, USA) in cases of maternal Rh-negative status and steroids for foetal lung maturation are important considerations.
- Damage control surgery may include the need to deliver the foetus urgently through Caesarean section (especially in cases with massive maternal abdominopelvic trauma or maternal cardiac arrest).

Pitfall

- Diagnostic imaging should not be delayed or deferred due to foetal radiation exposure concerns.
- Undertake necessary imaging but use non-ionizing methods if possible.[15]

14.4 NON-BENEFICIAL (FUTILE) CARE

In every environment, there are circumstances where the provision of adequate healthcare may not alter the outcome, but there may be a significant drain on the resources available, and denial to others of adequate care as a result. This 'rationing' of healthcare may be the result of operating theatres being in use and consequently not available, inadequate numbers of ICU beds, or financial restrictions.

It must be stressed, however, that all patients are entitled to an aggressive initial resuscitation and careful comprehensive diagnosis. The magnitude of their injuries should be assessed within their wider health context, and only then can the appropriateness and aggressiveness required in their care be determined. In addition, this must all be fully discussed with the associated staff and family. All resources are ultimately finite, and one should consider the implications of exhausting a single resource at the expense of the next patient. There will always be a next patient. An example includes blood utilization, where effort cessation should be considered beyond certain thresholds. Although mandatory cutoffs are not suggested, it is unlikely that supranormal transfusion practices lead to successful outcomes.

Inevitably, occasions arise in the management of older patients (as in any age group) when it is abundantly clear to the clinician that intervention is no longer beneficial. Prolongation of obviously futile care should prompt ethical considerations and discussions independently of resources available.

Sometimes, continued treatment can be justified by the wish to prolong the life until relatives arrive at the hospital. Local and national legislation needs to be adhered to. The clinician must be guided by basic ethical principles, and it is essential to be humane, and not to prolong life without definite and realistic therapeutic goals and without realistic expectations of any possibility of a positive outcome. Opting to allow the patient a death which is comfortable and dignified may be more positive as an outcome than a futile surgical intervention.[38]

REFERENCES AND RECOMMENDED READING

References

Paediatric Trauma

1. Tracya ET, Englumb BR, Barbasb AS, Foleyc C, Riced HE, Shapiro ML. Pediatric injury patterns by year of age. *J Pediatr Surg.* 2013 June;**48(6)**:1384–8. doi: 10.1016/j.jpedsurg.2013.03.041.

2. Goldstick JE, Cunningham RM, Carter PM. Current causes of death in children and adolescents in the United States. *N Engl J Med.* 2022;**386**:1955–6. doi: 10.1056/NEJMc2201761.

3. Weber AD, Nance ML. Clearing the pediatric cervical spine. *Curr Trauma Rep.* 2; 2016:210–5. doi: 10.1007/s40719-016-0059-6.

4. Kuppermann N, Holmes JF, Dayan PS, Hoyle JD Jr, Atabaki SM, Holubkov R, et al. Identification of children at very low risk of clinically-important brain injuries after head trauma: a prospective cohort study. *Lancet.* 2009. Oct 3;**374(9696)**:1160–70. doi: 10.1016/S0140-6736(09)61558-0. Epub 2009 Sep 14.

5. Nystrup KB, Stensballe J, Bøttger M, Johansson PI, Ostrowski SR. Transfusion therapy in paediatric trauma patients: a review of the literature. *Scand J Trauma Resusc Emerg Med.* 2015 Feb 15;**23**:21. doi: 10.1186/s13049-015-0097-z.

6. Eckert MJ, Wertin TM, Tyner SD, Nelson DW, Izenberg S, Martin MJ. Tranexamic acid administration to pediatric trauma patients in a combat setting: the pediatric trauma and tranexamic acid study (PED-TRAX). *J Trauma Acute Care Surg.* 2014 Dec;**77(6)**:852–8; discussion 858. doi: 10.1097/TA.0000000000000443.

7. Theodorou CM, Trappey AF, Beyer CA, Yamashiro KJ, Hirose S, Galante JM, et al. Quantifying the need for pediatric REBOA: A gap analysis. *J Pediatr Surg.* 2021 Aug;**56(8)**:1395–400. doi: 10.1016/j.jpedsurg.2020.09.011. Epub 2020 Sep 22.

8. Figaji AA, Graham Fieggen A, Mankahla N, Enslin N, Rohlwink UK. Targeted treatment in severe traumatic brain injury in the age of precision medicine. *Childs Nerv Syst.* 2017 Oct; **33(10)**:1651–61. 10.1007/s00381-017-3562-3.

9. Herbert JP, Venkataraman SS, Turkmani AH, Zhu L, Kerr ML, Patel RP, et al. Pediatric blunt cerebrovascular injury: the McGovern screening score. *J Neurosurg Pediatr.* 2018 Jun;**21(6)**:639–49. doi: 10.3171/2017.12.PEDS17498. Epub 2018 Mar 16.

10. Image Gently: The Image Gently Alliance. http://www.imagegently.org/. (accessed September 2023).

11. Adelson PD, Wisniewski SR, Beca J, Brown SD, Bell M, Muizelaar JP, et al. Paediatric Traumatic Brain Injury Consortium. Comparison of hypothermia and normothermia after severe traumatic brain injury in children (Cool Kids): a phase 3, randomised controlled trial. *Lancet Neurol.* 2013 Jun;**12(6)**:546–53. doi: 10.1016/S1474-4422(13)70077-2.

12. Kornblith AE, Addo N, Plasencia M, Shaahinfar A, Lin-Martore M, Sabbineni N, et al. Development of a Consensus-Based Definition of Focused Assessment With Sonography for Trauma in Children. *JAMA Netw Open.* 2022 Mar 1;**5(3)**:e222922. doi: 10.1001/jamanetworkopen.2022.2922.

13. Letton RW, Worrell V; APSA Committee on Trauma Blunt Intestinal Injury Study Group. Delay in diagnosis and treatment of blunt intestinal injury does not adversely affect prognosis in the pediatric trauma patient. *J Pediatr Surg.* 2010 Jan;**45(1)**:161–5; discussion 166. doi: 10.1016/j.jpedsurg.2009.10.027.

14. Naik-Mathuria BJ, Rosenfeld EH, Gosain A, Burd R, Falcone RA, Jr., Thakkar R, et al. Proposed clinical pathway for nonoperative management of high-grade pediatric pancreatic injuries based on a multicenter analysis: A pediatric trauma society collaborative. *J Trauma Acute Care Surg.* 2017;**83(4)**:589–96. doi: 10.1097/TA.0000000000001576.

15. Harbaugh CM, Lee JS, Hu HM, McCabe SE, Voepel-Lewis T, Englesbe MJ, et al. Persistent Opioid Use Among Pediatric Patients After Surgery. *Pediatrics.* 2018 Jan;**141(1)**. pii: e20172439. doi: 10.1542/peds.2017-2439.

Trauma in the Elderly

16. Ageing. *The United Nations Report.* 2017. Available from: https://www.un.org/en/global-issues/ageing (accessed online January 2018).

17. Peachey K, Kowal P. *Indicators for the Minimum Data Set Project on Ageing: A Critical Review in sub-Saharan Africa. WHO.* 2001 June; Available from https://cdn.who.int/media/docs/default-source/immunization/sage/sage-pages/ageing_mds_pub02.pdf. (accessed online January 2019).

18. Herron J, Hutchinson R, Lecky F, Bouamra O, Edwards A, Woodford M, et al. The Trauma Audit & Research Network 2017 (Manchester Academic Health Science Centre, University of Manchester). *Major Trauma in Older People. Bone Joint J.* 2017 Dec;**99-B(12)**:1677–80. doi: 10.1302/0301-620X.99B12.BJJ-2016-1140.R2.

19. Kirshenbom D, Ben-Zaken Z, Albilya N, Niyibizi E, Bala M. Older Age, Comorbid Illnesses, and Injury Severity Affect Immediate Outcome in Elderly Trauma Patients. *J Emerg Trauma Shock.* 2017 Jul-Sep;**10(3)**:146–50. doi: 10.4103/JETS.JETS_62_16.

20. Kozar RA, Arbabi S, Stein DM, Shackford SR, Barraco RD, Biffl WL, et al. Injury in the aged: Geriatric trauma care at the crossroads. *J Trauma Acute Care Surg.* 2015 Jun; **78(6)**:1197–209. doi: 10.1097/TA.0000000000000656.

21. Isaacs, B. The Giants of geriatric Medicine. *The Challenge of Geriatric Medicine.* Oxford. Oxford University Press, 1992.

22. Gustavsen I, Bramness JG, Skurtveit S, Engeland A, Neutel I, Mørland J. Road traffic accident risk related to prescriptions of the hypnotics zopiclone, zolpidem, flunitrazepam and nitrazepam. *Sleep Med.* 2008; **9(8)**:818–22.

23. Oakley R, Tharakan B. Vascular hyperpermeability and aging. *Aging Dis.* 2014; **5(2)**:114–25. 2014.

24. Rosenfeldt F, Wilson M, Lee G, Kure C, Ou R, Braun L, de Haan J. Oxidative stress in surgery in an ageing population: pathophysiology and therapy. *Exp Gerontol.* 2014;**48(1)**:45–54. Epub 2012 Mar 23.

25. Mukherjee K, Schubl SD, Tominaga G, Cantrell S, Kim B, Haines KL, Kaups KL, et al. Non-surgical management, and analgesia strategies for older adults with multiple rib fractures: A systematic review, meta-analysis, and joint practice management guideline from the Eastern Association for the Surgery of Trauma and the Chest Wall Injury Society. *J Trauma Acute Care Surg.* 2023 Mar 1;94**(3)**:398–407. doi: 10.1097/TA.0000000000003830. Epub 2022 Nov 15.

26. Banks SE, Lewis MC. Trauma in the elderly: considerations for anesthetic management. *Anesthesiol Clin.* 2013 Mar;**31(1)**:127–39. doi: 10.1016/j.anclin.2012.11.004.

Trauma in Pregnancy

27. Mendez-Figueroa H, Dahlke JD, Vrees RA, Rouse DJ. Trauma in pregnancy: an updated systematic review. *Am J Obstet Gynecol.* 2013;**209(1)**:1–10. doi: 10.1016/j.ajog.2013.01.021.

28. LA Rosa M, Loaiza S, Zambrano MA, Escobar MF. Trauma in Pregnancy. *Clin Obstet Gynecol.* 2020 Jun;**63(2)**:447–54. doi: 10.1097/GRF.0000000000000531.

29. Cahill AG, Bastek JA, Stamilio DM, Odibo AO, Stevens E, Macones GA. Minor trauma in pregnancy–is the evaluation unwarranted? *Am J Obstet Gynecol.* 2008 Feb;**198(2)**:208.e1–5. doi: 10.1016/j.ajog.2007.07.042. PMID: 18226625.

30. Gilet AG, Dunkin JM, Fernandez TJ, Button TM, Budorick NE. Fetal radiation dose during gestation estimated on an anthropomorphic phantom for three generations of CT scanners. *AJR Am J Roentgenol.* 2011 May;**196(5)**:1133–7. doi: 10.2214/AJR.10.4497.

Non-Beneficial Care

31. Ardagh M. Futility has no utility in resuscitation medicine. *J Med Ethics.* 2000 Oct;**26(5)**:396–9.

Recommended Reading

Paediatric Trauma

The Paediatric Trauma Manual. Royal Children's Hospital, Melbourne, Australia. Available from: https://www.rch.org.au/trauma-service/manual/. (accessed online September 2023).

Wesson D, Naik-Mathuria B. *Pediatric Trauma – Pathophysiology, Diagnosis and Treatment* – Second edition. CRC Press. 2017

Trauma in the Elderly

Bonne S, Schuerer DJ. Trauma in the older adult: epidemiology and evolving geriatric trauma principles. *Clin Geriatr Med.* 2013 Feb;**29(1)**:137–50. doi: 10.1016/j.cger.2012.10.008.

Adams SD, Holcomb JB. Geriatric trauma. *Curr Opin Crit Care.* 2015 Dec;**21(6)**:520–6. doi: 10.1097/MCC.0000000000000246.

Richardson J, Bresland K. The management of postsurgical pain in the elderly population. *Drugs Aging.* 1998 Jul;**13(1)**:17–31. doi: 10.2165/00002512-199813010-00003.

Principi T, Schonfeld D, Weingarten L, et al. Update in Pediatric Emergency Medicine: Pediatric Resuscitation, Pediatric Sepsis, Interfacility Transport of the Pediatric Patient, Pain and sedation in the Emergency Department, Pediatric Trauma. *Update Pediatr.* 2018; **17**:223.

Soles GL, Tornetta P 3rd. Multiple trauma in the elderly: new management perspectives. *J Orthop Trauma*. 2011;**Suppl 2**:S61–5.

Lai MM, Lin CC, Lin CC, Liu CS, Li TC, Kao CH. Long-term use of zolpidem increases the risk of major injury: a population-based cohort study. *Hum Factors*. 2012; **54**(**3**):303–15.

Dong XS, Wang X, Daw C. Fatal falls among older construction workers. *Injury*. 2014; **45**(**9**):1412–9. Epub 2014 Feb 28.

Rubinfeld I, Thomas C, Berry S, Murthy R, Obeid N, Azuh O, Jordan J, Patton JH. Octogenarian abdominal surgical emergencies: not so grim a problem with the acute care surgery model? *J Trauma*. 2009; **67**(**5**):983–9. doi: 10.1097/TA.0b013e3181ad6690.

Gosain A, DiPietro LA. Aging and wound healing. *World J Surg*. 2004;**28**(**3**):321–6. Epub 2004 Feb 17

Trauma in Pregnancy

Non-Beneficial Care

Deborah LK. When is medical treatment futile? A guide for students, residents, and physicians. *J Gen Intern Med*. 2004 Oct;**19**(**10**):1053–6. doi: 10.1111/j.1525-1497.2004.40134.x.

Part 4

Modern therapeutic and diagnostic technology

Minimal Access Surgery in Trauma **15**

Minimally invasive access techniques, such as laparoscopy and thoracoscopy, have a definite role to play in the management of trauma patients. Laparoscopy is now considered an acceptable alternative to laparotomy in haemodynamically stable penetrating and blunt abdominal trauma.[1] However, the decision to use laparoscopy is highly dependent on the clinical context, the physiological state of the patient, and the surgeon's laparoscopic skills in the trauma patient.

15.1 LAPAROSCOPY

The following definitions are useful when discussing laparoscopy in trauma.

15.1.1 Screening/Diagnostic Laparoscopy

Although the sensitivity and specificity of laparoscopy in detecting blunt small bowel injuries have improved considerably over the past years, sensitivity is still problematic for hollow viscus injury.

15.1.1.1 BLUNT TRAUMA[2]

Almost all patients with blunt abdominal trauma who do not have an indication for urgent surgery will undergo a computed tomography (CT) scan of the abdomen with vascular contrast as an initial examination, and laparoscopy is not indicated as a *primary* diagnostic tool.

15.1.1.2 PENETRATING TRAUMA – STAB WOUNDS[3]

Laparoscopy is used to ascertain whether the peritoneum has been breached following an abdominal stab wound. If the peritoneum has not been breached, then no further action is required. If the peritoneum has been breached, then the abdomen should be explored.

15.1.1.3 PENETRATING TRAUMA – GUNSHOT WOUNDS

The examination of choice is the CT scan (also using markers for the skin wounds). If the abdominal cavity is felt to have been breached, then a laparotomy is indicated, as the rate of missed injuries can be high, and there may be multiple injuries to multiple structures and not just a single-organ injury.

Pitfalls

Laparoscopy should only be considered in the haemodynamically stable patient!

Laparoscopy should not be considered in the patient who is haemodynamically stable but extended focussed assessment with sonography for trauma (eFAST) or CT scan shows significant intraperitoneal fluid.

15.1.2 Diagnostic Laparoscopy

The most common indication for diagnosis is in blunt trauma patients in whom isolated free intra-peritoneal fluid has been identified on imaging. There may be clinical uncertainty as to the origin of this fluid, and laparoscopy may well help confirm the source of the fluid. Is it a mesenteric tear, or an enteric injury, or fluid from a solid viscus?

Pitfall

Generally, it is difficult to adequately visualize retroperitoneal structures such as the duodenum, and great caution must be exercised in terms of excluding or confirming an injury to this structure laparoscopically.

DOI: 10.1201/9781003258124-19

15.1.3 Non-Therapeutic Laparoscopy

Laparoscopy is regarded as a non-therapeutic procedure where no injuries are identified, or injuries that do not require repair are identified.

Pitfall

Laparoscopy will make the abdomen more difficult to assess, both clinically and via patient history. Is the increase in abdominal discomfort due to the procedure rather than the pathology?

15.1.4 Therapeutic Laparoscopy

Laparoscopy is regarded as therapeutic when an advanced manoeuvre is performed to repair an identified injury. Simple manoeuvres such as organ mobilization or evacuation of a clot are **not** considered therapeutic. Therapeutic laparoscopy can only be performed in patients who are stable and in whom the injury complex is well defined.

Pitfall

Therapeutic laparoscopy is not advised in the presence of haemodynamic instability, extensive bleeding complex injuries, limited visibility, or inadequate equipment or an inexperienced operator.

15.1.5 Technique

Correct positioning and preparation of the patient for trauma laparoscopy are essential.

- The patient is placed supine (dorsal decubitus), legs spread apart on a beanbag and firmly strapped, because adequate abdominal organ exposure relies on dependency obtained with table rotation and tilting, rather than with retractors.
- Skin prep and draping should allow for rapid conversion to a complete laparotomy if necessary.
- Appropriate laparoscopic instruments as well as those for a traditional trauma laparotomy (and vascular surgery) must be available.
- One or more (flat) high-resolution screens should be placed opposite each surgeon. Monitors should be mobile and moved accordingly so that the surgeon always has the screen in front of his eyes without turning his head.
- The operating table should be adapted to the height of the surgeon's arms to ensure proper ergonomics for exploration as well as for advanced techniques of haemostasis and suturing. The surgeon can stand between the legs of the patient ('French' position) or opposite the target organ once this is recognized.
- Insertion of a bladder catheter is advised.
- Pneumoperitoneum should be:
  - Obtained with low flow to allow timely detection of a tension pneumothorax, leading to immediate stopping in insufflation and insertion of a thoracic drain.
  - Maintained at low pressures (8–12 mmHg) to avoid gas embolism if a large vein is injured.
- Trocar insertion should avoid all previous scars (incisions or drainage sites).
  - The first trocar should always be inserted with an open technique. Ideally, the trocar set-up should allow for triangulation; the optic should ideally be placed midway between the working trocars (equal azimuth angles). When performed for diagnostic purposes in a patient with an unclear abdomen, the optic trocar should be in the centre of the abdomen (i.e. at the level of the navel).
  - Next, two trocars should be inserted along the anterior axillary line in either flank: on the right slightly above the navel line and on the left slightly lower, so that both the upper and lower abdomen can easily be accessed.
  - Port positioning is governed by the indication for the operation, and monitors must be in direct line of view.
  - In specific indications, the trocars are located according to the organ involved, as determined by appropriate preoperative imaging.
- A straight or 30°10 mm scope can be used according to surgeon preferences. Ten millimetre scopes are better than 5 mm, as blood absorbs white light and darkens the optical field. Adequate tissue handling requires 5 mm atraumatic bowel graspers.

15.1.6 Risks

Laparoscopy in abdominal trauma entails four specific risks:

- Missed injuries, mainly intestinal, with their attending high morbidity and mortality

- Gas embolism, supposedly higher when mesenteric and hepatic (venous) lesions have occurred, but apparently as rare as in any laparoscopic procedure today
- Impeded venous return (because of elevated intra-abdominal pressure)
- Increased intracranial pressure

Pitfalls

These last two make physiological instability and severe head injury absolute contraindications to the creation of the pneumoperitoneum, which is necessary for most minimally invasive techniques.

Caution is warranted as well in the presence of abdominal compartment syndrome or diaphragmatic tears.[6] Whilst laparoscopy may rarely detect and treat the cause of the former, the risk of tension pneumothorax if there is a co-existing diaphragmatic tear requires that a large-bore needle – or, better still, a chest tube – be inserted into the thorax.

15.1.7 **Applications**

15.1.7.1 BOWEL INJURY

Laparoscopic examination for penetrating injury of the bowel is unreliable, as it is easy to miss occult or small lesions – especially in low-volume trauma environments – and can be very time-consuming. Laparoscopy can confirm the presence of peritoneal breach and may allow for the active exclusion and management of an intra-abdominal injury.[3]

In general, the safest approach is to use laparoscopy to exclude or confirm peritoneal breach. If there is no peritoneal breach, then there is no need to proceed further. If there is peritoneal breach, then formal laparotomy will exclude any intra-abdominal injuries. Laparoscopy can be successfully employed to repair small bowel injuries and fashion a colostomy. However, primary colon repair without colostomy is generally preferable.[4]

15.1.7.2 SPLENIC INJURY

Although laparoscopic splenic preservation and partial splenectomy have been reported after trauma using fibrin glue, argon beam coagulator, as well as splenic-wrapping with mesh, the role of minimal access techniques is limited in splenic injury. Independent of injury grade on CT scan, stable patients should be treated non-operatively. Laparoscopy is contraindicated in the unstable patient, who should be treated per trauma laparotomy.

15.1.7.3 LIVER INJURY

Patients failing a trial of non-operative management for hepatic injury have been managed successfully using minimally invasive surgery, including laparoscopic application of fibrin glue as a haemostatic agent.[5] Haemoperitoneum may be drained, and biliary leaks, with or without peritonitis, can be controlled via the laparoscope usually combined with endoscopic retrograde cholangiopancreatography (ERCP).[6]

15.1.7.4 DIAPHRAGMATIC INJURY

In asymptomatic patients with stab wounds of the *left* thoraco-abdominal area (ribcage below the fifth intercostal space), the risk of an occult diaphragmatic injury is about 7%.

Since imaging cannot reliably demonstrate a diaphragmatic defect (where no herniation has occurred), suspected diaphragmatic injury due to either blunt or penetrating injury can be diagnosed by direct inspection. Either video-assisted thoracoscopy (VATS) or laparoscopy may be employed in this setting. If there is no indication for exploration of the pleural cavity, most surgeons prefer laparoscopy, whilst VATS is preferable when there is a specific indication for it, such as a chest collection which needs to be evacuated simultaneously. If VATS is employed, there must be no suspicion of intra-abdominal injuries needing laparoscopy or laparotomy.

Laparoscopy is especially helpful to exclude occult diaphragmatic injury in a setting where non-operative management of penetrating thoracoabdominal injuries is employed.[7] After a period of observation, if the patient has no abdominal signs of concern, laparoscopy can be performed with the diaphragm as the main focus, whereas if laparoscopy is employed in the acute setting, a complete diagnostic laparoscopy needs to be performed and identified intra-abdominal injuries need to be dealt with either laparoscopically or via exploratory laparotomy.

Diaphragmatic injuries can be repaired laparoscopically or thoracoscopically. It is theoretically easier to repair the diaphragm from above (i.e. on the convex side of the muscle); however, it is imperative to place one's working ports in such a position as to facilitate easy access to the injury. The ribs are not pliable and do not allow working at acute angles without great difficulty.[8]

Finally, repair of longstanding post-traumatic diaphragmatic herniation may be possible with either laparoscopy or VATS.

15.1.7.5 BLADDER INJURY

In cases of isolated intraperitoneal rupture post blunt trauma, laparoscopic repair is eminently feasible and should be considered, provided the correct equipment and skills are available.

Pitfall

All of the above assume significant laparoscopic experience on the behalf of the operator, as unfamiliarity with the anatomy and techniques required leads to missed injury, sometimes with catastrophic results.

15.2 VIDEO-ASSISTED THORACOSCOPIC SURGERY[9]

Thoracic injuries may be managed by VATS in lieu of thoracotomy in selected circumstances.[10]

15.2.1 Technique

Double-lumen endotracheal intubation is essential, to facilitate lung collapse on the operative side. Positioning depends on the indication for the procedure; for most cases, a lateral position (injured side up) is appropriate with either a sandbag under the chest or the table broken to facilitate splaying of the ribs and allowing easy access to the intercostal spaces. The arm is secured overhead, and the patient is secured to the table. The first port is placed via the open technique, and further ports are placed as appropriate. Ports are positioned in such a way as to triangulate towards the working area, with the monitor directly in line.

Pitfall

Care must be taken not to accidentally place ports below the diaphragm.

15.2.2 Applications

In the acute trauma setting in stable patients, VATS may be employed to:

- Pinpoint and manage persistent, non-exsanguinating haemorrhage (> 300 cc within 3 hours).
- Perform a pericardial window in suspected penetrating cardiac trauma.[11]

In the post-acute or semi-elective setting, VATS can be utilized for:

- Evacuation of a clotted haemothorax
- Direct visualization and stapling of persistent or recurrent air leaks, with aspiration of associated haemothorax
- Ligation (rare) of thoracic duct injuries (when conservative medical management fails to reduce chyle leakage)
- Foreign body extraction

15.2.3 Summary

Although minimally invasive surgery still plays a minor role in trauma surgery relative to general surgery, it is being employed ever increasingly. Surgeons should be encouraged to incorporate laparoscopy and VATS into their trauma protocols and gain familiarity and expertise with their use. It should, however, in the light of current knowledge, still be regarded as suitable only for carefully selected stable patients.

15.3 RESUSCITATIVE ENDOVASCULAR BALLOON OCCLUSION OF THE AORTA (REBOA)

The use of modern endovascular bleeding treatment modalities started with the treatment of aortic aneurysmal disease and has since spread into trauma care. The evolution of modern endovascular devices (embolization and endografts), as well as improved diagnostic tools (CT, ultrasound, and angiography), have resulted in a wide increase in endovascular resuscitation and trauma management (EVTM). The use of endovascular tools alone or in combination with open surgery (hybrid procedures) is now part of standard treatment for trauma. In the past few years, there has been an increasing interest in REBOA, which, by definition, is an endovascular tool in hybrid or endovascular procedures to achieve temporary haemodynamic stability.[12]

REBOA is one of the most actively researched fields in EVTM and has been implemented in clinical use in several institutes as an adjunct for *temporary* control of massive non-compressible torso haemorrhage. REBOA is a balloon catheter for proximal aorta flow control, which is usually inserted into the aorta via the common femoral artery, but can be used through other vessels, like the brachial, axillary, or iliac vessels, or even the aorta directly.

REBOA does not stop bleeding: It is for source control and is only a bridge to definitive treatment.

15.3.1 **Anatomy**

In REBOA placement, the aorta is divided into three zones. Zone I (supracoeliac) is from the ascending thoracic aorta to the level of the coeliac axis. Zone II (pararenal) is the abdominal aorta from the coeliac axis to the renal vessels and is considered as a no-go zone for balloon occlusion, and Zone III (infrarenal) is from the infrarenal aorta down to bifurcation into the iliac arteries. The method can also be used for flow control in other vessels, like the subclavian artery or the inferior vena cava, but in that case, it is not referred to as REBOA. (See **Figure 15.1**.)

Zone I REBOA has been gaining acceptance as a feasible and less invasive resuscitation alternative to

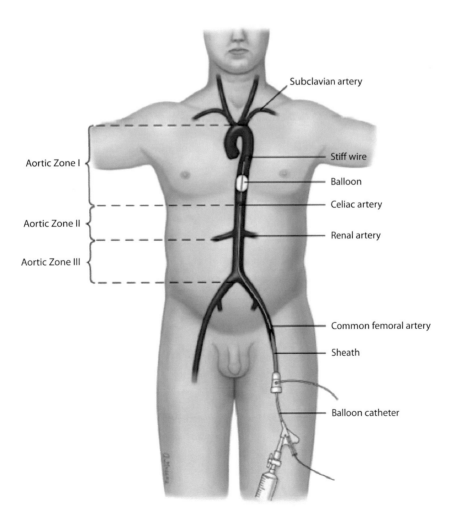

Figure 15.1 Resuscitative endovascular balloon occlusion of the aorta (REBOA) landing zones. Zone II is considered a 'no-go' zone.

resuscitative thoracotomy and aortic clamping.[13] Zone III REBOA is used to control pelvic haemorrhage.

REBOA can be used for total occlusion, partial occlusion, or intermittent occlusion and can be modified actively to control the haemodynamic status and organ perfusion in unstable patients.

Pitfalls

- REBOA does not stop the bleeding and is not a bleeding control procedure as such.
- REBOA requires a simultaneous plan for definitive bleeding control.
- REBOA can buy time for the team to stabilize the patient and catch up with the resuscitation.
- Despite rapidly expanding use of REBOA in trauma and other non-traumatic bleedings, solid evidence of its indications, methods, or benefits has still to be clarified. There are some data to encourage use of partial REBOA (pREBOA) as much as possible to hold the heart and central nervous system (CNS) perfusion pressure whilst avoiding ischaemia to the lower body, as described later in this chapter (see Section 15.3.5).

15.3.2 Physiology

Aortic occlusion will increase the central systolic blood pressure proximal to the occlusion, resulting in increased blood flow to coronary and cerebral arteries, and is used in critical cases as a part of the resuscitation. Blood pressure elevation of around 20%–30%–40% is often observed but is heavily dependent on the REBOA level (Zone I vs. Zone III), cardiac output, total remaining blood volume, resuscitation volumes versus blood product infusions, and vasoconstrictor effects.[14]

The effects are highly dynamic and depend on the REBOA method used (e.g., partial REBOA, described in Section 15.3.5). In addition to a resuscitative support, aortic occlusion will decrease the arterial bleeding distal to the occlusion; however, tissues with poor perfusion before balloon occlusion will become almost completely non-perfused. Liver and kidneys are the most vulnerable, but also the spinal cord poorly tolerates extended

thoracic aortic occlusion, increasing the risk of paraplegia. In Zone III occlusion (infrarenal aorta), the effect on central blood pressure is relatively small but has an impact on pelvic bleeding as a proximal control. It is important to remember that REBOA affects arterial pressure and bleeding, and does not have a *direct* effect on venous bleeding.

> *The REBOA occlusion time needs to be as limited as possible, preferably not more than 30 minutes in Zone I and 60 minutes in Zone III.*

In reperfusion after the balloon is deflated, there is a sudden decrease of blood volume due to arterial blood flow distribution to the previously closed area. Also, the reperfusion results in a large challenge of cold, acidotic, and hyperkalaemic venous blood back to the heart and circulation. This has a sudden direct effect on the cardiac output but will also have a later effect on capillary leakage and increase the risk of multiple organ failure.

Occlusion will not stop arterial back bleeding or venous bleeding, even though it might decrease perfusion pressure to visceral organs and thereby decrease bleeding pressure. Depending on the level of occlusion, organ ischaemia will follow an occlusion time of some length (even 10–20 minutes), and an ischaemia–reperfusion reaction will always follow to some degree. Acidosis and ischaemic metabolism with systemic effects will follow even if a short occlusion time is used due to the metabolic acidosis that has already affected the trauma patient.

> *It is particularly important to communicate with the anaesthesia team during REBOA use, since the patient will receive parallel massive transfusion, to prevent a hypertensive state during late resuscitation.*

15.3.3 Insertion Technique

The main limiting stage is vascular arterial access, which can be achieved by ultrasound (the method of choice), surgical cut-down, or using anatomical landmarks. Modern REBOA catheters need sheaths of around 7–8 French gauge (FG) for insertion, and proper sheath insertion is essential to the whole REBOA procedure. The change to smaller catheters, from current 7–8 FG to 4 FG Cobra-OS® Catheters (Frontline Medical Technologies, London, ONT, Canada), has made the method simpler to use, and it results in fewer complications. Specific centres continue to recommend the larger (8 FG) catheter, to allow parallel blood pressure monitoring from the access site as well as blood gas tests.

REBOA should be used in Zone I or III but can be used for short periods in Zone II (although not recommended). Before insertion of the REBOA balloon, one can measure the length to Zone I or III using external body landmarks (mid-sternum for Zone I, or umbilicus for Zone III) or use fluoroscopy (or other techniques as described in the *Top Stent Manual* – see Recommended Reading). In general, with blunt trauma and an unclear bleeding source, Zone I is used first, whilst different methods should be applied to minimize ischaemia time. REBOA can be changed to Zone III if the source of bleeding is pelvic, for example.

Femoral artery cannulation should be done in experienced hands, as part of the EVTM concept, already on arrival, and during the primary survey if possible. Once the needle is in the vessel, a guidewire is inserted and then a sheath of the proper size (7–8 FG), followed by the REBOA balloon (**Figure 15.2**). A femoral arterial line (4–5 FG) might be upgraded to a proper sheath and used for REBOA (different types exist).

The intraluminal location and proper function of the sheath must be verified by ultrasound and/or aspiration. It can be used as a distal arterial line parallel to the REBOA line.

In patients *in extremis,* parallel bilateral arterial access (venous at times) might be beneficial. Vascular access should not delay any other life-saving procedure.

On insertion, the REBOA catheter is carefully advanced (no resistance to wire or catheter) and positioned. When at its designated location, slow inflation of the balloon follows, with careful monitoring of central pressure if available, carotid pulses, or contralateral femoral pressure via the sheath, when using pREBOA or intermittent REBOA (iREBOA) (see Section 15.3.5). In general, it can be claimed that if blood pressure is not elevated when using REBOA:

- The REBOA is not in the aorta.
- The balloon is damaged or malfunctioning.

Pitfall

New data supports the concept of a 'REBOA responder' – if the patient does not respond with blood pressure elevation to REBOA, the chance of survival is extremely low, if at all.

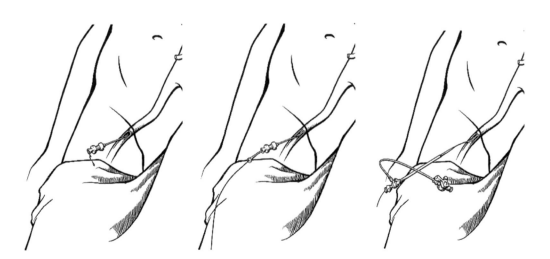

Figure 15.2 Puncture of the femoral artery, followed by a guidewire and sheath. These are the basic steps to be followed by the REBOA (resuscitative endovascular balloon occlusion of the aorta) catheter. Puncture by ultrasound is preferred, but this depends on the experience of the operator.

15.3.4 **Monitoring**

There are several ways to follow the haemodynamic effects of REBOA. The most obvious is measurement of central pressure, radial/brachial/subclavian artery pressure, carotid pulse, and possibly end-tidal CO_2, which decreases with total occlusion of the aorta. It is important to follow the clinical effects of REBOA and the simultaneous surgical management, and adjust them during resuscitation as well as in the direct postoperative period. Due to coagulopathy followed by massive transfusions and coagulation factors, thrombosis might occur, especially in the iliac–femoral vessels and lower extremities. It may occur during resuscitation or in the direct postoperative period.

15.3.5 **Total, Partial, and Intermittent Occlusion, and Targeted Blood Pressure**

Balloon occlusion can be *total* (no flow below the balloon – total REBOA, or tREBOA) or *partial* (balloon is not inflated totally, resulting in partial flow below the balloon – pREBOA). iREBOA is done by alternately inflating and deflating the balloon, resulting in intermittent partial flow below the balloon. In a critically unstable patient, total occlusion is normal at the start, but as soon as some stability has been gained, there should be attempts to transfer into partial or intermittent occlusion. This is done in balance with the haemodynamic stability and the tolerance to balloon deflation. The goal is to minimize the occlusion time. It also is possible to continuously work with the partial balloon inflation volume and aim for some targeted blood pressure. This prevents blood pressure peaks that are too high and allows some distal perfusion.

15.3.6 **Perioperative and Postoperative Care**

The vascular access and REBOA catheter should always be held by the REBOA operator, since it is a 'living entity', and can and should be modified to the haemodynamic need and situation of the patient. When the REBOA balloon is deflated (slowly, due to possible circulatory collapse), one should consider if it will be needed again. It might be best to leave the sheath for some time (6–12 hours), using a saline flush to prevent clotting.

Pitfall

All REBOA procedures should be considered as invasive, with the potential to cause thrombosis of the femoral artery. Accordingly, distal lower extremity status must be controlled during the first 24 hours on an hourly basis. REBOA might also cause aorta or iliac intimal damage, so vascular and distal clinical and radiological evaluation after its use is crucial.

Removal of the sheath can be done by manual compression, open cut-down and suture, or closure devices. The choice depends heavily on the experience of the operator.

15.3.7 **Indications**

The main indication is blunt trauma with non-compressible torso bleeding. It could be visceral organ bleeding, but the most documented and recognized indication is traumatic (blunt) pelvic bleeding. It should be noted that REBOA has been used successfully for penetrating trauma, even during cardiopulmonary resuscitation (CPR). In general, a hypotensive patient (with a systolic blood pressure of less than 80 mmHg) or a non-responsive bleeder might benefit from REBOA as a bridge to definitive care. In this sense, it is a form of intraluminal aorta clamping, which should be used carefully to increase and maintain an acceptable blood pressure, preferably by partial or intermittent occlusion of the aorta. The main advantage of REBOA use in these situations is to avoid opening another cavity for aortic clamping.

Recent large focussed empirical studies have shown that Zone I REBOA is at least as effective as emergency resuscitative thoracotomy (ERT),[15] and has significantly reduced mortality and provides better end-tidal CO_2 compared to ERT, thanks to ongoing CPR whilst inserting the REBOA. This advantage applies to both blunt and penetrating trauma, including patients with head injuries. New large studies suggest REBOA should be practised earlier, with a clear survival advantage with pre-hospital REBOA, including cases with pre-hospital CPR in trauma, and would be of benefit to a significant proportion of trauma patients if used early.

Recent studies have also proven the advantage of Zone III REBOA over preperitoneal packing in survival and complication.[16]

At times, REBOA has been used late when the patient has been in deep shock for a long time, a factor to be considered when evaluating the survival of these patients and well known in ruptured abdominal aorta patients. REBOA has been used as a time-winning tool in an austere environment, when there are no proper resources available, in transport, and in multiple-casualty scenarios. REBOA has been used successfully in military and pre-hospital scenarios, but there is much to investigate about its use and indications.

15.3.8 Contraindications

The peak increase in blood pressure after REBOA balloon deployment can be hazardous in cases of intracranial or thoracic bleeding, neck bleeding, or major hepatic injury, which are commonly considered as contraindications for REBOA. In cases of blunt thoracic aortic injury, the expanding balloon itself or sudden peak increase in blood pressure may deliver too much tension on the injured aortic wall, resulting in catastrophic consequences. A widened mediastinum and suspicion of blunt aortic a injury are also contraindications for REBOA.

15.3.9 Complications

Even being minimally invasive, REBOA has risks of potentially devastating complications. The vascular access is usually done via the common femoral artery (CFA) and there is a risk of intimal injury resulting in thrombus and inferior extremity ischaemia. The modern balloon catheters (4FG) are compatible with smaller sheath sizes and thus carry a relatively lower risk of thromboembolic complications, and damage to vessels.[17] Blind catheter deployment carries the risk of wrong landing zone. Also, when deploying in Zone I, the unnoticed balloon migration may lead to faulty positioning.[18]

The recently published UK REBOA trial,[19] cast doubts on many aspects of REBOA: The primary outcome was all-cause mortality at 90 days. Ten secondary outcomes included mortality at 6 months, while in the hospital, and within 24 hours, 6 hours, or 3 hours; the need for definitive hemorrhage control procedures; time to commencement of definitive hemorrhage control procedures; complications; length of stay; blood product use; and cause of death. Of the 90 patients included in the trial, over a 5 year period, all-cause mortality was higher in the REBOA group. Among the 10 secondary outcomes, all were increased in the REBOA versus the standard care group, and the Odds Ratios (OR) was increased with earlier mortality end points. There were more deaths due to bleeding in the REBOA and standard care group than in standard care alone group and most occurred within 24 hours. The trial concluded that "in trauma patients with exsanguinating hemorrhage, a strategy that includes REBOA, when used in the Emergency Department, does not reduce, and may increase mortality, compared with standard Major Trauma care. Other analyses differed slightly[20] and with the arrival of smaller (4FG) cannulae, the risks may diminish.

There are no "free lunches!" As with all other invasive procedures, the "perceived" benefits must be carefully balanced against the "justified" risks

15.3.10 Summary

REBOA is one component of the Damage Control Resuscitation effort. It is no substitute for excellent surgical care or surgical haemorrhage control, but might aid surgical, hybrid, or endovascular procedures. It is a minimally invasive procedure that might be useful as a bridge to definitive treatment in a bleeding trauma patient. It remains a widely accessible and rapid resuscitation adjunct with a relatively low complication profile. It should be regarded as part of the EVTM toolbox and used wisely. Great care should be taken to use it on patients who might benefit from its use and to avoid complications. Current evidence-based recommendations are shown in **Table 15.1**[21] and **Figure 15.3**.[22]

Table 15.1 Evidence-Based Recommendations for REBOA[19]

Level of Evidence	Recommendations
I	None
II	None

III	• Consider early placement of a common femoral artery catheter in the hypotensive trauma patient (SBP < 90 mmHg) to facilitate rapid upsizing to a 7-French sheath to accommodate a REBOA catheter if necessary.
	 • REBOA should be considered in patients with haemorrhagic shock and the following:
	   ○ Penetrating or blunt abdominopelvic trauma patients who are hypotensive (SBP < 90 mmHg)
	   ○ Transient responders to fluid resuscitation, or receiving a massive transfusion protocol (MTP)
	   ○ Positive FAST examination
	   ○ Suspected pelvic or lower extremity trauma with haemorrhage
	 • The REBOA device may also be considered for the following alternative indications:
	   ○ Prophylactic use in women undergoing surgery for abnormal placentation
	   ○ Severe gastrointestinal bleeding

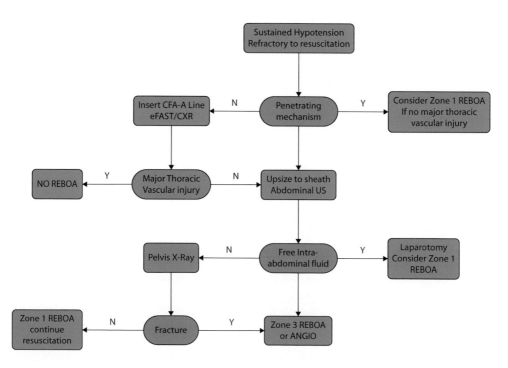

Figure 15.3 Western Trauma Association (WTA) algorithm for use of resuscitative endovascular balloon occlusion of the aorta (REBOA).

Table 15.2 Anaesthetic Considerations

LAPAROSCOPY

- Severe head injury mandates special attention and communication between surgeons and anaesthesiologists during the creation of the pneumoperitoneum. Monitoring of intracranial pressure (ICP) (or at least pupil reactivity) during the operation, possibly insufflating the abdomen at a lower pressure (10 instead of 14–15), and repeating the CT scan after the operation, are just a few of the precautions to be recommended in patients with head trauma.
- Caution is warranted as well, in the presence of abdominal compartment syndrome or diaphragmatic tears. Whilst laparoscopy may rarely detect and treat the cause of the former, the risk of tension pneumothorax if there is a co-existing diaphragmatic tear requires a chest tube inserted into the thorax.

REBOA

- REBOA, especially deployed in Zone I, will have a major impact on the need of ventilation. The perfused tissue volume will decrease dramatically when closing the aorta, meaning that if the respirator settings are not adjusted to the new circulated and perfused blood volume, that will result in severe hyperventilation.
- The dramatically increased perfused volume after the balloon deflation will result in hypoventilation if no ventilator adjustment is done. This must not happen, especially in combined head injury patients, and it rewards close communication and cooperation between surgeons and anaesthesiologists.
- Due to coagulopathy followed by massive transfusions and coagulation factors, the coagulation status changes quickly, and monitoring with VHA is very helpful.
- **It is very important for surgery and anaesthesiology teams to communicate during REBOA use, since the patient will receive parallel massive transfusion, and to prevent a hypertensive state during late resuscitation.**

Pitfall

- REBOA will cause an increase in bleeding from the liver, due to increased intrathoracic pressure with occlusion in Zone I, and back bleeding. Eighty-five per cent of bleeding from the liver is venous, and this will therefore be substantially increased. REBOA is contraindicated in liver injuries.

CT, Computed tomography
ICP, intracranial pressure
REBOA, resuscitative endovascular balloon occlusion of the aorta
VHA, viscoelastic haemostatic assay

REFERENCES AND RECOMMENDED READING

References

LAPAROSCOPY

1. Cirocchi R, Birindelli A, Inaba K, Mandrioli M, Piccinini A, Tabola R, et al. Laparoscopy for trauma and the changes in its use from 1990 to 2016: a current systematic review and meta-analysis. *Surg Laparosc Endosc Percutan Tech.* 2018 Feb;**28(1)**:1–12. doi: 10.1097/SLE.0000000000000466.

2. Koto MZ, Mosai F, Matsevych OY. The role of laparoscopy in blunt abdominal trauma: diagnostic, therapeutic or both? *S Afr J Surg.* 2017 Jun;**55(2)**:60.

3. Bain K, Meytes V, Chang GC, Timoney F. Laparoscopy in penetrating abdominal trauma is a safe and effective alternative to laparotomy. *Surg Endosc.* 2018 Sep 12. doi: 10.1007/s00464-018-6436-1.

4. Kong, L, Kong V, Christey G, Ah Yen D, Amey J, Denize GB, Marsden G, et al. Clinical decision making for abdominal stab wounds in high resourced but low volume centers require structured guidelines to be effective. *Surg Pract Sci.* 2022 Sep;**10**:100087. doi: 10.1016/j.sipas.2022.100087.

5. Chen RJ, Fang JF, Lin BC, Hsu YB, Kao JL, Kao YC, et al. Selective application of laparoscopy and fibrin glue in the failure of nonoperative management of blunt hepatic trauma. *J Trauma.* 1998 Apr;**44**:691–5. doi: 10.1097/00005373-199804000-00024.

6. Griffen M, Ochoa J, Boulanger BR. A minimally invasive approach to bile peritonitis after blunt liver injury. *Am Surg.* 2000;**66**:309–12.

7. Mjoli M, Oosthuizen G, Clarke D, Madiba T. Laparoscopy in the diagnosis and repair of diaphragmatic injuries in left-sided penetrating thoracoabdominal trauma: laparoscopy in trauma. *Surg Endosc.* 2015;**29(3)**:747–52. doi: 10.1007/s00464-014-3710-8.

8. Freeman RK, Al-Dossari G, Hutcheson KA, Huber L, Jessen ME, Meyer D, et al. Indications for using video-assisted thoracoscopic surgery to diagnose diaphragmatic injuries after penetrating chest trauma. *Ann Thorac Surg.* 2001 Aug;**72**:342–7.

Thoracoscopy (VATS)

9. Lowdermilk GA, Naunheim KS. Thoracoscopic evaluation and treatment of thoracic trauma. *Surg Clin North Am.* 2000 Oct;**80(5)**:1535–42. Review.

10. Lang-Lazdunski L, Mouroux J, Pons F, Grosdidier G, Martinod E, Elkaim D, et al. Role of videothoracoscopy in chest trauma. *Ann Thorac Surg.* 1997 Feb;**63**:327–33.

11. Morales CH, Salinas CM, Henao CA, Patino PA, Munoz CM. Thoracoscopic pericardial window and penetrating cardiac trauma. *J Trauma.* 1997 Feb;**42(2)**:273–5.

REBOA

12. Horer T. Resuscitative endovascular balloon occlusion of the aorta (REBOA) and endovascular resuscitation and trauma management (EVTM): a paradigm shift regarding hemodynamic instability. *Eur J Trauma Emerg Surg.* 2018 Aug;**44(4)**:487–9. doi: 10.1007/s00068-018-0983-y.

13. Brenner M, Inaba K, Ailofi A, DuBose JJ, Fabian T Bee, T, et al. Resuscitative endovascular balloon occlusion of the aorta and resuscitative thoracotomy in select patients with Haemorrhagic shock: early results from the American Association for the Surgery of Trauma's Aortic Occlusion in Resuscitation for Trauma and Acute Care Surgery Register. *J Am Coll Surg.* 2018 May;**226(5)**:730–40. doi: 10.1016/j.jamcollsurg.2018.01.044.

14. Qasim ZA, Sikorski RA. Physiologic considerations in trauma patients undergoing resuscitative endovascular balloon occlusion of the aorta. *Anesth Analg.* 2017;**125(3)**:891–4. doi: 10.1213/ANE.0000000000002215.

15. Cralley AL, Vigneshwar N, Moore EE, Dubose J, Brenner M, Sauaia A, et al. Zone 1 endovascular balloon occlusion of the aorta vs resuscitative thoracotomy for patient resuscitation after severe haemorrhagic shock. *JAMA Surgery.* 2023 Feb 1;**158(2)**:140–50. doi: 10.1001/jamasurg.2022.6393.

16. Bini JK, Hardman C, Morrison J, Scalea TA, Moore Lj, Podbielsi JM, et al. Survival benefit for pelvic trauma patients undergoing Resuscitative Endovascular Balloon Occlusion of the Aorta: Results of the AAST Aortic Occlusion for Resuscitation in Trauma Acute Care Surgery (AORTA) Registry. *Injury.* 2022 Jun;**53(6)**:2126–32. doi: 10.1016/j.injury.2022.03.005. Epub 2022 Mar 12.

17. Manzano-Nunez R, Orlas CP, Herrera-Escobar JP, Galvagno S, DuBose J, Melendez JJ, et al. A meta-analysis of the incidence of complications associated with groin access after the use of resuscitative endovascular balloon occlusion of the aorta in trauma patients. *J Trauma Acute Care Surg.* 2018 Sep;**85(3)**:626–34. doi: 10.1097/TA.0000000000001978.

18. Davidson AJ, Russo RM, Reva VA, Brenner ML, Moore LJ, Ball C, et al. The pitfalls of resuscitative endovascular balloon occlusion of the aorta: risk factors and mitigation strategies. *J Trauma Acute Care Surg.* 2018 Jan;**84(1)**:192–202. doi: 10.1097/TA.0000000000001711.

19. Jansen JO, Hudson J, Cochran C, MacLennan G, Lendrum R, Sadek S, et al. Emergency Department Resuscitative Endovascular Balloon Occlusion of the Aorta in Trauma Patients with Exsanguinating Hemorrhage: The UK-REBOA Randomized Clinical Trial. *JAMA.* 2023 Nov 21;**330(19)**:1862–1871. doi: 10.1001/jama.2023.20850.

20. Brede, J.R., Rehn, M. The end of balloons? Our take on the UK-REBOA trial. *Scand J Trauma Resusc Emerg Med.* 2023;**31(69)**. https://doi.org/10.1186/s13049-023-01142-5.

21. A Western Trauma Association critical decisions algorithm: resuscitative endovascular balloon occlusion of the aorta. *J Trauma Acute Care Surg.* 2022 Apr 1;**92(4)**:748–53. doi: 10.1097/TA.0000000000003438.

22. Inaba K, Alam HB, Brasel KJ, Brenner M, Brown CVR, Ciesla DJ, et al. A Western Trauma Association critical decisions algorithm: Resuscitative endovascular balloon occlusion of the aorta. *J Trauma Acute Care Surg.* 2022 Apr 1;**92(4)**:748–753. doi: 10.1097/TA.0000000000003438.

Recommended Reading

LAPAROSCOPY

Hajibandeh S, Hajibandeh S, Gumber AO, Wong CS. Laparoscopy versus laparotomy for the management of penetrating abdominal trauma: a systematic review and meta-analysis. *Int J Surg.* 2016;**34**:127–36. doi: 10.1016/j.ijsu.2016.08.524.

Li Y, Xiang Y, Wu N, Wu L, Yu Z, Zhang M, et al. A comparison of laparoscopy and laparotomy for the management of abdominal trauma: a systematic review and meta-analysis. *World J Surg.* 2015;**39(12)**:2862–71. doi: 10.1007/s00268-015-3212-4.

Thoracoscopy

Wu N, Wu L, Qiu C, Yu Z, Xiang Y, Wang M, et al. A comparison of video-assisted thoracoscopic surgery with open thoracotomy for the management of chest trauma: a systematic review and meta-analysis. *World J Surg*. 2015 Apr;**39(4)**:940–52. doi: 10.1007/s00268-014-2900-9.

REBOA

Brenner M, Bulger EM, Perina DG, Henry S, Kang CS, Rotondo MF, et al. Joint statement from the American College of Surgeons Committee on Trauma (ACS COT) and the American College of Emergency Physicians (ACEP) regarding the clinical use of Resuscitative Endovascular Balloon Occlusion of the Aorta (REBOA). *Trauma Surg Acute Care Open*. 2018 Jan 13;**3(1)**:e000154. doi: 10.1136/tsaco-2017-000154.

DuBose JJ, Rasmussen TE, Davis MR. Letter to the editor regarding the joint statement from the American College of Surgeons' Committee on Trauma (ACS-COT) and the American College of Emergency Physicians (ACEP) regarding the clinical use of resuscitative endovascular balloon occlusion of the aorta (REBOA). *Trauma Surg Acute Care Open*. 2018 Mar 2;**3(1)**:e000167. doi: 10.1136/tsaco-2018-000167.

Brenner M, Perina DG, Bulger EM, Winchell RJ, Kang CS, Henry S, et al. Response to letter to the editor from Dubose and colleagues regarding the Joint statement from the American College of Surgeons Committee on Trauma (ACS COT) and the American College of Emergency Physicians (ACEP) regarding the clinical use of Resuscitative Endovascular Balloon Occlusion of the Aorta (REBOA). *Trauma Surg Acute Care Open*. 2018 Mar 2;**3(1)**:e000170.

Brenner M, Inaba K, Aiolfi A, DuBose J, Fabian T, Bee T, et al. Resuscitative Endovascular Balloon Occlusion of the Aorta and Resuscitative Thoracotomy in Select Patients with Haemorrhagic Shock: early Results from the American Association for the Surgery of Trauma's Aortic Occlusion in Resuscitation for Trauma and Acute Care Surgery Registry. *J Am Coll Surg*. 2018 May;**226(5)**:730–40. doi: 10.1016/j.jamcollsurg.2018.01.044.

Hörer TM MJ, DuBose JJ, Reva VA, Matsumoto J, Matsumura Y, Falkenberg M, et al. Top Stent Manual, The art of EndoVascular hybrid Trauma and bleeding Management. In Hörer T, ed. *The REBOA Manual*. 1st Edn. Örebro University Hospital, Örebro, Sweden. 2017. Available from: http://www.jevtm.com/top-stent/ (accessed online September 2023).

Imaging in Trauma **16**

During the course of the past two to three decades, the main advancements that have been made with regard to imaging in trauma have included the following:

Ultrasound (US)

- Extended focussed assessment with sonography for trauma (eFAST) has become reliable in diagnosing haemothorax, pneumothorax, and pericardial tamponade and is the primary screening test for abdominal injury.
- Multiple other useful US techniques have emerged.

> *Whilst readily available, any algorithm should start from the physiology of the patient and not from ultrasound findings.*

Computed tomography (CT)

- Pan CT has revolutionized our ability to comprehensively diagnose multiple injuries in a polytrauma patient.[1]
- CT scanning of the cervical spine has largely replaced X-rays of the neck.
- CT has become a reliable tool for identifying a bullet track or trajectory, which helps determine whether vital structures have been injured, especially in injuries of the trunk.
- CT angiography (CTA) has become easily accessible, is reliable, and has largely replaced diagnostic catheter-directed angiography, especially since the introduction of hybrid theatres.
- Whilst CT currently plays a major role in trauma, providing excellent diagnostic information, there is major concern regarding the risks of radiation to our patients – especially since all other medical disciplines also rely heavily on CT for diagnosis and management, making it likely that any one patient may receive several CT investigations during the course of

their life. Up to 2% of all cancers may be secondary to CT investigation.[5]

Pitfalls

- Modern CTs are very fast, and the trauma bay is near the CT, which enables transient responders who used to bypass CT to go through Imaging first. The time-consuming moment is transportation and the positioning of the patient on the CT table, along with dealing with tubes, lines, monitoring equipment, and other external devices.
- *Radiology should never delay an emergency procedure.* Patients who are haemodynamically unstable despite resuscitation may be directed to the operating room (OR) for immediate operative treatment after the initial workup in the emergency room (ER).
- Patients who are mentally alert, are not intoxicated, and do not show signs of other than minor injuries do not benefit from CT and may be managed with repeated clinical evaluation combined with specific CT exams if needed.
- A correct diagnosis is vital in the care of polytrauma patients, and fear of radiation should not prevent adequate imaging.

16.1 **RADIATION DOSES AND PROTECTION FROM RADIATION**

Ionizing radiation affects the human cells. In high doses or with repeated exposure, it may be harmful. Trying to estimate morbidity and mortality due to medical imaging is extremely difficult and should be accompanied by estimates of the benefits of the procedures.

DOI: 10.1201/9781003258124-20

There is no evidence to suggest at which exact dose the harmful effects begin; they are random and unpredictable. Therefore, healthcare normally acts from the assumption that there is **no safe threshold dose.**

ALARA – Doses 'As Low As Reasonably Achievable'

All efforts must be made to minimize the effect of ionizing radiation on the human body.

'Any decision that alters the radiation exposure situation should do more good than harm' – ICRP (International Committee for Radiation Protection)

Sievert (Sv) and Gray (Gy) are both units of measurement for radiation, but they measure different things:

- The Sievert (Sv) is used in setting radiological protection standards and contains 1000 milliSieverts (mSv). It measures the biological effect of ionizing radiation on the human body.
- The Gray (Gy) is the SI-derived unit of absorbed radiation dose. It measures the amount of energy deposited in a material by ionizing radiation. The Gray is used to quantify the amount of radiation absorbed by an object or material, such as the human body.

The average annual natural background radiation worldwide is 2.4 mSv, ranging from 1 to 20 mSv, mainly due to terrestrial and airborne radiation, and radiation from building materials. The World Health Organisation (WHO) and the IRCP recommend a maximum annual radiation dose of 50 mSv.[2]

- The current maximum *whole-body dose* is recommended *not to exceed 50 mSv* per annum.
- In 250 flying hours, aircrew receive 50 mSv per year.
- Maximum annual dose for radiation workers is 20 mSv averaged over 5 years, not exceeding 50 mSv per year.
- For therapeutic oncological radiation of single organ targets, the dose may reach 500 mSv (e.g., irradiation of a breast tumour).

Modern CTs will customize radiation according to the density and size of the patient. The transfer itself, as well as the neck collar and the headrest of the CT, will add to the dose required. The dose will also vary widely with the equipment; the dose examples are estimations.

Table 16.1 Dose Examples of Common Diagnostic Radiological Procedures

Examination	Effective Dose (mSv)
Chest X-ray: Bedside AP view	0.02–0.1
Chest CT	6–10
Routine trauma 'pan CT', also called WBCT: Brain, face, neck, torso including pelvis, and proximal femur	20–40 (*2× WBCT will exceed maximum annual dose)
Chest X-ray	2
Pelvic X-ray	5

The younger the patient, the greater the risk of a radiation-induced malignancy due to the impact on proliferating cells and the longer life expectancy. In these cases, observation and repeated clinical exams combined with specific CT exams should be considered as an option.

With pregnant patients, the health of the mother is always the first priority. If possible, specific CT scans instead of whole-body CT (WBCT) may be discussed. If local criteria for WBCT are fulfilled, however, this should be performed. A hospital physicist can calculate the foetus dose after the examination. The 64-MDCT (64-slice multidetector CT) scanner is the most dose-efficient machine when the foetus is outside the direct scan volume, as in the case of pulmonary angiograms. For abdominal examinations, the 64-MDCT scanner imparts the highest foetal dose.[3]

Two percent of all malignant disease now being recorded in the United States and Australia can be attributed directly to medical radiation.[5]

It is therefore important not to overuse the ionizing radiological diagnostic and therapeutic techniques available to us, unless benefits available exceed the risks incurred.[4]

16.2 PRINCIPLES OF TRAUMA IMAGING

- A short but comprehensive medical history on the referral will facilitate correct imaging and speed up reading.
- Position the patient accurately in the gantry. Repositioning is time-consuming.

- Artefacts from external devices (e.g., monitors) as well as from arms positioned beside the body may impede correct diagnosis of injuries, mainly to the liver and the spleen. Lifting the arms above the head or securing them on a pillow in front of the torso, and removing as many objects like drains and monitoring devices as possible from the scan field, will therefore help to optimize image quality and may even reduce the radiation dose.
- A trauma protocol should be robust and fast, and as far as possible eliminate the need for additional CTs because the first one was inadequate. For severely injured patients who need a WBCT, this means:
  - Always scan thorax and abdomen – the impact of the trauma doesn't stop at the diaphragm.
  - Never scan only the vertebral column – if there is risk of a vertebral injury, there may well be injuries to the abdomen and thorax as well.
  - There is seldom need for additional plain films of the pelvis or proximal extremities – these may be included in the scan, and CT offers better imaging than plain films.
- Intravenous (IV) contrast is essential for diagnosing injury to solid organs and vessels.
- In blunt cerebral injury, a CT angiogram of the vessels of the neck and head is now regarded as essential to exclude blunt cerebrovascular injury (BCVI).[6]

Sometimes the question of impaired kidney function arises. If a trauma patient needs an emergency examination, it must never be delayed waiting for a creatinine level – postponing the CT or diverging from the contrast protocol may cause greater harm than the contrast itself.[7] In patients who require repeated CTs during their hospital stay, however, it is important to monitor the creatinine level. Repeated IV contrast administration in a short time span may be harmful, especially in patients with impaired kidney function.

- If needed, the protocol can be adjusted to look for vessel injuries or distal extremity fractures; however, all adjustments will add to the time spent in the radiology department.
- Specific examinations, like triple-contrast CT for intestinal evaluation, or contrast infusion to examine the urine bladder, are in many trauma centres not part of the initial workup.

Communicate with the radiologist to set up the best possible protocol and speedy examination, reading, and reporting.

16.2.1 Extended Focused Assessment by Sonography for Trauma (eFAST)

The basic application of US in trauma is eFAST, which aims to answer the following simple questions:

- Is there free fluid (blood) in the abdomen, pleural spaces, and pericardium?
- Is there free air (pneumothorax) in the pleural cavities?

Four areas of the abdomen are scanned for the detection of free fluid (the eFAST protocol):

- Pericardial
- Perihepatic
- Perisplenic
- Pelvic

The cranial extension of the perihepatic and perisplenic views, obtained by simply sliding the probe upwards, allows a check for haemothorax.

Parasternal sagittal views on the anterior thoracic wall are used to search for the physiologic sliding of the visceral pleura (the so-called 'sliding lung'). The absence of the sliding lung and the recognition of the contact of the lung with the thoracic wall ('lung point') are US signs of pneumothorax. Lung point is not detectable in complete pneumothorax.

Sensitivity and specificity of US in the detection of haemothorax are similar to that of the portable chest X-rays. Sensitivity of US for the detection of pneumothorax in supine position is twice that of chest X-rays and approximates that of CT.

eFAST is not organ-specific, so organ injuries (liver, spleen, etc.) are not the goal and must not be included in the eFAST protocol.

eFAST is non-invasive and repeatable. Whenever the physical assessment and/or the physiology of the patient require it, eFAST could be used to answer clinical questions.

Repeated scans have been shown to increase sensitivity for abdominal views in haemodynamically normal patients. Repetition of eFAST is even more important when no further diagnostic investigations are available.

The amount of free fluid detected can be estimated according to some available scores in the abdomen, and at a glance in the thorax. In the abdomen, immediate and easy detection of fluid in all three views means that more than 800 mL of blood is present in 85% of cases.

Correlation with potential or already established injuries and with the physiological status allows the best clinical decision (observation, definitive treatment, further investigation) to rapidly be made.

- eFAST should be performed:
  - During the primary survey in physiologically unstable patients.
  - At the end of the primary survey in normal and stable patients.
  - During the secondary survey and whenever needed by changes in patient clinical status.
- eFAST refers to the B and C steps of the primary survey, as well as adjuncts to the primary survey.

16.2.2 Indications and Results

16.2.2.1 PENETRATING THORACIC TRAUMA

Detection of pneumothorax and haemothorax by US cannot delay obvious indications for immediate thoracic drainage or surgery.

US (subxiphoid or parasternal view) has replaced pericardiocentesis for the diagnosis of pericardial effusion. Penetrating precordial or transthoracic wounds suspicious for cardiac injury demonstrated accuracy in the detection of pericardial fluid of more than 97%. If it is decided that a pericardiocentesis is required, either as a bridge to surgery or for monitoring, US can help in performing a safer and easier procedure.

16.2.2.2 BLUNT THORACIC TRAUMA

Accuracy of US in detection of haemothorax and pneumothorax is well established. Detection of occult 'small' pneumothorax by US has similar accuracy as CT and can anticipate the need for drainage in mechanically ventilated patients.

16.2.2.3 PENETRATING ABDOMINAL TRAUMA

There is no role for US in hypotensive patients with abdominal penetrating trauma, except for those with thoracoabdominal injuries, when eFAST could help in prioritizing the surgical approach (thorax vs. abdomen first).

A positive FAST after penetrating injury in a haemodynamically normal patient is a strong predictor of significant injury (high positive predictive value). If negative, a different approach (additional diagnostic studies, clinical observation, diagnostic laparoscopy) may be required to rule out occult injury.

16.2.2.4 BLUNT ABDOMINAL TRAUMA

Even if a positive FAST exam is defined by the detection of fluid in one or more views, the meaning of positivity depends on the clinical setting, mechanism of trauma, and associated lesions. FAST significantly shortens the time to definitive treatment.

A small amount of fluid in the perisplenic view in a hypotensive patient suggests other sources of shock (retroperitoneal, pelvic, thoracic, long bones bleeding; tension pneumothorax; neurogenic shock). The same small amount of free fluid in a normotensive trauma patient, with a seatbelt sign, entails a high index of suspicion for hollow viscus injury.

A negative or slightly positive FAST gives information for the decision-making process which may be as useful as a grossly positive one, according to the clinical status.

16.2.2.5 PELVIC TRAUMA

Ultrasound plays a relevant role in hypotensive patients with haemorrhagic pelvic fractures. A grossly positive exam is a marker of intraperitoneal bleeding and associated abdominal injuries, and mandates surgical exploration. A negative or slightly positive FAST exam suggests pelvic bleeding is the major cause of shock. These two findings allow for a better therapeutic strategy, according to institutional resources. If the patient's stability allows it, CT with CTA is preferable.

16.2.3 Other Applications of Ultrasound in Trauma

- In an ABCDE (airway, breathing, circulation, disability, and exposure) sequence, US could be used for assessing proper orotracheal intubation (tracheal and lung views), to speed recognition of landmarks for cricothyroidotomy or tracheostomy, and for assessing the presence and evolution of pulmonary contusions.
- Inferior vena cava diameter and collapsibility help in evaluation of volume status and shock management,[8] together with the subxiphoid assessment of cardiac chambers' repletion and contractility.
- Bone fracture edges can be easily detected by US (sternum, ribs, long bones).

- A more advanced application of US is contrast-enhanced US (CEUS), which could be used both for the detection of solid organ injuries in selected groups of patients (e.g., haemodynamically normal paediatric patients sustaining blunt abdominal trauma) and for the follow-up of non-operative management of parenchymatous organs (liver, spleen, kidney).

16.2.4 Training

US, like any technical skill, is operator dependent. Formal training is needed for getting competence in acquisition and interpretation of US findings. Hands-on courses and proctored practice are needed. Due to its clinical value and relative ease of learning, eFAST training still represents the suggested first step for beginners.

16.3 PITFALLS AND PEARLS

- Use external wound markers for all visible entry sites (e.g., vitamin E capsules or paper clips) to facilitate wound tracking and to enhance the speed of the reading of images. In the case of gunshot wounds, counting entry and exit wounds and projectiles will also help to localize any missing bullets.
- Use the planning overview image (also known as the scout image) to look for foreign bodies, fractures, and large pneumo- and haemothoraces.
- If it is not possible to insert an IV needle, the contrast may be given in an intraosseous (IO) needle. High pressure is needed, and power injection is possible, although very little studied. Humeral placement is the preferred site of access. The procedure is painful, and a local anaesthetic should be given if the patient is not sedated. The arm must be kept still when the humeral IO needle is in place and must therefore not be lifted above the head.
- Notoriously difficult areas include the diaphragm and the oesophagus; a negative examination does not exclude injury, even with modern MDCT.
- CT after damage control surgery is an entity which involves the most badly wounded, unstable patients who go to the OR before CT, and it needs special attention. It can be difficult to differentiate between traumatic injuries and postoperative findings. Vessels may be ligated, organs removed, and bowels stapled, and foreign objects like packings and

thrombus-generating cellulose (e.g., Surgicel®) may cause confusion.

- Dual-energy imaging is a relatively new CT application which may facilitate the diagnosis of bleeding, metal fragments, bone oedema, and injuries to the bowel wall.
- It is of great value to practice trauma management regularly. Ideally, this is done together with the other departments who are involved in trauma care. In addition to initial resuscitation and radiological procedures, safe transportation and transfer of the patient also need to be practiced regularly. This includes making sure the anaesthetic team is well acquainted with the surroundings and limited space in the CT lab.
- Quality is improved by regular multidisciplinary morbidity and mortality conferences, where all involved disciplines discuss trauma cases together.

Key success factors in trauma management include:

- A well-known trauma routine which is practiced regularly.
- A robust protocol for WBCT.
- Communication, evaluation, and feedback.
- Subcutaneous emphysema makes deep structures undetectable and is a contraindication to the use of US.
- Organ injuries are in general out of the scope of clinical US in trauma patients (except CEUS-FAST). Diagnoses of bowel injury, diaphragmatic rupture, retroperitoneal lesions and haematomas, and solid organ injury could be considered based on direct/indirect B-mode US findings, but they need to be assessed with other methods when suspected.
- Free abdominal fluid is not always blood (e.g., enteric/bile aspiration in a suspected hollow viscus injury, or urine in a stable patient with a pelvic fracture). When in doubt, aspiration under US guidance can enhance the decision-making process.

16.4 LOW-DOSE X-RAY (LODOX®)[9,10]

First developed for the diamond mines in South Africa, the low-dose X-ray (LODOX) is an X-ray unit (not a scanner) capable of performing a whole-body digital X-ray in 13 seconds at very high quality. Relative digital radiation doses compared to conventional ones varied from 72% (chest) to 2% (pelvis), with a simple average of 6% of the equivalent conventional X-ray dose. It has replaced X-rays in many units in South Africa and elsewhere, ideally placed at the entrance to the ER. The time taken for the X-ray including loading and unloading onto the resuscitation stretcher is < 120 seconds, so it is suited to multiple patients and has military applications as well for multiple projectiles. It removes the need for any other X-rays, allowing almost immediate resuscitation. It is not a substitute for the CT scanner. See **Figure 16.1**.

16.5 CT IN TRAUMA

Judicious use of CT can make a significant difference to the management of a trauma patient. Several CT applications and trauma settings are considered in this section.

16.5.1 Pan CT

Pan CT, also sometimes referred to as whole-body CT (WBCT), is often contrast-enhanced (CECT; see below) and provides diagnostic detail in each of the mentioned body regions, which is infinitely useful in terms of guiding further management. The cranial component allows examination of the brain, skull, and facial bones; the cervical component demonstrates the cervical spine; and the thoracic component scans the spine, ribs, bony elements, lungs, heart, great vessels, and posterior mediastinum. In the abdomen, certain injuries may be safely selected for non-operative management, such as injuries to the solid organs, whilst free intra-abdominal air warrants laparotomy. Three phases (arterial, venous, and delayed) provide all the necessary information, and CT cystography may be added in the delayed phase if bladder injury is suspected.

The radiation dose of this extensive scan is high, and therefore it should not be used inappropriately. Universally accepted indications include:

- Significant injuries on both sides of the diaphragm (e.g., traumatic brain injury and fractured femur), to exclude injury in between
- Dangerous mechanism of injury (e.g., fell from a height or ejected from a vehicle)
- Unable to assess clinically (e.g., decreased Glasgow Coma Score or spinal cord injury)

There is a concern among clinicians that patients who undergo pan CT in the acute trauma setting may develop contrast-induced acute kidney injury (AKI). The balance of literature, however, seems to indicate that whilst AKI is common in trauma patients, CECT is not an independent risk factor for its development.[7]

16.5.2 CT Angiography

Modern multi-slice CT scanners provide the ability to perform angiography rapidly and with high diagnostic accuracy. CTA can be performed in any body region where vascular injury is suspected, and injuries can be selected for conservative management (e.g., minor intimal injuries), operative management, or endovascular management.

16.5.3 CT in Specific Body Regions

16.5.3.1 CT OF THE NECK

In most trauma centres, CTA has largely replaced X-rays in diagnosis of suspected cervical spine injury, the sensitivity of CT being far superior to that of X-rays.[7]

In patients with traumatic brain injury from a blunt mechanism, it is advisable to perform CT not only of the brain but also of the cervical spine. Uncontrasted CT may be sufficient for this purpose in the acute trauma setting; however, patients presenting with significant injuries to the head, face, neck, and upper chest (i.e., the presence of 'extended Denver screening criteria') are at risk of having blunt cerebrovascular injury, and in such a case, contrasted CT is becoming mandatory.[8]

In penetrating injury of the neck, apart from looking for a vascular injury, it should also be noted whether there is free air in the deep cervical fascia, suggestive of oesophageal injury. In the absence of such free air, there is evidence to suggest that it may not be mandatory to follow up with oesophageal imaging or endoscopy (negative predictive value approaching 100%).[11]

16.5.3.2 CT OF THE CHEST

CT imaging of the chest outlines bony injuries very well, and three-dimensional reconstructions can be helpful in delineating multiple rib fractures when planning operative rib fracture fixation.

CT is highly sensitive for demonstrating haemo- or pneumothorax, and lung contusions can be assessed for extent and severity. Aortic arch injury must always be

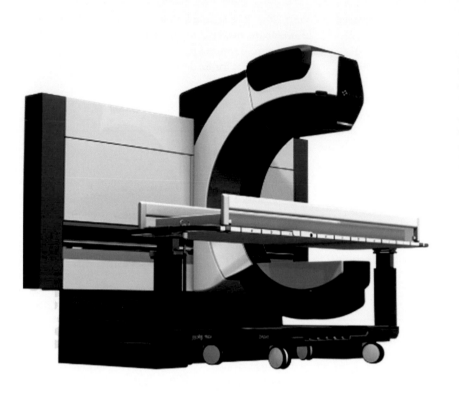
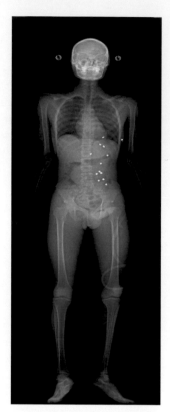

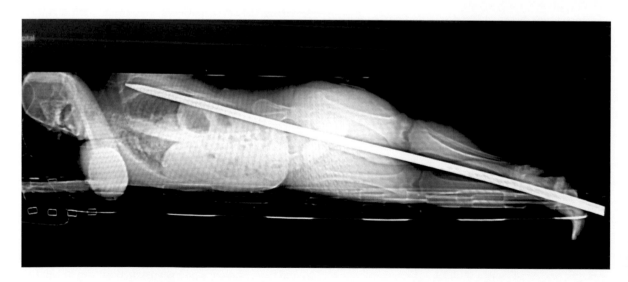

Figure 16.1 Low-dose X-ray (LODOX®).

carefully excluded in patients with blunt chest trauma, and the pericardial space should be assessed for the presence of pericardial effusion.

It is important to pay specific attention to the posterior mediastinum on the chest CT. In rare cases, blunt force trauma to the abdomen can displace gastric contents upwards (retrograde) and cause an oesophageal blow-out injury. This will manifest as free air in the posterior mediastinum (surrounding the oesophagus) with or without accompanying pleural effusion. The oesophageal rupture most commonly occurs just above the diaphragm on the left (Boerhaave syndrome) but may occasionally occur above the azygos vein on the right, in the superior mediastinum. If this injury is missed on initial presentation, it can culminate in deadly mediastinitis within the next 48 hours.

Finally, CT of the chest is imperative in haemodynamically stable patients with transmediastinal penetrating injuries, such as a gunshot which has traversed the midline. CT in this instance will show the bullet track and either demonstrate or strongly suggest which mediastinal structures may have been injured. *Don't forget the skin markers!*

16.5.3.3 CT OF THE ABDOMEN

For blunt trauma, solid organ injury can be diagnosed and graded, and most can be managed non-operatively, unless there is an indication for laparotomy, such as the presence of free air.

A diagnostic dilemma arises when no abnormality is seen other than free fluid. Such fluid may represent any of the following body fluids:

- Blood (e.g., from a mesenteric injury)
- Bile (e.g., from a gall bladder/bile duct/liver/duodenal injury)
- Bowel content (injury of any part of the intra-abdominal gastrointestinal [GI] tract)
- Pancreatic fluid (injury to the main pancreatic duct)
- Urine (bladder injury)

In this case, it is important to carefully re-examine the patient as well as the CT images and rule out any of the above-mentioned possibilities that would warrant laparotomy. In the absence of any of these, the patient may be observed. The majority of these patients will settle without further intervention.[12]

For penetrating trauma, CT of the abdomen has a limited role. Patients who are unstable or peritonitic, have free air under the diaphragm on erect chest X-ray, or have eviscerated bowel or evidence of abdominal penetration need laparotomy.

CT, however, is helpful in two specific instances in penetrating trauma:

- To avoid surgery:
  - In a patient with penetrating injury limited to the right upper quadrant, CT can confirm that the track is confined to the liver and no other structures have been injured. Such a liver injury, if it meets the criteria for non-operative management, can then be managed without laparotomy.[13]
  - In a very obese patient with a gunshot track suspicious of having only traversed extra-abdominal adipose tissue (i.e., tangential injury), CT can confirm the track and prevent the need for laparotomy. See **Figure 16.2**.

- To guide surgery:
  - In a stable patient with an existing indication for laparotomy (e.g., peritonitis) and with frank haematuria suggestive of a renal injury (based on the bullet trajectory), it is helpful to obtain CT of the abdomen prior to laparotomy. The current trend regarding renal injuries is to manage these non-operatively as much as possible (e.g., catheter-directed embolization for intrarenal pseudo-aneurysm and/or ureteric stent for urinary extravasation). CT in this instance provides the opportunity to grade the renal injury and plan whether it should be explored during laparotomy or managed separately (i.e., Gerota's fascia not opened during laparotomy).
  - In a stable patient with a trans-pelvic gunshot wound, CT prior to laparotomy can be infinitely helpful. There are many structures packed together within a small space in the pelvis, and to explore all of them to rule out injury can be not only difficult and time-consuming, but also more destructive than necessary. CT will outline the ureters, blood vessels, bladder, female organs, and rectum, and guide the surgeon as to which areas should be explored and which can be safely left alone. Free air in the para-rectal tissues should warrant on-table sigmoidoscopy and possibly de-functioning sigmoid loop colostomy.

In most cases, thanks to the detail provided by modern multi-slice CT scanners, it is no longer necessary to use oral contrast and/or rectal contrast (i.e., request double- or triple-contrasted CT) routinely. Single-contrast

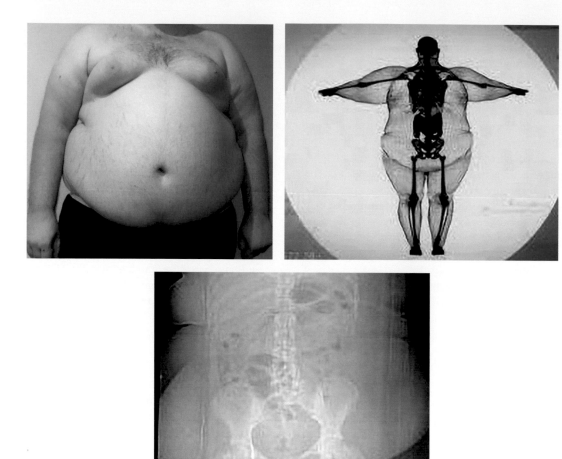

Figure 16.2 'Urban armour' in the obese patient.

(i.e. IV contrast only) will suffice for most trauma scans, unless the addition of GI contrast is specifically indicated (e.g., looking to outline a duodenal injury or rectal injury in particular).[14]

16.5.3.4 CT ANGIOGRAPHY OF THE LIMBS

A single stab or gunshot to the thigh or to the arm above the elbow, accompanied by an absent distal pulse, warrants no angiography unless endovascular management is being considered. In these anatomical areas, there is only one main vessel, and surgical exploration will easily pinpoint the injury.

CTA is, however, indicated in the following cases with absent distal pulses:

- Multiple penetrating wounds (i.e., it is not clear where the vessel is injured along its course)

- Longitudinal bullet track, running alongside the axis of the vessel in question (i.e., it is not clear as to where the vessel is injured along this track)
- Blunt trauma (fracture/dislocation)
- Penetrating injury to forearm or leg below knee (more than one vessel need to be assessed)

CTA is indicated in cases where endovascular management is anticipated, as well as in the following scenarios:

- Distal pulse present, but weak ankle-brachial index (below 0.9)
- Audible bruit over the injury site, suggesting arteriovenous fistula
- Posterior knee dislocation or tibial plateau fracture (always rule out popliteal artery injury!)

16.6 CATHETER-DIRECTED ANGIOGRAPHY (CDA)

CDA can be utilized as a diagnostic and/or therapeutic modality but has been largely replaced by CTA.

16.6.1 Diagnostic

When CTA is unavailable or unhelpful, CDA can be used as a diagnostic modality. An example is a patient who has been injured by birdshot, with multiple small metal pellets lodged in an area of interest, causing scatter on CT or simply obscuring the necessary vascular detail. In such a case, CDA with digital subtraction can diagnose even small injuries that may have been missed on CTA.

16.6.2 Therapeutic

CDA is commonly used in two trauma scenarios:

- *Catheter-directed angioembolization*: For example, for a splenic injury diagnosed on abdominal CT, with a central 'blush' suggesting pseudo-aneurysm.
- *Stenting of a vascular injury*: This has become widespread as a trauma treatment modality, with arteries from the neck all the way down to the popliteal arteries being stented, sparing patients the need for vascular exploration. This is especially of benefit when *major* exploration is avoided (e.g., aortic arch injury or subclavian artery injury) and when there are other injuries adding to the patient's overall injury burden.

16.7 RETAINED WEAPONS

When a blade is retained in a patient's body (e.g., neck) on presentation to the hospital, it poses the question as to whether it can safely be extracted. Any blade that is suspected (based on X-ray imaging) to be in the vicinity of a known artery should be left *in situ* and CTA conducted. If there is scatter, or if it is not clear as to whether there is a vascular injury, CDA should be performed.

If there is no obvious injury to an artery, the knife can be extracted in the OR, ready to perform exploration in case of torrential bleeding. If the blade, however, is shown to be situated in an artery, one of two methods may be employed for blade removal:

- *Operative*: Formal vascular exploration is done, proximal and distal control obtained, and the blade extracted, followed by vascular repair.
- *Endovascular*: A stent is positioned radiologically in the area where the knife has breached the arterial wall, the blade is removed, and the stent is deployed in real time under fluoroscopic guidance, covering the defect in the vessel wall.

16.8 SUMMARY

eFAST remains the basic diagnostic application.

- eFAST is a good initial screening tool for blunt abdominal injury and shortens the time to definitive treatment in hypotensive patients.
- Ultrasound is a highly reliable method for detecting haemothorax and pneumothorax in trauma patients.
- Many procedural manoeuvres could be realized under US guidance, increasing decisional process and safety.
- The clinically integrated use of US in trauma requires specific training.

CT currently plays a major role in trauma, and this role continues to evolve.

- Radiation is a serious concern, and therefore all CT examinations should be carefully considered.

REFERENCES AND RECOMMENDED READING

References

1. Huber-Wagner S, Lefering R, Qvick LM, Körner M, Kay MV, Pfeifer KJ, et al. Effect of whole-body CT during trauma resuscitation on survival: a retrospective, multicentre study. Lancet. 2009 Apr 25;**373**(**9673**):1455–61. doi: 10.1016/S0140-6736(09)60232-4.
2. The 2007 Recommendations of the International Commission on Radiological Protection. ICRP publication 103. Ann ICRP. 2007;**37**(**2–4**):1–332. doi: 10.1016/j.icrp.2007.10.003.

3. Gilet AG, Dunkin JM, Fernandez TJ, Button TM, Budorick NE. Foetal radiation dose during gestation estimated on an anthropomorphic phantom for three generations of CT scanners. AJR Am J Roentgenol. 2011 May;**196(5)**:1133–7. doi: 10.2214/AJR.10.4497.

4. Linder F, Mani K, Juhlin C, Eklöf H. Routine whole body CT of high energy trauma patients leads to excessive radiation exposure. Scand J Trauma Resusc Emerg Med. 2016 Jan 27;**24**:7. doi: 10.1186/s13049-016-0199-2.

5. de Gonzalez, AB, Mahesh M, Kim, KP, Bhargavan M, Lewis R, Mettler F, et al. Projected cancer risks from computed tomographic scans performed in the United States in 2007. Arch Int Med. 2009 Dec 14:**169(22)**:2071–7. doi: 10.1001/archinternmed.2009.440

6. Brommeland T, Helseth E, Aarhus M, Moen KG, Dyrskog S, Bergholt B, Olivecrona Z, Jeppesen E. Best practice guidelines for blunt cerebrovascular injury (BCVI). Scand J Trauma Resusc Emerg Med. 2018 Oct 29;**26(1)**:90. doi: 10.1186/s13049-018-0559-1.

7. Ehrmann MR, Mitchell J, Levin S, Smith A, Menez S, Hinson JS, Klein EY. Renal outcomes following intravenous contrast administration in patients with acute kidney injury: a multi-site retrospective propensity-adjusted analysis. Intensive Care Med. 2023 Jan 30. doi: 10.1007/s00134-022-06966-w.

8. Stawicki, SP, Adkins EJ, Eiferman DS, Evans DC, Ali NA, Njoku C, et al. Prospective evaluation of intravascular volume status in critically ill patients: does inferior vena cava collapsibility correlate with central venous pressure? J Trauma Acute Care Surg, 2014 Apr;**76(4)**:956–63; discussion 963–4. doi: 10.1097/TA.0000000000000152.

9. Boffard KD, Goosen J, Plani F, Degiannis E, Potgieter. The use of low dosage X-ray (Lodox/Statscan) in major trauma: comparison between low dose X-ray and conventional X-ray techniques J Trauma. 2006 Jun;**60(6)**:1175–81; discussion 1181–3. doi:

10. LODOX® Exemplar-dr Whole body Low Dose X-ray. https://www.lodox.com (accessed September 20–23).

11. Madsen AS, Oosthuizen G, Laing GL, Bruce JL, Clarke DL. The role of computed tomography angiography in the detection of aerodigestive tract injury following penetrating neck injury. J Surg Res. 2016 Oct;**205(2)**:490–8. doi: 10.1016/j.jss.2016.06.044.

12. Bekker W, Smith M, Kong VY, Bruce JL, Laing G, Manchev V, et al. Isolated free fluid on computed tomography for blunt abdominal trauma. Ann R Coll Surg Engl. 2019 Nov;**101(8)**:552–7. doi: 10.1308/rcsann.2019.0078.

13. Navsaria P, Nicol A, Krige J, Edu S, Chowdhury S. Selective nonoperative management of liver gunshot injuries. Eur J Trauma Emerg Surg. 2019 Apr;**45(2)**:323–8. doi: 10.1007/s00068-018-0913-z.

14. Ramirez RM, Cureton EL, Ereso AQ, Kwan RO, Dozier KC, Sadjadi J, et al. Single-contrast computed tomography for the triage of patients with penetrating torso trauma. J Trauma. 2009 Sep;**67(3)**:583–8. doi: 10.1097/TA.0b013e3181a39330.

Recommended Reading

International Commission for Radiological Protection (ICRP) Publications. Available from: http://www.icrp.org/page.asp?id=5 (accessed online August 2023).

Royal College of Radiologists. Standards of practice and guidance for trauma radiology in severely injured patients. 2015. Available from: https://www.rcr.ac.uk/our-services/all-our-publications/clinical-radiology-publications/standards-of-practice-and-guidance-for-trauma-radiology-in-severely-injured-patients-second-edition/

Horer T. The Hybrid OR and Hybrid Options for Trauma and Bleeding Patients. In: DuBose JJ, Horer T eds. Top Stent. Orebro University Hospital, Orebro, Sweden. 2017. ISBN 978-91-639-2522-1.

Part 5

Specialized aspects of total trauma care

Critical Care of the Trauma **17** Patient 2024

17.1 INTRODUCTION

Most trauma admissions to the intensive care unit (ICU) occur as a result of haemorrhagic shock, hypoxic respiratory failure, or refractory severe traumatic brain injury (TBI), some of them preventable deaths. Trauma ICU care is best provided by a multidisciplinary team focussed on resuscitation, monitoring, and life support.

Fundamental early goals are restoration and maintenance of tissue oxygenation, diagnosis and treatment of occult injuries, and prevention and treatment of infection and multiple organ failure (MOF). In the ICU, those who take care of a patient admitted with lethal brain injury play a vital role in the identification and support of potential organ donors and their families.

17.2 PHASES OF ICU CARE

17.2.1 Resuscitative Phase (First 24 Hours Post-Injury)[1]

Management is focussed on haemostatic resuscitation, with maintaining adequate tissue perfusion the goal of treatment. Simultaneously, occult life-threatening or limb-threatening injuries are carefully sought and addressed.

Inadequate tissue oxygenation must be recognized and treated immediately.

Deficient tissue oxygen delivery in the acutely traumatized patient is usually caused by impaired perfusion, severe hypoxaemia, or impaired oxygen delivery. Although several different types of shock can be present, inadequate resuscitation from hypovolaemia and blood loss is the most common.

After major trauma, some patients experience considerable delay before *organ perfusion* is fully restored, despite apparently adequate systolic blood pressure (SBP) and apparently normal urine output. This phenomenon has been called *occult hypoperfusion*.[2] A clear association has been identified between occult hypoperfusion or persistent hypovolaemia after major trauma and increased rates of infection, length of stay, days in the surgical/ trauma ICU, hospital charges, multiple organ dysfunction syndrome (MODS), and mortality.[3] Rapid control of bleeding and early identification and aggressive resuscitation aimed at correcting hypovolaemia have been shown to improve survival and reduce complications in severely injured trauma patients.

A positive fluid balance alone is an independent risk factor for acute respiratory distress syndrome (ARDS) and MOF. Currently, a more balanced approach utilizes an initial restricted or controlled volume resuscitation (SBP approx. 90 mmHg) until surgical bleeding is controlled. (See Chapter 6: 'Damage Control'.)

17.2.1.1 'TRADITIONAL' ENDPOINTS OF RESUSCITATION

The optimal single endpoint to determine the adequacy of resuscitation remains elusive. Markers of inadequate global oxygen delivery, such as base deficit, lactate level, or mixed venous oxygen saturation, are used. These include the following to try to assess microcirculation and microcirculatory changes to guide in the resuscitation:

- *Clinical endpoints*: Restoration of a normal blood pressure, pulse rate, capillary refill, and temperature, and adequate urine output. The neurology should be improving, and no clinical features on coagulopathy should be noted. Important that these are shown to be improving with less transfusion, fluid,

DOI: 10.1201/9781003258124-22

and vasopressor support. Overall condition should improve with less support than required.

- *Biochemical endpoints*:
  - Assuring that the clinical endpoints are objectively assessed. This includes a decreasing lactate level and improving coagulation parameters. Base deficit and failure to clear lactic acidosis in 24 hours comprise an ominous sign.
  - An improving base excess level and other surrogates of perfusion, like central venous saturations above 70%. Glucose level stabilization with less variability and acceptable haemoglobin and platelets function. Base deficit and lactate should reduce by 30% in the first hour.
  - The shock index, obtained by dividing the heart rate by the systolic pressure, where a value of > 0.7–0.9 detects hypovolaemia and shock and is a prognostic factor.
  - Central venous pressure is not of value in determining fluid requirements.[4]
- *Cardiac function assessment*: Invasive or non-invasive monitoring of cardiac output or cardiac index, total peripheral resistance, and stroke volume variations. This allows for evaluation of fluid status and response to resuscitations. It further assists in the selection of an appropriate vasopressor to assist with output.[5]
- *Organ-specific parameters*: These include assessment of specific organ regions. Gastric tonometry was an example of such systems, but it is not commonly used. The local measurement of jugular venous saturation or intracranial partial pressures is another example in head injury cases.

Pitfall

Blood pressure, central venous pressure, heart rate, arterial partial pressure of oxygen (PaO_2), and so on can be helpful but may **not** identify occult hypoperfusion. Current practice involves an assimilation of multiple endpoints of resuscitation into an overall assessment.

17.2.1.2 POST-TRAUMATIC ACUTE LUNG INJURY

Aetiology:

- Chest trauma
- Fluid overload
- Distributive shock
- Aspiration
- Fat embolism syndrome
- Acute insult with pre-existing respiratory disease

17.2.1.3 RESPIRATORY ASSESSMENT AND MONITORING[6]

- Work of breathing and use of accessory muscles (if spontaneously breathing).
- Respiratory rate and minute volume (if spontaneously breathing).
- Arterial blood gases – including repeat measurement of base deficit (BD) and lactate.
- Oxygen delivery (DO_2) and consumption (VO_2).
- The PaO_2/fraction of inspired oxygen (FiO_2) (PF) ratio is used to assess the degree of lung injury, where:
  - *400–500*: Normal
  - *< 300*: Mild lung injury/ARDS
  - *< 200*: Moderate lung injury/ARDS
  - *< 100*: Severe lung injury/ARDS
- Bronchoscopy may be necessary if aspiration or a foreign body is suspected.

17.2.1.4 MECHANICAL VENTILATION (MV)

Ventilatory support should be instituted earlier rather than later; select a mode of ventilation tailored to the patient's need using 6–8 mL/Kg tidal volumes and sufficient positive end-expiratory pressure (PEEP) to optimize oxygenation and compliance.

Pitfalls

Failure to respond *early* to indications for ventilatory support:

- Apnoea or severe chest pathology
- Tachypnoea (in the adult, > 30 or < 10/min; or child, respiratory rate [RR] > 40 or < 15/min)
- Mechanical ventilatory compromise (such as severe flail chest and pulmonary contusion)
- Hypoxaemia (pO_2 < 8 kPa/60 mmHg on a reservoir mask [FiO_2 = 0.6] or a saturation that is decreasing)
- Hypercarbia (partial pressure of carbon dioxide [pCO_2] > 6.5 kPa/50 mmHg, especially in the context of associated TBI or where it is associated with an acidosis)
- Mental compromise (GCS < 9/15)
- Haemodynamic instability/cardiac arrest

17.2.1.5 VENTILATORY MODE (ACTUAL MODE IS UNIMPORTANT)

- Lung-protective ventilation (LPV), **from the beginning**, with low tidal volume and higher rate, tolerating higher than normal $PaCO_2$ (sometimes up to 50–70 mmHg, without detriment) if required. Use adequate volumes despite the frequent requirement for higher pressures.
- Limit the peak pressure (pressure modes) and the plateau (pause) pressure (volume modes) to < 30 cm H_2O.
- **Limit the driving pressure (plateau pressure – PEEP) to < 15 cm H_2O.**[7]
- High PEEP (> 10 up to 14 cm H_2O may be required) to recruit alveoli.
- ECMO (extracorporeal membrane oxygenation) may be considered where appropriate (see Section 17.3).
- Non-invasive ventilatory support in selected cases only.

The most commonly used mode is volume or pressure assist–control, or if the patient is conscious and initiating breaths, pressure support ventilation (PSV) and PEEP are the most synchronous mode. Recruitment manoeuvres may be necessary if there is atelectasis, which in the acute setting usually consists of application of a positive pressure of 40 cm H_2O for 30–40 seconds.[8]

17.2.2 Early Life Support Phase (24–72 Hours Post-Injury)

During this phase, treatment is focussed on the management of post-traumatic respiratory failure and a progressive intracranial pressure (ICP) rise in patients suffering from severe head injury. Usually, diagnostic evaluation for occult injuries has been completed. Evidence of early MOF may become apparent during this time.

Problems that may develop at this time include intracranial hypertension (ICH), systemic inflammatory response syndrome (SIRS), early MODS, and continued respiratory insufficiency. The main priorities of the early life support phase are the maintenance of tissue oxygenation, the control of ICH, an ongoing search for occult injuries, the institution of nutritional support, venous thromboembolism (VTE) prophylaxis, and withdrawal or replacement of trauma resuscitation lines or devices that may have been placed in less-than-ideal conditions.

17.2.2.1 PRIORITIES

- Gas exchange and ventilatory support
- Haematological parameters
- Fluid and electrolyte balance
- ICP monitoring and control
- Identification of occult injuries
- Identification of delayed intracranial haematoma formation using repeated computed tomography (CT) of the head, as required
- Identification of intra-abdominal injuries with CT or ultrasound of the abdomen
  - Identification or exclusion of spinal injury
  - Extremity injury, using selective radiography as indicated by clinical examination
- Identification of nerve injuries sometimes delayed until patients regain consciousness

17.2.3 Prolonged Life Support (> 72 Hours Post-Injury)

The duration of the prolonged life support phase depends on the severity of the injury and its associated complications. Many of those who are critically injured can be successfully weaned from life support early, whilst the more seriously injured enter a phase in which ongoing life support is necessary to prevent or treat organ system failure. Infectious complications are the commonest cause of late MOF or death.

The main objective of the management of patients developing MODS is to provide support for failing organ systems whilst attempts are made to isolate and eliminate inflammatory foci. In addition, prolonged immobility can cause problems with muscle wasting, joint contractures, and skin compromise in pressure areas. Physiotherapy should be commenced early, with the proper use of splints, early exercise, and ambulation when possible.

17.2.3.1 RESPIRATORY FAILURE

- Unexplained persisting respiratory failure.
  - Look for occult infection or necrotic tissue.
  - Consider early tracheostomy at approximately day 7 in patients who can be anticipated to have persisting airway compromise from early in their ICU course – those with neurological injuries in the high-thoracic/low-cervical level.
  - Trials show no advantage for earlier tracheostomy in other critically ill patients.

17.2.3.2 INFECTIOUS COMPLICATIONS

- Nosocomial pneumonia.[9]
- There should be new X-ray infiltrates and evidence of worsening systemic inflammation as measured by elevated procalcitonin (PCT), and an indication that this is infection related by the presence of purulent secretions. Serial PCT measurements can be useful in this regard.[10]
- Lung abscess and empyema.
- Surgical site infection:
  - Superficial incisional surgical site infection (e.g., wound infection).
  - Deep incisional surgical site infection.
  - Organ/space surgical site infection (e.g., intra-abdominal abscess).
- Intravenous catheter-related sepsis.
- Bloodstream infections.
- Urinary tract infection.
- Acalculous cholecystitis.
- Sinusitis and otitis media.
- Ventriculitis and meningitis.

Pitfalls

- Antibiotic therapy in life-threatening infection should be broad when empirically treating, then narrowed to a limited spectrum when permitted by positive cultures.
- Duration of antibiotics should be as short as possible, determined by clinical resolution and not arbitrary time periods.
- De-escalation strategy clearly defined.
- Remember the risk of antibiotic-associated colitis.

17.2.3.3 NON-INFECTIOUS CAUSES OF FEVER

- Metabolic response to tissue trauma
- Medications (esp. phenytoin, tricyclic antidepressants, dexmedetomidine, and antimicrobials)
- Pulmonary embolus (PE)
- Deep venous thrombosis (DVT)

17.2.3.4 PERCUTANEOUS TRACHEOSTOMY[11]

Percutaneous tracheostomy has been shown to have fewer perioperative and postoperative complications compared with conventional tracheostomy and is now the technique of choice in critically ill patients with favourable anatomy. Various techniques are described, with dilatation by forceps or multiple or single dilators. Patient selection is important.

Pitfalls

- Percutaneous tracheostomy should not be attempted if the procedure is non-elective, the landmarks are obscure in the neck, or the patient has a coagulopathy.
- Caution should be exercised if the patient has a known cervical spine injury.
- Confirmation of correct placement by fibre-optic bronchoscopy is valuable and mandated in the practice standards of some professional bodies.
- Percutaneous tracheostomy is not suitable for children.

17.2.3.5 WEANING FROM VENTILATORY SUPPORT

During the recovery phase, the most important transition made is that from mechanical ventilation to unassisted breathing, known as *weaning*. Weaning begins as soon as the causes of respiratory failure have resolved.

17.2.3.6 EXTUBATION CRITERIA ('SOA2P')

S *Secretions*: Minimal
O *Oxygenation*: Good (typically requiring FiO_2 of less than 35%)
A *Alert*
A *Airway*: Without injury or compromise
P *Pressures or parameters*: Measurements of tidal volume, vital capacity, negative inspiratory force, and so on

17.2.4 Recovery Phase (Transition from the ICU)

During the recovery phase, the patient is weaned from full ventilatory support until breathing spontaneously, and invasive monitoring devices can be removed. The patient and family are prepared for the transition from the ICU to a general patient or intermediate care unit, and plans for further convalescence and rehabilitation are developed. (See 'The ABCDEF ICU Liberation Bundle'[12] – **Table 17.1**.)

Table 17.1 The ABCDEF ICU Liberation Bundle

Symptoms	Monitoring Tools		Care	Done
Pain	Critical-Care Pain Observation Tool (CCPOT) Numeric Rating Scale (NRS) Behavioural Pain Scale (BPS)	A	Assess, prevent, and manage pain	☐
		B	Both Spontaneous Awakening Trials (SATs) and Spontaneous Breathing Trials (SBTs)	☐
Agitation	Richmond Agitation-Sedation Scale (RASS) Sedation-Agitation Scale (SAS)	C	Choice of analgesia and sedation	☐
		D	Delirium: Assess, prevent, and manage	☐
Delirium	Confusion Assessment Method for the Intensive Care Unit (CAM-ICU) Intensive Care Delirium Screening Checklist	E	Early mobility and exercise	☐
		F	Family engagement and empowerment	☐

17.3 EXTRACORPOREAL MEMBRANE OXYGENATION (ECMO)[13–15]

17.3.1 Overview

ECMO is an expensive therapy, so outcome should be unequivocally improved to justify its use. It is a technology that has been shown to be efficient in improving oxygenation but has substantial cost implications and limited evidence of survival benefit, depending on patient selection. In a recent review of 58 publications reporting 548 trauma patients undergoing ECMO, bleeding (22.9%) and thrombosis (19%) were the most common complications, with an overall hospital mortality of 30.3%. It is envisaged, however, that as ECMO is more frequently employed and expertise is improved, new indications and exclusions may become apparent.[16]

Modern circuit coatings reduce the requirement for systemic anticoagulation, so unlike intraoperative cardiopulmonary bypass, it is not mandatory to fully anticoagulate a trauma patient undergoing ECMO. However, at least some anticoagulation is desirable, as thrombosis is a common complication. Consensus guidelines in trauma recommend anticoagulation may be withheld for 5 days to an entire run, so long as there is minimal evidence of oxygenator clot formation, but that at least some systemic anticoagulation is desirable if the patient's overall condition allows.[17]

This is a living science that will develop along with new technical developments.

17.3.2 Modes of ECMO

Three types of ECMO are available.

17.3.2.1 VENO-VENOUS ECMO (VV-ECMO)

Blood is extracted from the vena cava/right atrium and returned to the right atrium, providing respiratory but no cardiac support. Indications:

- Primary ARDS with refractory hypoxaemia (particularly viral, but any pneumonia without MOF), contusion, gas or smoke inhalation, and aspiration.
- Status asthmaticus or reversible airway obstruction not able to be ventilated conventionally.
- Massive pulmonary embolism (if haemodynamically stable).
- Pulmonary contusion, gas inhalation, aspiration, and smoke inhalation. Hypoxic respiratory failure with a PF ratio < 70–100 mmHg despite optimum ventilator settings.
- Hypercapnic respiratory failure with pH < 7.2.
- Ventilatory support as a bridge to lung transplantation.
- Pneumonia (particularly viral, but any pneumonia without MOF).
- ARDS if the PF ratio < 70 (Berlin consensus statement).

VV-ECMO is the most commonly employed mode in trauma patients, used primarily to treat refractory hypoxaemia.

17.3.2.2 VENO-ARTERIAL ECMO (VA-ECMO)

In VA-ECMO – which is effectively cardiopulmonary bypass, performed over a longer period and often via peripherally inserted cannulae rather than lines placed surgically through a thoracic incision – blood is extracted from the right atrium and returned to the arterial system.

It allows haemodynamic support and is indicated for cardiac failure, with or without respiratory failure.

- Weaning from cardiopulmonary bypass after cardiac surgery
- As a bridge to cardiac transplantation
- Reversible cardiac disease, such as contusion and acute myocarditis
- Pulmonary hypertension (after pulmonary endarterectomy or following surgery on congenital heart defects)

The potential for improvement in oxygenation with VV-ECMO is less than that with VA-ECMO and is due to an increase in the central venous oxygen saturation, such that the shunted blood elevates overall arterial saturation despite a potential increase in shunt fraction from loss of hypoxic pulmonary vasoconstriction (HPV). VV-ECMO may, however, reduce pulmonary pressures and right ventricular strain through correction of HPV.

VV-ECMO has a lower risk of thrombo-embolic complications, and because the lung is perfused, in contrast to VA-ECMO, pulmonary endocrine function remains normal. This allows for extracorporeal removal of CO_2 whilst providing lung rest, avoiding ventilator-induced lung injury. In addition, the dual-chamber cannula (Avalon Laboratories, Rancho Dominguez, CA, USA) drains the inferior and superior vena cava, returning the blood to the region of the tricuspid valve without significant re-recirculation (drainage of oxygenated blood injected by the return cannula when dual-catheter systems are utilized) and allowing better patient mobilization.

17.3.2.3 ARTERIOVENOUS ECMO (AV-ECMO), MORE COMMONLY TERMED EXTRACORPOREAL CARBON DIOXIDE REMOVAL (ECCO2R)

ECCO2R facilitates CO_2 removal by using the patient's own arterial pressure to pump blood through the extracorporeal circuit. It is more efficient at CO_2 removal than it is at correcting hypoxaemia. Disappointingly, the 412-patient REST trial of ECCO2R versus standard lung protective ventilation was terminated early for futility and potential harm associated with ECCO2R.[18] The place of ECCO2R in trauma, and critical care in general, is currently not clear.

ECMO for respiratory failure results are better if instituted within 7 days of intubation.

17.3.3 ECMO Exclusion Criteria

It is recommended that the following should be overall exclusions for ECMO:

- Non-recoverable injury.
- Severe comorbid or intercurrent illness that will significantly impact life expectancy (e.g., a severe neurological injury, or overwhelming sepsis or any pre-existing condition which is incompatible with recovery).
- Established MOF from severe sepsis.
- Non-availability of a trained multidisciplinary team with access to specialized intensive care and cardiothoracic and vascular surgical services.
- Major vascular disease precluding deployment of ECMO.
- Pulmonary oedema from myocardial dysfunction, unless ECMO is a holding measure before transplantation or the patient has acute myocarditis and is likely to recover.
- Exacerbations of chronic obstructive pulmonary disease with respiratory failure.
- Technical difficulty associated with the procedure.
- Where systemic anticoagulation is contraindicated, although this is less problematic with special pre-heparinized catheters and tubing.
- Patients mechanically ventilated for longer than 7 days, as underlying lung damage might be irreversible.
- Age > 75 years.

Pitfall

Despite VA-ECMO improving oxygenation more than VV-ECMO, and the fact that there is no loss of HPV, there are higher risks associated with this method. The technique requires arterial cannulation with large catheters and therefore has the potential for limb ischaemia, and if blood is returned to a femoral artery, brain oxygenation cannot be guaranteed.

17.4 **COAGULOPATHY OF MAJOR TRAUMA**[19,20]

(See also Chapter 4: 'Transfusion in Trauma'.)

Trauma patients are susceptible to the early development of trauma-induced coagulopathy (TIC), which is associated with increased mortality, bleeding, and transfusions, due to a thrombomodulin-dependent activation of protein C. Thirty per cent of the most severely injured patients are coagulopathic on hospital admission.

This acute traumatic coagulopathy (ATC) is worsened by:

- Tissue damage combined with haemorrhagic shock, with a vicious cycle of bleeding and worsening of shock.
- Disruption of the endothelial glycocalyx, with expression of endothelial tissue factor promoting coagulation.
- Inflammation due to damage-associated molecular patterns (DAMPs) released from dying cells, cell-free DNA, histones, and high-mobility group box protein 1 (HMGB1)
- Dysfunctional platelets despite normal numbers, with clinically significant reductions of platelet function and coagulation factor activity. This starts at temperatures less than 36 °C and worsens dramatically at temperatures less than 33 °C.
- Depletion of coagulation factors from consumption at the wound site and from disseminated intravascular coagulation (DIC).
- Many components of the coagulation system require calcium, which is consumed as a co-factor, and also it is inactivated by citrate in blood products.
- Dilutional thrombocytopenia is the most common coagulation abnormality in trauma patients.
- Hypothermia and acidosis, both of which interfere with coagulation reactions (although evidence for this is lacking). A pH drops from 7.4 to 7.2 reduces the activity of each of the coagulation proteases by more than half.
- Haemodilution.
- The thrombin–thrombomodulin complex activates protein C which inactivates co-factors V and VIII, inhibiting the coagulation pathway. Activated protein C also inactivates plasminogen activator inhibitor type 1, increasing fibrinolysis. The thrombin–thrombomodulin complex also binds thrombin-activated fibrinolysis inhibitor (TAFI), reducing the inhibition of fibrinolysis.

- Excess plasmin generation is reflected by reduced plasma levels of fibrin and elevated levels of fibrin degradation products, with abnormal concentrations being found in 85% of patients.[21]
- Hypocalcaemia is another mechanism by which haemorrhagic shock can impair coagulation. Calcium has an important role in the formation and stabilization of fibrin polymerization sites, and, consequently, it affects all platelet-dependent functions.

The importance of hypocalcaemia has been sufficiently emphasized that the 'triad of death' has become known as the 'deadly diamond'.

Whereas a coagulopathy is defined by a prothrombin ratio of ≥ 1.2, the complexity of the process cannot be defined by one parameter. As such, other parameters are utilized, such as fibrinogen levels < 1.5 g/L and a low platelet count. However, because of this problem, viscoelastic haemostatic assays (VHAs) have become more commonly used (rotational thromboelastometry [ROTEM] or thromboelastography [TEG]) which provide information as to platelet function, fibrinogen activity, and clot formation or lysis within 5–20 minutes.

Excess plasmin generation is reflected by reduced plasma levels of fibrin and elevated levels of fibrin degradation products, with abnormal concentrations being found in 85% of patients. In addition, tranexamic acid may have a major role in clot stabilization[22] and reversal of the coagulopathy if given early (i.e. within 3 hours of injury). Despite the increased use of tranexamic acid, the gathering and validity of the data have been called into question in a major trauma centre environment.[23]

17.4.1 **Management**

The management of diffuse bleeding after trauma relies on haemorrhage control, active re-warming, and replacement of blood products using a haemostatic resuscitation as a central part of damage control resuscitation (DCR). The condition will not resolve until the underlying cause has been corrected; whilst this is being achieved, component therapy is indicated.

Identification of TIC within a cohort of massively bleeding patients can be augmented by laboratory testing. The conventional tests include a platelet count,

Clauss assay to measure fibrinogen level, prothrombin time (PT), and activated partial thromboplastin time (aPTT). Major limiting factors with these assays are the time to obtain results from multiple tests and the inability to identify hyperfibrinolysis.

The rapid availability of the comprehensive information provided by VHAs (TEG and RoTEM) has led to the recommendation that VHAs should replace conventional coagulation testing in TIC assessment, although their additional costs limit their accessibility in underresourced settings. Early VHA (no later than commencement of the need for blood transfusion) is strongly recommended. See Section 4.5.2: Viscoelastic Haemostatic Assays (VHA).

Among bleeding patients who require active correction of coagulopathy, use of a red cells/plasma/platelets ratio of 1:1:1 results in more rapid haemostasis and decreased mortality (the PROPPR trial).[24] The use of fresh whole blood, when available, may be the ideal resuscitation product in the immediate resuscitation setting.[25] Low anti-A and anti-B titre, group O whole blood (LTOWB) became the standard for trauma resuscitation, and it has been shown to be feasible and safe as initial fluid in many trauma centres.

17.5 HYPOTHERMIA

Whilst hypothermia may itself cause cardiac arrest, it is also protective to the brain through a reduction in metabolic rate and thus reduced oxygen requirements. Oxygen consumption is reduced by 50% at a core temperature of 32 °C. The American Heart Association guidelines recommend that the hypothermic patient who appears dead should not be considered so until a near-normal body temperature is reached.

Hypothermia is, on balance, extremely harmful to trauma patients, especially by virtue of the way it alters oxygen delivery and promotes coagulopathy.

Primary hypothermia is common after immersion injury, and re-warming must take place with intensive monitoring. Patients who have spontaneous respiratory effort and whose hearts are beating, no matter how severe the bradycardia, should not receive unnecessary resuscitation procedures. Patients with a core temperature of less than 28 °C are at high risk of ventricular arrhythmias,

and below 25 °C asystole may occur; they should be re-warmed as rapidly as possible. Therefore, further heat loss should be minimized at all costs, and the patient must be warmed as soon as possible. Recent studies have not shown any increase in ventricular arrhythmias with rapid re-warming. Resuscitation should not be abandoned whilst the core temperature is subnormal, since it may be difficult to distinguish between cerebro-protective hypothermia and hypothermia resulting from brainstem death.

Secondary hypothermia occurs secondary to the metabolic derangements from trauma, and for this group of patients rapid re-warming is far more important for haemostasis. The same methods are used; however, these must be even more aggressive, whilst controlling haemorrhage and securing the airway, giving warmed blood products, and preparing for surgical intervention.

External:

- Removal of wet or cold clothing, and drying of the patient
- Infrared (radiant) heat
- Electrical heating blankets
- Warm air heating blankets

Pitfall

In the presence of hypothermia, 'space blankets' are ineffective, since there is minimal intrinsic body heat to reflect!

Internal:

- Heated, humidified respiratory gases to 42 °C
- Intravenous fluids warmed to 37 °C
- Gastric lavage with warmed fluids (usually saline at 42 °C)
- Continuous bladder lavage with water at 42 °C
- Peritoneal lavage with potassium-free dialysate at 42 °C (20 ml/kg every 15 minutes)
- Intrapleural lavage
- Extracorporeal (ECMO) re-warming

Intraoperative surgical irrigation of the abdomen or thorax with warmed fluids, if these cavities have been explored as part of overall trauma management, is also particularly effective.

The **ICE score** is a useful tool in the triage of hypothermic patients (see **Table 17.2**), and patients who scored > 12 had a 0% chance of survival.[26]

Table 17.2 The ICE Score

Characteristics	Points
Male	0
Female	−3
Asphyxia	5
No asphyxia	0
Potassium < 5 mmol/L	0
Potassium 5–10 mmol/L	5
Potassium > 10 mmol/L	10
Total score	

17.6 MULTISYSTEM ORGAN DYSFUNCTION SYNDROME

MODS is characterized by the progressive failure of multiple and interdependent organs. The 'dysfunction' identifies a phenomenon in which organ function is not capable of maintaining homeostasis, so it occurs along a continuum of progressive organ failure, rather than absolute failure. The lungs, liver, and kidneys are the organs primarily affected; however, failure of the cardiovascular and central nervous system may be prominent as well. The main inciting factors in trauma patients are haemorrhagic shock and infection. As life support and resuscitation techniques have improved, so the incidence of MODS has increased.

MODS/MOF develops because of local inflammation with activation of the innate immune system and a subsequent uncontrolled or inappropriate systemic inflammatory response to inciting factors called DAMPs, released in response to severe tissue injury (e.g., brain, lung, or soft tissue), hypoperfusion, or infection.[26] The early development of MODS (< 3 days post-injury) is usually a consequence of extensive tissue injury exacerbated by shock and inadequate resuscitation or, more commonly, overly aggressive resuscitation with fluid overload. Later onset is usually a result of severe infection. (See Chapter 3 on the physiology of trauma.)

Specific therapy for MODS is currently limited, apart from providing adequate and full resuscitation (without overload), treatment of infection, and general ICU organ-supportive care. Strategies to prevent MODS include adequate fluid resuscitation to establish and maintain tissue oxygenation, debridement of devitalized tissue, early fracture fixation and stabilization (24–72 hours), early enteral nutritional support, when possible, the prevention and treatment of nosocomial infections, and early mobility and resumption of exercise.

17.7 SYSTEMIC INFLAMMATORY RESPONSE SYNDROME (SIRS)

(See also Chapter 3 on the physiology of trauma.)

Fifty per cent of patients with 'sepsis' do not have bacteria isolated from blood cultures. Whilst some of these patients will have occult infections, others have sterile causes of inflammation: burns, pancreatitis, and significant soft tissue injuries, particularly when associated with shock. The common theme through all these various injuries and types of sepsis is that the inflammatory cascade has been initiated and runs amok. Once the inflammatory response has been initiated, it leads to systemic symptoms that may or may not be beneficial or harmful.

Patients who have two or more specified features of inflammation are defined as having SIRS. The features of SIRS include:

- Temperature < 36 °C or > 38 °C
- Heart rate > 90 beats per minute
- Respiratory rate > 20 breaths per minute
- *Deranged arterial gases*: Partial pressure of carbon dioxide ($PaCO_2$) < 32 mmHg (4.2 kPa)
- White blood count > 12.0×10^9/L or < 4.0×10^9/L, or 0.10% immature neutrophils

The utility of this definition of SIRS has been questioned, as it is highly non-specific, encompassing many ICU patients who are not especially unwell. SIRS was once a component of the definition of sepsis but was replaced in the Sepsis-3 criteria in 2016.[27] In trauma, the physiological thresholds defining SIRS retain some utility in identifying patients with systemic as well as local effects of injury.[28]

17.8 SEPSIS

17.8.1 Definitions

International consensus definitions for sepsis and septic shock were reviewed in 2021.[29]

Table 17.3 The SOFA Score

Score	GCS	Cardiovascular System Mean Arterial Pressure *or* Administration of Vasopressors Required	Respiratory System PaO₂/FiO₂ (mmHg/kPa)	Coagulation Platelets (×10³/μl)	Liver Bilirubin (mg/dl) [μmol/L]	Renal Function Creatinine (mg/dL) [μmol/L] (or Urine Output)
+0	15	MAP ≥ 70 mmHg	≥ 400 (53.3)	≥ 150	< 1.2 [< 20]	< 1.2 [< 110]
+1	13–14	MAP ≤ 70 mmHg	< 400 (53.3)	< 150	1.2–1.9 [20–32]	1.2–1.9 [110–170]
+2	10–12	Dopamine < 5 μg/kg/min **or** dobutamine (any dose)	< 300 (40)	< 100	2.0–5.9 [33–101]	2.0–3.4 [171–299]
+3	6–9	Dopamine > 5 μg/kg/min **or** epinephrine ≤ 0.1 μg/kg/min **or** norepinephrine ≤ 0.1 μg/kg/min	< 200 (26.7) and mechanically ventilated including CPAP	< 50	6.0–11.9 [102–204]	3.5–4.9 [300–440] or < 500 ml/day
+4	< 6	Dopamine > 15 μg/kg/min **or** epinephrine > 0.1 μg/kg/min **or** norepinephrine > 0.1 μg/kg/min	< 100 (13.3) and mechanically ventilated including CPAP	< 20	> 12.0 [> 204]	> 5.0 [440] or < 200 ml/day

CPAP, Continuous positive airway pressure
FiO₂, fraction of inspired oxygen
GCS, Glasgow Coma Scale score
MAP, mean arterial pressure
PaO₂, arterial partial pressure of oxygen
SOFA, Sequential Organ Failure Assessment

17.8.1.1 SEPSIS

Sepsis is defined as life-threatening organ dysfunction in SIRS plus documented infection (**Table 17.3**).

- *Life-threatening organ dysfunction* is defined as an *increase* in the Sequential [sepsis-related] Organ Failure Assessment (SOFA) score of 2 points or more *due to infection.*
- The SOFA score allocates points on a scale of 0–4, according to dysfunctions in parameters of the respiratory, coagulation, hepatic, cardiovascular, central nervous, and renal systems.
- Baseline SOFA is assumed to be 0 if no pre-existing organ dysfunction exists.

It was recognized that application of this scoring system would be impractical for most clinicians, so a Quick SOFA (qSOFA) score with acceptable sensitivity and specificity was also defined, incorporating only three elements:

- Respiratory rate ≥ 22/min
- Altered mentation
- Systolic blood pressure ≥ 100 mmHg

The presence of these three criteria in the context of suspected infection now forms the operational definition of sepsis (**Table 17.4**).

17.8.1.2 SEPTIC SHOCK[27]

Septic shock was redefined in 2016 (Sepsis-3) as the subset of sepsis patients with particularly profound circulatory,

Table 17.4 The qSOFA Score

Assessment	qSOFA Score
Low blood pressure (SBP ≤ 100 mmHg)	1
High respiratory rate (≥ 22 breaths/min)	1
Altered mentation (GCS ≤ 14)	1

Note: qSOFA scores of 2–3 are associated with a 3- to 14-fold increase in in-hospital mortality. Assess for evidence of organ dysfunction with blood testing including serum lactate and calculation of the full SOFA score. Patients meeting these qSOFA criteria should have infection considered, even if it was previously not.

cellular, and metabolic abnormalities. Patients with septic shock can be clinically identified by:

- Persistent hypotension requiring vasopressors to maintain a **mean arterial pressure** (MAP) ≥ 65 mmHg
- Lactate > 2 mmol/L (> 18 mg/dL)
- Despite adequate volume resuscitation

With these criteria, in-hospital mortality is > 40%.

17.8.2 'Surviving Sepsis' Guidelines

Updated 'Surviving Sepsis Campaign: International Guidelines for Management of Severe Sepsis and Septic Shock' guidelines were published in 2004, 2008, 2012, 2016, and 2021.[29] A full summary of the guidelines in appears in table form (**Table 17.5**).

Table 17.5 Surviving Sepsis Campaign: 2021 Recommendations and Changes

Recommendations 2021	Recommendation Strength and Quality of Evidence	Changes from 2016 Recommendations
1. For hospitals and health systems, we recommend using a performance improvement program for sepsis, including sepsis screening for acutely ill, high-risk patients and standard operating procedures for treatment	**Strong**, *moderate-quality evidence (For screening)* **Strong**, *very low-quality evidence (For standard operating procedures)*	**Changed from *Best practice statement*** 'We **recommend** that hospitals and hospital systems have a performance improvement program for sepsis including sepsis screening for acutely ill, high risk patients'
2. We recommend against using qSOFA compared with SIRS, NEWS, or MEWS as a single screening tool for sepsis or septic shock	**Strong**, *moderate-quality evidence*	**NEW**
3. For adults suspected of having sepsis, we suggest measuring blood lactate	**Weak**, *low quality of evidence*	
Initial Resuscitation		
4. Sepsis and septic shock are medical emergencies, and we recommend that treatment and resuscitation begin immediately	***Best practice statement***	
5. For patients with sepsis-induced hypoperfusion or septic shock, we suggest that at least 30 mL/kg of IV crystalloid fluid should be given within the first 3 hours of resuscitation	**Weak**, *low quality of evidence*	**DOWNGRADE** from **Strong**, *low quality of evidence* 'We **recommend** that in the initial resuscitation from sepsis-induced hypoperfusion, at least 30 mL/kg of IV crystalloid fluid be given within the first 3 hr'
6. For adults with sepsis or septic shock, we suggest using dynamic measures to guide fluid resuscitation, over physical examination or static parameters alone	**Weak**, *very low quality of evidence*	

(Continued)

Table 17.5 (*Continued*) Surviving Sepsis Campaign: 2021 Recommendations and Changes

Recommendations 2021	Recommendation Strength and Quality of Evidence	Changes from 2016 Recommendations
7. For adults with sepsis or septic shock, we suggest guiding resuscitation to decrease serum lactate in patients with elevated lactate level, over not using serum lactate	*Weak*, *low quality of evidence*	
8. For adults with septic shock, we suggest using capillary refill time to guide resuscitation as an adjunct to other measures of perfusion	*Weak*, *low quality of evidence*	**NEW**
Mean Arterial Pressure		
9. For adults with septic shock on vasopressors, we recommend an initial target mean arterial pressure (MAP) of 65 mmHg over higher MAP targets	*Strong*, *moderate-quality evidence*	
Admission to Intensive Care		
10. For adults with sepsis or septic shock who require ICU admission, we suggest admitting the patients to the ICU within 6 hours	*Weak*, *low quality of evidence*	
Infection		
11. For adults with suspected sepsis or septic shock but unconfirmed infection, we recommend continuously re-evaluating and searching for alternative diagnoses and discontinuing empiric antimicrobials if an alternative cause of illness is demonstrated or strongly suspected	*Best practice statement*	
12. For adults with possible septic shock or a high likelihood for sepsis, we recommend administering antimicrobials immediately, ideally within 1 hour of recognition	*Strong*, *low quality of evidence* (*For septic shock*) *Strong*, *very low quality of evidence* (*For sepsis without shock*)	**CHANGED from previous:** 'We recommend that administration of intravenous antimicrobials should be initiated as soon as possible after recognition and within one hour for both a) septic shock and b) sepsis without shock' *Strong recommendation*, *moderate quality of evidence*

(Continued)

Table 17.5 (*Continued*) Surviving Sepsis Campaign: 2021 Recommendations and Changes

Recommendations 2021	Recommendation Strength and Quality of Evidence	Changes from 2016 Recommendations
13. For adults with possible sepsis without shock, we recommend rapid assessment of the likelihood of infectious versus non-infectious causes of acute illness	*Best practice statement*	
14. For adults with possible sepsis without shock, we suggest a time-limited course of rapid investigation and, if concern for infection persists, the administration of antimicrobials within 3 hours from the time when sepsis was first recognized	*Weak, very low quality of evidence*	**NEW from previous:** 'We recommend that administration of IV antimicrobials should be initiated as soon as possible after recognition and within 1 hr for both a) septic shock and b) sepsis without shock' *Strong recommendation, moderate quality of evidence*
15. For adults with a low likelihood of infection and without shock, we suggest deferring antimicrobials whilst continuing to closely monitor the patient	*Weak, very low quality of evidence*	**NEW from previous:** 'We recommend that administration of IV antimicrobials should be initiated as soon as possible after recognition and within 1 hr for both a) septic shock and b) sepsis without shock' *Strong recommendation, moderate quality of evidence*
16. For adults with suspected sepsis or septic shock, we suggest against using procalcitonin plus clinical evaluation to decide when to start antimicrobials, as compared to clinical evaluation alone	*Weak, very low quality of evidence*	
17. For adults with sepsis or septic shock at high risk of MRSA, we recommend using empiric antimicrobials with MRSA coverage over using antimicrobials without MRSA coverage	*Best practice statement*	**NEW from previous:** 'We recommend empiric broad-spectrum therapy with one or more antimicrobials for patients presenting with sepsis or septic shock to cover all likely pathogens (including bacterial and potentially fungal or viral coverage' *Strong recommendation, moderate quality of evidence*

(Continued)

Table 17.5 (*Continued*) Surviving Sepsis Campaign: 2021 Recommendations and Changes

Recommendations 2021	Recommendation Strength and Quality of Evidence	Changes from 2016 Recommendations
18. For adults with sepsis or septic shock at low risk of MRSA, we suggest against using empiric antimicrobials with MRSA coverage, as compared with using antimicrobials without MRSA coverage	*Weak*, *low quality of evidence*	**NEW from previous:** 'We recommend empiric broad-spectrum therapy with one or more antimicrobials for patients presenting with sepsis or septic shock to cover all likely pathogens (including bacterial and potentially fungal or viral coverage' *Strong recommendation*, *moderate quality of evidence*
19. For adults with sepsis or septic shock and at high risk for multidrug-resistant (MDR) organisms, we suggest using two antimicrobials with Gram-negative coverage for empiric treatment over one Gram-negative agent	*Weak*, *very low quality of evidence*	
20. For adults with sepsis or septic shock and at low risk for MDR organisms, we suggest against using two Gram-negative agents for empiric treatment, as compared to one Gram-negative agent	*Weak*, *very low quality of evidence*	
21. For adults with sepsis or septic shock, we suggest against using double Gram-negative coverage once the causative pathogen and the susceptibilities are known	*Weak*, *very low quality of evidence*	
22. For adults with sepsis or septic shock at high risk of fungal infection, we suggest using empiric antifungal therapy over no antifungal therapy	*Weak*, *low quality of evidence*	**NEW from previous:** 'We recommend empiric broad-spectrum therapy with one or more antimicrobials for patients presenting with sepsis or septic shock to cover all likely pathogens (including bacterial and potentially fungal or viral coverage' *Strong recommendation*, *moderate quality of evidence*

(Continued)

Table 17.5 (*Continued*) Surviving Sepsis Campaign: 2021 Recommendations and Changes

Recommendations 2021	Recommendation Strength and Quality of Evidence	Changes from 2016 Recommendations
23. For adults with sepsis or septic shock at low risk of fungal infection, we suggest against empiric use of antifungal therapy	*Weak*, *low quality of evidence*	**NEW from previous:**
		'We recommend empiric broad-spectrum therapy with one or more antimicrobials for patients presenting with sepsis or septic shock to cover all likely pathogens (including bacterial and potentially fungal or viral coverage)'
		Strong recommendation, *moderate quality of evidence*
24. We make no recommendation on the use of antiviral agents	*No recommendation*	
25. For adults with sepsis or septic shock, we suggest using prolonged infusion of beta-lactams for maintenance (after an initial bolus) over conventional bolus infusion	*Weak*, *moderate-quality evidence*	
26. For adults with sepsis or septic shock, we recommend optimizing dosing strategies of antimicrobials based on accepted pharmacokinetic/pharmacodynamic (PK/PD) principles and specific drug properties	*Best practice statement*	
27. For adults with sepsis or septic shock, we recommend rapidly identifying or excluding a specific anatomical diagnosis of infection that requires emergent source control, and implementing any required source control intervention as soon as medically and logistically practical	*Best practice statement*	
28. For adults with sepsis or septic shock, we recommend prompt removal of intravascular access devices that are a possible source of sepsis or septic shock after other vascular access has been established	*Best practice statement*	
29. For adults with sepsis or septic shock, we suggest daily assessment for de-escalation of antimicrobials over using fixed durations of therapy without daily reassessment for de-escalation	*Weak*, *very low quality of evidence*	

(Continued)

Table 17.5 (*Continued*) Surviving Sepsis Campaign: 2021 Recommendations and Changes

Recommendations 2021	Recommendation Strength and Quality of Evidence	Changes from 2016 Recommendations
30. For adults with an initial diagnosis of sepsis or septic shock and adequate source control, we suggest using a shorter over longer duration of antimicrobial therapy	*Weak*, very low quality of evidence	
31. For adults with an initial diagnosis of sepsis or septic shock and adequate source control where optimal duration of therapy is unclear, we suggest using procalcitonin **and** clinical evaluation to decide when to discontinue antimicrobials over clinical evaluation alone	*Weak*, low quality of evidence	
Haemodynamic Management		
32. For adults with sepsis or septic shock, we recommend using crystalloids as the first-line fluid for resuscitation	*Strong*, moderate-quality evidence	
33. For adults with sepsis or septic shock, we suggest using balanced crystalloids instead of normal saline for resuscitation	*Weak*, low quality of evidence	**CHANGED from *Weak* recommendation**, low quality of evidence 'We suggest using either balanced crystalloids or saline for fluid resuscitation of patients with sepsis or septic shock'.
34. For adults with sepsis or septic shock, we suggest using albumin in patients who received large volumes of crystalloids	*Weak*, moderate-quality evidence	
35. For adults with sepsis or septic shock, we recommend against using starches for resuscitation.	*Strong*, high-quality evidence	
36. For adults with sepsis and septic shock, we suggest against using gelatine for resuscitation	*Weak*, moderate-quality evidence	**UPGRADE from *Weak* recommendation**, low quality of evidence 'We suggest using crystalloids over gelatins when resuscitating patients with sepsis or septic shock'

(Continued)

Table 17.5 (*Continued*) Surviving Sepsis Campaign: 2021 Recommendations and Changes

Recommendations 2021	Recommendation Strength and Quality of Evidence	Changes from 2016 Recommendations
37. For adults with septic shock, we recommend using norepinephrine as the first-line agent over other vasopressors	*Strong*	
	Dopamine: *High-quality evidence*	
	Vasopressin: *Moderate-quality evidence*	
	Epinephrine: *Low quality of evidence*	
	Selepressin: *Low quality of evidence*	
	Angiotensin II: *Very low-quality evidence*	
38. For adults with septic shock on norepinephrine with inadequate mean arterial pressure levels, we suggest adding vasopressin instead of escalating the dose of norepinephrine	*Weak*, *moderate-quality evidence*	
39. For adults with septic shock and inadequate mean arterial pressure levels despite norepinephrine and vasopressin, we suggest adding epinephrine	*Weak*, *low quality of evidence*	
40. For adults with septic shock, we suggest against using terlipressin	*Weak*, *low quality of evidence*	
41. For adults with septic shock and cardiac dysfunction with persistent hypoperfusion despite adequate volume status and arterial blood pressure, we suggest either adding dobutamine to norepinephrine or using epinephrine alone	*Weak*, *low quality of evidence*	
42. For adults with septic shock and cardiac dysfunction with persistent hypoperfusion despite adequate volume status and arterial blood pressure, we suggest against using levosimendan	*Weak*, *low quality of evidence*	*NEW*
43. For adults with septic shock, we suggest invasive monitoring of arterial blood pressure over non-invasive monitoring, as soon as practical and if resources are available	*Weak*, *very low quality of evidence*	

(Continued)

Table 17.5 (*Continued*) Surviving Sepsis Campaign: 2021 Recommendations and Changes

Recommendations 2021	Recommendation Strength and Quality of Evidence	Changes from 2016 Recommendations
44. For adults with septic shock, we suggest starting vasopressors peripherally to restore mean arterial pressure rather than delaying initiation until a central venous access is secured	*Weak, very low quality of evidence*	*NEW*
45. There is insufficient evidence to make a recommendation on the use of restrictive versus liberal fluid strategies in the first 24 hours of resuscitation in patients with sepsis and septic shock who still have signs of hypoperfusion and volume depletion after the initial resuscitation	*No recommendation*	NEW
		'We suggest using either balanced crystalloids or saline for fluid resuscitation of patients with sepsis or septic shock'
		Weak recommendation, low quality of evidence
		'We suggest using crystalloids over gelatins when resuscitating patients with sepsis or septic shock'
		Weak recommendation, low quality of evidence
Ventilation		
46. There is insufficient evidence to make a recommendation on the use of conservative oxygen targets in adults with sepsis-induced hypoxic respiratory failure	*No recommendation*	
47. For adults with sepsis-induced hypoxic respiratory failure, we suggest the use of high-flow nasal oxygen over non-invasive ventilation	*Weak, low quality of evidence*	*NEW*
48. There is insufficient evidence to make a recommendation on the use of non-invasive ventilation in comparison to invasive ventilation for adults with sepsis-induced hypoxic respiratory failure	*No recommendation*	
49. For adults with sepsis-induced ARDS, we recommend using a low tidal volume ventilation strategy (6 mL/kg) over a high tidal volume strategy (> 10 mL/kg)	*Strong, high-quality evidence*	

(Continued)

Table 17.5 (*Continued*) Surviving Sepsis Campaign: 2021 Recommendations and Changes

Recommendations 2021	Recommendation Strength and Quality of Evidence	Changes from 2016 Recommendations
50. For adults with sepsis-induced severe ARDS, we recommend using an upper limit goal for plateau pressures of 30 cm H_2O over higher plateau pressures	**Strong**, *moderate-quality evidence*	
51. For adults with moderate to severe sepsis-induced ARDS, we suggest using higher PEEP over lower PEEP	**Weak**, *moderate-quality evidence*	
52. For adults with sepsis-induced respiratory failure (without ARDS), we suggest using low tidal volume as compared with high tidal volume ventilation	**Weak**, *low quality of evidence*	
53. For adults with sepsis-induced moderate to severe ARDS, we suggest using traditional recruitment manoeuvres	**Weak**, *moderate-quality evidence*	
54. When using recruitment manoeuvres, we recommend against using incremental PEEP titration/ strategy	**Strong**, *moderate-quality evidence*	
55. For adults with sepsis-induced moderate to severe ARDS, we recommend using prone ventilation for greater than 12 hours daily	**Strong**, *moderate-quality evidence*	
56. For adults with sepsis-induced moderate to severe ARDS, we suggest using intermittent NMBA boluses over NMBA continuous infusion	**Weak**, *moderate-quality evidence*	
57. For adults with sepsis-induced severe ARDS, we suggest using VV-ECMO when conventional mechanical ventilation fails in experienced centres with the infrastructure in place to support its use	**Weak**, *low quality of evidence*	**NEW**

(Continued)

Table 17.5 (*Continued*) Surviving Sepsis Campaign: 2021 Recommendations and Changes

Recommendations 2021	Recommendation Strength and Quality of Evidence	Changes from 2016 Recommendations
Additional Therapies		
58. For adults with septic shock and an ongoing requirement for vasopressor therapy, we suggest using IV corticosteroids	*Weak*, *moderate-quality evidence*	**UPGRADE from *Weak recommendation*, *low quality of evidence*
		'We suggest against using IV hydrocortisone to treat septic shock patients if adequate fluid resuscitation and vasopressor therapy are able to restore hemodynamic stability (see goals for Initial Resuscitation). If this is not achievable, we suggest IV hydrocortisone at a dose of 200 mg/day'
59. For adults with sepsis or septic shock, we suggest against using polymyxin B haemoperfusion	*Weak*, *low quality of evidence*	**NEW from previous:** 'We make no recommendation regarding the use of blood purification techniques'
60. There is insufficient evidence to make a recommendation on the use of other blood purification techniques	*No recommendation*	
61. For adults with sepsis or septic shock, we recommend using a restrictive (over liberal) transfusion strategy	*Strong*, *moderate-quality evidence*	
62. For adults with sepsis or septic shock, we suggest against using IV immunoglobulins	*Weak*, *low quality of evidence*	
63. For adults with sepsis or septic shock, and who have risk factors for gastrointestinal (GI) bleeding, we suggest using stress ulcer prophylaxis	*Weak*, *moderate-quality evidence*	
64. For adults with sepsis or septic shock, we recommend using pharmacologic venous thromboembolism (VTE) prophylaxis unless a contraindication to such therapy exists	*Strong*, *moderate-quality evidence*	
65. For adults with sepsis or septic shock, we recommend using low-molecular-weight heparin over unfractionated heparin for VTE prophylaxis	*Strong*, *moderate-quality evidence*	

(Continued)

Table 17.5 (*Continued*) Surviving Sepsis Campaign: 2021 Recommendations and Changes

Recommendations 2021	Recommendation Strength and Quality of Evidence	Changes from 2016 Recommendations
66. For adults with sepsis or septic shock, we suggest against using mechanical VTE prophylaxis, in addition to pharmacological prophylaxis, over pharmacological prophylaxis alone	*Weak, low quality of evidence*	
67. In adults with sepsis or septic shock and acute kidney injury (AKI), we suggest using either continuous or intermittent renal replacement therapy	*Weak, low quality of evidence*	
68. In adults with sepsis or septic shock and AKI, with no definitive indications for renal replacement therapy, we suggest against using renal replacement therapy	*Weak, moderate-quality evidence*	
69. For adults with sepsis or septic shock, we recommend initiating insulin therapy at a glucose level of > 180 mg/dL (10 mmol/L)	*Strong, moderate-quality evidence*	
70. For adults with sepsis or septic shock, we suggest against using IV vitamin C	*Weak, low quality of evidence*	*NEW*
71. For adults with septic shock and hypoperfusion-induced lactic acidaemia, we suggest against using sodium bicarbonate therapy to improve haemodynamics or to reduce vasopressor requirements	*Weak, low quality of evidence*	
72. For adults with septic shock and severe metabolic acidaemia (pH ≤ 7.2) and AKI (AKIN score 2 or 3), we suggest using sodium bicarbonate therapy	*Weak, low quality of evidence*	
73. For adult patients with sepsis or septic shock who can be fed enterally, we suggest early (within 72 hours) initiation of enteral nutrition	*Weak, very low quality of evidence*	
Long-Term Outcomes and Goals of Care		
74. For adults with sepsis or septic shock, we recommend discussing goals of care and prognosis with patients and families over no such discussion	*Best practice statement*	

(Continued)

Table 17.5 (*Continued*) Surviving Sepsis Campaign: 2021 Recommendations and Changes

Recommendations 2021	Recommendation Strength and Quality of Evidence	Changes from 2016 Recommendations
75. For adults with sepsis or septic shock, we suggest addressing goals of care early (within 72 hours) over late (72 hours or later)	*Weak*, *low quality of evidence*	
76. For adults with sepsis or septic shock, there is insufficient evidence to make a recommendation on any specific standardized criterion to trigger a goals-of-care discussion	*No recommendation*	
77. For adults with sepsis or septic shock, we recommend that the principles of palliative care (which may include palliative care consultation, based on clinician judgement) be integrated into the treatment plan, when appropriate, to address patient and family symptoms and suffering	*Best practice statement*	
78. For adults with sepsis or septic shock, we suggest against routine formal palliative care consultation for all patients over palliative care consultation based on clinician judgement	*Weak*, *low quality of evidence*	
79. For adult survivors of sepsis or septic shock and their families, we suggest referral to peer support groups over no such referral	*Weak*, *very low quality of evidence*	
80. For adults with sepsis or septic shock, we suggest using a handoff process of critically important information at transitions of care over no such handoff process	*Weak*, *very low quality of evidence*	
81. For adults with sepsis or septic shock, there is insufficient evidence to make a recommendation on the use of any specific structured handoff tool over usual handoff processes	*No recommendation*	
82. For adults with sepsis or septic shock and their families, we recommend screening for economic and social support (including housing, nutritional, financial, and spiritual support), and make referrals where available to meet these needs	*Best practice statement*	

(Continued)

Table 17.5 (*Continued*) Surviving Sepsis Campaign: 2021 Recommendations and Changes

Recommendations 2021	Recommendation Strength and Quality of Evidence	Changes from 2016 Recommendations
83. For adults with sepsis or septic shock and their families, we suggest offering written and verbal sepsis education (diagnosis, treatment, and post-ICU/post-sepsis syndrome) prior to hospital discharge and in the follow-up setting	**Weak**, *very low quality of evidence*	
84. For adults with sepsis or septic shock and their families, we recommend the clinical team provide the opportunity to participate in shared decision-making in post-ICU and hospital discharge planning to ensure discharge plans are acceptable and feasible	**Best practice statement**	
85. For adults with sepsis and septic shock and their families, we suggest using a critical care transition program, compared with usual care, upon transfer to the floor	**Weak**, *very low quality of evidence*	
86. For adults with sepsis and septic shock, we recommend reconciling medications at both ICU and hospital discharge	**Best practice statement**	
87. For adult survivors of sepsis and septic shock and their families, we recommend including information about the ICU stay, sepsis and related diagnoses, treatments, and common impairments after sepsis in the written and verbal hospital discharge summaries	**Best practice statement**	
88. For adults with sepsis or septic shock who developed new impairments, we recommend hospital discharge plans include follow-up with clinicians able to support and manage new and long-term sequelae	**Best practice statement**	
89. For adults with sepsis or septic shock and their families, there is insufficient evidence to make a recommendation on early post-hospital discharge follow-up compared with routine post-hospital discharge follow-up	**No recommendation**	

(Continued)

Table 17.5 (*Continued*) Surviving Sepsis Campaign: 2021 Recommendations and Changes

Recommendations 2021	Recommendation Strength and Quality of Evidence	Changes from 2016 Recommendations
90. For adults with sepsis or septic shock, there is insufficient evidence to make a recommendation for or against early cognitive therapy	*No recommendation*	
91. For adult survivors of sepsis or septic shock, we recommend assessment and follow-up for physical, cognitive, and emotional problems after hospital discharge	*Best practice statement*	
92. For adult survivors of sepsis or septic shock, we suggest referral to a post–critical illness follow-up program if available	***Weak**, very low quality of evidence*	
93. For adult survivors of sepsis or septic shock receiving mechanical ventilation for > 48 hours or an ICU stay of > 72 hours, we suggest referral to a post-hospital rehabilitation program	*Weak, very low quality of evidence*	

Source: Surviving Sepsis Campaign: International Guidelines for Management of Sepsis and Septic Shock 2021, Laura Evans, Andrew Rhodes, Waleed Alhazzani, Et Al, Critical Care Medicine 49(11): e1063-e1143, November 2021. | DOI: 10.1097/CCM.0000000000005337. Reprinted with permission.

17.9 ANTIBIOTICS

The goal of antibiotic treatment is to improve survival; however, preventing the emergence of antibiotic resistance is also important. Appropriate antimicrobial stewardship (AMS) is essential. Antibiotics should not be used prophylactically and should be guided by the presence and duration of wound contamination and documented infection, as well as biomarkers such as PCT.[30]

> *Note that C-reactive protein (CRP) rises with the trauma insult and should **not** be used to screen for sepsis.*
>
> *There must be a clear distinction between prophylaxis and treatment.*
>
> *There is good evidence to **limit** the use of antibiotics in the critically ill trauma patient.[31]*

For thoracoabdominal injuries requiring operation, a single dose of broad-spectrum antibiotics at the time of surgery is indicated. Prolonged courses of antibiotics, extending beyond 24 hours, are not indicated in most patients.[32] There is conflicting evidence regarding the need for routine antibiotics with tube thoracostomy.

For patients with hollow viscus injuries or closed-space infections, with major contamination, once the patient has surgical source control obtained, antibiotics can be limited to a short course. For patients with gross intra-abdominal contamination, a short course of antibiotics (e.g., 4 days from date of source control) is appropriate and superior to a longer course.

Patients with open fractures are frequently treated with both Gram-negative and Gram-positive prophylaxis for long periods. There is no evidence for this practice, nor for whether management should be any different from that for torso injury.[33]

Patients in the ICU undergoing mechanical ventilation, with or without known aspiration, have no indication for antibiotics to prevent pneumonia. This practice has hastened the onset of antibiotic resistance worldwide.

17.9.1 Criteria

According to the US Centers for Disease Control and Prevention, a diagnosis of ventilator-associated pneumonia (VAP) must meet the following criteria (as per **Table 17.6**):[34]

- Rales or dullness to percussion AND any of the following:
  - New purulent sputum or a change in sputum
  - Culture growth of an organism from blood or tracheal aspirate, bronchial brushing, or biopsy

- Radiographic evidence of new or progressive infiltrate, consolidation, cavitation, or effusion

And any of the following:

- Isolation of virus or detection of viral antigen in respiratory secretions
- Diagnostic antibody titres for pathogen
- Histopathological evidence of pneumonia

VAP is defined by:[35]

- Pneumonia that occurs 48–72 hours or thereafter following endotracheal intubation
- The presence of a new or progressive infiltrate
- Signs of systemic infection (e.g., fever or altered white blood cell count)
- Changes in sputum characteristics
- Detection of a causative agent

Table 17.6 CDC Ventilator-Associated Event Guidelines

Two or More Serial Radiographs with At Least One of the Following	One of the Following	Two of the Following
New or progressive and persistent infiltrate, cavitation, effusion, or consolidation	Fever (> 38 °C)	Rales or bronchial breath sound Worsening gas exchange (e.g., oxygen desaturation, increased oxygen requirements, or increased ventilator demand)
	OR	**AND ANY OF THE FOLLOWING**
	Leukopenia (> 4000 WBC/μL) or Leukocytosis (> 12,000 WBC/μL)	New onset of purulent sputum or change in character of sputum or increased respiratory secretions or increased suctioning requirements
	For adults ≥ 70 years old, altered mental status with no other recognized cause	New onset of worsening cough or dyspnoea, or tachypnoea
	AND ANY OF THE FOLLOWING	Culture growth of an organism from blood or tracheal aspirate, bronchial brushing, or biopsy
	Isolation of virus or viral antigen in respiratory secretions	
	Diagnostic antibody titres for pathogen	
	Histopathological evidence of pneumonia	

VAP interventions should include:

- Early chest X-ray with expert interpretation within 1 hour
- Immediate reporting of respiratory secretion Gram-stain findings, including cells
- Immediate antibiotic treatment after microbiological sampling
- Empirical therapy based on a knowledge of local pathogens and an assessment of risk factors
- De-escalation of antibiotics in responding patients once culture results are available
- Assessment of response to treatment within 72 hours
- Short duration (5–8 days; 10 days for *Pseudomonas aeruginosa*) and **guided by PCT if possible**

Given the variations in antibiotic susceptibility profiles of VAP pathogens, both in location and with respect to changes over time, it is inappropriate to specify the use of specific antibiotic regimens.

17.10 ABDOMINAL COMPARTMENT SYNDROME (ACS)

17.10.1 Introduction

Raised intra-abdominal pressure (IAP) has far-reaching consequences for the physiology of the patient. There have been major developments in our understanding of IAP and intra-abdominal hypertension (IAH). The syndrome that results when organs fail as a result is known as ACS.

The formation of the World Society of the Abdominal Compartment Syndrome[36] has been a major advance, with the production of consensus definitions, the formation of a research policy, multicentre trials, and the publication of the consensus guidelines on ACS. The first World Congress on ACS was held in 2004, and an internal consensus agreement relating to definitions was updated in 2009 and 2013. Various aspects were defined (see **Table 17.7**).[36]

17.10.2 Definition

The concept of IAP measurement, and its significance, is important in the ICU. It is less common since there has been a better understanding of fluid (particularly crystalloid) administration, especially with DCR (see Chapter 6). Patients with raised IAP require close and careful monitoring, aggressive resuscitation, and a low index of suspicion for the requirement of surgical abdominal decompression.

- *Primary ACS* develops due to conditions associated with injury or illness in the abdominopelvic region. This includes conditions requiring emergency surgical or angio-radiological intervention, including damage control laparotomy, bleeding pelvic fractures, massive retroperitoneal haematomas, and failed non-operative management of solid organ injuries, and following disease processes such as severe acute pancreatitis.
- *Secondary ACS* develops from causes originating outside the abdomen, such as sepsis, capillary leak, major burns, and fluid over-resuscitation.

17.10.3 Pathophysiology

The causes of acutely increased IAP are usually multifactorial (**Table 17.8**). Raised IAP occurs commonly with fluid over-resuscitation, and the incidence has fallen dramatically following the adoption of lower-volume, blood-based resuscitation in preference to crystalloids (DCR). In addition to the direct causes shown, hypothermia, acidosis, and overall injury severity will further exacerbate the problem.

17.10.4 Effect of Raised IAP on Individual Organ Function

17.10.4.1 CARDIOVASCULAR

Increased IAP reduces cardiac output as well as increasing central venous pressure, systemic vascular resistance, pulmonary artery pressure, and pulmonary artery wedge pressure. Cardiac output is affected mainly by a reduction in stroke volume, secondary to a reduction in preload and an increase in afterload. This is further aggravated by hypovolaemia. Paradoxically, in the presence of hypovolaemia, an increase in IAP can be temporarily associated with an increase in cardiac output. It has been identified that venous stasis occurs in the legs of patients with abdominal pressures above 12 mmHg. In addition, recent studies of patients undergoing laparoscopic cholecystectomy show up to a fourfold increase in renin and aldosterone levels.

Table 17.7 Final 2013 Consensus Definitions of the World Society of the Abdominal Compartment Syndrome

2006 Consensus Statements	
Definition 1	Intra-abdominal pressure (IAP) is the steady-state pressure concealed within the abdominal cavity
Definition 2	The reference standard for intermittent IAP measurement is via the bladder with a maximal instillation volume of 25 mL of sterile saline
Definition 3	IAP should be expressed in mmHg and measured at end-expiration in the complete supine position after ensuring that abdominal muscle contractions are absent and with the transducer zeroed at the level of the mid-axillary line
Definition 4	Normal IAP is approximately 5–7 mmHg in critically ill adults
Definition 5	IAH is defined by a sustained or repeated pathological elevation of IAP ≥ 12 mmHg
Definition 6	ACS is defined as a sustained IAP ≥ 20 mmHg (with or without an APP < 60 mmHg) that is associated with new organ dysfunction/failure
Definition 7	IAH is graded as follows: • *Grade I*: IAP 12–15 mmHg • *Grade II*: IAP 16–20 mmHg • *Grade III*: IAP 21–25 mmHg • *Grade IV*: IAP ≥ 25 mmHg
Definition 8	Primary ACS is a condition associated with injury or disease in the abdominopelvic region that frequently requires early surgical or interventional radiological intervention
Definition 9	Secondary ACS refers to conditions that do not originate from the abdominopelvic region
Definition 10	Recurrent ACS refers to the condition in which ACS redevelops following previous surgical or medical treatment of primary or secondary ACS
Definition 11	Abdominal perfusion pressure (APP) = Mean arterial pressure (MAP) – Intra-abdominal pressure (IAP)
2013 New Definitions Accepted by the Consensus Panel	
Definition 12	A polycompartment syndrome is a condition where two or more anatomical compartments have elevated compartmental pressure
Definition 13	Abdominal compliance is a measure of the ease of abdominal expansion, which is determined by the elasticity of the abdominal wall and diaphragm. It should be expressed as the change in intra-abdominal volume per change in IAP
Definition 14	The open abdomen is one that requires a temporary abdominal closure due to the skin and fascia not being closed after laparotomy
Definition 15	Lateralization of the abdominal wall is the phenomenon where the musculature and fascia of the abdominal wall, most exemplified by the rectus abdominus muscles and their enveloping fascia, move laterally away from the midline with time

ACS, Abdominal compartment syndrome
APP, abdominal perfusion pressure
IAH, intra-abdominal hypertension

IAP, intra-abdominal pressure
MAP, mean arterial pressure

Table 17.8 Causes of Raised Intra-abdominal Pressure (IAP)

- Massive fluid resuscitation
- Major intra-abdominal and retroperitoneal haemorrhage
- Tissue oedema secondary to insults such as ischaemia and sepsis
- Secondary to generalized oedema (e.g., from burns resuscitation)
- Paralytic ileus
- Ascites

17.10.4.2 RESPIRATORY

In association with increased IAP, there is diaphragmatic splinting, exerting a restrictive effect on the lungs, with a reduction in ventilation, decreased lung compliance, an increase in airway pressures, and a reduction in tidal volumes.

In critically ill, mechanically ventilated patients, the effect on the respiratory system can be significant, resulting in reduced lung volumes, impaired gas exchange, and high ventilatory pressures. Hypercarbia can occur, and the resulting acidosis can be exacerbated by simultaneous cardiovascular depression as a result of raised IAP. The effects of raised IAP on the respiratory system in ICU can sometimes be life-threatening, requiring urgent abdominal decompression. Patients with true ACS undergoing abdominal decompression demonstrate a remarkable change in their intraoperative vital signs.

17.10.4.3 VISCERAL PERFUSION

There is an association between IAP and visceral perfusion as measured by gastric pH. This has recently been confirmed in 18 patients undergoing laparoscopy, in whom a reduction of between 11% and 54% in blood flow was seen in the duodenum and stomach, respectively, at an IAP of 15 mmHg. Animal studies suggest that the reduction in visceral perfusion is selective, affecting intestinal blood flow before, for example, adrenal blood flow. Early decreases in visceral perfusion are related to levels of IAP as low as 15 mmHg.

17.10.4.4 RENAL

The most likely direct effect of increased IAP is an increase in the renal vascular resistance, coupled with a moderate reduction in cardiac output. Pressure on the ureter has been ruled out as a cause, as investigators have placed ureteric stents with no improvement in function. Other factors that may contribute to renal dysfunction include humeral factors and intraparenchymal renal pressures.

17.10.4.5 INTRACRANIAL PRESSURE

Raised IAP can have a marked effect on intracranial pathophysiology and cause severe rises in ICP.

17.10.5 Measurement of IAP

IAP is not a static condition and should be measured continuously. In addition, whether IAP is measured intermittently or continuously, consideration should be given to abdominal perfusion measurement.

The gold standard for IAP measurement involves using a urinary catheter. The patient is positioned flat on the bed. A standard urinary catheter is used. The size of the urinary catheter does not matter. Elevation of the catheter and measuring the urine column provide a rough guide and are simple to perform. A T-piece bladder pressure device connected to a pressure transducer on-line to the monitoring system can be used. The pressure transducer is placed in the mid-axillary line, and the urinary tubing is clamped. If the patient is not lying flat, IAP can be measured from the pubic symphysis. Approximately 25 mL isotonic saline is inserted into the bladder via a three-way stopcock. After zeroing, the pressure on the monitor is recorded. Commercial direct transducers are available.

Pitfalls

A strict protocol and staff education on the technique and interpretation of IAP are essential.

Very high pressures (especially unexpected ones) are usually caused by a blocked urinary catheter and should be repeated.

17.10.5.1 MEASUREMENT OF ABDOMINAL PERFUSION PRESSURE (APP)

As with the concept of cerebral perfusion pressure, calculation of APP, which is defined as MAP minus IAP, assesses not only the severity of IAP present but also the adequacy of the patient's abdominal blood flow.

17.10.6 **Management**[37]

17.10.6.1 PREVENTION

To avoid ACS developing in the first place, in the emergency department, concepts of DCR coupled with adequate pre-hospital information will help identify patients at high risk even before they arrive in the emergency room, and avoiding excessive fluid resuscitation is an important factor in reducing the risk of developing subsequent ACS. In patients undergoing damage control laparotomy, it is mandatory to leave the abdomen open to prevent ACS and in anticipation of a second operation.

17.10.6.2 TREATMENT

There are several key principles in the management of patients with potential ACS:

- Regular appropriate monitoring of IAP in the ICU
- Optimization of systemic perfusion, circulating volume, and organ function in the patient with IAH grade I and grade II (i.e. ≤ 20 mmHg)
- Institution of specific medical procedures to reduce IAP and the end-organ consequences of IAH/ACS, including diuretics, and removing excess ascites if present by percutaneous puncture
- In patients with grade III–IV IAH (IAP > 20 mmHg) with evidence of new-onset organ failure not responding to non-operative management, a decompressive laparostomy performed as soon as possible

The decompressed abdomen should be closed using a low-vacuum (< 50 mmHg) sandwich technique.

17.10.6.3 REVERSIBLE FACTORS

The second aspect of management is to correct any reversible cause of ACS, such as intra-abdominal bleeding. Massive retroperitoneal haemorrhage is often associated with a fractured pelvis, and consideration should be given to measures that would control haemorrhage, such as pelvic fixation or vessel embolization. In some cases, severe gaseous distension or acute colonic pseudo-obstruction can occur in ICU patients. This may respond to drugs such as neostigmine, but if it is severe, surgical decompression may be necessary. A common cause of a raised IAP in ICU is related to the ileus. There is little that can be actively done in these circumstances apart from optimizing the patient's cardiorespiratory status and serum electrolytes and inserting a nasogastric tube.

17.10.7 **Surgery for Raised IAP**

There are few guidelines for exactly when surgical decompression is required in the presence of raised IAP. The indications for abdominal decompression are related to correcting pathophysiological abnormalities as much as achieving a precise and optimum IAP.

In general, temporary abdominal closure is superior to conventional techniques for dealing with intra-abdominal sepsis. Indications for performing temporary abdominal closure include:

- Abdominal decompression
- When re-exploration is planned
- To facilitate re-exploration in abdominal sepsis
- Inability to close the abdomen
- Prevention of ACS

Many different techniques have been used to facilitate a temporary abdominal closure, including intravenous bags, Velcro, silicone, zips, and vacuum-assisted wound closure dressings. Whatever technique is used, it is important that effective decompression be achieved with adequate incisions. ACS can recur even after apparent decompression if the temporary closure devices permit re-accumulation of pressure.

17.10.7.1 TIPS FOR SURGICAL DECOMPRESSION FOR RAISED IAP

- There should be early investigation and correction of the cause of raised IAP.
- Ongoing abdominal bleeding with raised IAP requires urgent operative intervention.
- Reduction in urinary output is a late sign of renal impairment. Gastric tonometry may provide earlier information on visceral perfusion.
- Abdominal decompression requires a full-length abdominal incision.
- The surgical dressing should be closed using a sandwich technique using two suction drains placed laterally to facilitate fluid removal from the wound.

17.10.8 **Management Algorithm**

Suggested management of IAH and ACS, including medical management algorithms, is in **Tables 17.9** and **17.10**.[37]

Table 17.9 Intra-abdominal Hypertension (IAH) and Abdominal Compartment Syndrome (ACS) Management Algorithm

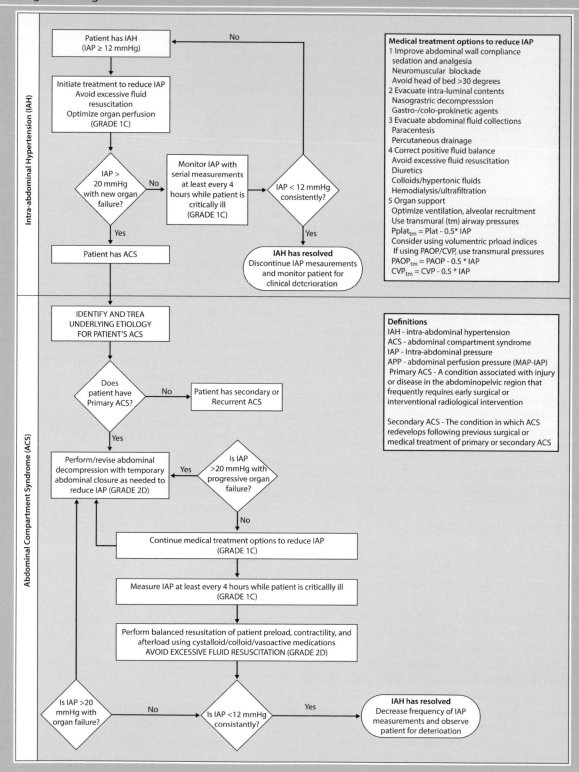

Table 17.10 Intra-abdominal Hypertension/Abdominal Compartment Syndrome Medical Management Algorithm

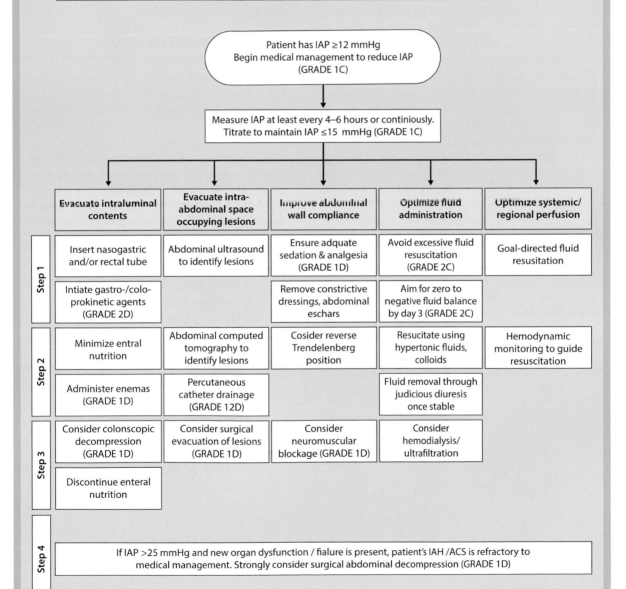

IAH/ACS MEDICAL MANAGMENT ALGORITHM

- *The choice and (success) of the medical management strategies listed below is stongly related to both the etiology of the patient's IAH/ACS and the patient's clinical situation. The appropriateness of each intervention should always be considered prior to implementing these interventios in any individual patient.*
- *The interventions should be applied in a stepwise fashion until the patients intra-abdominal pressure (IAP) decreases.*
- *If there is no response to particular intervention, therapy should escalated to the next step of the algorithm*

Patient has IAP ≥12 mmHg
Begin medical management to reduce IAP
(GRADE 1C)

Measure IAP at least every 4–6 hours or continiously.
Titrate to maintain IAP ≤15 mmHg (GRADE 1C)

	Evacuate intraluminal contents	Evacuate intra-abdominal space occupying lesions	Improve abdominal wall compliance	Optimize fluid administration	Optimize systemic/regional perfusion
Step 1	Insert nasogastric and/or rectal tube	Abdominal ultrasound to identify lesions	Ensure adquate sedation & analgesia (GRADE 1D)	Avoid excessive fluid resuscitation (GRADE 2C)	Goal-directed fluid resusitation
Step 1	Intiate gastro-/colo-prokinetic agents (GRADE 2D)		Remove constrictive dressings, abdominal eschars	Aim for zero to negative fluid balance by day 3 (GRADE 2C)	
Step 2	Minimize entral nutrition	Abdominal computed tomography to identify lesions	Cosider reverse Trendelenberg position	Resucitate using hypertonic fluids, colloids	Hemodynamic monitoring to guide resuscitation
Step 2	Administer enemas (GRADE 1D)	Percutaneous catheter drainage (GRADE 12D)		Fluid removal through judicious diuresis once stable	
Step 3	Consider colonscopic decompression (GRADE 1D)	Consider surgical evacuation of lesions (GRADE 1D)	Consider neuromuscular blockage (GRADE 1D)	Consider hemodialysis/ ultrafiltration	
Step 3	Discontinue enteral nutrition				

Step 4
If IAP >25 mmHg and new organ dysfunction / fialure is present, patient's IAH /ACS is refractory to medical management. Strongly consider surgical abdominal decompression (GRADE 1D)

17.11 ACUTE KIDNEY INJURY[38]

Whilst the frequency of acute kidney injury (AKI) is relatively low, injured patients are at high risk.[39] Several indicators of the severity of physiological injury, including the lowest body temperature, the highest lactate level, and the need for packed red blood cell and cryoprecipitate transfusions, were independently associated with a higher risk of developing AKI. Other factors included tissue damage and necrosis, hypotension, rhabdomyolysis, ACS, DIC, and endothelial injury, and pre-existing conditions such as diabetes. The development of AKI complicates ICU management, increases the length of stay, and is associated with a mortality of approximately 60%. Approximately one-third of acute post-traumatic AKI cases are caused by inadequate or over-resuscitation, whilst the remainder develop as part of MODS.

One quarter of the patients developed AKI within the first week; 26% of these patients received continuous renal replacement therapy. None of the surviving AKI patients had developed end-stage renal disease 1 year after injury. Diabetes mellitus, male sex, age, ISS greater than 40, massive transfusion, and fluid resuscitation with starches (e.g., hydroxyethyl starch [HES]) were independently associated with the development of post-injury AKI in the ICU, whereas sepsis was not.

The clinician should look for and manage these common causes:

- Hypovolaemia.
- Rhabdomyolysis.
- Abdominal compartment syndrome.

- Obstructive uropathy.
- Avoid nephrotoxic dyes, when possible, although there is evidence that CT contrast is unlikely to be harmful, and if indicated should not be delayed.[40,41]

Guidelines for AKI include the Kidney Disease Improving Global Outcomes (KDIGO) guidelines shown in **Table 17.11**.[42]

17.12 RHABDOMYOLYSIS

The Eastern Association for the Surgery of Trauma (EAST) Practice Management Guidelines for the Management of Rhabdomyolysis make the following recommendations:

The treatment of rhabdomyolysis remains controversial. Although there is no question that any associated compartment syndrome needs to be identified and released, debate persists regarding the benefit of further therapy including aggressive intravenous fluid resuscitation (IVFR), urine alkalization with bicarbonate, and the use of mannitol. The goal of this practice management guideline was to evaluate the effects of bicarbonate, mannitol, and aggressive intravenous fluids on patients with rhabdomyolysis.[43]

Table 17.11 Kidney Disease Improving Global Outcomes (KDIGO) Guidelines for Acute Kidney Injury

Stage	Serum Creatinine	Urine Output
1	Increase by 1.5–1.9 times baseline within 7 days **or** Increase by ≥ 0.3 times mg/dL (26.5 μmol/L) within 48 hours	Less than 0.5 mL/Kg/h for 6–12 hours
2	Increase by 2–2.9 times baseline	Less than 0.5 mL/Kg/h for ≥ 12 hours
3	Increase by ≥ 3 times baseline **or** Increase to ≥ 4 mg/dL (353.6 μmol/L) **or** Renal replacement therapy initiation **or** In patients younger than 18 years, decrease in estimated GFR to < 35 mL/min/1.73 m²	Less than 0.3 mL/Kg/hr for ≥ 24 hours **or** Anuria for ≥ 12 hours

KDIGO: Kidney Disease Improving Global Outcomes
AKI: Acute Kidney Injury
GFR: Glomerular Filtration Rate

Table 17.12 The Eastern Association for the Surgery of Trauma (EAST) Practice Management Guidelines for the Management of Rhabdomyolysis

P	**P**atient, **P**opulation, or **P**roblem	How would I describe the patient group?
I	**I**ntervention, Prognostic factor, or Exposure	Which main intervention, prognostic factor, or exposure is considered?
C	**C**omparison or Intervention (if appropriate)	What is the main alternative to compare with the intervention?
O	**O**utcome you would like to measure or achieve	What can be accomplished, measured, improved, or affected?
PICO		**Recommendation**
PICO Question 1		
Recommendation for the use of bicarbonate		Based on the analysis of included studies, the effect of bicarbonate on the selected outcomes, and the very low level of evidence; we **conditionally recommend against** the use of bicarbonate in patients with rhabdomyolysis versus routine medical care without bicarbonate to improve outcomes of ARF or need for dialysis.
PICO Question 2		
Recommendation for the use of mannitol		Based on the available evidence, the effect of mannitol on the selected outcomes, and the very low level of evidence; we conditionally recommend against the use of mannitol in patients with rhabdomyolysis versus routine medical care without mannitol to improve outcomes of ARF or need for dialysis.
PICO Question 3		
Recommendation for the use of aggressive intravenous fluids		Based on the analysis of included studies, the effect of IV fluids on the selected outcomes, and the very low level of evidence, **we conditionally recommend for** the use of aggressive IVFR in patients with rhabdomyolysis, versus usual medical care, to improve outcomes of ARF or need for dialysis.

In patients with rhabdomyolysis, to improve the outcomes of acute renal failure (ARF) and lessen the need for dialysis:

- We conditionally recommend for aggressive intravenous fluid resuscitation.
- We conditionally recommend against treatment with bicarbonate or mannitol.
- We conditionally recommend for the use of aggressive IVFR in patients with rhabdomyolysis.

Systematic review of the literature for treatment of rhabdomyolysis reveals a paucity of data and overlapping treatment effects (**Table 17.12**).

17.13 METABOLIC DISTURBANCES

Disturbances in acid–base and electrolyte balance can be anticipated in patients in shock, those who have received massive transfusions, and the elderly with comorbid conditions.

Typical abnormalities may include:

- Acid–base disorders
- Electrolyte disorders:
    - Hypokalaemia
    - Hyperkalaemia
    - Hypocalcaemia
    - Hypomagnesaemia
    - Hypophosphataemia

Metabolic acidosis is a frequent event in patients following major trauma. Physicians have at their disposal numerous plasma and urine tests to characterize metabolic acidosis and determine its aetiology. Acute metabolic acidosis may accompany various diseases and be associated with organ failure, in particular respiratory (increased ventilatory demand) and cardiovascular (arterial vasodilatation, decreases in cardiac inotropism and cardiac output, and ventricular arrythmia).

In acid–base disorders, one must identify and correct the aetiology of the disturbance, for example metabolic acidosis caused by hypoperfusion secondary to occult pericardial tamponade.

Pitfalls

Bicarbonate therapy in severely acidotic trauma patients increases mortality.

Sodium bicarbonate is **contraindicated** for correction of acidosis in acute trauma, as this is best corrected with improvement of tissue oxygenation.[44]

17.14 NUTRITIONAL SUPPORT[45,46]

Trauma patients are hypermetabolic and have increased nutritional needs due to the immunological response to trauma and the requirement for accelerated protein synthesis for wound healing. Early enteral feeding has been shown to reduce postoperative septic morbidity after trauma. A meta-analysis of several randomized trials has demonstrated a twofold decrease in infectious complications in patients treated with early enteral nutrition compared with total parenteral nutrition. In general, protein administration should be limited for the first 3 days to 0.8 g/kg and then increased to 1.3–1.5 g/kg (with adjustments for obesity, i.e., a BMI > 30) and administer 18–20 Kcal per gram of protein).[47] Thereafter, the nutrition is based on status. (See **Table 17.13**.)

TBI patients appear to have similar outcomes whether fed enterally or parenterally. A Cochrane review has confirmed that early (either parenteral or enteral) feeding is associated with a trend towards better outcomes in terms of survival and disability compared with later feeding.[48] Patients with a TBI exhibit protein wasting and gastrointestinal

Table 17.13 Recommendations for Nutritional Management by Nutritional Status and Phase of Critical Illness

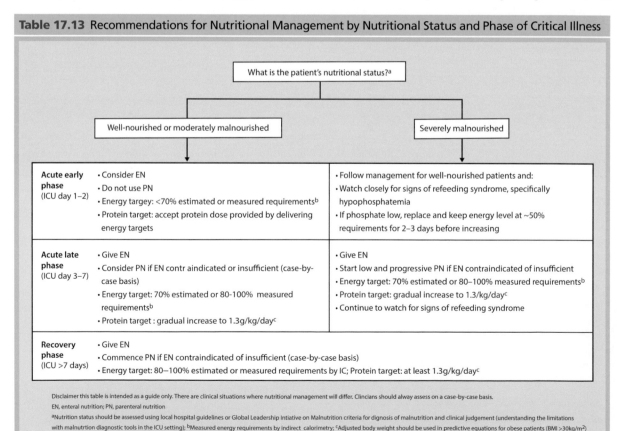

Disclaimer this table is intended as a guide only. There are clinical situations where nutritional management will differ. Clincians should alway assess on a case-by-case basis.

EN, enteral nutrition; PN, parenteral nutrition

[a]Nutrition status should be assessed using local hospital guidelines or Global Leadership Intiative on Malnutrition criteria for dignosis of malnutrition and clinical judgement (understanding the limitations with malnutrtion diagnostic tools in the ICU setting); [b]Measured energy requirements by indirect calorimetry; [c]Adjusted body weight should be used in predictive equations for obese patients (BMI >30kg/m²)

dysfunction, which may be risk factors for a septic state. However, standard nutritional support may not allow restoration of the nutritional state of TBI patients.[49]

Enteral nutrition is superior and should be the first choice, when the gut is accessible and functioning. Enteral nutrition is not invariably safer and better than parenteral nutrition, but a mix of the two modalities can be used safely.

Patients at risk for malnutrition include those with:

- Major trauma
- Burns

In severely injured blunt/penetrating trauma patients, there appears to be no outcome advantage to initiating enteral feedings within 24 hours of admission as compared with 72 hours after admission. In burn patients, intragastric feedings should be started as soon after admission as possible, because delayed enteral feeding (> 18 hours) results in a high rate of gastroparesis and need for intravenous nutrition. Patients with severe head injury who do not tolerate gastric feedings within 48 hours of injury should be switched to post-pyloric feedings, ideally beyond the ligament of Treitz, if feasible and safe for the patient. In severely injured patients undergoing laparotomy for blunt and penetrating abdominal injuries, direct small bowel access should be obtained (via a nasojejunal feeding tube, gastrojejunal feeding tube, or feeding jejunostomy) and enteral feedings begun as soon as is feasible after resuscitation from shock.

It is critical to:

- Determine energy and protein requirements.
- Determine and establish a route of administration.
- Set a time to begin nutritional support.

17.14.1 Access for Enteral Nutrition

17.14.1.1 SIMPLE

- Nasogastric tube
- Nasoduodenal tube
- Nasojejunal tube

Most critically ill trauma patients should be started on early enteral nutrition. The majority do not require prolonged tube feeding (beyond 10–14 days). For patients who have prolonged tube-feeding requirements, nasoenteric tubes are inconvenient, as they tend to dislodge, worsen aspiration, and are uncomfortable.

17.14.1.2 MORE COMPLICATED, LONGER TERM

- *Percutaneous endoscopic gastrostomy* (PEG): This does not interfere with swallowing, is easy to nurse, and has target feeding rates that are more likely to be achieved compared with nasoenteric tubes. However, it is an invasive procedure with some risk.
- *Jejunostomy*: A jejunostomy can be placed endoscopically or during laparotomy. Rates of major complications should be less than 5%.[50]

17.14.2 Monitoring Nutritional Support

Multiple diagnostic tests have been proposed to monitor the response to nutritional support.

- Body measurements (e.g., weight change, anthropometric determinations)
- Body composition studies (e.g., determinations of body fat, lean body mass, total body water)
- Urine analyses for metabolic byproducts (e.g., urea, creatinine)
- Immunologic tests (e.g., antibody production, delayed hypersensitivity skin tests)
- Functional tests (e.g., handgrip strength)
- Serum chemistry analyses (e.g., albumin, prealbumin)

17.15 PROPHYLAXIS IN THE ICU

17.15.1 Stress Ulceration[51]

Stress ulceration and associated upper gastrointestinal bleeding have been on the decline in most ICUs. This is, in great part, due to improved resuscitation efforts in the pre-hospital environment, emergency department, and operating room, as well as earlier feeding. In addition, the use of acid-blocking and cytoprotective therapies has become commonplace.

Those patients at greatest risk for stress ulcer development are those with a previous history of ulcer disease and those *not* enterally fed. Burn patients have also been labelled as high risk in historical studies.

The simplest and safest method of stress ulcer prevention is adequate resuscitation and early intragastric enteric nutrition.

During the early resuscitative phase, and whilst vaso-active drugs are used to elevate blood pressure, it is not always prudent to provide nutrition enterally. It is in these circumstances that the use of acid blockade, cyto-protective agents, or both is necessary.

Proton pump inhibitors (PPIs) have replaced H_2 block-ade as the mainstay of therapy; however, they should not be administered routinely, as they may increase Gram-negative colonization of the pharynx and increase the potential for VAP.

Pitfall

Most studies demonstrating the efficacy of PPIs in stress ulcer prevention do not attempt to fully neutralize gastric pH.

Cytoprotective agents (e.g., sucralfate) as a preventive measure have been shown to be the most cost-effective in ventilated trauma patients, as there is a marked decrease in the rate of development of VAP (especially *Candida* spp.) seen in the sucralfate population compared to the use of PPIs, which does make this therapeutic option quite attractive.

See Surgical Critical Care.net's guidelines for 2023.[52]
- Level 1
  - No recommendations
- Level 2
  - Chemoprophylaxis for stress ulcer prevention is indicated in patients with acute risk factors.
  - Discontinue therapy when patients no longer have acute risk factors.
  - Consider discontinuing therapy when a patient is tolerating full enteral feeding.
  - Sucralfate is an acceptable alternative to a hista-mine type 2 receptor antagonist (H2RA) and may decrease the incidence and severity of VAP.
  - A PPI is an alternative to a H2RA or sucralfate in situations where these agents cannot be used.
- Level 3
  - Stress ulcer prophylaxis should be continued in patients with any of the following risk factors for stress ulceration:
    - Mechanical ventilation (> 48 hours) without enteral nutrition
    - Coagulopathy
    - Hypoperfusion (shock, or organ dysfunction)
    - High-dose corticosteroids (> 250 mg/day hydrocortisone or equivalent)

- Significant burn injury (total body surface area ≥ 20%)
- Acute spinal cord injury
- Severe TBI

17.15.2 Deep Venous Thrombosis and Pulmonary Embolus[53]

Pulmonary embolus from DVT, or pulmonary thrombo-sis developed *in situ*, continues to be a leading preventable cause of death in the injured patient. Recognizing the risk factors for the development of DVT and instituting an aggressive prophylactic regimen can reduce this risk from DVT in the ICU with little added morbidity. The incidence of DVT in trauma patients is 12%–32%, and those at high-est risk of fatal PE include those with spinal cord injuries, weight-bearing pelvic fracture, and combined long bone fracture/TBI or long bone fracture/pelvic fracture.

Recent evidence in trauma suggests reductions in DVT and PE with weight-based prophylaxis, rather than stan-dardized doses.[54] All high-risk patients should be proac-tively monitored with VHA or factor Xa.

There is a separate guideline for paediatric patients.[55]

A high index of suspicion in severely injured patients should result in preventative therapy and diagnostic screening measures in the ICU.

Unless haemorrhagic TBI or spinal cord epidural haematoma precludes the use of low-molecular-weight heparin therapy, these patients should all receive fractionated low-molecular-weight subcutaneous heparin within 24 hours of injury, or within 6–12 hours of bleeding control.

Unfractionated heparin is not as effective in this severely injured population.

Unless extremity injury precludes their use, graded pneumatic compression devices should be used on all such patients. Foot pumps may also be of some benefit. Standard compression stockings ('TED stockings') have no role in the non-ambulant patient.

Most patients can be initiated on prophylactic antico-agulation within 24 hours of cessation of haemorrhagic shock, *even in the presence of solid organ injury*. For those with acute traumatic brain or spinal injury, prophylac-tic VTE therapy can be initiated within 24–48 hours of a stable head injury as prophylaxis against VTE after major trauma. Similarly, unless extremity injury precludes their use, graded elastic compression stockings should be used on all such patients. Foot pumps or intermittent calf-compression devices may also be of some benefit. See also the Western Trauma Association's algorithm for early anticoagulant reversal after trauma.[56]

Screening for the presence of DVT – which, if present, would necessitate more aggressive anticoagulant therapy – should also be implemented in these patients. The easiest and safest screening tool is venous Doppler ultrasound or duplex scanning. This is a portable, readily available, repeatable, and cost-effective procedure with no side effects for the patient. These modalities are, however, operator-dependent and can fail to diagnose DVT in the deep pelvic veins. Contrast ultrasound might overcome this weakness. This screening should be performed whenever clinical suspicion of DVT arises.[57]

In the highest-risk patients previously mentioned, consideration for prophylactic placement of an inferior vena cava (IVC) filter may be made. However, prophylactic IVC filter placement has been associated with an increased incidence of DVT (odds ratio [OR] = 1.83; 95% confidence interval [CI] = 1.15–2.93). Furthermore, prophylactic IVC filter placement has not been effective in reducing trauma patient mortality.[58] The combination of aggressive prevention measures, screening by duplex, and VTE chemoprophylaxis can result in a fatal PE rate of significantly less than 1% of the trauma ICU population.

17.15.3 Tetanus Prophylaxis

In patients with any open wounds from trauma, it is imperative that the tetanus immunization status of the patient is addressed. For those patients immunized within the previous 5 years, no additional treatment is generally needed, whilst booster tetanus toxoid should be administered to those who have previously received the initial tetanus series but have not been reimmunized in the preceding 5–10 years. Tetanus immune globulin should be administered to those patients who lack any previous history of immunization.

Patients undergoing splenectomy require immunization for *Haemophilus influenza* type B, meningococcus, and pneumococcus. (See Section 9.7 on splenic injury.) Debate continues regarding the timing of administration of these vaccines in trauma patients, but adult patients do not benefit from the antibacterial chemoprophylaxis needed in paediatric patients post splenectomy. Due to the multiple strains of each organism, immunization is not foolproof in preventing overwhelming post-splenectomy infection (OPSI). Therefore, patients must be carefully counselled to seek medical attention immediately for high fevers, and healthcare providers must be aggressive in the use of empirical antibiotics in patients who may have OPSI upon presentation in the outpatient setting.

17.15.4 Line Sepsis

Thrombophlebitis and sepsis from intravenous cannulae are significant considerations, as these intravenous lines are frequently placed under less-than-optimal circumstances and technique in the field and in resuscitation areas. Whilst routine changes of central lines are no longer advocated, peripheral cannulae and lines should be changed at least every 72–96 hours.

17.16 PAIN AND DELIRIUM CONTROL[58]

17.16.1 Pain Control

If the patient can cooperate, visual analogue pain scores may be helpful. Several adverse consequences result when pain is inadequately treated. These include increased oxygen consumption, increased minute volume demands, psychic stress, increased delirium, sleep deprivation, and impaired lung mechanics with associated pulmonary complications. Subjective pain assessment is best documented objectively and, after initiation of treatment, requires serial re-evaluation. Inadequate pain relief can be determined objectively by the failure of the patient to achieve adequate volumes on incentive spirometry, persistently small radiographic lung volumes, or a reluctance to cough and cooperate with chest physiotherapy.

Early pain control in the ICU is primarily achieved using intravenous opiates, although there is emerging evidence for the use of ketamine infusion as an opioid-sparing option. Other techniques are employed and tailored to the individual patient and injury:

- Bolus analgo-sedation opioids and non-opioids.
  - Morphine, fentanyl, or ketamine titrated intravenously.
- Multimodal therapies activating heterogeneous receptors (e.g., non-steroidal anti-inflammatory drugs, GABA-adrenergic receptor agonists).
- Patient-controlled analgesia (PCA).

- Fentanyl patches.
- Fentanyl 'lollipops'.
- Inhalational analgesia with pentoxyflurane 'whistles' are useful options for initial pain control and during dressing changes.
- Epidural or paraspinal analgesia (continuous infusion or patient-controlled).
- Intrapleural anaesthesia.
- Extrapleural analgesia.
- Intercostal nerve blocks.
- Catheter techniques for peripheral nerve blocks (e.g., femoral nerve, brachial plexus, popliteal nerve, and paravertebral nerve blocks).

17.16.2 Delirium[58]

Delirium is a recognized complication in patients in the ICU. A breakdown of treatment strategies is beyond the scope of this chapter, but identification of causative factors, re-establishing a day–night rhythm, and medical strategies should be attempted.

17.17 ICU TERTIARY SURVEY[59]

The tertiary survey is a complete re-examination of the patient, plus a review of the history and all available results and imaging. Missed injuries are a potent cause of morbidity, and the majority will be identified by a thorough tertiary survey. A systematic review of 10 studies found the overall incidence of missed injuries identified by tertiary survey was 4.3%, with one hospital reporting 65%.[60] A tertiary trauma survey has much to recommend it in minimizing the delay in the ultimate diagnosis of missed injury. Nevertheless, it is not a complete solution, and an ongoing analysis of errors should be undertaken at any major trauma centre.

17.17.1 Evaluation for Occult Injuries

Factors predisposing to missed injuries:

- Mechanism of injury – re-verify the events surrounding the injury.
- Unresponsive victim who cannot participate in an examination.

High-priority occult injuries:

- Brain, spinal cord, and peripheral nerve injury
- Thoracic aortic injury
- Intra-abdominal or pelvic injury
- Vascular injuries to the extremities
- Cerebrovascular injuries – occult carotid/vertebral artery injury
- Cardiac injuries
- Aerodigestive tract injuries – ruptured bowel
- Occult pneumothorax
- Compartment syndrome – foreleg, thigh, buttock, or arm
- Eye injuries (remember to remove the patient's contact lenses)
- Other occult injuries – hands, feet, digits, or joint dislocations
- Vaginal tampons

17.17.2 Assess Comorbid Conditions

- Medical history (including drugs and alcohol).
- Contact the patient's personal physicians.
- Check pharmacy records.

17.17.3 ICU Summary

Complete a **FAST HUGS BID** protocol for all patients (see **Table 17.14**).[61]

"In addition, the tertiary survey is an excellent time to review initial cross-sectional imaging and other studies with attention to any incidental findings identified. These need to be review[ed] with the patient/family, communicated to a primary physician if able, and documented in the medical record."[62]

17.18 FAMILY CONTACT AND SUPPORT

(See Chapter 22: 'Psychology of Trauma'.)

It is very important to establish early contact with family members to explain the injuries, clinical condition, and prognosis of the patient. This provides family members with essential information and establishes a relationship between the ICU care team and the family. Utilization of

Table 17.14 'FAST HUGS BID' Medical Mnemonic for a Surgical Patient

	Medical Patient	**Surgical Patient**
F	Feeding	Feeding (NPO, enteral, TPN)
A	Analgesia	Analgesia (VAS score)
S	Sedation	Sensorium (GCS, Ramsay sedation score)
T	Thromboprophylaxis	Thromboprophylaxis, temperature, tubes
H	Head-up position	Head-up position, haemodynamics
U	Ulcer prophylaxis	Ulcer prophylaxis, urine output
G	Glycaemic control	Glycaemic control
B	Bowel movement	Bowel (ileus, gastroparesis, distension, movement)
I	Indwelling catheter	Indwelling lines (catheter, A-line, CVC, epidural, Foley) Imbalance (electrolyte, cumulative fluid)
D	Drug de-escalation	Drugs (de-escalation, delirium, number of days)

TPN, Total Parenteral Nutrition
VAS, Visual Analog Scale
GCS, Glasgow Coma Scale

NIV, Non-invasive ventilation
CVC, Central Venous Catheter
NPO, *Nil per os* (Nil by mouth)

tools such as the best-case/worst-case can be very effective in such communication. Administrative facts, such as ICU procedures, visiting hours, and available services, should also be explained. When patients lose their decisional capacity, it is incumbent to identify the medical-legal decision maker. Especially in older patients, identifying the existence of advanced directives, living wills, or other predetermination documents is important. Patients and their families should be familiar with the multidisciplinary approach to patient care in the ICU as well.

"The involvement of a Palliative Care Service, if available, may well help with symptom management and family interface for those with functional dependency and advanced care needs."[63]

REFERENCES AND RECOMMENDED READING

References

1. Hardcastle TC, Maier R, Muckart DJ. Ventilation in trauma patients – the first 24 hours is different! *World J Surg*. 2017 May;**41(5)**:1153–58. doi: 10.1007/s00268-016-3530-1.

2. Claridge JA, Crabtree TD, Pelletier SJ, Butler K, Sawyer RG, Young JS. Persistent occult hypoperfusion is associated with a significant increase in infection rate and mortality in major trauma patients. *J Trauma*. 2000 Jan;**48(1)**:8–14.

3. Blow O, Magliore L, Claridge JA, Butler K, Young JS. The golden hour and the silver day: detection and correction of occult hypoperfusion within 24 hours improves outcome from major trauma. *J Trauma*. 1999 Nov;**47(5)**:964–9.

4. Hernandez G, Messina A, Kattan E. Invasive arterial pressure monitoring: much more than mean arterial pressure! *Intensive Care Med*. 2022 Oct;**48(10)**:1495–7. Epub 2022 Jul 8. doi: 10.1007/s00134-022-06798-8.

5. Rali AS, Butcher A, Tedford RJ, Sinha S, Mekki P, Van Spall H, et al. Contemporary review of hemodynamic monitoring in the critical care setting. *US Cardiol Rev*. 2022;**16**:e12. doi: 10.15420/usc.2021.34.

6. Richards GA, Hardcastle TC, Hodgson RE. *Ventilation in the Trauma Patient: A Practical Approach*. Springer-Verlag, Berlin Heidelberg. 2021.

7. Amato MB, Meade MO, Slutsky AS, Brochard L, Costa EL, Schoenfeld DA, et al. Driving pressure and survival in the acute respiratory distress syndrome. *N Engl J Med*. 2015 Feb 19;747–55. doi: 10.1056/NEJMsa1410639.

8. Santos RS, Silva PL, Pelosi P, Rocco PR. Recruitment maneuvers in acute respiratory distress syndrome: the safe way is the best way. *World J Crit Care Med*. 2015;**4(4)**:278–86. doi: 10.5492/wjccm.v4.i4.278.

9. Garner JS, Jarvis WR, Emori TG, Horan TC, Hughes JM. CDC definitions for nosocomial infections, 1988. *Am J Infect Control*. 1988 Jun;**16(3)**:128–40.

10. Gutiérrez-Pizarraya A, León-García MDC, De Juan-Idígoras R, Garnacho-Montero J, Clinical impact of procalcitonin-based algorithms for duration of antibiotic treatment in

critically ill adult patients with sepsis: a meta-analysis of randomized clinical trials *Rev Anti-Infect.* 2022;**20**(**1**):103–12. doi: 10.1080/14787210.2021.1932462.

11. Mallick A, Bodenham AR. Tracheostomy in critically ill patients. *Eur J Anaesthesiol.* 2010 Aug;**27**(**8**):676–82. doi: 10.1097/EJA.0b013e32833b1ba0. Review.

12. Ely EW. The ABCDEF bundle: science and philosophy of how ICU liberation serves patients and families. *Crit Care Med.* 2017 Feb;**45**(**2**):321–30. doi: 10.1097/CCM.0000000000002175.

13. Zonies D, Merkel M. Advanced extracorporeal therapy in trauma. *Curr Opin Crit Care.* 2016 Dec;**22**(**6**):578–83. Review.

14. Zonies D. ECLS in trauma: practical application and a review of current status. *World J Surg.* 2017 May;**41**(**5**):1159–64. doi: 10.1007/s00268-016-3586-y.

15. Swol J, Brodie D, Napolitano L, Park PK, Thiagarajan R, Barbaro RP, et al. Extracorporeal Life Support Organization (ELSO). *J Trauma Acute Care Surg.* 2018 Jun;**84**(**6**):831–7. doi: 10.1097/TA.0000000000001895.

16. Wang C, Lei Zhang L, Qin T, Xi Z, Sun L, Wu H, et al. Extracorporeal membrane oxygenation in trauma patients: a systematic review. *World J Emerg Surg.* 2020 Sep 11;**15**(**1**):51. doi: 10.1186/s13017-020-00331-2.

17. Zonies D, Codner P, Park P, Martin ND, Lissauer M, Evans S, et al. AAST critical care committee clinical consensus: ECMO, nutrition. *Trauma Surg Acute Care Open.* 2019 Apr 3;**4**(**1**):e000304. doi: 10.1136/tsaco-2019-000304. eCollection 2019.

18. McNamee JJ, et al. Effect of lower tidal volume ventilation facilitated by extracorporeal carbon dioxide removal vs standard care ventilation on 90-day mortality in patients with acute hypoxemic respiratory failure: the REST randomized clinical trial. *JAMA.* 2021 Sep 21; **326**(**11**):1013–23.

19. Tieu BH, Holcomb JB, Schreiber MA. Coagulopathy: its pathophysiology and treatment in the injured patient. *World J Surg.* 2007 May;**31**(**5**):1055–64. Review.

20. Ganter MT, Pittet JF. New insights into acute coagulopathy in trauma patients. *Best Pract Res Clin Anaesthesiol* 2010 Mar;**24**(**1**):15–25. Review.

21. Moore HB, Moore EE, Gonzales E, Chapman MP, Chin TL, Silliman CC, et al. Hyperfibrinolysis, physiologic fibrinolysis, and fibrinolysis shutdown: The spectrum of post injury fibrinolysis and relevance to antifibrinolytic therapy. *J Trauma Acute Care Surg.* 2014 Dec;**77**(**6**):811–7; discussion 817. doi: 10.1097/TA.0000000000000341.

22. CRASH-2 Trial Collaborators. Effects of tranexamic acid on death, vascular occlusive events, and blood transfusion in trauma patients with significant haemorrhage (CRASH-2): a randomised, placebo-controlled trial. *Lancet.* 2010;**376**:27–32.

23. Karl V, Thorn S, Mathes T, Hess S, Maegele M. Association of tranexamic acid administration with mortality and thromboembolic events in patients with traumatic injury: a systematic review and meta-analysis. *JAMA Network Open.* 2022;**5**(**3**):e220625. doi: 10.1001/jamanetworkopen.2022.0625.

24. Holcomb JB, Tilley BC, Baraniuk S, Fox EE, Wade CE, Podbielski JM, et al. Transfusion of plasma, platelets, and red blood cells in a 1:1:1 vs a 1:1:2 ratio and mortality in patients with severe trauma: the PROPPR randomized clinical trial. *JAMA.* 2015 Feb 3;**313**(**5**):471–82. doi: 10.1001/jama.2015.12.

25. Cap AP, Beckett A, Benov A, Borgman M, Chen J, Corley JB, et al. Whole blood transfusion. *Mil Med.* 2018 Sep 1;**183**(**suppl_2**):44–51. doi: 10.1093/milmed/usy120.

26. Relja B, Land WG. Damage associated molecular patterns in trauma. *Eur J Trauma Emerg Surg.* 2020;**46**:751–75. doi: 10.1007/s00068-019-01235-w.

27. Singer M, Deutschman CS, Seymour CW, Shankar-Hari M, Annane D, Bauer M, et al. The third international consensus definitions for sepsis and septic shock (Sepsis-3). *JAMA.* 2016;**315**(**8**):801–10. doi: 10.1001/jama.2016.0287.

28. Napolitano LM. Sepsis 2018: definitions and guideline changes. *Surg Infect (Larchmt).* 2018 Feb/Mar;**19**(**2**): 117–25. doi: 10.1089/sur.2017.278.

29. Evans L, Rhodes A, Alhazzani W, Antonelli M, Coopersmith CM, French C, et al. Surviving sepsis campaign: international guidelines for management of sepsis and septic shock 2021. *Intensive Care Med.* 2021;**47**:1181–247. doi: 10.1007/s00134-021-06506-y.

30. AlRawahi AN, AlHinai FA, Doig CJ, Ball CG, Dixon E, Xiao Z, Kirkpatrick AW. The prognostic value of serum procalcitonin measurements in critically injured patients: a systematic review. *Crit Care.* 2019;**23**:390. doi: 10.1186/s13054-019-2669-1.

31. Spellberg B, Rice LB. Duration of antibiotic therapy: shorter is better. *Ann Int Med.* 2019 Aug 6;**171**(**3**):210–1. doi: 10.7326/M19-1509. Epub 2019 Jul 9.

32. Velmahos GC, Toutouzas KG, Sarkisyan G, Chan LS, Jindal A, Karaiskakis M, et al. Severe trauma is not an excuse for prolonged antibiotic prophylaxis. *Arch Surg.* 2002 May;**137**(**5**):537–41. doi: 10.1001/archsurg.137.5.537.

33. Hoff WS, Bonadies JA, Cachecho R, Dorlac WC. Eastern Association for the Surgery of Trauma. Eastern Association for the Surgery of Trauma. Practice Management Guidelines Workgroup: Update to practice management guidelines for prophylactic antibiotic use in open fractures. *J Trauma.* 2011;70(3):751–4. doi: 10.1097/TA.0b013e31820930e5.

34. Klompas, M. Advancing the science of ventilator-associated pneumonia surveillance. *Crit Care.* 2012;**16**:165. doi: 10.1186/cc11656

35. National Healthcare Safety Network; Centres for Disease Control: Ventilator-Associated Event (VAE). January 2022. https://www.cdc.gov/nhsn/pdfs/pscmanual/10-vae_final.pdf (accessed September 2023).

36. Abdominal Compartment Syndrome. World Society for Abdominal Compartment Syndrome. Available from www.wsacs.org (accessed online September 2023).

37. De Laet IE, Malbrain MLNG, De Waele JJ. A clinician's guide to management of intraabdominal hypertension and abdominal compartment syndrome in critically Ill patients. *Critical Care.* 2020;**24**:97. doi: 10.1186/s13054-020-2782-1.

38. Messerer DAC, Halbgebauer R, Nilsson B, Pavenstädt H, Radermacher P, Huber-Lang M. Immunopathophysiology of trauma-related acute kidney injury. *Nat Rev Nephrol.* 2021;**17**:91–111. doi: 10.1038/s41581-020-00344-9.

39. Hatton GE, Harvin JA, Wade CE, Kao LS. Importance of duration of acute kidney injury after severe trauma: a cohort study. *Trauma Surg Acute Care Open.* 2021;**6**:e000689.

40. Aycock RD, Westafer LM, Boxen JL, Majlesi N, Schoenfeld EM, Bannuru RR. Acute kidney injury after computed tomography: a meta-analysis. *Ann Emerg Med.* 2018 Jan;**71(1)**:44–53.e4. doi: 10.1016/j.annemergmed.2017.06.041.

41. Giles T, Weaver N, Varghese A, Way TL, Abel C, Choi P, et al. Acute kidney injury development in polytrauma and the safety of early repeated contrast studies: a retrospective cohort study. *J Trauma Acute Care Surg.* 2022 Dec 1;**93(6)**:872–81. doi: 10.1097/TA.0000000000003735. Epub 2022 Jul 7

42. Clinical Practice Guidelines for Acute Kidney Injury https://kdigo.org/guidelines/acute-kidney-injury/ (accessed online August 2023).

43. Sawhney JS, Kasotakis G, Goldenberg A, Abramson S, Dodgion C, Patel N, et al. Management of rhabdomyolysis: a practice management guideline from the Eastern Association for the Surgery of Trauma. A*m J Surg.* 2021 Nov 22:S0002-9610(21)00681–4. doi: 10.1016/j.amjsurg.2021.11.022. Epub ahead of print

44. Wilson RF, Spencer AR, Tyburski JG, Dolman H, Zimmerman LH. Bicarbonate therapy in severely acidotic trauma patients increases mortality. *J Trauma Acute Care Surg.* 2013 Jan;**74(1)**:45–50; discussion 50. doi: 10.1097/TA.0b013e3182788fc4.

45. Jacobs DO, Kudsk KA, Oswanski MF, Sacks GS, Sinclair KE. Practice management guidelines for nutritional support of the trauma patient. In *Eastern Association for the Surgery of Trauma. Practice Management Guidelines. J Trauma.* 2004 Sep;**57(3)**:660–78; discussion 679. Available from www.east.org (accessed online January 2019).

46. Kreymann KG, Berger MM, Deutz NE, Hiesmayr M, Jolliet P, Kazandjiev G, et al. ESPEN (European Society for Parenteral and Enteral Nutrition). ESPEN Guidelines on Enteral Nutrition: intensive care. *Clin Nutr.* 2006 April;**25(2)**:210–23.

47. Lambell KJ, Tatucu-Babet OA, Chapple L-A, Gantner D, Ridley EJ. Nutrition therapy in critical illness: a review of the literature for clinicians. *Crit Care.* 2020;**24**:35. doi: 10.1186/s13054-020-2739-4.

48. Perel P, Yanagawa T, Bunn F, Roberts I, Wentz R, Pierro A. Nutritional support for head-injured patients. *Cochrane Database Syst Rev.* 2006 Oct 18;(**4**):CD001530. Review. doi: 10.1002/14651858.CD001530.pub2.

49. Cook AM, Peppard A, Magnuson A. Nutrition considerations in traumatic brain injury. *Nutr Clin Pract.* 2008 Dec–2009 Jan;**23(6)**:608–20. doi: 10.1177/0884533608326060.

50. Holmes JH 4th, Brundage SI, Yuen P, Hall RA, Maier RV, Jurkovich GJ. Complications of surgical feeding jejunostomy in patients. *J Trauma.* 1999 Dec;**47(6)**:1009–12. doi: 10.1097/00005373-199912000-00004.

51. Guillamondegui OD, Gunter OL Jr, Bonadies JA, Coates JE, Kurek SJ, De Moya Mae, et al. Practice management guidelines for stress ulcer prophylaxis. In *Eastern Association for the Surgery of Trauma. Practice Management Guidelines.* Available from https://www.east.org/education-resources/practice-management-guidelines/details/stress-ulcer-prophylaxis (accessed August 2023).

52 Guidelines for Stress Ulcer Prophylaxis. Updated 7 February 2023. *Surgical Critical Care.net.* https://surgicalcriticalcare.net/Guidelines/Stress%20Ulcer%20Prophylaxis%202023.pdf (accessed September 2023).

53. Ley EJ, Brown CVR, Moore EE, Sava JA, Peck K, Ciesla DJ, et al. Updated guidelines to reduce venous thromboembolism in trauma patients: a Western Trauma Association critical decisions algorithm. *J Trauma Acute Care Surg.* 2020;**89**:971–81 doi: 10.1097/TA.0000000000002830.

54. Kay AB, Majercik S, Sorensen J, Woller SC, Stevens SM, White T, et al. Weight-based enoxaparin dosing and deep vein thrombosis in hospitalized trauma patients: a double-blind, randomized, pilot study. *Surgery.* 2018;**23**. pii: S0039-6060(18)30094-1. doi: 10.1016/j.surg.2018.03.001

55. Mahajerin A, Petty JK, Hanson SJ, Thompson AJ, O'Brien SH, Streck CJ, et al. Prophylaxis against venous thromboembolism in pediatric trauma: a practice management guideline from the Eastern Association for the Surgery of Trauma and the Pediatric Trauma Society. *J Trauma Acute Care Surg.* 2017;**82(3)**:627–36. doi: 10.1097/TA.0000000000001359.

56. Peck KA, Ley EJ, Brown CV, Moore EE, Sava JA, Ciesla DJ, et al. Early anticoagulant reversal after trauma: a Western Trauma Association critical decisions algorithm. *J Trauma Acute Care Surg.* 2021 Feb 1;**90(2)**:331–6. doi: 10.1097/TA.0000000000002979.

57. Stevens SM, Woller SC, Kreuziger LB, Bounameaux H, Doerschug, Geersing G-J, et al. Executive summary: antithrombotic therapy for VTE disease: second update of the CHEST guideline and expert panel report. *Chest.* 2021;**160**(6):e545–e608. doi: 10.1016/j.chest.2021.07.055.

58. Devlin JW, Skrobik Y, Gélinas C, Needham DM, Slooter A, Pandharipande PP, et al. Executive summary: clinical practice guidelines for the prevention and management of pain, agitation/sedation, delirium, immobility, and sleep disruption in adult patients in the ICU. *Crit Care Med.* 2018 Sept;**46**(9):1532–48. doi: 10.1097/CCM.0000000000003259.

59. Janjua KJ, Sugrue M, Deane SA. Prospective evaluation of early missed injuries and the role of the tertiary trauma survey. *J Trauma.* 1998 Jun;**44**(6):1000–6; discussion 1006–7.

60. Keijzers GB, Giannakopoulos GF, Del Mar C, Bakker FC, Geeraedts LM Jr. The effect of tertiary surveys on missed injuries in trauma: a systematic review. *Scand J of Scand J Trauma Resusc Emerg Med.* 2012 Nov 29;**20**:77. doi: 10.1186/1757-7241-20-77.

61. Nair AS, Naik VM, Rayani BK. FAST HUGS BID: modified mnemonic for surgical patient. *Indian J Crit Care Med.* 2017 Oct;**21**(10):713–4. doi: 10.4103/ijccm. IJCCM_289_17.

62. Smith LM, King SA, Shealy JA, Heidel RE, Morin-Ducote G, Husband LD, et al. Incidental findings in the trauma population: interdisciplinary approach and electronic medical record reminder association with pre-discharge reporting and medicolegal risk. *J Am Coll Surg.* 2021 Apr;**232**(4):380–5.e1. doi: 10.1016/j.jamcollsurg.2020.11.028.

63. Zimmermann CJ, Zelenski AB, Buffington A, Baggett ND, Tucholka JL, Weis HB, et al. Best case/worst case for the trauma ICU: development and pilot testing of a communication tool for older adults with traumatic injury. *J Trauma Acute Care Surg.* 2021 Sep 1;**91**(3):542–51. doi: 10.1097/TA.0000000000003281.

Trauma Anaesthesia **18**

18.1 INTRODUCTION

Trauma anaesthesiologists are an essential part of the trauma team working in close collaboration with the surgeon. Trauma anaesthesia participates in the entire chain of trauma care, from pre-hospital to the emergency room (ER), often multiple operating room (OR) episodes, intensive care, and pain management. Strategies that work in elective cases may not be appropriate for trauma patients. The trauma anaesthesiologist participates in and contributes to the decision making process during the initial resuscitation and provides resuscitation and anaesthesia in the perioperative setting.

Because of this comprehensive involvement and the frequent multiple surgeries for some severely injured patients, trauma anaesthesiologists may be a consistent asset throughout the entire treatment process.

In this chapter, we will cover the aspects of trauma anaesthesia related to damage control in trauma. Anaesthetic involvement in specific situations, such as head trauma, is dealt with in the relevant other chapters. Special skills are also described in those chapters.

18.2 PLANNING AND COMMUNICATING

Preparation for the treatment of the trauma patient is best started before arrival. This way, it is possible to activate the team and make a briefing, contact other services, and prepare all necessary drugs, blood products, and equipment so that the approach of the polytrauma patient is made quickly but safely. Although the composition of trauma teams varies between countries and institutions, the presence of an anaesthesiologist in the trauma team is an asset because of their contribution to the management of the airway, oxygenation, and ventilation, as well as the patient's neurological condition and temperature. The presence of the anaesthesiologist in the trauma team ensures continuity of care, prevents loss of information, and facilitates the transfer process to the operating theatre by reducing the time to control the haemorrhage.

Closest to the patient's head, they are often best placed to elicit a history from a conscious patient, and to provide explanation and reassurance.

The trauma team should then decide the optimal process of care for that individual.

Pitfalls

Interventions in the ER should be limited to those that are essential for survival. Ensuring adequate venous access and perhaps an extra-large-bore intravenous (IV) cannula may make an important difference; however, delaying moving the patient for an arterial line may not be worthwhile. Keep in mind that difficult vascular access is likely an indicator of physiologic *extremis* in the trauma patient. Decisive action by experienced clinicians is crucial to avoid lost time.

The anaesthesiologist has a crucial role in optimizing the physiology to match the surgical strategies. The assessment of ongoing dynamic changes and reaction to treatment is an essential contribution to the decision-making process.

The planned strategy for resuscitation and surgery should be communicated closely between surgeon, anaesthesiologist, and team, coordinated by the trauma team leader.

(See also Chapter 2 on non-technical skills.)

DOI: 10.1201/9781003258124-23

18.3 DAMAGE CONTROL RESUSCITATION (DCR)[1]

Damage control includes damage control anaesthesia, damage control resuscitation (haemostatic trauma resuscitation), and damage control surgery, aiming to rapidly stop bleeding, restore blood volume and homeostasis, and aggressively prevent and correct coagulopathy, hypothermia, hyperkalaemia, hypercalcaemia, and acidosis.[2] (See Chapter 6: 'Damage Control'.)

Additional knowledge of damage control radiology is of great assistance@.[3]

The five principal pillars of DCR are:

- Limiting or omitting fluid administration; early use of components
- Permissive hypotension
- Targeting coagulopathy
- Preventing and treating hypothermia
- Early use of tranexamic acid (TXA), where indicated

DCR aims to treat and prevent conditions which exacerbate haemorrhagic shock and the ensuing systemic inflammatory response. DCR addresses the pathophysiologic consequences of tissue trauma and blood loss, and reduces the risks of overly aggressive fluid resuscitation, whilst targeting correction of metabolic derangements and coagulopathy. DCR supports the concept of limiting operative stress by delaying definitive repair until after control of haemorrhage and after physiology improves. The importance of an early transfer to an intensive care unit (ICU) for subsequent normalization of microcirculation, correction of coagulopathy, and re-warming is stressed.

With early haemorrhage control and optimal resuscitation, some patients may rapidly improve their haemodynamic state. Therefore, even if initially considered for the DCR pathway, they might then be suitable for definitive treatment. Constant reassessment is crucial, and the role of the anaesthesiologist in providing continued information about the patient's haemodynamic and organ perfusion is key for joint decision-making.

18.3.1 Limited Fluid Administration

Aggressive fluid resuscitation to restore normal circulatory function was once the mainstay of the initial approach for haemorrhagic shock. In 2004, Moore et al. coined the term 'bloody vicious cycle', showing that crystalloid administration leads to a transient rise in blood pressure, followed by increased haemorrhage, which requires further fluid administration, leading to the sequence of hypotension, fluid bolus, re-bleeding, and deeper hypotension. It is currently accepted that administration of high volumes of fluid before achieving definitive haemostasis increases the rate of bleeding by raising cardiac output, increased blood pressure counteracting local vasoconstriction, and reopening spontaneously clotted vessels. In addition to dilutional coagulopathy, large volumes of crystalloid fluids have deleterious effects on organ function, the endothelium, and immunological and inflammatory mediators. All of these are associated with poor outcome. Recent studies have shown that high volumes of crystalloids increase reperfusion injury and leukocyte adhesion, resulting in an increased incidence of infectious complications and multiple organ failure (**Table 18.1**).

During ongoing surgical bleeding, clear fluids should be limited to minimal amounts or even omitted until definitive control of haemorrhage has been achieved. Early use of blood or targeted blood components (equivalent to whole blood) in this critically bleeding group of trauma patients reduces crystalloid administration and is the mainstay of modern resuscitation in damage control. Some even recommend limiting the use of crystalloids in trauma-related haemorrhagic shock to a function of carrier of drugs. Preferred types of crystalloids are balanced solutions such as Ringer's lactate solution or buffered electrolyte solutions. Sodium chloride 0.9% solution ('normal saline') can contribute to hyperchloraemic acidosis.

Pitfalls

- Synthetic colloids containing starches have been shown to interfere with fibrin polymerization, coating of platelets, and blocking of fibrinogen receptor (GPIIb-IIIa) and von Willebrand type 1–like syndrome and cause coagulopathy (colloid-induced coagulopathy), increased bleeding and transfusion requirements. Starch solutions have also been associated with an increased risk of renal failure, and increased mortality in the critically ill.[6]
- Infusion of human albumin is not recommended in trauma, as it is associated with worse outcome.

Limiting fluid administration raises the question of how to maintain blood pressure. The use of vasopressors for haemodynamic support during resuscitation after injury is controversial. Whilst arginine vasopressin and

Table 18.1 Consequences of Aggressive Crystalloid Resuscitation[4,5]

Respiratory	↑ Capillary permeability
	Pulmonary oedema, which also results in ALI and ARDS
Gut	↑ Intestinal permeability
	Bacterial translocation
	Paralytic ileus
	ACS
	Anastomotic dehiscence
Heart	↓ Myocyte action potential
	Ventricular dysfunction
	Arrhythmia
	↓ Membrane polarization
	Disruption of phosphorylation
	Cellular oedema
	Apoptysis
Blood	Dilution of coagulation factors
	Increased blood loss
	Counteracting vasoconstriction
	↓ Oncotic pressure
Vessels	↓ Catecholamine release
	↑ Vascular resistance to catecholamines
Inflammatory pathways	Activation of inflammation (TNFα, interleukins, SIRS)
	Early vasoplegia
Endothelium	Damage to endothelial integrity and loss of the endothelial glycocalyx
	↑ Capillary leak

Source: Adapted from Refs. [4,17].

phenylephrine have shown to provide some beneficial effects in patients with traumatic brain injury or lung contusion, or in animal models with haemorrhagic shock, a prospective multicentre study on blunt trauma patients has shown an increased mortality in patients with early vasopressors use.[7] Therefore, hypovolaemic shock should be treated primarily by volume replacement, but low doses of vasopressors such as noradrenaline might be useful to counteract the sympatholytic and cardiovascular depressant effects of anaesthetic agents.

Subsequent to the question around maintaining blood pressure is: what blood pressure goal should be aimed for during the acute resuscitation of bleeding trauma patients? The current European Guidelines state[8]:

Recommendation 12: We recommend permissive hypotension with a target systolic blood pressure of 80–90 mmHg (mean arterial pressure 50–60 mmHg) until major bleeding has been stopped in the initial phase following trauma without brain injury. (Grade 1C)

In patients with severe TBI (GCS ≤ 8), we recommend that a mean arterial pressure ≥ 80 mmHg be maintained. (Grade 1C)

18.3.2 Targeting Coagulopathy

Early identification of patients with acute coagulopathy of trauma (ACoT), now referred to as acute trauma coagulopathy (ATC) or trauma-induced coagulopathy (TIC), is crucial for timely initiation of haemostatic resuscitation.[9,10] Early blood gases to identify abnormal base deficit (BD) or raised lactate provide a reliable correlation with the need for massive transfusion and risk of death. A BD > 2 mmol/l correlates with class II shock, and a BD > 6 mmol/l with class III shock, according to the Advanced Trauma Life Support (ATLS®) definitions.[11] Lactate > 2.5 mmol/L indicates hypoperfusion of tissue. Early initiation of haemostatic resuscitation is indicated before biologic or viscoelastic confirmation of TIC. The implementation of a massive transfusion protocol (MTP) is recommended, which will allow the ready availability of blood products and has been associated with a reduction in mortality and overall blood product use. MTPs are changing from fixed ratios to administration guided by viscoelastic methods.[12]

In severe trauma patients, plasma fibrinogen concentrations decrease earlier and more frequently than other coagulation factors; hypofibrinogenaemia is associated with increased transfusion requirements and worse outcomes. Fibrinogen reaches critically low values earlier than other coagulation factors or platelets. Replacement is generally necessary to support a plasma concentration of 150–200 mg/dl, and its early use (in the form of cryoprecipitate or fibrinogen concentrate) has been integrated in many massive haemorrhage protocols (MHPs) and MTPs, even though convincing evidence supporting this is lacking. A recent study indicated that most severely injured patients have a fibrinolysis shutdown, and therefore TXA may have no effect.[13] Standard preparation fresh frozen plasma (FFP) contains 2.0 g/L of fibrinogen (equivalent to 0.6 g in a 300 mL unit), so plasma administration alone will not be enough to correct the fibrinogen levels.

Fibrinolysis is a key feature of the TIC. A bolus of 1 or 2 g of TXA, followed by an infusion of 1 g over 8 hours, has become used within many MHPs/MTPs. It should be given as early as possible to bleeding trauma patients; if treatment is not given until 3 hours or later after injury, it is less effective and could even be harmful.

The CRASH-2 trial[14] showed a 15% relative and 1.5% absolute mortality reduction after the administration of TXA in trauma patients at risk of significant haemorrhage *in the environments in which the trial took place*. Many environments mandate the routine pre-hospital administration of TXA within the first 3 hours. However, TXA is not universally used routinely, with several nations undertaking further randomized trials.

Pitfall

A low calcium concentration should be corrected, often several times during resuscitation. It is usually a result of the use of citrate in blood products. It is important to correct hyperkalaemia, which increases with the transfusion of red blood cells and tissue damage.

18.3.3 Prevent and Treat Hypothermia

Hypothermia adversely affects coagulation as well as cardiac output and function in most bodily organs. Hypothermia and acidosis compromise thrombin generation kinetics via different mechanisms. Hypothermia primarily inhibits the initiation phase, whereas acidosis severely inhibits the propagation phase of thrombin generation. Similarly, hypothermia and acidosis affect fibrinogen metabolism differently. Hypothermia inhibits fibrinogen synthesis, whereas acidosis accelerates fibrinogen degradation, leading to a potential deficit in fibrinogen availability. Thus, the specific steps related to hypothermia prevention and treatment are:

- The OR temperature should be warm (26 °C or higher). Maintaining a warm OR on patient arrival helps keep patients warm.

- Have additional warming devices available, including a forced-air device system, fluid warmers on the IV line, warm IV solutions, and warm blankets.
- Have a system to warm all irrigation solutions that are to be used in the surgical field.

Pitfalls

- Limit crystalloid fluid resuscitation.
- Do not use synthetic colloids or starches.
- Assess arterial blood gases on every trauma patient to aid decision-making.
- Commence blood products and goal-directed haemostatic resuscitation early, before surgical control of haemorrhage.
- Allow blood pressure to be lower than normal (hypotensive resuscitation) during early haemorrhage control.
- Arrange early transfer to ICU and effective multidisciplinary communication.

18.4 DAMAGE CONTROL SURGERY

Damage control surgery (DCS) describes the strategy of limiting surgical intervention in haemodynamically compromised trauma patients by restricting procedures to early control of haemorrhage and contamination and postponing the definitive anatomical repair until the patient is more stable. (See also Chapter 6: 'Damage Control'.)

18.4.1 Anaesthetic Procedures

Being able to predict surgical requirements is a key skill for the trauma anaesthesiologist and is derived from experience. The anaesthesiologist should be able to predict how the patient physiology will evolve over a brief period of time, and the required response to treatment. The anaesthesiologist should anticipate the treatment the patient will receive and the route the patient will need to take to get to a stable state.

18.4.1.1 AIRWAY

In order to be able to correct hypoxia, manage CO_2, protect the airway, and facilitate interventions, most severe trauma patients will require intubation. Anaesthesiologists who deal with airway management daily are probably the best group to perform this task. If other groups are to perform this, they should be trained to perform it to the same standards and quality. Intubation in patients with possible neck trauma is a recognized difficult airway management situation. There are difficult airway algorithms available to assist decision-making for situations. An oral tube may be impossible, a laryngeal mask not suitable, and a surgical airway the only and fastest option viable in the time required. This decision needs to be made before the patient decompensates, and it requires skills and experience to make the decision in a timely manner. The anaesthesiologist may need to rely on their own skills rather than wait for another individual. The skill of establishing a surgical airway needs to be taught and practised to be retained.

Intubation and induction may have great repercussions in a patient with a physiology *in extremis*, and therefore the best timing and place to perform it should be considered.[15] These decisions must consider the clinical situation of the patient but also the organizational and architectural structure of each hospital. The operating theatre usually has more trained resources and more equipment for complex situations. In cases where the indication for intubation is an A or B problem, intubation should be performed as early as possible. On the other hand, when the patient has a C problem, the decision to intubate must consider that a collapse may occur during induction and an emergent thoracotomy may be required. Therefore, in institutions where the operating theatre is close to the ER, early transfer of the patient to the operating theatre for intubation should be considered.

18.4.1.2 BREATHING

Mechanical ventilation is a life-saving treatment but also has greater dangers for trauma patients than in elective patients. Trauma patients are at increased risk of volume and barotrauma and acute respiratory distress syndrome (ARDS) from mechanical ventilation. The injured lung is more susceptible to maldistribution of pressure between healthy and injured parts, leading to collapse in some areas with overdistension in others even at lower tidal volumes. The anaesthesiologist needs to apply judicious amounts of positive end expiratory pressure (PEEP) and a ventilation strategy aimed at minimizing overdistension of the lung.

Damage to the thoracic wall and to the lung increases the risks of pneumothorax and air embolism, adding to the original acute lung injury. During ventilation, the anaesthesiologist needs to be aware of these potential complications and the options for treatment. Again, if a tension pneumothorax is suspected, pleural decompression, either by needle thoracocentesis or preferably by finger thoracostomy, needs to be performed swiftly, either by the anaesthesiologist or by a dedicated and clearly allocated member of the surgical team.

Pitfall

In blunt thoracic injury, decreased air entry and dullness to percussion are usually due to pulmonary contusion. Do not do a needle thoracocentesis, as the needle may lacerate the lung and cause the pneumothorax. Screening should be done by eFAST.

Whilst ventilating the patient, the anaesthesiologist also needs to consider associated injuries and the influence of ventilation on injury. For example, PEEP, $PaCO_2$ (arterial blood CO_2 pressure), and PaO_2 (arterial oxygen pressure) are important in traumatic brain injury treatment strategies. PEEP may reduce blood pressure, especially in the presence of hypovolaemia. Furthermore, PEEP at high levels (> 12 mmHg / > 12 cm H_2O) may increases intracranial pressure (ICP). Ventilator driving pressure (plateau pressure – PEEP) above 15 cm H_2O has been recognized as a significant determinant for lung injury. Nevertheless, it has also been demonstrated that in brain-injured patients during mechanical ventilation, the application of moderate levels of PEEP (up to 8 cm H_2O) provided protection against the occurrence of lung injury, probably by restoring lung volume and reducing atelectasis, airway closure, and tidal expiratory flow limitation. Mean arterial pressure (MAP) and ICP monitoring, and prevention of hypoxia, are essential for prevention of secondary brain injury. $PaCO_2$ also affects ICP, and the aim is to achieve normocarbia ($PaCO_2$ = 35–4.5 mmHg/4.6–6 kPa). Hypocarbia increases cerebral vasoconstriction, leading to decreased cerebral blood flow (CBF), which may decrease ICP but also cause ischaemia. Decreasing $PaCO_2$ (by hyperventilating the patient) is a treatment strategy that should be limited to short-duration management of critically raised ICP, for example en route to an intervention for reducing the ICP (e.g., surgery). Hypercarbia increases CBF by vasodilatation and increases ICP in severe brain injury with the risk of decreasing cerebral perfusion pressure and causing or worsening secondary brain injury.

18.4.1.3 CIRCULATION

Control of exsanguinating bleeding takes priority over the airway, breathing, and circulation, changing the ABC mnemonic to 'control of catastrophic bleeding (C)-ABC', certainly in the pre-hospital and military settings.

18.4.1.4 VASCULAR ACCESS

Vascular access is required for the administration of resuscitation drugs and blood. The ATLS approach calls for two large-bore IV cannulae. The rationale is to have redundancy when required. With a second IV, there is also separate access for medications that cannot be Intravenous catheter gauge mixed.

If one of the IVs is a small-calibre one, there is the option to change it to a larger one using a wire Seldinger technique that will allow exchange for a rapid infusion catheter. Another way to gain better IV access is to apply a tourniquet above the small catheter, infuse 60 mL of IV fluid, and insert a larger-bore IV catheter above the small catheter in the now-distended vein. Consider intraosseous access as a temporizing measure and the early use of ultrasound to establish peripheral access.

Pitfall

Be wary of short cannulae in deep veins – it is easy for them to slip or pull out.

If the need for a rapid infusor system is foreseen, at least a 14 G catheter will be needed to allow high flow (500–800 mL/min). The IV lines used for the rapid infusor should not have one-way valves, such as are sometimes used in the ICU or operating theatre, and three-way stopcocks only if unavoidable. Medication should have a separate line from the high-flow system. A central venous line allows multiple ports, central venous pressure measurement, and high-flow fluid administration as well as venous blood gas measurements.

The larger the bore of the IV cannula, the greater the flow, see **Figure 18.1**.

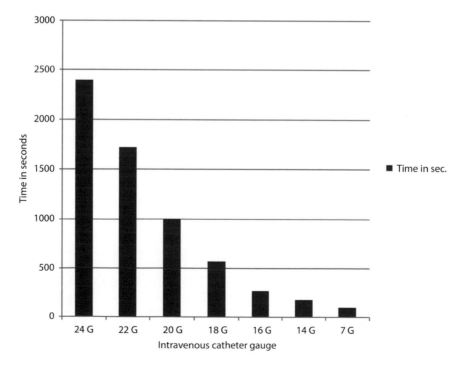

Figure 18.1 Time (in seconds) to infuse 1 L of clear fluids versus intravenous catheter gauge.

18.4.2 **Monitoring**

Besides standard anaesthesia monitoring, a five-lead electrocardiogram (ECG) in case of thoracic injury is advisable. Blunt cardiac injury can be detected by changes in ECG and elevated troponin I levels, and it is treated with supportive therapy. Ventilation should be monitored with pulse oximetry for adequate oxygenation and end-tidal CO_2 (ETCO$_2$) compared with arterial blood gases to assess adequate respiratory minute volume and V/Q mismatch. ETCO$_2$ further informs about cardiac output decreasing in case of circulatory collapse.

An arterial line provides the opportunity for beat-to-beat blood pressure monitoring, blood sampling, and physiological status, but should not delay time to surgery or intervention. An arterial line should be inserted in the upper part of the body in the majority of cases.

Pitfalls

- A central venous pressure (CVP) line through the femoral should not be used in any situation where the cava may have sustained injury (e.g., penetrating injury of the pelvis or abdomen).
- In patients where an aortic clamp is considered, an arterial line below the clamp is useless….
- In peri-arrest scenarios, central arterial monitoring may be a more reliable indicator of perfusion.

In the OR, haemodynamic status can be evaluated by accessing cardiac output. The purpose is to evaluate the status of the blood volume and cardiac function in order to secure normovolaemia and adequate perfusion, meanwhile avoiding hypo- as well as hypervolaemia. However, in the dramatic early phase of management of severe trauma, the patient's pulse, blood pressure, pulse oximetry, and ETCO$_2$ provide the minimum necessary monitoring required for a damage control approach; when more control is achieved, haemodynamic monitoring can be intensified according to the clinical condition.

Haemodynamic monitoring – means of cardiac output and volume estimation:

- Pulse and blood pressure
- CVP or central venous saturation ($S_{cv}O_2$) accessed via a central line

- Transthoracic or transoesophageal echocardiogram – focus-assessed transthoracic echocardiography (FATE)
- Mixed venous oxygen saturation via pulmonary artery catheter (rarely indicated in damage control)
- Minimally invasive cardiac output estimation via arterial line

Monitoring urine output may give some indication of the volume status. Due care should be given whilst inserting a urinary catheter in case of suspected urethra injury, but suprapubic catheterization is not commonly required.

Temperature monitoring is essential in trauma management. Intraoperative normothermia is an important quality performance measure for patients undergoing surgery, as it should be in trauma management. See also below.

18.5 **ANAESTHESIA INDUCTION IN HYPOVOLAEMIC SHOCK**

18.5.1 **Introduction**

Anaesthetizing a severely injured patient requires a thorough knowledge of the medications used and their altered pharmacokinetics and pharmacodynamics in the hypovolaemic, acidotic, and hypothermic trauma patient. The principal goal of anaesthesia for trauma patients is to provide analgesia, unconsciousness, and amnesia and eventually muscle relaxation without further deteriorating the deranged physiology and haemodynamic situation. In traumatic brain injury, systolic blood pressure < 90 mmHg and PaO$_2$ < 60 mmHg are independently associated with increased morbidity and mortality.

The pharmacokinetics (absorption, distribution, metabolism, and elimination) change significantly with hypovolaemic shock. The severely injured patient is in a condition of increased sympathetic tone in attempts to redistribute the circulation to brain and heart. In shock, the body becomes the equivalent of a single compartment model, a blood–brain circuit, at the expenses of the perfusion of gut, liver, kidneys, and muscles. IV drugs will be almost instantaneously distributed to heart and brain, resulting in a more rapid onset, higher brain concentrations, and more profound effects. Furthermore, many anaesthesia induction agents show a high protein binding. Hence, in hypovolaemic shock and especially after fluid resuscitation, reduced plasma protein binding leads to increased availability of free drug with higher effect site concentration and concomitantly increased adverse haemodynamic effects.

Anaerobic metabolism and metabolic acidosis will alter the distribution of ionizable drugs, leading to an enhanced brain concentration. Furthermore, in shock, hepatic and renal blood flow is markedly decreased, impairing the intrinsic metabolic capacity and leading ultimately to an increase in the free fraction of drugs and prolonged action. Drugs with a high hepatic extraction rate, such as propofol, ketamine, and morphine and synthetic opioids, will show a prolonged duration of action.

During the induction of anaesthesia, there is a substantial risk of cardiovascular collapse; therefore, the operative field is prepped and draped, and the surgical team should be gowned, gloved, and ready to start.

18.5.2 Drugs for Anaesthesia Induction

The effect site equilibration constant, cited as *t1/2Keo*, represents the time necessary for an administered drug to reach an appropriate anaesthetic concentration in the brain. The longer the t1/2Keo of a drug, the higher the initial plasma concentration will be needed to achieve an effective anaesthetic concentration. Hence, IV anaesthetic agents with the shortest t1/2Keo are generally best suited for a rapid induction in the severely injured, hypovolaemic patient (**Table 18.2**).

Commonly used anaesthetic drugs have a direct depressant effect on the cardiovascular system, inhibit compensatory mechanisms, and carry a substantial risk to further deteriorate the haemodynamic status of trauma patients. Subsequent positive pressure ventilation will impair venous return and contribute to further haemodynamic impairment. Recognition of masked hypovolaemia and an accurate estimation of its extent are crucial in the choice of type and dose of anaesthetic drugs.

For induction of general anaesthesia, the most commonly used drugs include ketamine, thiopental, etomidate, midazolam, and propofol. For the choice of the

Table 18.2 Effects of Anaesthetic Induction Agents

Induction Agent	Effector Site Equilibration (t½Keo)	Haemodynamic Effects	Comments
Propofol	< 20 min	↔ Heart rate unchanged (↔) ↓ Cardiac output ↓ Blood pressure ↓ Laryngeal reflexes Vagotonic	Dose reduction for rapid induction in haemodynamic compromise. Potential increase in intracranial pressure outweighs maintenance of haemodynamics.
Ketamine	± 2 min	↑ Heart rate ↑ Cardiac output ↑ Blood pressure Sympathomimetic	Minimal dose adjustment needed in hypovolaemic shock.
Etomidate	± 2.5 min	↔ Cardiac output ↔ Blood pressure ↓ Steroid synthesis ↔ Heart rate ↓ Inotropy ↔ Laryngeal reflexes	Possible adrenocortical suppression.
Thiopental	± 1.5 min	Vasodilatation	Dose reduction required, ideally < 3 mg/kg.
Benzodiazepines	± 9 min	↓ Cardiac output ↓ Systemic vascular resistance ↓ Sympathetic tone	Time to reach effector site is slow.

most suitable induction agent, the patient's physiology and comorbidities, and the anaesthesiologist's experience, should be taken into consideration. All anaesthetic induction agents can be vasodepressors and have potential to cause hypotension. The skill and experience of the anaesthesiologist are the most important determinants for a good outcome. Short-term use of a vasopressor can reverse vasodepressor effects, but it must be emphasized that continued need for vasopressors in the trauma patient population is associated with poor outcomes.

> ## Pitfall
>
> Dose reduction of the induction agent is crucial in shock.

18.5.2.1 KETAMINE

Ketamine is a highly lipid-soluble drug. At a physiologic pH, almost 50% is dissociated and only 12% is bound to plasma proteins. This ensures a rapid blood–brain equilibration and fast clinical onset.

Ketamine is the least likely agent to cause cardiovascular depressant effects. Its direct negative inotrope effect is counteracted by a stimulatory effect on the cardiovascular system, probably by a centrally mediated sympathetic response and inhibition of noradrenaline reuptake. In the severely shocked patient with a state of catecholamine exhaustion or resistance to further catecholamine effect, the direct effects of ketamine on myocardial depression may outweigh the indirect sympathetic effects, and haemodynamic collapse may still occur. A reduction of the induction dose to 0.25 to 0.5 mg/kg or less IV may be indicated in shock. Ketamine has further shown to provide anti-inflammatory proprieties; however, its clinical impact in trauma patients remains to be determined. Ketamine has reportedly both raised and lowered ICP. In traumatic brain injury, the cerebral autoregulation is impaired, and the CBF is directly dependent on the cerebral perfusion pressure. Maintenance of haemodynamic stability may, therefore, outweigh potential risks. Furthermore, ketamine reduces cerebral oxygen consumption, and the cerebral vasodilatation due to hypercapnoea observed in spontaneously breathing patients may be reduced by prevented ventilation. Ketamine has the added advantage that it can also be used for the maintenance of anaesthesia at 2–4 mg/kg/hour in adults, particularly before proximal control of bleeding has been established.

> ## Pitfall
>
> Ketamine is a dissociative anaesthetic, and a common side effect is hallucinations.

18.5.2.2 PROPOFOL

Propofol has a long $t1/2Keo$ of up to 20 minutes, indicating that for rapid induction, a higher initial dose is required. However, in shocked patients, propofol shows an increased end-organ sensitivity (e.g., lower C50) and a slower intercompartmental clearance. Haemorrhagic shock has demonstrated to shift the concentration–effect relationship to the left, demonstrating a 2.7-fold decrease in the effect site concentration required to achieve 50% of the maximal effect in the Bispectral Index (BIS) Scale. In shock, the potency of propofol is increased, and the dose required to reach effect site concentration is 5.4-fold reduced. Therefore, rapid induction can be performed with propofol, but a high dose is required in patients exhibiting increased organ sensitivity. This, in the view of the important concomitant negative effects on haemodynamics, makes propofol a poor choice for the trauma setting, but if used, **dose reduction to approximately one-third of a standard induction dose is highly recommended**.

18.5.2.3 ETOMIDATE

Haemorrhagic shock produces minimal changes in the pharmacokinetics and pharmacodynamics of etomidate. Etomidate preserves the pressor response to intubation, and shock affects only minimally its ability to reach rapidly the effector site. Its central and peripheral volumes are only lightly decreased in acute hypovolaemia, increasing its blood levels by about 20%. Therefore, unlike as with other hypnotics, only minimal adjustments in induction dose are required to achieve the same drug effect in haemorrhagic shock. As compared to propofol, no increased drug sensitivity had been demonstrated for etomidate. These points provide etomidate with a good safety profile as an induction agent in trauma patients.

However, in many countries, etomidate has been withdrawn after the CORTICUS study, and it was found that in septic patients, even a single dose may suppress the cortico-adrenal axis for up to 67 hours.[16] In the nonseptic trauma patients, suppression of steroid synthesis does not seem to be associated with worse outcome, such as increased mortality or prolonged length of stay.

18.5.2.4 THIOPENTAL

Thiopental exhibits several desirable properties in the shocked patient, such as a short t1/2Keo (1.5 min) and a tendency to preserve autonomic responsiveness as a reflex tachycardia and the pressor response to laryngoscopy. However, its usefulness in the setting of hypovolaemic shock is compromised by the important negative inotropy and arteriolar vasodilatation, leading to severe hypotension in shocked patients. Doses must therefore be carefully adapted to values, if possible, below the usual range of 3 mg/kg.

18.5.2.5 MIDAZOLAM

Midazolam in induction dose has shown to significantly decrease plasma norepinephrine concentration and alters baroreflex control of the heart rate. It also causes reduction of systemic vascular resistance and left ventricular stroke work index. Hence, in hypovolaemic patients, it may further decrease blood pressure and prevent compensatory tachycardia. In addition, midazolam is highly protein bound, inhibiting a rapid entry into the brain effector site. The half-life for closure of its imidazol-ring, which enhances lipid solubility and brain entry, is long (10 min), making this agent of little value for rapid sequence induction (RSI).

There is no hard outcome evidence supporting one induction agent over the other, but whatever agent is chosen, induction doses must be adapted and most often reduced, according to the patient's physiology. Many use a combination of induction drugs, combining their different effects. Normalization of haemodynamic parameters with aggressive fluid resuscitation prior to induction has not proven to completely reverse the increase in induction drug potency.

Maintenance of anaesthesia during damage control procedures in the haemodynamically compromised patient needs a careful choice and titration of drugs. Ketamine is a suitable option for induction and also maintenance of anaesthesia. Perioperative awareness is well recognized during emergency anaesthesia, often because of dose reduction. A comparison of patients treated by ketamine induction and maintenance with volatiles versus no maintenance drug showed a perioperative awareness rate of 11% versus 43%. The choice of the optimal maintenance drug is influenced by the patient's physiology and injury profile.

For traumatic brain injury and trauma to the spinal cord, IV anaesthesia with propofol is recommended, whilst in other settings, inhalational anaesthesia might be more suited. A BIS measure might be a valuable help in preventing awareness in the severely shocked patient with altered dose requirements.

18.6 BATTLEFIELD ANAESTHESIA

(**See also** Chapter 19: 'Austere Environments'.)
(**See also** Chapter 20: 'Military Environments'.)

Battlefield anaesthesia is both an anaesthetic as well as an operational problem. It is not an exclusive medical problem.

Battlefield anaesthesia presents many challenges, including the need to maintain airway control, hypothermia of the casualty, restricted drug availability, lack of supplementary oxygen, and the possible requirement for prolonged postoperative mechanical ventilation. Mass casualty situations are also a constant possibility in the military arena. Surgery requires both adequate analgesia and anaesthesia. No single agent can provide an appropriate level of both anaesthesia and analgesia; hence, a combination of drugs and techniques is required. The choices of anaesthetic are narrowed in austere conditions; these are limited to general anaesthesia (either IV or inhalational), regional anaesthesia, local anaesthesia, or none at all. For surgical exploration of body cavities, general anaesthesia is most frequently chosen, whilst a regional anaesthetic may be more appropriate for injuries of the extremities or perineum. In the field, RSI is the norm, using fast-acting hypnotic and neuromuscular blocking agents to facilitate rapid airway control. In the absence or limitation of supplemental oxygen supplies, RSI becomes even more crucial as pre-oxygenation of the patient's lungs is often not possible. There are several RSI cocktails used in the pre-hospital setting, most using a combination of induction agent, paralyzing agent, and analgesia. Sedation, amnesia, and analgesia can then be maintained with IV agents such as ketamine, benzodiazepines, and opiates.

For long procedures or surgical sites involving the abdomen or thorax, a combination anaesthetic that includes an inhalation agent such as isoflurane may be used. British surgical teams use the portable DiaMedica DPA0$_2$ 'draw-over' device (DiaMedica Therapeutics, Minneapolis, MN, USA), which does not require a compressed gas source, and have gained much experience with this technique of field anaesthesia. This draw-over type of vaporizer is currently also in use by several other countries in austere settings. The draw-over configuration places the ventilator distal to the vaporizer, entraining ambient air and vapour across the vaporizer in the same manner as the spontaneously breathing patient.

Regional anaesthesia remains an important option in battlefield anaesthesia, as it provides both patient comfort and surgical analgesia, whilst maintaining patient consciousness and spontaneous ventilation. With the relatively large number of extremity wounds in modern conflicts, and certainly in the mass casualty setting with a limited anaesthesia capability, regional aesthetic techniques should not be overlooked. Continuous infusion nerve blocks provide excellent analgesia for postoperative casualties during evacuation.

18.6.1 Damage Control Anaesthesia in the Military Setting

Anaesthesia for damage control procedures and major cavity injury is really a fusion of continuing resuscitation and critical care. This requires optimization of haemodynamic status, re-warming of the casualty, and pain relief. One of the biggest challenges will be reversing the hypothermia that is almost universal in haemorrhagic patients in these conditions. As well as warming all IV fluids and ventilator circuits, an active re-warming device will be required. If a return to the operating theatre for more definitive surgery is not planned in the forward location, critical care must be maintained throughout the aeromedical evacuation.

18.6.2 Battlefield Analgesia

Relief of pain is an important consideration for both the wounded and the military caregiver. Provision of effective analgesia is humane but also attenuates the adverse pathophysiological responses to pain and is likely to aid evacuation from the battlefield and maintain morale. Analgesia may be given at self and buddy-aid levels; protocols to guide medical and paramedical staff in the provision of safe and effective analgesia are available.

Analgesia methods used in recent conflicts include:

- Simple non-pharmacological reassurance
- Splinting of fractures
- Cooling of burns
- Oral analgesics:
  - Non-steroidal anti-inflammatory drugs
  - Paracetamol
- Nerve blocks and infiltration of local anaesthesia
- Intramuscular and IV opiates
- Fentanyl lollipops
- Methods under development including intranasal ketamine, fentanyl, and inhalation analgesics (e.g., methoxyflurane inhalation)

REFERENCES

1. Holcomb JB, Jenkins D, Rhee P, Johannigman J, Mahoney P, Mehta S, et al. Damage control resuscitation: directly addressing the early coagulopathy of trauma. *J Trauma.* 2007;**62**(**2**):307–10. doi: 10.1097/TA.0b013e3180324124.

2. Moore FA, McKinley BA, Moore EE. The next generation in shock resuscitation. *Lancet.* 2004;**363**(**9425**):2088–96. doi: 10.1016/S0140-6736(04)16415-5.

3. Chakraverty S, Zealley I, Kessel D. Damage control radiology in the severely injured patient: what the anaesthetist needs to know. *Brit J Anaesth.* 2014 Aug;**113**(**2**):250–7. doi: 10.1093/bja/aeu203.

4. Cotton BA, Guy JS, Morris JA, Jr., Abumrad NN. The cellular, metabolic, and systemic consequences of aggressive fluid resuscitation strategies. *Shock.* 2006 Aug;**26**(**2**):115–21. doi: 10.1097/01.shk.0000209564.84822.f2.

5. Kasotakis G, Sideris A, Yang Y, de Moya M, Alam H, King DR, et al. Inflammation, host response to injury I: aggressive early crystalloid resuscitation adversely affects outcomes in adult blunt trauma patients: an analysis of the Glue Grant database. *J Trauma Acute Care Surg.* 2013 May;**74**(**5**):1215–21; discussion 1221–2. doi: 10.1097/TA.0b013e3182826e13.

6. Zarychanski R, Abou-Setta AM, Turgeon AF, Houston BL, McIntyre L, Marshall JC, et al. Association of hydroxyethyl starch administration with mortality and acute kidney injury in critically ill patients requiring volume resuscitation: a systematic review and meta-analysis. *JAMA: J Amer Med Assoc.* 2013 Feb 20;**309**(**7**):678–88. doi:10.1001/jama.2013.430.

7. Sperry JL, Minei JP, Frankel HL, West MA, Harbrecht BG, Moore EE, Maier RV, Nirula R. Early use of vasopressors after injury: caution before constriction. *J Trauma.* 2008 Jan;**64**(**1**):9–14. doi: 10.1097/TA.0b013e31815dd029.

8. Spahn DR, Bouillon B, Cerny V, Duranteau J, Filipescu D, Hunt BJ, et al. The European guideline on management of major bleeding and coagulopathy following trauma: fifth edition. *Crit Care.* 2019 Mar 27;**23**(**1**):98. doi: 10.1186/s13054-019-2347-3.

9. Brohi K, Singh J, Heron M, Coats T. Acute traumatic coagulopathy. *J Trauma.* 2003 Jun;**54**(**6**):1127–30. doi: 10.1097/01.TA.0000069184.82147.06.

10. Brohi K, Cohen MJ, Ganter MT, Matthay MA, Mackersie RC, Pittet JF. Acute traumatic coagulopathy: initiated by hypoperfusion: modulated through the protein C pathway? *Ann Surg.* 2007May;**245(5)**:812–18. doi: 10.1097/01.sla.0000256862.79374.31.

11. Mutschler M, Nienaber U, Brockamp T, Wafaisade A, Fabian T, Paffrath T, et al. TraumaRegister DGU®: renaissance of base deficit for the initial assessment of trauma patients: a base deficit-based classification for hypovolemic shock developed on data from 16,305 patients derived from the TraumaRegister DGU®. *Crit Care.* 2013 Mar 6;**17(2)**:R42. doi: 10.1186/cc12555.

12. Stensballe J, Ostrowski SR, Johansson PI. Viscoelastic guidance of resuscitation. *Curr Opin Anesthesiol.* 2014 Apr;**27(2)**:212–8. doi: 10.1097/ACO.0000000000000051. Review.

13. Moore HB, Moore EE, Gonzales E, Chapman MP, Chin TL, Silliman CC, et al. Hyprinofibrinolysis, physiologic fibrinolysis, and fibrinolysis shutdown: the spectrum of post injury fibrinolysis and relevance to antifibrinolytic therapy. *J Trauma Acute Care Surg.* 2014 Dec;**77(6)**:811–7; discussion 817. doi: 10.1097/TA.0000000000000341.

14. Shakur H, Roberts I, Bautista R, Caballero J, Coats T, Dewan Y, et al. Effects of tranexamic acid on death, vascular occlusive events, and blood transfusion in trauma patients with significant haemorrhage (CRASH-2): a randomised, placebo-controlled trial. *Lancet.* 2010;**376(9734)**:23–32. doi: 10.1016/S0140-6736(10)60835-5. Epub 2010 Jun 14.

15. Hudson AJ, Strandenes G, Berkvig CK, Svanevik M, Glassberg M. Airway, and ventilation management strategies for hemorrhagic shock. To tube, or not to tube, that is the question! *J Trauma Acute Care Surg.* 2018 Jun;**84(6S Suppl 1)**:S77–S82. doi: 10.1097/TA.0000000000001822.

16. Jabre P, Combes X, Lapostolle F, Dhaouadi M, Ricard-Hibon A, Vivien B, et al. Etomidate versus ketamine for rapid sequence intubation in acutely ill patients: a multicentre randomised controlled trial. *Lancet.* 2009 Jul 25;**374(9686)**:293–300. doi: 10.1016/S0140-6736(09)60949-1. Epub 2009 Jul 1

17. Kozar RA, Peng Z, Zhang R, Holcomb JB, Pati J, Park S, et al. Plasma restoration of endothelial glycocalyx in a rodent model of hemorrhagic shock. *Anesth Analg.* 2011 Jun;**112(6)**:1289–95. doi: 10.1213/ANE.0b013e318210385c. Epub 2011 Feb 23.

Austere Environments 19

19.1 DEFINITION

Austere: Severely simple, morally strict, harsh

Harsh: Unpleasantly rough or sharp, severe, cruel

Multiple casualties: More than one patient, but can be dealt with within existing resources

Mass casualties: Many patients with demands beyond the resources available

19.2 OVERVIEW

Austerity is characterized by deficiency and inadequacy. Even within a First World setting, a person can find themselves in an austere environment. Frequently, the support may arrive much later than the surgical team. There may be inadequacies such as lack of knowledge and experience, and the deficiency is in the absence of immediate senior backup or equipment availability.

In certain situations, as for example in the early aftermath of a major natural disaster or in war situations, limited resources mandate the care that can be given. However, these situations can be enhanced by better preparedness and organization of medical/surgical teams and their equipment.

Therefore, it is important to understand where deficiencies and inadequacies lie, and how to deal with them.

The underpinning mantra needs to be 'Improvise, adapt, overcome'.

The need to improve and standardize humanitarian medical and surgical care became obvious after the Haiti earthquake in 2010, when many medical teams and 44 field hospitals were delivered, all with different medical policies and capacities to fulfil their missions as needed. Concerns were raised about legal rights to deliver care, the lack of coordination and professional standards, as well as the wrong type of care offered. This led to relief expert meetings and the creation of the Forward Medical Team (FMT) group. Under the auspices of the Global Health Cluster and the World Health Organisation (WHO), the document 'Classification and Minimum Standards for Foreign Medical Teams in Sudden Onset Disasters'[1] was published in 2013 in order to limit situations where 'futile care in resources limited circumstances' would be delivered. A minimum of standards should always be met, and preparedness is key. Nevertheless, this chapter briefly touches on hospital and surgical minimum standards, and solutions available when hospital system and equipment or logistic support fail for unexpected reasons.

The perspective of working in an austere environment is quite different from the training paradigm, an academic practice with multi-tiered care, or an elective private practice. Austere surgery requires a thoughtful approach to realistic surgical care within the context of the environment in which the surgical team must alter their perspective.

Humanitarian surgical care operates within the framework of a staged systematic approach to care. The role of the team is not to merely operate on the individual patient, but to make every attempt at preserving lives and returning the patient back to his or her home. This can only be realized within the framework of environment and contingencies. In the response to a natural or man-made disaster, this also implies that medical aid workers should protect their own life, health, and work stamina, and not become casualties of austere circumstances themselves. This includes not only infrastructure, resources, sutures, and drugs, but also sleep discipline and self-protection against sleep disturbances. Flexibility and capability beyond one's conventional speciality are also required: surgeons do not often service generators, and anaesthetists do not often sterilize water, but they may have to.

DOI: 10.1201/9781003258124-24

19.3 INFRASTRUCTURE AND TEAM COMPOSITION

The WHO defines levels of emergency medical teams as:

- Level one, which is a primary healthcare facility.
- Level two, which is emergency medical care including surgery and obstetrics.
- Level three, which is a hospital focussed upon rehabilitation and reconstructive osteoplastic surgery.

Austere surgical care in response to humanitarian crises can be delivered by either:

1. *Non-governmental organizations* such as the International Committee of the Red Cross (ICRC) and Médecins Sans Frontières (MSF). Their model of care centres around smaller teams, with often a single surgeon expected to manage all aspects of surgery, orthopaedics, and obstetrics. They have advantages in manoeuvrability and sustainability.
2. *Government-based emergency medical teams*, which can be civilian or military. These are usually larger, with more specialists available, but are slower to move and more suited to the initial surge response.

Infrastructure requirements include shelter, power for lighting and temperature control, and water for hygiene and cooking purposes. Waste needs to be disposed of properly, with medical waste disposal (particularly sharps) always being problematic. Resources include medical gases, food, drugs, fluids, and other consumables such as gloves and gowns.

Following a natural disaster, or in a conflict or post-conflict environment, supply chains and systems will be disrupted and vulnerable. Lack of security may enable looting or vandalism of medical aid facilities. No delivery can ever be guaranteed, and the team may have only what they carried with them initially.

19.3.1 Location

The location of a field hospital should be in a 'safe place' where all parties in the conflict are aware of its purpose. It should be protected by walls, sandbags, adhesive plastic on glass windows, and so on against damage from explosions. Security guards speaking the common language should check all entering people.

19.3.2 Hospital Structures

19.3.2.1 WATER SUPPLY

Trauma and surgical/obstetrical emergency care consumes approximately 60–100 L minimum of water/patient/day and is therefore dependent on a continuous secured water supply. That supply is essential when the hospital location is decided. However, extra water storage facilities should be installed, as it is difficult to supply water by other means (e.g., water trucks).

19.3.2.2 ENERGY

Electrical or energy support needs robustness which may necessitate parallel systems, such as electricity from a local supplier or from fuel/kerosene generators, or backup electricity from car batteries in operating rooms (ORs). A surgical hospital of 50 beds requires 100 KVA for OR lights, heating or air conditioning, sterilization, X-ray, and refrigeration.

19.3.2.3 WASTE DISPOSAL

A waste disposal system needs an efficient incinerator for contaminated solid waste and a septic tank for the main sewage.

19.3.2.4 STERILIZATION DEPARTMENT

This should be located close to the ORs and be divided into a 'dirty area', where used instruments are collected and washed, and a 'clean area' where the same instruments are packed before being sent to the 'sterilization area'. The autoclave system needs to be robust and can depend on electric- or gas-heated steam/pressure autoclaves, but the same type of steam/pressure autoclaves heated by open fire can be sufficient when energy supplies are unreliable. Commercial pressure cookers can be utilized for sterilization in the absence of electricity, with acceptable results.

19.3.2.5 SURGICAL EQUIPMENT

Surgical instruments are subject to wear and tear when specially used for severe injuries to the extremities including bone. For example, Gigli saws do break, and in rare situations other sterilizable tools (e.g., a hacksaw, for amputations) bought from the market can be used.

The main principle is to use tools/instruments which do not cause any further harm (e.g., to soft tissues during amputations). It is recommended to keep instruments packaged in smaller, flexible groups rather than the large trays traditionally utilized in mainstream hospital practice.

19.3.2.6 BLOOD BANK

Set-up of a blood bank takes time, and it demands special equipment and trained laboratory technicians. It also needs established routines to find blood donors, to test and preserve the donated blood, and so on. Autotransfusion may be the only alternative, and the technique of collecting non-contaminated blood from the chest and/or the abdomen, filtering it, and intravenously re-infusing the blood should be well known. New portable and user-friendly devices have been developed and should be in the equipment. This, in addition to a total focus on blood-sparing surgical techniques, may be life-saving.

19.3.3 Health Protection of the Deployed Surgical Team

Psychological and physical stamina are preconditions *sine qua non*: psychologically, some doctors do not work well out of their normal hospital or workplace, and some cannot adapt easily. The inability to deliver a standard of care that personnel would consider the standard in their own nation is a major psychological stressor for deployed personnel. The availability of a volunteer does not imply the ability or even the affability required to work in a small team. All members of a surgical team need to understand this and have a realistic expectation of what they can – or cannot – provide in the situation in which they find themselves.

19.3.3.1 VECTOR-BORNE DISEASE

In 2003, in Liberia, nearly 20% of 225 deployed US Marines developed malaria; it was subsequently found that only 10% of the population at risk had been compliant with chemoprophylaxis, and none had slept under mosquito nets. Attention must be paid to the existing threats, and simple measures are effective: anti-malarial prophylaxis, long sleeves at dawn and dusk, repellent, sleeping under nets, and mosquito control measures.

19.3.3.2 ENTERIC ILLNESS

The incidence of diarrhoea among deployed military personnel from industrialized countries to lesser developed countries is typically 30% per month overall, with clinical incidence between 5 and 7 per 100 person-months. The risk appears to be higher early during deployment and is associated with poor hygiene conditions and contaminated food sources. Meticulous attention to hand-washing and food source management mitigates this risk.

19.3.3.3 ROAD TRAUMA

Globally, many road trauma deaths now occur in the developing world, and 50% of these deaths occur among vulnerable road users, such as pedestrians, cyclists, or motorcyclists. The risks of speeding, weak adherence to seatbelt discipline, and cavalier driving are not only to the vehicle occupants, but also to host nation road users. A deployed Westerner causing injury or death to a local child would not only be a personal tragedy for the child, the family, and the driver, but could also ruin a mission!

19.3.3.4 PHYSICAL, SEXUAL, AND MENTAL HEALTH

Surgeons wishing to deploy need to have high health status; diabetics, for example, are unlikely to do well without their cold-chain controlled insulin. An unfit surgeon could become a liability rather than an asset to the mission. Deployments away from home, time away from duty, availability of alcohol, interaction of deployed workers with local women prepared to undertake transactional sex, and the non-use of condoms increase the risks of sexually transmitted infections.

All members of a surgical team need to have a realistic expectation of what they can – or cannot – provide in the situation in which they find themselves.

19.4 CASELOAD AND SURGICAL TECHNIQUES TO HAVE IN MIND

19.4.1 Caseload

The type of cases received will depend upon the type of crisis responded to and the timing of the response. Humanitarian response to war will unsurprisingly provide severely wounded persons, requiring the skill of an experienced trauma surgeon to manage. Other responses, such as after natural disasters, will have differing caseloads such as fractures in earthquakes, foot injuries, and infected wounds in inundations. Surgeons responding to a natural disaster often arrive several days after the event, by which time all of the major trauma patients have either survived or succumbed. The majority of this work will be wound and limb salvage and dealing with advanced infections due to lack of, or inappropriate, initial care. Secondly, as local health infrastructure is usually affected and often restricted by the disaster, care of routine surgical, paediatric, and obstetric conditions can be anticipated.

19.4.2 Bleeding Control

All surgeons should be able to operate whilst limiting blood loss to a minimum, whether diathermy is available or not. Each millilitre of extra blood loss may be difficult to replace. An early decision to perform laparotomy or thoracotomy for suspect bleeding is necessary, particularly for penetrating trauma (e.g., anterolateral thoracotomy when chest drains yield 1100 mL or more).

Thorough control of haemostasis before closure or packing of an abdomen, chest, or wound may take extra time but is even more important when blood is missing. Ligation of a large vessel may be the only life-saving possibility when shunting or repair is unfeasible.

19.4.3 Control of Contamination

Bowel injuries should be treated according to damage control when indicated. Control of contamination needs to be followed by primary repair or restoration of bowel continuity as early as possible, because stomas are poorly tolerated in this setting.

19.4.4 Treatment of Wounds

19.4.4.1 DELAYED/NEGLECTED WOUNDS

Non-combat wounds in the austere environment have similar management principles as for war wounds (see Section 19.4.4.2, below). It is best to surgically debride/excise such wounds and leave them open, planning for delayed primary closure around day 4–5. Potable water is acceptable for wound irrigation. Delayed closure can be by direct suture, skin graft, or random pattern flap, but keep things as simple as possible. Consider the increasing prevalence of diabetes in many low- and middle-income countries.

19.4.4.2 WAR WOUNDS

Thorough examination, cleaning, and debridement of war wounds are critical, as these actions reduce the number of re-operations and infectious complications. Remove all dead tissue and loose bone fragments that do not have any blood supply. Be very conservative with skin removal, and when amputations are needed, skin can be harvested from the amputated part and spared in refrigerators. The wounds should be left open for delayed closure. Only do packing of the wounds for haemostasis, but dressings of wounds should allow some drainage. Dressing change can be performed every third or fourth day unless signs of infection force the patient back to the OR earlier.

19.4.5 Amputations

It is strongly preferable to only perform amputation with consent from the patient and/or family, and second opinion is important when possible. Avoid guillotine amputations and aim for preserving length. Use a pneumatic tourniquet to avoid bleeding from vessels before they have been ligated. Leave the wound of the stump open for delayed closure. Liaison with rehab providers is ideal, but not always possible.

19.4.6 Stabilization of Fractures

Stabilization of fractures can be achieved satisfactorily with plaster of Paris or, if available, external fixators. When strict sterile conditions are questionable, internal – and sometimes also external – fixation should not be applied. Traction is an option for certain fractures of the femurs, although ideally only for a limited time whilst waiting for better surgical circumstances. For the upper limb, mobility is a priority over stability, in opposition to the lower limb where stability is a priority before mobility. Generally speaking, internal fixation of fractures is contraindicated in the austere environment.

19.4.7 Obstetrics

Obstetrical problems are frequently encountered in war situations, and knowledge of the Caesarean section technique is mandatory. Listen to midwife suggestions if they are available, and always prioritize the health of the mother.

19.4.8 **Anaesthesia**[2,3]

Anaesthesia is always a significant medical intervention, and the anaesthesiologist must ideally be a qualified, registered specialist, or have significant experience. The drug of choice for major surgery is, for the ICRC, still Ketamine®, as it is safe and possible to administer intravenously and intramuscularly. A draw-over apparatus for anaesthesia is an important option when supply of compressed gases is unavailable. The use of regional or peripheral nerve blockade with ultrasound guidance can be of great value, although care needs to be taken not to mask signs of compartment syndrome. Lack of a recovery area can be a disaster for a field hospital, and consideration should be given to utilizing techniques that favour a brisk, safe recovery, so the operating theatre can be utilized for the next case.

19.5 **POSTOPERATIVE CARE AND DOCUMENTATION**

The field hospital level II (WHO classification) does not allow advanced postoperative care with ventilator support which implicates that indications for surgery need to be adapted. Pain relief is based on paracetamol and anti-inflammatory medication, tramadol, and oral morphine if needed (intravenous should be avoided). A minimum pre- and postoperative standard includes pulse oximetry and a postoperative care protocol. Patient documentation should include an admission number and an individual patient file on paper. In mass casualty situations and when hospitals are overloaded, patient reports stay short and can be completed by written information on bandages (e.g., date for the next change of dressing).

It is recommended that the patient keep the record themselves upon discharge, as it will facilitate reintegration into the local health system once the humanitarian team departs.

19.6 **SUMMARY**

Although futile care in resource-limited circumstances should be avoided by good preparedness, all medical personnel may have to rapidly adapt when situations are extreme or deteriorate. Acceptable levels of care can still be preserved by remaining thorough and adapting equipment and surgical and anaesthesiologic techniques to more basic levels (**Table 19.1**).

When the surgical team is placed in a position where they are aware that they are likely to be challenged professionally, it is imperative that they take stock of what they, personally, are capable of in terms of expertise in surgical care. This requires a hard, honest look in the mirror, without pride or ego fogging the reflected image. And there are not always guidelines....

Table 19.1 Questions to Ask Yourself

Questions to Ask Yourself: This List Is Clearly Not Exhaustive.
• Do I have what it takes to be working solo in a surgical team in the bush/on a rescue mission/at an earthquake site/in a war zone/where the nearest qualified help may be over 1000 km away/with no communication or re-supply for at least 10 days?
• If I have enough surgical skills to tackle most problems, will the situation allow it?
• Is there even a hospital? Has it been destroyed by tsunami, earthquake, bombing? What shelter will I have to work in – if any? What can I do on the floor of a school-room with only a headlight and no anaesthetist?
• What equipment is available to me? Do I have any surgical instruments, or must I take my own? Are there any disposables – sutures, syringes, needles, drugs, drapes, gowns, gloves, etc.? If not, how can I get around these problems? Is it possible to make up my own intravenous fluids – do I know how? Where can I get clean water from? What 'disposables' can I re-use?
• If I can deal with all these deficiencies, can I relate to those who I will be working with and/or my patients? Can I speak the language – or one that will allow communication?
• What – if any – arrangements can be made for a higher level of care or transfer out of my working environment? How long could I reasonably manage a patient postoperatively – with or without ventilation?
• What drugs do I have for dealing with pain, infection, anaesthesia, and intercurrent illnesses? What antiseptics do I have for cleaning wounds and surgical site preparation?

These uncomfortable questions often must be dealt with in a hurry, on the spot, and when we are least prepared for them. It is therefore vital that we have prepared ourselves as best we can by our training and by having thought out beforehand just what we would need if asked to pick up a grab-bag and go to a remote and possibly dangerous spot, where little or no support will be on hand for several days.

Along with our professional armamentarium and competence, we will need good interpersonal skills to deal with the stresses of facing a scenario where others may also be finding themselves in an isolated position and well out of their comfort zones, both professionally and personally. Those we are asked to work with may have been significantly traumatized, both physically and emotionally, due to loss of property and loved ones. They may not be seeing priorities in the same way, and their normal skill levels may be affected by grief and anger. It is important to recognize that their emotions are probably not directed at you, but their level of control over them in crisis is not normal.

It is not the purpose of this section to provide the surgical team with all the answers when exposed to an austere environment for the first time, but rather to make them think of what can go wrong.

If it can go wrong, it will – and in the worst way possible.

However, whatever does go wrong can usually be mitigated by prior preparation and imaginative thought. In these uncomfortable situations, it is important to realize and accept that you will not achieve the standard that your usual working environment allows you, such that sterilization of equipment may not be 100% certain, valves on cylinders of gases may malfunction or not work at all, washed bandages and gloves may have to be recycled after drying on a cactus or thorn bush, and water may have to be drawn from a well to scrub up with, using a piece of soap that has been getting smaller and dirtier for a week. Instruments may have to be improvised or made up. Scissors and knives from a kitchen may need to be called into service, and wooden spoons and clothes pegs cut to a curve to use as vascular clamps or occluders.

There are no easy answers to such working environments, but the challenges are as exciting as they are demanding. In such scenarios, no-one will expect miracles (though they sometimes occur!), and you will have to accept at the outset that you will not be able to save all

that you could in a more replete and protected setting, so blaming yourself when you have tried your best is not sensible or intelligent.

But giving up is not an option either.

REFERENCES AND SELECTED READING

References

1. Norton I, Von Schreeb J, Aitken P, et al. *Classification and Minimum Standards for Foreign Medical Teams in Sudden Onset Disasters.* World Health Organisation, Geneva. 2013.

2. Merry AF, Cooper JB, Soyannwo O, Wilson IH, Eichhorn JH. International standards for a safe practice of anaesthesia. *Can J Anaesth.* 2010 Nov;**57**(**11**):1027–34. doi: 10.1007/s12630-010-9381-6.

3. Mahoney P.F, Jeyanathan J, Wood P, et al. *Anaesthesia Handbook.* International Committee of the Red Cross, February 2017. https://www.icrc.org/en/publication/anaesthesia-handbook

Recommended Reading

Chackungal S, Nickerson JW, Knowlton LM, Black L, Burkle FM, Casey K, et al. Best practice guidelines on surgical response in disasters and humanitarian emergencies: report of the 2011 Humanitarian Action Summit Working Group on Surgical Issues within the Humanitarian Space. *Prehosp Disaster Med.* 2011 Dec;**26**(**6**):429–37. doi: 10.1017/S1049023X12000064.

Chu K, Trelles M, Ford N.P. Quality of care in humanitarian surgery. *World J Surg.* 2011 Jun;35(6):1169–72; discussion 1173–4. doi: 10.1007/s00268-011-1084-9.

Giannou C, Baldan M. War Surgery: Working with Limited Resources in Armed Conflict and Other Situations of Violence. In: *War Surgery Vol. 1 & 2.* ICRC Publication. 2009 ref. 0973.

Geneva: International Committee of the Red Cross icrc.org.

Hayward-Karlsson, J. Jeffery Herard P, Boillot F. Amputation in emergency situations: indications, techniques and Médecins sans Frontières experience in Haiti. *Int Orthop.* 2012 Oct;**36**(**10**):1979–81. doi: 10.1007/s00264-012-1552-3. Epub 2012 May 15.

International Committee of the Red Cross. 2018 *Anaesthesia Handbook* https://www.google.com/url?sa=t&rct=j&q=&esrc=s&source=web&cd=&ved=2ahUKEwjHuNrozbz8AhWQ5KQKHfKTDuUQFnoECCAQAQ&url=https%3A%2F%2

Fshop.icrc.org%2Fdownload%2Febook%3Fsku%3D4270%2F002-ebook&usg=AOvVaw3x4vYJp6cjhLTXYHqD53uC (accessed online August 2023).

Kerr A, Schmidt H. *Hospitals for War-Wounded*. ICRC, Geneva. 2005. Available at https://shop.icrc.org/catalogsearch/result/?q=Hospitals+for+War-Wounded (accessed online August 2023) or https://www.icrc.org/en/publication/0714-hospitals-war-wounded-practical-guide-setting-and-running-surgical-hospital-area

World Health Organization, *The Clinical Use of Blood in Medicine, Obstetrics, Paediatrics, Surgery & Anaesthesia, Trauma & Burns*. WHO, Geneva. Available from: https://apps.who.int/iris/handle/10665/42397 (accessed online August 2023).

World Health Organisation - International Committee of the Red Cross. 2018 Basic Emergency Care: approach to the acutely ill and injured. https://www.who.int/publications/i/item/basic-emergency-care-approach-to-the-acutely-ill-and-injured (accessed online August 2023).

Wren SM, Wild HB, Gurney J, Amirtharajah M, Brown ZW, Bulger EM, et al. A consensus framework for the humanitarian surgical response to armed conflict in 21st century warfare. *JAMA Surg*. 2020;**155(2)**:114–21. doi: 10.1001/jamasurg.2019.454.

20.1 **INTRODUCTION**

The four 'humanitarian principles' are humanity, neutrality, impartiality, and independence.

> *Military surgery is related to, but distinct from, surgery performed by teams affiliated with humanitarian aid organizations.*

Military clinicians are usually designated by their armed forces as *non-combatants*, as defined by Additional Protocol I of the Geneva Conventions, meaning that they must not participate directly in hostile acts and must provide medical assistance to any person solely on the basis of clinical need. However, they are not prohibited from acting in other ways to the benefit of their own side. As such, they are not *neutral*, *impartial*, or *independent*. The primary purpose of the armed force deploying military surgical capability is to maintain the health, morale, and combat power of its own troops, even if this differs from the ethical obligations of the clinicians themselves. Understanding the implications of these complexities is the responsibility of all clinicians who serve in military forces.

Military surgery operates within the framework of a staged or echeloned system of care. In many operational circumstances, abbreviated initial wound surgery is ideally conducted as close as possible to the point of injury, followed by rapid evacuation: 'treating to evacuate' rather than 'evacuating to treat'. This system requires clinicians at every level to understand the limitations of austere forward surgery, and, most importantly, the patient transport system (including critical care patient transport) available and able to move patients rapidly to appropriate higher levels of care, both for the benefit of individual patients and to ensure that forward treatment facilities are not overwhelmed.

Infrastructure requirements for the most basic life-saving forms of military surgery are fundamentally very simple, and can be provided in 1–2 highly mobile tents or (often better) using commandeered buildings. These include shelter, power (for lighting, monitors, syringe drivers, and ideally diathermy and temperature control of certain medications and blood products), and water for hygiene. Medical waste disposal (particularly sharps) is often problematic; burn pits appear expedient but have substantial health concerns. Resupply of medical gases is particularly challenging, as these are classified as dangerous goods for flight, restricting other cargo that can be carried. Medications, fluids including blood, and other consumables such as gloves and gowns should have a documented cold chain, and an agreed policy for shelf life if ideal temperatures are exceeded. In the civilian setting, these materials and resources are provided by a series of complex supply chains that generally ensure rapid resupply. Achieving and maintaining this supply standard in a deployed environment can prove difficult, as supply chains are notoriously vulnerable in times of crisis (as demonstrated during the coronavirus disease 2019 [COVID-19] pandemic) and may even be specifically targeted during conflict.

Thus, no delivery can ever be guaranteed, so the deployed surgical team may have only what they carry. Appreciating the risk this entails, and deciding what, if any, clinical service should be delivered, is a task for a senior health officer with a technical understanding of all the relevant factors. Adverse clinical outcomes will always occur; minimizing these requires a global understanding of risk, not merely risk aversion from the perspective of an institution alone.

Modern militaries ensure that small surgical teams train together prior to deployment in order to prepare the team members for work that is well beyond normal civilian experience and their zone of comfort. Training permits assessment and refinement of interpersonal dynamics such that individuals meld into an effective team. It enables instillation of a thoughtful approach to realistic surgical care that acknowledges the context of

DOI: 10.1201/9781003258124-25

the environment. The forward surgical team must alter their perspective from definitive management towards a staged approach to surgical care in which they occupy only one part. However, many members of such teams are reserve officers, whose civilian job and skill set are vastly different from those into which they have been placed in the military context.

Maturation of an integrated system approach to military trauma care was remarkably successful in the conflicts in Iraq and Afghanistan that began in the early 2000s. Small improvements in clinical care at every point, combined with improved casualty triage and speed of transport through echelons of care, translated into dramatic improvements in overall performance. In one study of critically injured service personnel between 2003–2004 and an injury-matched cohort in 2007–2008, the case fatality rate was reduced from 47% to 20%. This association likely resulted from rapid transport and excellent pre-hospital care leading to increased arrival of mortally wounded casualties to combat hospitals.[1] This observation further underscores the importance of highly functioning surgical teams to further minimize combat mortality rates. Whilst true, much of the magnitude of this fall in case fatality rate also reflects system-based improvements dependent on stabilizing theatres of operations with medical resources that took time to adapt to emerging requirements.

Additional threats loom as asymmetric combat operations in the Middle East have subsided:

1. A time of relative peace that can lead to complacency and decreased combat readiness (including staffing) among military medical units.
2. The threat of a near-peer conflict in the future like the current combat operations in Ukraine.
3. Civilian surgeons are seeing 'military wounds' in urban hospitals.
4. As army medical establishments are depleted in 'peace', much greater reliance is placed on reserve officers, who may have little or no experience of combat or the wounds which result.
5. It is sometimes lamented that the medical and surgical 'lessons' underpinning this improvement risk being lost as experienced clinicians leave.

Lessons learnt in every war are forgotten in every peace.

Ensuring optimal readiness amid these threats will require a multifaceted strategy including collaboration

with civilian institutions and inclusion of team training into readiness exercises. The remainder of this chapter addresses many of the aspects that military trauma surgical team members must master to maintain a high level of combat readiness.[2]

20.2 INJURY PATTERNS

In the nineteenth century, warfare was infantry-based. In the twentieth century, it became mechanized and airborne, whilst in the early part of the twenty-first century, combat became asymmetric, with only one side in uniform. To quote General Sir Rupert Smith, author of *The Utility of Force*,[3] the battlefield became 'amongst the people'. The war in Ukraine has seen a return to large-scale combat operations and high civilian and military casualties. At the time of writing, Ukraine has had upwards of 20,000 amputees[4] as a result of the conflict, a scale unseen since World War I. Increasing political instability makes future predictions unwise. By the end of 2023, according to the BBC, across Ukraine's vast expanse, there are thought to be 174,000 square kilometres which are contaminated by landmines.[5]

Weapons of mass destruction in slow motion.

What does appear clear is that wounds sustained in contemporary combat are inflicted on combatant and non-combatant alike: in a recent review of activity at a coalition hospital in Afghanistan, 60% of casualties were local nationals, including women and children.

Similarly, in an urban setting of Somalia,[6] casualty distribution in military personnel was like that of the Vietnam War.[3] Over the 20-plus years of conflict in Iraq and Afghanistan since 2001, US and Coalition military deaths exceeded 4879 (Iraq) and 3540 (Afghanistan).[7] One thousand four hundred and seventy-two deaths were due to disease, non-battle injury, and other causes, and over 52,000 troops were wounded in action.

The leading causes of injury among casualties in the Afghanistan and Iraq wars were explosive devices and gunshot wounds. Over two-thirds of casualties died within 10 minutes of wounding without any realistic opportunity for advanced medical intervention; head injuries were the most common cause of these immediate deaths. However, the commonest cause of *preventable* death was haemorrhage; it is estimated that more than one-third of these casualties might have survived with better pre-hospital haemorrhage control.[8]

Injuries can be sustained by gunshot or the effect of conventional explosive munitions (air-delivered bombs, artillery shells, rocket-propelled grenades, or hand grenades). Wounding patterns are modified by the presence or absence of modern ballistic protection (armour) and the pre-hospital timeline. The availability of personal protection devices for the chest, head, and eyes (ballistic vests, Kevlar helmets, and full eye protection) has changed wound patterns significantly, dramatically reducing deaths from head and torso trauma. Extremity injuries predominate. Many fatal penetrating injuries are likely to be caused by missiles entering through areas not protected by body armour, such as the face and junctional areas in the neck, groin, and buttocks.

During 20th-century conflicts, the case fatality rate for gunshot wounds was approximately 33%. Amongst US casualties in Iraq, one study found it was 4.6%, with a nearly two-thirds reduction in the incidence of thoracic injuries in particular.

In the US Role 2 and UK Role 3 (multispeciality surgical) hospitals in Afghanistan during 2006–2014, the overall survival rates were 95.1% and 93.2%, respectively (see **Table 20.1**). The survival rate was influenced by the nationality of the patient, with a reduced rate amongst the Afghan population attributed to the lower use of personal protective equipment (PPE) and a higher prevalence of comorbidities. Hospital statistics in isolation can, however, be misleading, as 80%–90% of deaths occurred pre-hospital. Air evacuation was more available than ever before, and many critically injured patients, who would previously have died, reached hospital alive. For example, the proportion of patients who died in US military hospitals in the Iraq and Afghanistan wars was higher (4.8%) than in either the Vietnam War (3.2%) or World War II (3.5%).[8]

The defining injury pattern in recent counterinsurgency operations is that caused by improvised explosive devices (IEDs): the combination of bilateral lower limb amputation with pelvic fracture and perineal injury has been described as the 'signature injury' of the conflicts in Afghanistan and Iraq.[9] The leading causes of death and injury were blast, followed by gunshot wounds.

Protocols for casualty assessment, tourniquet application, the use of haemostatic wound dressings, and the direct transfer of casualties from ambulance to operating theatre are designed to recognize that exsanguination remains the main cause of preventable battlefield death. In a recent review of deaths of servicemen after combat injury, half of those who were potentially survivable were the result of intracavity haemorrhage. Multiple teams operating simultaneously on several body parts are an efficient use of theatre time, and they can minimize physiological compromise and expedite onward evacuation.

Military medical practitioners have been described as 'working at the interface of two dynamic technologies, warfare and trauma management'. In addition to the problems of dispersed battlefields, highly mobile front lines, extended lines of logistics, and a delay in evacuation, the modern military surgical team is likely to be called upon to treat civilians, females (including obstetric care), and children, as well as service personnel, with a requirement to offer immediate care well away from their speciality. Also, problems in ophthalmology; maxillofacial surgery; ear, nose, and throat medicine; paediatrics; gynaecology; tropical medicine; and even public health will fall under the remit of the military surgeon. These challenges are magnified by the nature of modern surgical training, with its accent on early training in subspecialities, combined with the non-operative trends in the management of trauma surgery. Military surgical teams therefore must be trained in a variety of specialities and undergo multiple training courses including team training – before they deploy. Blended learning (digital interactive education, and theoretical and skills training) before deployment has become increasingly important.

Table 20.1 Outcomes of Admissions to a US Role 2 and a UK Role 3 Hospital in Afghanistan

	Survivors	Deaths	Recovery Rate
US Role 2			
US military	3461	117	97%
Coalition military	371	13	97%
Afghan	5260	335	94%
Totals	9092	465	95%
UK Role 3			
UK military	1906	58	97%
Coalition military and entitled civilians	1206	42	97%
Afghan	3250	367	90%
Totals	6362	467	93%

Everything should be as simple as possible ... but not simpler.

Modern all-arms battle presents a vast array of potential wounding agents, from high-energy military rifles to fragments from mortars or mines, blast from any explosive, and chemical, biological, radiological, and nuclear exposure (e.g., depleted uranium in tank munitions and armour). In many operational theatres, motor vehicle crashes are the most common cause of injury. As observed in Syria recently, it is imperative that military medical personnel become familiar with the medical consequences of toxin exposure, the illnesses caused by these agents, and the measures required to protect military healthcare providers themselves.

20.3 MILITARY TRAUMA SYSTEMS

20.3.1 The Echelons of Medical Care

The patient presenting to the trauma surgical team in a civilian hospital often does so in the context of a well-coordinated trauma system. Considering the victim of a motor vehicle crash summoning help: this requires the existence of an intact telephone or radio system, appropriately trained individuals arriving in suitable equipped vehicles, and an unimpeded journey, delivering an appropriately 'packaged' patient to the hospital. In the deployed environment, this pre-hospital chain is particularly vulnerable. Patients may experience delays of hours or days getting to care, which will in turn influence how they present to the surgical team, as has been seen in Ukraine. During such dynamic care, detailed pre-hospital protocols and training of their providers are critically important to optimize outcome. Similar *prolonged field care* is likely to be required during future large-scale combat operations.

Deployed military medical systems usually consist of an echeloned series of levels (roles) of care in military medical treatment units, traditionally called medical treatment facilities (MTFs), and divided by the North Atlantic Treaty Organization (NATO) into Role 1 to Role 4.

Close to the point of injury, a casualty either applies self-aid or receives aid such as a field dressing or tourniquet application ('buddy care').

20.3.1.1 ROLE 1

The next stage is care by a military paramedical provider, then by a doctor or nurse at an aid post (Role 1 facility). The Role 1 MTF provides primary healthcare, specialized first aid, triage, resuscitation, and stabilization. Generally, Role 1 medical support must be readily and easily available to all force personnel.

20.3.1.2 ROLE 2

A Role 2 MTF is a structure, usually nearby where the conflict is taking place, capable of the reception and triage of casualties, as well as being able to perform resuscitation and treatment of shock to a higher level than Role 1 (damage control resuscitation [DCR]). In the armed forces of some nations, Role 2 MTFs incorporate the ability to perform damage control surgery (DCS); in others (unless augmented by a surgical team), this is not the case. (This leads to confusion when reading historical accounts and can necessitate questioning during international planning.) Role 2 MTFs may include a limited facility for the short-term holding of casualties until they can be returned to duty or evacuated, or they may be little more than surgical facilities providing immediate postoperative care.

In an effort to reduce this confusion, NATO now further divides Role 2 MTFs into Role 2 Light Manoeuvre (R2LM) and Role 2 Enhanced (R2E).

20.3.1.2.1 Role 2 Basic (R2B) / Role 2 Light Manoeuvre (R2LM)

A R2B/R2LM MTF can conduct triage and advanced resuscitation including DCR and DCS. It will usually evacuate its post-surgical cases to Role 3 (or R2E) for stabilization and further surgery *before* evacuation to Role 4. It is light and mobile, with 12–20 personnel, and must be resupplied frequently if undertaking clinical work.

20.3.1.2.2 Role 2 Enhanced (R2E)

R2E MTFs are effectively small field hospitals. They provide basic secondary healthcare, built around general and orthopaedic surgery, an intensive care unit (ICU), and nursed beds. A R2E MTF can stabilize post-surgical cases for evacuation to Role 4 without routing through a Role 3 MTF first. CT scanning, laboratory services, sterilization, and even basic rehabilitation may be available.

20.3.1.3 ROLE 3

Role 3 MTFs are designed to provide combat theatre secondary healthcare. Role 3 medical support is deployed hospitalization and the elements required to support it. The feature distinguishing a R3 from R2E MTF is the presence of surgical and medical specialities other than general and orthopaedic surgery: for example, neurosurgery, maxillofacial surgery, vascular surgery, ophthalmology, interventional radiology, and specialist internal medicine.

20.3.1.4 ROLE 4

Role 4 medical support provides definitive care of patients for whom the treatment required is longer than the theatre evacuation policy or for whom the capabilities usually found at Role 3 are inadequate. This would normally comprise specialist surgical and medical procedures, reconstruction, rehabilitation, and convalescence. This level of care is usually specialized, time-consuming, and normally provided outside the area of operations, often in the 'home' country.

The NATO system described above has evolved to support an expeditionary concept of operations. It is recognized that not all conflicts are fought in remote areas of operations, especially in Europe. Integration with civilian hospital infrastructure in support of local active combat operations is fortunately not a challenge most Western military forces have faced for many decades. To do so requires appropriate allocation of resources at a whole-of-government level, informed by an accurate appreciation of both military and civilian requirements.

Pitfall

The situation becomes complicated when casualties move between systems (e.g., military to host nation, or non-governmental organization to military) having received surgery in the first system. Because standards of care can vary enormously between systems, these casualties need a thorough examination and re-evaluation.

Soldiers have been trained and issued their equipment before the disaster or injury occurs, to perform immediate aid on themselves or each other. Civilians, however, generally have no such training. It is critically important that full documentation accompanies the patient to prevent overtreatment.

20.3.2 Incident Management and Multiple Casualties

At incidents involving explosive devices, the '4 Cs' provide a suggested approach (see **Table 20.2**).

20.3.2.1 CONFIRM

Incident commanders must be clear about what is happening, and about the risk and position of further hazards. Factors that must be considered are clearance priorities, cordon locations, safe areas, access and egress routes, and rendezvous points.

Table 20.2 The Four Cs of Incident Management

- Confirm
- Clear
- Cordon
- Control

20.3.2.2 CLEAR

The scene should be cleared to a safe distance. This distance will vary depending on the terrain and the size of the threat. The method and urgency of clearance will depend on the incident.

20.3.2.3 CORDON

Cordons establish the area in which the rescue effort is taking place and define safe zones and tiers of command. An outer cordon should be established as a physical barrier preventing accidental or unauthorized access to the site. An inner cordon may be set up around wreckage, especially if hazards still exist.

20.3.2.4 CONTROL

Once cordons are set up, the control of the cordons and scene is maintained by clear rendezvous and access points.

Once the '4 Cs' have been established, medical management and support can begin (see **Table 20.3**).

20.3.3 Incident Command and Control

If effective command and control are not established early at the scene, the initial chaos will continue, and the injured will suffer regardless of how well some individual casualties are treated. Command implies the overall responsibility for the mission, as well as authority to establish procedures and to direct tasks, whereas control refers to the implementation of directions

Table 20.3 Medical Management and Support

Command and control
Safety
Communication
Assessment
Triage
Treatment
Transport

including modification for unanticipated circumstances if required. Command usually overrides control.

20.3.3.1 SAFETY

Healthcare workers must remember that their own safety is paramount, and that they *must* not become casualties themselves. Considerations may include infectious agents that can occur coincidently during a natural disaster.

20.3.3.2 COMMUNICATION

Communication is the transmission between a sender and a receiver, preferably such that the receiver is in no doubt about the intent and need of the sender. Every major incident inquiry has identified failings in communications. Without good communication, command and control are impossible. When a formal medical record system may not exist, simply writing instructions over wound bandages may suffice.

20.3.3.3 ASSESSMENT

This is a constant process. Commanders should always consider the current situation, what resources are required, and where these can be obtained.

20.3.3.4 TRIAGE

In any situation when there is more than one casualty and insufficient resources to treat all simultaneously, a system of triage (allocating patients to resources) must be used (see Section 20.4: 'Triage'). The US Centers for Disease Control and Prevention (CDC) sponsored a working group that developed the following SALT triage tool for use in mass casualty situations[10] (see **Figure 20.1**).

- **S**ort.
- **A**ssess.
- **L**ife-saving interventions.
- **T**ransport and/or treat.

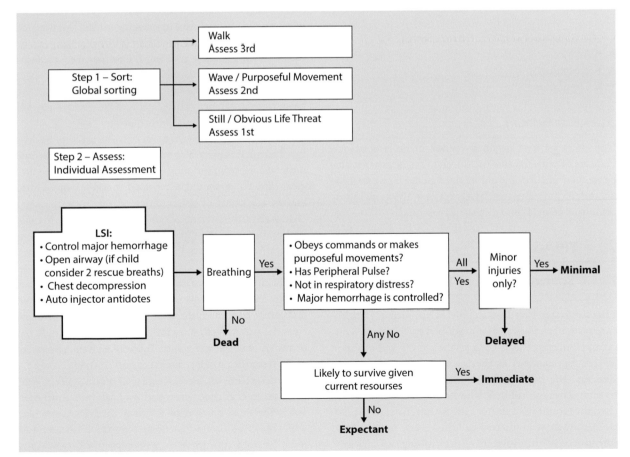

Figure 20.1 SALT (sort, assess, life-saving interventions, and transport and/or treat) multi-casualty assessment scheme.

Table 20.4 Triage Categories

	Label Colour	Description
T1	Red	Immediate
T2	Yellow	Urgent
T3	Green	Delayed
Dead	White or black	Dead
T4	Blue (not standard)	Expectant

By sorting and then assessing patients, treatment priorities can be quickly assigned based on local resources using a standard colour scheme. There are many different systems in use (**Table 20.4**).

20.3.3.5 TREATMENT

At the scene of any blast or ballistic incident, treatment teams are likely to be faced with casualties with multiple serious injuries. Treatment must follow the <C>A-B-C paradigm:

- <**C**> Catastrophic haemorrhage control
- **A** Airway
- **B** Breathing
- **C** Circulation

20.3.3.6 TRANSPORT

Not every patient needs to travel in an ambulance. Vehicles of opportunity, including buses or other multipassenger vehicles, should be used to move the walking wounded. Judicious use of scarce resources, including armoured vehicles and aircraft, is essential.

20.4 TRIAGE

20.4.1 Source and Aim of Triage

Effective triage is crucial in an efficient military healthcare system, and it was first described by Napoleon's surgeon, Dominique Jean Larrey, who introduced a system of sorting casualties as they presented to field dressing stations. His priority, and the aim of the system, was to identify those soldiers who had minor wounds, and therefore could with minor treatment return to the battle. Although we might now call this reverse triage, he had introduced a formal system of prioritizing casualties.

Triage remains a fundamental principle in modern military and disaster medicine. It is dynamic and can be applied at all levels of medical care, from the point of wounding to definitive surgical care. Ultimately, critical 'bottlenecks' must be managed to ensure the optimal care of the largest number of patients including (1) emergency department beds, (2) cross-sectional imaging resources (i.e. CT scan, if available), (3) operating rooms, and (4) blood products.

The system for 'surgical triage' may be slightly different from the triage system used in resuscitation, but the same principles apply. Those requiring life-saving surgical intervention (with the prospect of a successful outcome) take priority over patients requiring limb-saving surgery in forward locations, and considering all the other factors, the key questions will be: if there is limited surgical space available forward, 'Who goes on first?' and 'Do they need to go on at all?'

Overtriage is a feature of all mass casualty situations; however, a high rate of overtriage is acceptable to avoid missing patients who really did require an intervention. In a series of 1350 laparotomies from the Vietnam War, based on the clinical assessment of wounded soldiers, the rate of negative laparotomy was 19.2%. The philosophy of selective non-operative management (SNOM) was not available at that time. In a modern military setting, accurate screening tools (e.g., using CT or focussed abdominal sonography for trauma [FAST]) may aid SNOM; nevertheless, such time-consuming procedures may not be appropriate in busy surgical situations, where a quick laparotomy yields definite information.

Effective triage is crucial in an efficient military healthcare system. It is dynamic and can be applied at all levels of medical care, from the point of wounding to definitive surgical care. Triage should be repeated at every point of care, and at any point of deterioration. Patients compensate, change condition, and deteriorate without warning. In civilian practice, 'expectant' patients are rare because resources are relatively unlimited. In the military environment, care is often 'rationed'. The needs of the dying, who will require significant resources of a surgical team, must be balanced against the needs of the next wave of patients who arrive and can be saved with the same effort. **Table 20.5** summarizes the patterns of injury for non-survivors in a military or austere environment, whilst **Table 20.6** gives an overview of the resource considerations that impact triage.

Transfer time will also dictate who requires life-saving interventions at that point, and who can wait until they reach the next echelon of medical care. Consumables will always be limited in these forward locations and must be used appropriately, as resupply will take time. The flow of casualties in a fast-moving battle will also influence how many and what type of casualties should

Table 20.5 Patterns of Injury for Non-Survivors in an Austere Environment

- Long bone amputations*
- Open-skull fracture
- Full-thickness burns > 50%
- Inhalation injury
- Head injury with GCS < 8
- Arrival in cardiac arrest

*Amputations with a reasonably long stump may be closed with a tourniquet if available, which can be left until further surgical capacity is available.

be operated on. The prospect of incoming serious casualties will change triage decisions for the wounded already at the medical facility.

Ultimately, an awareness of the overall tactical picture on the part of the senior clinician is paramount. It may be wise to remember that triage, including surgical triage, means doing the 'best for the most', and expectant treatment for some may eventually benefit the 'most'.

20.4.2 **Forward Surgical Teams and Triage**

Forward surgical teams must be light, mobile, and rapidly deployable to allow them to respond in an uncertain battlefield (see Section 20.6). Restrictions and constraints within these teams are many, and include limitations of space and equipment, poor lighting, and the need to achieve some degree of climate control for the human resources and, particularly, for blood and medications. Some re-sterilization of surgical tools may be possible, but disposable equipment, water, and especially oxygen will all be limited.

Human factors of physical and emotional fatigue will also affect how long the surgical team can endure the challenges of operating in austere and dangerous environments without reinforcement or resupply. The teams will often have to function independently but may also deploy as augmentation of an existing medical facility during a casualty surge. Even in wartime, the best

Table 20.6 Factors Affecting Triage

- Patient load and severity
- Medical capability and supply
- Local situation and safety
- Available evacuation assets and flight times
- Theatre medical assets

surgical teams could not operate for more than 19 hours at a time over a sustained period without breaking after 3 days. A single team has no on/off duty cycle.

There is a difference between a well-equipped, relatively static 'field' (or combat support) hospital and a 'forward surgical team'. The *raison d'être* of the team is delivery of the life- and limb-saving surgery as far forward as possible without major evacuation delay, to a select group of potentially salvageable patients who would otherwise suffer due to delays in evacuation from the battlefield.

Triage is challenging, it requires difficult decisions to be made, but it remains crucial to the effective use and efficiency of the forward surgical teams. Different nations approach this in different ways, influenced by their medical and military organizational cultures. The most senior surgeon should always have input into what is, or is not, surgically possible. However, once operating, the senior surgeon is not then able to maintain situational awareness of what might be an evolving situation for tens or hundreds of other patients. Medics and even non-clinicians are able to apply simple vital signs–based triage tools, and medical rules of eligibility, so that clinicians only need to consider a fraction of patients presenting to a MTF. Furthermore, the most senior non-surgical clinician in a forward surgical team is often best placed to maintain oversight of the triage zone once operating has begun.

20.4.3 **Forward Surgical Team Decision-Making**

Small surgical teams can be expected to work in tactical environments where insecure lines of evacuation, minimal diagnostic infrastructure, and very constrained patient-holding make clear decision-making on *who* to operate on and *what* operation to execute critical functions (see Section 20.6). Surgical decision-makers must ensure that their choices do not unfairly reduce treatment options available for future patients and factor in likely predicted clinical states (and unlikely but impactful worst-case states) plus the capacity of the staged care system. Critically, the surgeon must avoid defaulting to judgements based purely on factors used in civilian practice that pay no heed to pressing operational realities. Whilst 'surgical' in nature, such decisions must be made in conjunction with other key stakeholders, and operational, physiological, ethical, and resource issues must be considered.

The surgical team should understand available clinical and human resources. Stock-taking cannot be left to the medical logistician; the surgical team must know what the current supply state is of key consumables (e.g., blood and oxygen) to anticipate potential shortages and to develop a contingency plan.

20.4.4 Selection of Patients for Surgery

The R2LM patient load consists of two categories: those who require DCR/DCS, and non–damage control cases. The former group require *immediate haemorrhage control*. The latter group are usually better served by rapid transport to a higher echelon of care for an operation *later*. The questions that the surgeon must ask of every patient who arrives in their small unit are therefore:

1. Does the patient need surgery?
2. Does this surgery need to be done here (*non-discretionary intervention*), or can the patient be transferred for surgery elsewhere (*discretionary intervention*)?

If the timelines to transfer a *non*-patient to Role 3 or Role 4 are prolonged – or the evacuation route becomes more tenuous – the surgeon may decide the risk of in-flight deterioration justifies *discretionary intervention* and surgery. The surgeon must balance the risks of each strategy: the excess individual patient morbidity incurred by a longer wait for surgery at a different location versus the impact on R2LM capacity if a greater proportion of patients are triaged into a *discretionary* pathway.[11]

20.5 MASS CASUALTIES

An estimate of the numbers and types of casualties, the resources required to deal with them per phase of battle, and their evacuation is the cornerstone of operational medical planning. Casualty estimates are major resource-drivers and will determine what capabilities are required. The medical support for a specific operation will therefore be planned considering the perceived threat.

Mass casualties, however, may occur for many reasons, and the cause of the major incident may not have been identified as one of the known 'threats'. The term *mass casualty* is, of course, relative, and for a small team, this number may be as low as three patients. Multiple motor vehicle crashes, downed helicopters, floods, and even earthquakes have recently produced mass casualty situations or major incidents for military forces. All these incidents have produced an unexpected surge in casualties, far greater than the casualty estimate that each operation had declared. The key in all these events was that the medical facilities were overwhelmed, and available resources could not meet the required demand.

> *The essence of military medicine is to realize that the overwhelming of key resources does not imply that the most important elements of treatment could not be delivered.*

When major incidents produce mass casualties in civilian situations, for example from rail crashes or as a result of urban terrorism events, there are often several receiving hospitals to choose from, to spread the load of casualties. This luxury is rarely available in the military environment. In some situations, other nations' medical facilities may be available, but often the only available 'receiving hospital' will be the forward surgical team. Triage remains the key to effective medical management of a mass casualty event, especially when large numbers of wounded arrive at the location in a short space of time. Equipment, people, and transport will be in short supply, so sound training and adherence to the principles of triage should ensure effective use of the limited resources available.

In civilian practice, advanced triage tools have been developed to predict workload capacity in mass casualties. Critically injured casualties at a rate of greater than one per hour may rapidly exceed the capability of competent trauma teams. Modelling mass casualty events indicate that about 5%–10% of patients die immediately, and 5%–10% of survivors have severe, potentially life-threatening injuries. In terms of patients presenting for medical treatment after a mass casualty event, typically 50% of total patient volume will occur by one hour of an incident, as shown in **Figure 20.2**. More than 75% of casualties will have arrived by the end of the second hour. Therefore, total patient volume and requisite staffing may be somewhat predictable in an isolated mass casualty event. These estimates are a useful guide in a permissive military context but are likely to be highly misleading if pre-hospital evacuation times are lengthened by adverse operational circumstances – for example, enemy activity.

After triage and treatment, transport remains the third key element of medical support in a mass casualty event. Unlike in a civilian environment, where there will be many options for both ground and air transport, transport is likely to be very limited in the military mass casualty situation. Regular and effective triage will

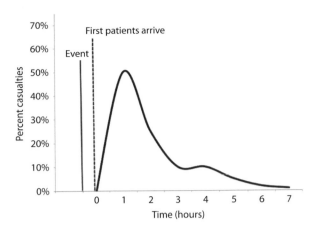

Figure 20.2 Percentage of casualties arriving at casualty reception.

determine who is transported first, and by what means, to ensure that the right patient arrives at the right time at the next level of medical care.

20.6 EVACUATION

Speed of evacuation from point of wounding to first surgical intervention is a critical determinant of outcome. The Korean War saw the introduction of helicopter evacuation of the wounded from the front line to mobile army surgical hospitals (MASH) – increasing the proportion of wounded reaching surgery on the day of wounding from 34% in 1950 to 73% in 1953 (US Department of the Army, Battle casualties and medical statistics: US Army experience in the Korean War, 1973: 790–800), with onward transport by fixed-wing aircraft to base hospitals. During the Vietnam conflict, the average pre-hospital time for combat casualties treated at a US Navy hospital was 80 minutes. Limited provision of aircraft in a combat setting has meant that medical evacuation has used assets earmarked for other purposes. During Operations Desert Shield and Desert Storm in 1991, many patients were successfully airlifted using converted cargo aircraft.

Three forward aeromedical evacuation platforms operated in the Afghanistan war: the UK Medical Emergency Response Team (MERT), the US Air Force Expeditionary Rescue Squadron (PEDRO – named after the call sign of the first US Air Force HH-43 rescue helicopters in the Vietnam conflict), and US Army Medical Evacuation Squadrons (DUSTOFF), each with a different clinical

capability. Recent evidence suggests that retrieval by a platform with a greater clinical capability (MERT), with physician capability, is associated with improved mortality in critical patients when compared with platforms with less clinical capability (PEDRO and DUSTOFF),[12] both of which paramedic-staffed platforms demonstrated superior clinical results compared to helicopters staffed by medics capable of only more basic interventions.[1] Since the introduction of a dedicated air asset, pre-hospital times from wounding to point of care have fallen to approximately 45 minutes. A recent study of more than 900 patients evacuated to a Role 4 facility demonstrated a <0.02% mortality rate with significantly injured soldiers (mean injury severity score of 23).[11]

Many military healthcare systems are now incorporating far-forward resuscitative surgery capabilities into mission planning. Although these forward surgical teams can provide trauma surgical capability for only a limited number of patients, they aim to provide life- and limb-saving surgery to the select group of potentially salvageable patients who would otherwise die or suffer permanent disability due to delays in evacuation. These teams provide life-saving thoracoabdominal haemorrhage control, control of contamination within body cavities, temporary limb or carotid revascularization, stabilization of fractures, and evacuation of major intracranial haematomas. Each nation has a slightly different balance and skill mix within their forward surgical capability, but most will normally provide the three main tenets of forward care: initial resuscitation, surgery, and postoperative critical care. Most nations 'mission-tailor' their teams in size to the specific operational environment. As part of the casualty estimate, military planners need to decide on the number of surgical tables required and the speed at which they can safely transfer patients to the next echelon of care. The size and sophistication of the attached critical care element will be determined by the capability of forward medical evacuation. If there is no such facility, either in- or out-country, then the first few patients will fill a facility and render it completely ineffective.

20.7 RESUSCITATION

20.7.1 Overview

Treatment and resuscitation available will alter with each echelon of care; resources and complexity of care generally increase as the casualty moves away from the battlefield. Exsanguinating haemorrhage remains the commonest preventable cause of death amongst those killed in action during military conflicts. Unlike in the urban setting, the military must consider weight of supplies that can be transported into forward locations. Large volumes of fluids at any stage in the resuscitation process are therefore not a feasible option. More importantly, recent conflicts have demonstrated improved

mortality with balanced haemostatic resuscitation. Early utilization of blood products, including low-titre group O stored or fresh whole blood, has been incorporated into Tactical Combat Casualty Care guidelines.[13] For patients with haemorrhagic shock in whom surgical intervention is not immediately available, the goal of maintaining a systolic arterial pressure of 80 mmHg (palpable radial pulse) is now generally accepted. See **Table 20.7**.

Table 20.7 Clinical Considerations in Penetrating Injury

Catastrophic Haemorrhage
Penetrating wounds to the groin, axilla, and neck. Consider temporary packing.
Penetrating wounds to major limb vessels/traumatic amputations. Consider early use of tourniquet.

Airway and C-Spine
Simple first: Jaw thrust, oral airway.
Airway at risk from:

- Burn injury
- Disruption from fragments
- Compression from penetrating vascular injury in the neck

Consider early anaesthesia and intubation (aided by fibre-optic scopes and diameter of endotracheal tubes) or early surgical airway, noting the difficulty of performing subsequent bronchoscopy through a < 7.5 mm endotracheal tube.
Cervical collars: These have a limited role in pure penetrating injury and may conceal developing haematoma in the neck. Consider (according to local protocols) in mixed injury as occurs in bombings.

Breathing
Needle decompression for tension pneumothorax.
Manage sucking chest wounds with Asherman (or similar) seals, and then consider chest drainage.

Circulation
Catastrophic bleeding should have been controlled early. Smaller external bleeds can be managed with simple first aid measures of compression and elevation. Ongoing internal bleeding from penetrating cavity injury needs to be suspected or recognized from history and clinical findings.
Difficulty in obtaining vascular access can be experienced in austere conditions, when hypotension, low ambient temperature, and tactical considerations, such as the presence of mass casualties or operating light restriction, can conspire to frustrate attempts at vascular access; intraosseous access is an attractive option in these scenarios.

Deficit
The majority of casualties who sustain a high-energy penetrating brain injury do not survive to medical care. Casualties who survive to care from penetrating injury are generally a preselected group, and in the absence of obvious devastating injury should be resuscitated as above to minimize secondary injury. There is an obvious conflict between hypotensive resuscitation for cavity bleeding and the need to maintain cerebral perfusion, and this becomes a judgement call at the time.

Environment
Hypothermia needs to be treated and managed with warm air blankets and environmental control. The temperature of any fluid given to trauma patients, particularly in a military or austere environment, is crucial. Any fluid used in resuscitation should be warmed to avoid further cooling of a haemorrhagic casualty. The actual process of warming the fluids remains a considerable challenge, and in most cases, it requires improvisation on behalf of the provider.

20.7.2 **Damage Control Resuscitation (DCR)**[13,14]

Approximately 90% of casualties are in a stable condition on arrival at hospital; however, about 10% of combat casualties will require massive transfusion, and it is in these maximally injured patients that major improvements in care have been achieved. The concept of DCR in the field implies that, rather than treating haemorrhage per se by replacement of fluid, efforts are primarily directed at stopping any bleeding, using local methods such as pressure, topical agents such as zeolite (QuikClot®, Teleflex, Morrisville, NC, USA) and chitosan (HemCon®, Tricol Biomedical, Portland, OR, USA), and regional haemostasis with the use of combat tourniquets. This is followed by rapid evacuation to a surgical facility where DCS can take place. Resuscitation fluids are minimized where possible, and the early transfusion of blood and blood products where available is encouraged. (See also Chapter 6: 'Damage Control'.)

In the severely injured casualty, DCR consists of two parts; first, pre-surgical fluid therapy is limited to keep blood pressure at approximately 80 mmHg, preventing renewed bleeding from recently clotted vessels (in practice, this means limiting crystalloid fluid infusion and using the level of consciousness and/or the presence of a radial pulse as a guide). Second, intravascular volume restoration is accomplished by using thawed plasma as a primary resuscitation fluid in at least a 1:1 or 1:2 ratio with packed red cells and empiric transfusion with platelets. An example of this is the UK Military Damage Control Resuscitation protocol (**Table 20.8**).

Difficulty in obtaining vascular access can be experienced in austere conditions, when hypotension, low ambient temperature, and tactical considerations, such as the presence of mass casualties or operating light restriction, can frustrate attempts at vascular access. Intraosseous access is an attractive option in these scenarios.[15]

Blood is the preferred fluid of choice in such casualties, particularly those in profound shock, and is now carried by many military resuscitation teams forward of the first surgical teams. However, in some military healthcare systems, blood is still not yet available, and other fluids need to be carried. Options available to resuscitation teams include isotonic crystalloids, colloids, hypertonic saline, and hypertonic saline plus colloid. The choice of fluid remains unresolved and may in fact be less important than the quantity and rate of fluid infused in patients with uncontrolled haemorrhage.

Table 20.8 UK Damage Control Resuscitation Protocol

1	For the first hour after injury, resuscitate to a palpable radial pulse, and after this (if not in surgery) resuscitate to a 'normal' blood pressure – an approach known as novel hybrid resuscitation and taught on the UK Battlefield Advanced Life Support (BATLS™) course.
2	For severely injured casualties, recognize they are likely to be coagulopathic early – and resuscitate with blood, thawed plasma, and platelets (blood and plasma initially in a 1:1 ratio) or whole blood.
3	Balance the need for volume replacement against the risk of over-transfusion – reassess constantly.
4	Early use of tranexamic acid.
5	Monitoring of blood gases, lactate, calcium, and potassium – with the active management of falling calcium or rising potassium.
6	With blast casualties, anticipate lung injury and ventilate using adult respiratory distress syndrome protocols.
7	The anaesthesia team and surgical team work closely together to ensure the correct sequencing of damage control procedures.

The temperature of any fluid given to trauma patients, particularly in a military or austere environment, is crucial. Any fluid used in resuscitation should be warmed to avoid further cooling of a haemorrhagic casualty. The actual process of warming the fluids remains a considerable challenge and, in most cases, requires improvisation on behalf of the provider. Locally available rewarming/protective devices, such as plastic bags, use of hot car engines, sunlight, and so on, may suffice.

20.7.3 **Damage Control Surgery (DCS) in the Military Setting**[16–18]

The typical civilian damage control patient is likely to require the direct attention of at least two surgeons and one nurse during the first 6 hours, full invasive monitoring, multiple operations, massive transfusion of blood and products, and a prolonged ICU stay, with a high mortality. The utility of this philosophy has been labelled as 'impractical for common use in a forward military unit during times of war'. However, experience in recent counterinsurgency conflicts has led to a widespread adoption of the philosophy of DCS in the military context as 'minimally acceptable care' with rapid procedures and pragmatic objectives. Current military surgical efforts are framed within a 'damage control' mindset, with temporary revascularization of limbs and damage control laparotomy providing good control, to enable early transport as soon as the military situation allows (see Section 6.3).

In the far-forward, highly mobile, austere military environment, it is quite likely that the surgeon will not have the luxury of being able to perform definitive surgery on every casualty. Short, focussed operative interventions can be used on peripheral vascular injuries, extensive bone and soft tissue injuries, and thoracoabdominal penetrations in patients with favourable physiology, instead of *definitive* surgery being provided for every injured soldier. This may conserve precious resources such as time, operating table space, and blood. Instead of applying these temporary abbreviated surgical control (TASC) manoeuvres to patients about to exhaust their physiological reserve, as in classic damage control, TASC is applied when the limitations of reserve exist outside the patient.

This philosophy relies heavily on the military medical system, with postoperative care and evacuation to the 'resource-replete environment' a priority. In the military, the key is triage (patient selection) and knowledge of one's own resources as well as the tactical and operational situation. The philosophy for the military surgical team exposed to numbers of casualties in the setting of limited resources remains to do the best for the most, rather than expend resources on limited numbers of critically wounded.

20.8 BATTLEFIELD ANALGESIA[19,20]

Relief of pain is an important consideration for both the wounded person and the military caregiver. Provision of effective analgesia is humane, but it also attenuates the adverse pathophysiological responses to pain, and is likely to aid evacuation from the battlefield and maintain morale. Analgesia may be given at self- and buddy-aid levels; protocols to guide medical and paramedical staff in the provision of safe and effective analgesia are available.

Analgesia methods used in recent conflicts include:

- Simple non-pharmacological
  - Reassurance
  - Splinting of fractures
  - Cooling of burns
- Oral analgesics
  - Non-steroidal anti-inflammatory drugs
  - Paracetamol/acetaminophen
- Nerve blocks using infiltration of local anaesthetic
- Intramuscular and intravenous opioids. Traditionally morphine, but more recently recognizing the superior kinetics of intravenous fentanyl and oxycodone
- Intramuscular and intravenous ketamine
- Fentanyl 'lollipops'
- Inhaled methoxyflurane

Methods under development include inhalational forms of analgesics and sedatives, such as fentanyl derivatives, dexmedetomidine, and ketamine.[21]

20.9 BATTLEFIELD ANAESTHESIA

Battlefield anaesthesia presents many challenges, including the need to maintain airway control, hypothermia of the casualty, restricted drug availability, potential lack of supplementary oxygen, and the possible requirement for prolonged postoperative mechanical ventilation. Mass casualty situations are also a constant possibility in the military arena.

Surgery requires both adequate analgesia and anaesthesia. No single agent can provide an appropriate level of both anaesthesia and analgesia; hence, a combination of drugs and techniques is required. The choices of anaesthetic are narrowed in austere conditions, being limited to general anaesthesia (either intravenous or inhalational), regional anaesthesia, or local anaesthesia. For surgical exploration of body cavities, general anaesthesia is most frequently chosen, whilst a regional anaesthetic may be more appropriate for injuries of the extremities or perineum.

In the field, rapid sequence induction (RSI) is the norm, using fast-acting hypnotic and neuromuscular blocking agents to facilitate rapid airway control. There are several RSI cocktails used in the pre-hospital setting, most using a combination of an induction agent, a paralysing agent, and analgesia. Sedation, amnesia, and analgesia can then be maintained with intravenous agents such as ketamine, benzodiazepines, and opioids.

For long procedures or surgical sites involving the abdomen or thorax, a combination anaesthetic that includes an inhalational agent such as isoflurane or sevoflurane may be used. British forward surgical teams use the Diamedica Portable Anaesthesia Machine, which does not require a compressed gas source, and have gained much experience with this technique of field anaesthesia. This low-resistance draw-over type of vaporizer is currently also in use by US forces in austere settings. An alternative means of delivering volatile anaesthesia is the Mobile Anaesthesia Delivery Module (MADM™, Thornhill Medical, Toronto, ONT, Canada), such as is used by the Australian Defence Force and elements of the US military. This is a direct-injection device relying on anaesthetic agent monitoring and which, when combined with a circle system such as the MOVES®SLC™ (Thornhill Medical) integrated oxygen concentrator/ventilator, efficiently conserves anaesthetic agent.

Total intravenous anaesthesia is a suitable alternative to volatile anaesthesia in almost all military circumstances. Propofol using target-controlled infusion (TCI) pumps is available in the military hospitals of most nations, although TCI is not registered for use in the United States. Ketamine, or a combination of ketamine plus propofol, during the maintenance phase of anaesthesia also produces acceptable results, especially in haemodynamically unstable casualties. The incidence of intraoperative awareness might be slightly higher than with volatile anaesthesia, but this uncommon complication might be considered an acceptable risk under the circumstances.

Peripheral regional anaesthesia remains an important option in battlefield anaesthesia, as it provides both patient comfort and surgical analgesia whilst maintaining patient consciousness and spontaneous ventilation. With the relatively large number of extremity wounds in modern conflicts, and certainly in the mass casualty setting with a limited anaesthesia capability, regional anaesthetic techniques should not be overlooked. Single-shot or catheter techniques are both valuable, ideally under ultrasound guidance. Continuous-infusion nerve blocks provide excellent analgesia for postoperative casualties during evacuation and, when properly monitored, have been shown not to increase the incidence or complications of compartment syndrome.

The pragmatic approach is to build systems around managing the severely injured patient and then adapt them to other situations when necessary.

20.9.1 Induction of Anaesthesia

RSI of anaesthesia is the accepted standard for the trauma casualty. Indications for RSI in the emergency department include:

- Casualties requiring immediate airway protection or mechanical ventilation.
- Uncontrollable agitation or Glasgow Coma Score (GCS) < 8.
- Severe uncontrollable pain.
- In cases of non-compressible haemorrhage such as intra-abdominal bleeding, RSI is usually more appropriately performed on the operating table with the casualty prepared for immediate surgery.

Prior to RSI, equipment and team preparation are paramount. A trained anaesthetic assistant should be available and ideally a second clinician whose role is to administer drugs and to monitor vital signs. A team member should be designated to perform thoracostomy should a tension pneumothorax become evident. In the event of cervical spine control being necessary, any cervical collar should be opened or removed and replaced with manual in-line stabilization by another team member. All equipment should be checked daily and again prior to casualty arrival. The minimum equipment immediately available includes:

- Self-inflating bag and correctly sized facemask
- Two sizes of laryngoscope (MAC 3 and 4 for adults)
- Appropriately sized endotracheal tubes
- Failed/difficult intubation equipment
- Bougie
- Oropharyngeal and nasopharyngeal airways
- Laryngeal mask airway (ideally second generation, e.g., ProSeal® and iGel®)
- Alternative laryngoscope (e.g., AirTraq® and Glidescope®, if available)
- Surgical airway equipment
- Working suction
- Monitoring including end-tidal CO_2, electrocardiogram (ECG), non-invasive blood pressure (NIBP), and SpO_2

Choice of induction agent(s) is not prescriptive. The aim is to preserve cardiac output as far as possible. For this reason, most military anaesthesiologists favour ketamine (1–2 mg/kg) in major trauma. In the most severely injured, a lower dose than that suggested may be required. The choice of muscle relaxant in RSI has long been suxamethonium (1.5 mg/kg), by virtue of its rapid onset and offset. An alternative to this is rocuronium (1.2 mg/kg), which provides good intubating conditions within 60 seconds. The much longer time to offset a neuromuscular blockade is argued as advantageous should the need for a surgical airway arise. Rocuronium is also the drug of choice for RSI in cases of hyperkalaemia, burns older than 24 hours, and spinal cord injuries older than 10 days. Immediate reversal is with sugammadex 16 mg/kg. This may not be available in the deployed environment.

Extreme care should be taken with RSI in hypovolaemic casualties. Severe hypovolaemia should be corrected prior to induction to avoid the risk of a pulseless electrical activity (PEA) cardiac arrest. The aim of resuscitation should be to achieve a normal blood pressure in controlled haemorrhage and a palpable radial pulse in uncontrolled haemorrhage. If immediate RSI is required, the dose of induction agent should be reduced accordingly. Ventilation should be established, minimizing the respiratory rate (e.g., 6 bpm) and airway pressures (avoid positive end expiratory pressure [PEEP]).

20.9.2 Maintenance of Anaesthesia

Anaesthesia can be maintained initially by use of intravenous agents. This is particularly useful if induction has taken place in the emergency department and further imaging is needed, or if there is a delay prior to transfer to the operating theatre.

Fentanyl (1–2 μg/kg initially) is used as an adjunct to blood product resuscitation by virtue of its effect as a sympatholytic countering the extreme vasoconstriction seen in extreme hypovolaemia. This permits further volume resuscitation and avoids rebound hypertension. Further doses are titrated during DCR/DCS up to 15 μg/kg.

Midazolam (0.02–0.05 mg/kg initially) can be used to maintain anaesthesia immediately following RSI in addition to fentanyl. Further boluses of 0.02 mg/kg can be titrated to anaesthetic effect. Anaesthesia for surgery is usually maintained with a volatile agent. In ongoing hypovolaemia, volatile use should be carefully titrated along with fentanyl according to physiological parameters. An alternative to volatile anaesthesia is total intravenous anaesthesia (TIVA). In its simplest form, this could be bolus administration of ketamine for short cases. Syringe drivers are now in common use and allow for a variety of TIVA drugs to be used.

Epidural anaesthesia is usually not undertaken in the most austere environments. This is due to difficulty in ensuring a consistently sterile environment for safe catheter placement, as well as the requirement for specialist equipment and the need for trained staff to escort in evacuation. In the mature deployment with a robust logistical and evacuation chain, epidural placement may be considered.

Spinal anaesthesia is a common technique in developing countries where there may be a lack of trained anaesthesia practitioners; the risk of airway complications associated with general anaesthesia can thus be avoided. Placement of a spinal block in the shocked casualty leads to catastrophic hypotension from loss of sympathetic tone. Spinal anaesthesia should be avoided in this situation. In patients where spinal anaesthesia may be appropriate, the risks of infection from placement in the field may outweigh any benefits.

20.10 CRITICAL CARE

(See also Chapter 17.)

If DCR/DCS is going to be the norm for the far-forward surgeon, a critical care capability must be a part of the forward surgical team structure. Postoperative priorities must therefore be optimization of haemodynamic status, rewarming, control of coagulopathy, pain relief, and preparation for return to the operating theatre or evacuation, depending on the situation.

20.11 TRANSLATING MILITARY EXPERIENCE TO CIVILIAN TRAUMA CARE[22–24]

Six aspects of military trauma care have been identified as contributing to recent good outcomes for patients wounded in combat.

20.11.1 Leadership

Current military trauma care systems are delivered by consultants. The deployed military hospital is led by a clinical director (or equivalent) with overall responsibility for all the clinical functions of the hospital, including triage, admission, decisions to operate, and discharge. Unlike a civilian hospital administrator, the clinical director has daily hands-on oversight of individual patient care, coordinating the team of hospital clinicians.

20.11.2 Front-End Processes

The treatment of patients wounded by military weapons is fundamentally geared towards the concept of damage control. Correction of deranged physiology is recognized as a greater priority than definitive anatomical repair. In addition, the key hospital infrastructure (emergency department, operating room, CT scanner, and ICU) is planned around the needs of the time-critical patient, ensuring that all key components are close to each other.

20.11.3 Common Training

The common military training model (from first aid to multidisciplinary field hospital simulation) facilitates effective teamworking and delivery of appropriate human and other resources at the right time for wounded patients.

20.11.4 Governance

Military trauma systems operate a robust and diligent framework that, through a vigorous review of injury data, clinical processes, and patients' outcomes, provides feedback to improve system performance.

20.11.5 Rehabilitation Services

Formal, dedicated rehabilitation specialists and facilities are recognized as being fundamental to favourable long-term outcomes.

20.11.6 Translational Research

Integrated basic and clinical research streams feed rapid improvements in all aspects of care to clinicians, and these improvements can then be introduced into clinical care.

20.12 SUMMARY

Geopolitical shifts have re-focussed the priorities for military planners, and surgical doctrines also must adapt to the emerging scenarios of future conflict. The latter include peer-on-peer conflict as well as asymmetric warfare set in low-density, dispersed battlefields; highly mobile operations, with extended lines of evacuation and logistic supply; the prospects of large and untreated populations of civilian wounded; and the possibility of chemical, biological, radiological, and

nuclear attack. All of these necessitate the retention of surgical adaptability and resourcefulness, as well as technical skill.

In summary, in the operational setting, resources are more limited, and the word 'finite' should underpin all clinical decision-making. Triage and intervention may be modified by an open or closed back door, or by open skies. Environmental protection is minimal when compared with civilian structures. Surgery must be tailored, taking into consideration operational realities. Procedures such as simple burr holes, evacuation of a retro-orbital haematoma compressing the optic nerve, damage control thoracotomy and laparotomy, shunting of vascular injuries, fasciotomies, and, above all, the extent of debridement required must be readily executable and within the skill set of a forward-deployed general surgeon.

The concentration of severely wounded patients in the hands of well-resourced, motivated clinicians provides the impetus for advances in the surgical and perioperative critical care of the wounded. Each mission will bring a new set of technical and personal challenges.

REFERENCES AND RECOMMENDED READING

References

1. Nessen SC, Gurney J, Rasmussen TE, Cap AP, Mann-Salinas E, Le TD, et al. Unrealized potential of the US military battlefield trauma system: DOW rate is higher in Iraq and Afghanistan than in Vietnam, but CFR and KIA rate are lower. *J Trauma Acute Care Surg.* 2018 Jul;**85(1S Suppl 2)**:S4–S12. doi: 10.1097/TA.0000000000001969.
2. Cannon JW, Holena DN, Geng Z, Stewart IJ, Huang Y, Yang W, et al. Comprehensive analysis of combat casualty outcomes in US service members from the beginning of World War II to the end of Operation Enduring Freedom. *J Trauma Acute Care Surg.* 2020 Aug;**89(2S Suppl 2)**:S8–S15. doi: 10.1097/TA.0000000000002789.
3. Smith R. *The Utility of Force: The Art of War in the Modern World.* Allen Lane. 2005.
4. Number of amputees in Ukraine. *Agence France-Presse (AFP).* 2023. https://apnews.com/article/ukraine-russia-war-amputees-wounded-soldiers-e2c5c47ea4b-8326d980e630d3df87b77 (accessed October 2023).
5. Landmines sown in the Ukraine. BBC News. https://www.bbc.com/news/world-europe-65204053 (accessed October 2023).

6. Mabry RL, Holcomb JB, Baker AM, Cloonan CC, Uhorchak JM, Perkins DE, et al. United States Army Rangers in Somalia: an analysis of combat casualties on an urban battlefield. *J Trauma*. 2000 Sep;**49(3)**:515–28.

7. iCasualties.org. Casualty Reports. Deaths in Iraq and Afghanistan. Available from: http://icasualties.org (accessed online August 2023). Hardaway RM III. Vietnam wound analysis. *J Trauma* 1978 Sept; **18(9)**: 635–42.

8. Webster S, Barnard EBG, Smith JE, Marsden MER, Wright C. Killed in action (KIA): an analysis of military personnel who died of their injuries before reaching a definitive medical treatment facility in Afghanistan (2004–2014). *BMJ Military Health*. 2021 Apr;**167(2)**:84–88. doi: 10.1136/bmjmilitary-2020-001490. Epub 2020 Jun 2.

9. Cannon JW, Hofmann LJ, Glasgow SC, Potter BK, Rodriguez CJ, Cancio LC, et al. Dismounted complex blast injuries: a comprehensive review of the modern combat experience. *J Am Coll Surg*. 2016 Oct;**223(4)**:652–64.e8. doi: 10.1016/j.jamcollsurg.2016.07.009. Epub 2016 Jul 30.

10. SALT mass casualty triage: concept endorsed by the American College of Emergency Physicians, American College of Surgeons Committee on Trauma, American Trauma Society, National Association of EMS Physicians, National Disaster Life Support Education Consortium, and State and Territorial Injury Prevention Directors Association. Disaster Med Public Health Prep. 2008 Dec;2(4):245–6. doi: 10.1097/DMP.0b013e31818d191e.

11. Ingalls N, Zonies D, Bailey JA, Martin K, Iddins BO, Carlton BK, et al. A review of the first 10 years of critical care aeromedical transport during operation Iraqi freedom and operation enduring freedom: the importance of evacuation timing. *JAMA Surg*. 2014;**149(8)**:807–13. doi: 10.1001/jamasurg.2014.621.

12. Apodaca AN, Morrison JJ, Spott MA, Lira JJ, Bailey J, Eastridge BJ, et al. Improvements in the hemodynamic stability of combat casualties during en route care. *Shock*. 2013 Jul;**40(1)**:5–10. doi: 10.1097/SHK.0b013e31829793d7.

13. Holcomb JB. Damage control resuscitation. *J Trauma*. 2007 Jun;**62(6 Suppl)**:S36–S37. doi: 10.1097/TA.0b013e3180654134.

14. Joint Trauma System Clinical Practice Guideline. https://jts.health.mil/index.cfm/PI_CPGs/cpgs (accessed online August 2023).

15. Cooper BR, Mahoney PF, Hodgetts TJ, Mellor A. Intraosseous access (EZ-IO) for resuscitation: UK military combat experience. *J R Army Med Corps*. 2007 Dec; **153(4)**:314–6.

16. Holcomb JB, Helling TS, Hirshberg A. Military, civilian, and rural application of the damage control philosophy. *Mil Med*. 2001 Jun;**166(6)**:490–317.

17. Rotondo MF, Zonies DH. The damage control sequence and underlying logic. *Surg Clin North Am*. 1997 Aug;**77(4)**:761–77. Review.

18. Granchi TS, Liscum KR. The logistics of damage control. *Surg Clin North Am*. 1997 Aug;**77(4)**:921–8. doi: 10.1016/s0039-6109(05)70594-6.

19. Stark TR, Davidson NL, Cannon JW, Polk TM, Shackelford SA, Stallings JD, et al. Battlefield Pain Research Steering Committee and Panel Discussion Members*. Battlefield pain summit 2022: expert consensus statements. *J Trauma Acute Care Surg*. 2022 Aug 1;**93(2S Suppl 1)**:S12–S15. doi: 10.1097/TA.0000000000003711. Epub 2022 Jun 2.

20. Clifford JL, Fowler M, Hansen JJ, Cheppudira B, Nyland JE, Salas MM, et al. State of the science review: advances in pain management in wounded service members over a decade at war. *J Trauma Acute Care Surg*. 2014 Sep;**77(3 Suppl 2)**:S208–36. doi: 10.1097/TA.0000000000000403.

21. Fisher AD, Rippee B, Shehan H, Conklin C, Mabry RL. Prehospital analgesia with ketamine for combat wounds: a case series. *J Spec Oper Med*. 2014 Winter;**14(4)**:11–7. doi: 10.55460/BO8F-KYQT.

22. Beekley AC, Starnes BW, Sebesta JA. Lessons learned from modern military surgery. *Surg Clin North Am*. 2007 Feb;**87(1)**:157–194, vii. doi: 10.1016/j.suc.2006.09.008.

23. Caterson EJ, Carty MJ, Weaver MJ, Holt EF. Boston bombings: a surgical view of lessons learned from combat casualty care and the applicability to Boston's terrorist attack. *J Craniofac Surg*. 2013 Jul; **24(4)**:1061–7. doi: 10.1097/SCS.0b013e31829ff967.

24. Dubose J, Rodriguez C, Martin M, Nunez T, Dorlac W, King et al. Preparing the surgeon for war: present practices of US, UK, and Canadian militaries and future directions for the US military. *J Trauma Acute Care Surg*. 2012 Dec;**73(6 Suppl 5)**:S423–30. doi: 10.1097/TA.0b013e3182754636. Review.

Recommended Reading

American College of Surgeons Military Clinical Readiness Curriculum https://www.facs.org/for-medical-professionals/education/programs/military-clinical-readiness-curriculum/ (accessed October 2023).

Battlefield Advanced Trauma Life Support BATLS. *J R Army Med Corps* Available from https://militaryhealth.bmj.com/content/jramc/146/2/110.full.pdf (accessed October 2023).

Bono R, Thomas RW, Peacock T, Cubano M, Elster E, Gurney J, et al. Eds. *Emergency War Surgery*. 5th Edn. U.S. Department of Defence. 2018. The Borden Institute.

Giannou C, Baldan M. *War Surgery: Working with Limited Resources in Armed Conflict and Other Situations of Violence*. War Surgery Vol. 1 & 2. ICRC Publication 2009 ref. 0973. Geneva: International Committee of the Red Cross.

Butler FK Jr, Hagmann JH, Richards DT. Tactical management of urban warfare casualties in special operations. *Mil Med.* 2000 Apr;**165**(**4 Suppl**):1–48.

Calderbank P, Woolley T, Mercer S, Schrager J, Kazel M, Bree S, et al. Doctor on board? What is the optimal skill-mix in military pre-hospital care? *Emerg Med J.* 2011 Oct;**28**(**10**): 882–3. doi: 10.1136/emj.2010.097642.

Cannon JW, Holena DN, Geng Z, Stewart IJ, Huang Y, Yang WY, et al. Comprehensive analysis of combat casualty outcomes in US service members from the beginning of World War II to the end of Operation Enduring Freedom. *J Trauma Acute Care Surg.* 2020 Aug;**89**(**2S Suppl 2**):S8–S15. doi: 10.1097/TA.0000000000002789.

Coupland RM. *War Wounds of Limbs: Surgical Management*. Butterworth Heinemann, Oxford. 2000.

Coupland R, Molde A, Navein J. *Care in the Field for Victims of Weapons of War*. International Committee of the Red Cross, Geneva. 2001.

Defence and Veterans Pain Management Initiative. *The Military Advanced Regional Anesthesia and Analgesia Handbook.* Available from ARAPMI which stands for Army Regional Anaesthesia & Pain Management Initiative, now Defense & Veterans Center for Integrative Pain Management (DVCIPM). https://www.dvcipm.org/ (accessed October 2023).

Department of the Army. *War Surgery in Afghanistan and Iraq: A Series of Cases, 2003–2007.* Textbooks of Military Medicine. Department of the Army, Washington DC USA. 2008.

Dufour D, Kromann Jensen S, Owen-Smith M, et al. *Surgery for Victims of War*. 3rd Edn. International Committee of the Red Cross, Geneva. 1998.

Greenfield RA, Brown BR, Hutchins JB, Iandolo JJ, Jackson R, Slater LN, et al. Microbiological, biological, and chemical weapons of warfare and terrorism. *Am J Med Sci.* 2002 Jun;**323**(**6**):326–40. Review. doi: 10.1097/00000441-200206000-00005.

Holcomb JB, McMullin NR, Pearse L, Caruso J, Wade CE, Oetjen-Gerdes L, Champion HR. Causes of death in US Special Operations Forces in the global war on terrorism: 2001–2004. *Ann Surg.* 2007 Jun;**245**(**6**):986–91. doi: 10.1097/01.sla.0000259433.03754.98.

Husum H, Gilbert M, Wisborg T. *Save Lives, Save Limbs: Life Support for Victims of Mines, Wars and Accidents*. Third World Network, Penang, Malaysia. 2000.

International Committee of the Red Cross. *First Aid in Armed Conflict and Other Situations of Violence*. ICRC, Geneva. 2006.

Lounsbury DE, Brengman M, Bellamy RF, eds. *Emergency War Surgery*, Third United States Revision. Borden Institute, Washington DC USA. 2004.

North Atlantic Treaty Organisation. Allied Joint Medical Support Doctrine. AJP-4.10(A). March 2006.

North Atlantic Treaty Organization. *Emergency War Surgery NATO Handbook.* The Borden Institute, Washington DC.

Reade MC. Whose side are you on? Complexities arising from the non-combatant status of military medical personnel. *Monash Bioethics Rev.* 2023 Jan 11. Online ahead of print.

Roberts P, ed. *The British Military Surgery Pocket Book*. AC No. 12552. HMSO, London. 2004.

Santry HP, Alam HB. Fluid resuscitation: past, present, and the future. *Shock.* 2010 Mar;**33**(**3**):209–41. doi: 10.1097/SHK.0b013e3181c30f0c

Ballistics and Blast Injuries **21**

21.1 **DEFINITION**

Balista (Latin) is from *ballein* (Greek).

Ballista: A military engine used in antiquity for hurling stones and other missiles – the first catapult (see **Figure 21.1**).

Ballistics: The science of the motion of projectiles (usually from a firearm). The study of a missile's dynamics as it travels through the barrel of the firearm, its subsequent trajectory through the air, and its final complicated effect after striking the target and transferring its energy to the tissue.

Blast: An explosion. A destructive wave of highly compressed air spreading outwards from an explosion.

21.2 **THE SCIENCE**

Energy is the capacity to perform 'work'.

Every object has *potential energy* (e.g., an object before it is dropped under gravity). It is only if the object moves that this energy is realized, and it has actual *kinetic energy* (KE) based on its mass and velocity.

- Potential energy: Available energy
- Kinetic energy: Delivered energy

> *Projectiles are classified by actual energy (not velocity).*

21.2.1 **Kinetic Energy**

Every moving projectile (e.g., a bullet) has been imparted some energy; by using gunpowder to drive it from the

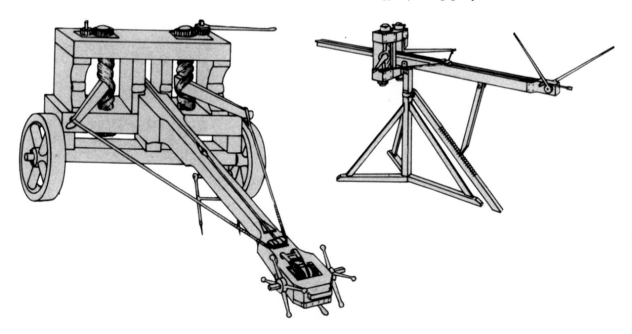

Figure 21.1 A ballista catapult.

DOI: 10.1201/9781003258124-26

barrel of a firearm. This energy, known as *kinetic energy*, is the energy of the body in motion, and it can be calculated according to this formula:

$$\textbf{Kinetic Energy}\,(\textbf{KE}) \;=\; \frac{\textbf{MV}^2}{2}$$

where *M* = mass, and *V* = velocity.

When a projectile (bullet) hits tissue (the human body), the energy is applied to the tissue. The mass of the projectile is not altered, but the resistance of the tissue to the movement causes the projectile to slow down. If the bullet stops, this implies that there is no more kinetic energy remaining (e.g., the entire energy has been imparted to the tissue).

21.2.2 **Wounding Energy**

If the bullet passes through the tissue and exits, the difference between potential energy on entrance and potential energy on leaving is known as *wounding energy*, and this is what will be imparted to the tissue and cause the damage. If the mass of the bullet is unchanged, the exit energy is determined entirely by how much the resistance of the tissue slows the bullet. Wounding energy can be calculated as follows:

$$\textbf{WE} \;=\; \frac{\textbf{Mass}\times\left(\textbf{Velocity}_{\text{entry}} - \textbf{Velocity}_{\text{exit}}\right)^2}{\textbf{Velocity}_{\text{entry}}}$$

The higher the mass of the bullet, the greater the energy. Twice the mass equates to two times the energy, but velocity is squared (twice the velocity equates to four times the energy). The bullet can be designed to deform, forming a greater cross-section and thus increasing the resistance to movement in tissue, slowing down more, and thus imparting more energy.

The ability to transfer energy is therefore based on the degree of retardation, which is dependent on:

- Velocity
- Bullet shape
- Tissue density

The effects can be:

- Direct laceration of tissue
- Displacement of tissue

- Breaking of bones
- Energy imparted to secondary fragments

21.3 **BULLETS**

Firearms ballistics is subdivided into:

- Internal ballistics
- External ballistics
- Terminal ballistics
- Wound ballistics

21.3.1 **Internal Ballistics**

This consists of a shell (usually brass) which is filled with gunpowder and the bullet. The quantity of gunpowder will determine the initial energy imparted to the bullet when it is fired from a gun. The velocity which the bullet will reach is dependent on both the mass of the bullet and the time during which the gunpowder explosion is applied – the shorter the barrel, the less time, since the bullet achieves its maximum velocity when it leaves the gun barrel.

The bullet is cylindrical. However, due to its shape, with most of the mass concentrated to the rear of the bullet, the bullet is inherently unstable, tending to wobble or tumble. To minimize this, most guns have spiral grooves or projections in their barrels to make the bullet spin, imparting stability. These imprint on the bullet, leaving a specific pattern that is unique to the weapon, which can be used to identify that specific weapon (**Figure 21.2**).

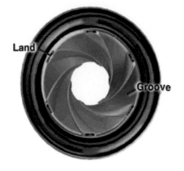 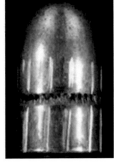

Figure 21.2 Rifling on the inside of a gun barrel, and corresponding marks on a bullet.

Pitfalls

- When retrieving a bullet from a patient, **never** handle it with metal forceps which can scratch it and destroy the pattern. Use plastic-shod (e.g., with a nasogastric tube) forceps to hold the bullet to extract it, wrap it in gauze, and store it in a bottle, labelled with the precise site from which it was removed.
- Store each bullet separately and label the position from which it was removed.
- If removing from under the skin, use local anaesthetic at least 5 cm from the bullet; otherwise, you will 'lose it' in the oedema which results, and it will no longer be palpable.
- Do **not** cut down on the bullet with a scalpel in case you groove the bullet. Cut down to one side, and then remove it laterally with shod forceps.
- Once the bullet is removed, it is critical that a *chain of custody* is begun to ensure that the bullet reaches a forensics laboratory, where it will become legal evidence.

21.3.2 **External Ballistics**

This is the study of the flight of the projectile from when it leaves the barrel until it hits a target, although bullets are inherently unstable whilst in flight (**Figure 21.3**). Once outside the gun, the bullet will in principle follow a straight line, although the bullet may rock, or even tumble, depending on the centre of gravity of the bullet.

Bullets from handguns typically used by civilians travel at about 300 m/sec.

21.3.3 **Terminal Ballistics**

The unstable movements will be exaggerated when the bullet hits the victim, or anything of a greater density (e.g., skin).

21.3.4 **Wound Ballistics**

This is what happens to the bullet when it causes wounds within the human body via:

- Dissipation of kinetic energy (slowing down due to tissue resistance)
- Damage from shock waves and cavitation
- Damage from secondary missiles
  - External (e.g., glass fragments)
  - Internal (e.g., bone fragments)
- The missile fragments themselves, if the bullet breaks up

21.3.4.1 PISTOL/LOW-ENERGY BULLETS

Different bullets can be designed for different purposes. When the bullet hits the target (victim), the bullet may have been designed to distort to offer a greater cross section in the tissue, making it slow down or stop in the body; it thereby imparts much greater energy or breaks

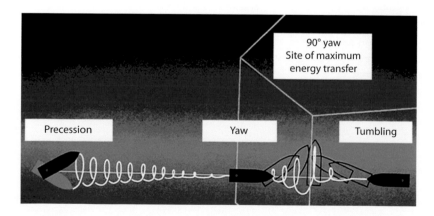

Figure 21.3 Bullets are inherently unstable: The front may 'wobble' (*precession*), the back may move (*yaw*), or the bullet may turn over (*tumble*).

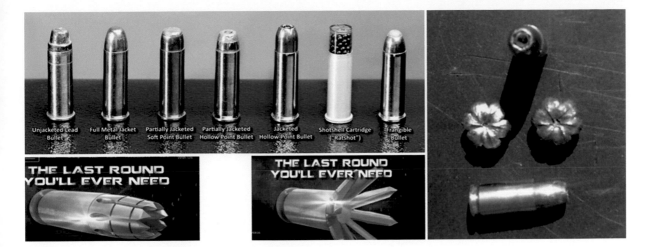

Figure 21.4 Different types of bullets and expanding bullets.

up into multiple lighter fragments which will remain in tissue, slowing completely, so that the entire energy is dissipated (**Figure 21.4**). (This is the principle of anti-hijacking frangible rounds used in the aircraft industry, so that neither the aircraft nor other passengers are impacted.)

The effects of both fragments and bullets on tissue (**Figure 21.5**) may be:

- Mechanical effects.
  - Breaking up of the bullet (frangible bullets).
  - Bullet hitting bone, causing:
    - Primary fragments of bone.
    - Secondary injuries by bone fragment being driven through organs or skin.

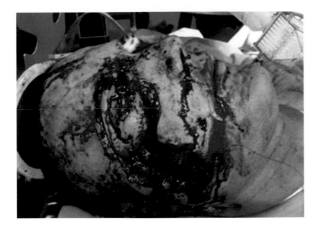

Figure 21.5 Facial injury, shattering maxilla, showing wounds due to secondary bony fragments from the maxilla expelled through the skin.

- The associated shock wave causes 'bursting' of solid organs such as the liver.

Pitfalls

- **Always** mark all wounds with a radiopaque material before X-ray. This will enable you to look at trajectory (one hole and internal bullet, or two wounds showing the bullet track). Items such as paper clips or vitamin E tablets are radiopaque. (Do not use electrocardiogram [ECG] dots, which can mimic small metal projectiles.)
- Never decide which is entrance or exit. You will be wrong half the time, and simply confuse the legal investigation. Leave that to the crime scene investigators!
- Count the bullet holes.
  - One hole = bullet is still inside. Look for it (may be tangential).
  - Two holes = In and out **or** two retained bullets. The holes and the bullets should add up to an even number. If they do not, there may be an unidentified bullet in the body.
- **Never** put your fingers into a wound. There may be razor-sharp remnants of bullet casing, or bone fragments.
- Bullets are generally 'clean' – although not sterile. The wounds are contaminated not by the bullet, but by skin surface contamination, clothing, or debris which may be pulled in. (See Section 21.3.5: 'Antibiotics'.)
- Do **not** suture bullet wounds closed (except sometimes on the face for haemostasis). Allow free drainage and an absorbent dressing.

- Bullets tend to maintain stability for some centimetres after impact; initiation of the yaw cycle produces a temporary cavity along the distal part of the track.
- High-'velocity' projectiles do not necessarily produce high-energy-transfer wounds.
- Small entry wounds and small exit wounds do **not** imply low energy transfer internally.

21.3.4.2 RIFLE/HIGH-ENERGY BULLETS

Rifle bullets have a much larger load, and often a much lighter bullet. The rifle bullet travels at approximately 3× the speed of a pistol bullet (about 800–900 m/sec, or > 2–3× the speed of sound), which implies up to nine times the energy available. As such, there is a shock wave ahead of the bullet (similar to the bow wave of a boat). This displaces the tissue ahead of the bullet, forming a moving temporary cavity containing a vacuum (the tissue is blown aside). All tissue affected by the shock wave will sustain damage, resulting from the high energy imparted by the bullet. There is wide dispersion of contaminants (**Figure 21.6**).

There is a vacuum from the dynamic temporary cavity behind the bullet, which has the effect of sucking in surface debris. If the bullet is unstable enough to turn over, the effect of the shock wave is magnified due to the increased resistance which results.

Pitfalls

- Damage control policies apply to all high-energy wounds.
- Irrigate all such wounds with a copious lavage of normal saline.

21.3.5 **Antibiotics**

Although for lower-energy wounds, antibiotics are not always required, if in doubt, prophylaxis is appropriate. Antibiotics are **not** a substitute for good wound toilet, including irrigation of a bullet track using intravenous (IV) drip tubing.

21.3.5.1 BACTERIAL CONTAMINATION – GENERAL: GRAM-NEGATIVE COVER

- *Streptococcus* spp.
- *Clostridium* spp.

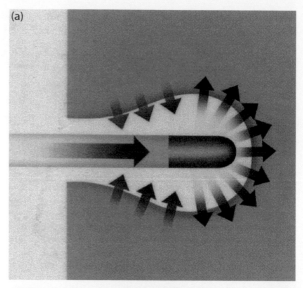

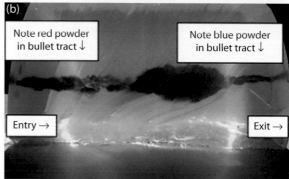

Figure 21.6 Bullet effects in tissue. (a) Bullet forming a temporary cavity. (b) Gelatine block, which has the same density as muscle, used for simulation. Small sachets of talcum powder were affixed to this block. Red is on the left, and blue on the right. Rifle bullet entry was through the sachet at left, and exit through the sachet on the right. The bullet passed through the powder. Note that the red powder has been 'sucked' along the greater length of the wound – not 'pushed' through by the bullet itself. The blue powder from the exit side has also been sucked into the wound by the vacuum. The greater cavity in the middle was caused by the unstable bullet 'turning over' in its trajectory through the gelatine.

Only a single dose of antibiotic is required. Low threshold for re-operation referes to:

- Augmentin/clavulanate 2.4 g IV
- Kefazolin 2 g IV

Note that the dose is double that of normal, due to the bruising and poorer blood supply to the wound.

21.3.5.2 BACTERIAL CONTAMINATION – ABDOMINAL CAVITY

- *Above plus Gram-negative organisms*
  Repeat up to 24 hours, or longer if contamination is present:
- Augmentin/Clavulanate 2.4 g IV
- Metronidazole 500 mg 8 hourly
- Fourth-generation cephalosporin (e.g., ceftazidime), 2 g initially, then 1 g 12 hourly

21.3.5.3 TETANUS TOXOID IF NOT PREVIOUSLY RECEIVED

21.3.6 General Treatment Principles

See the general principles for treating penetrating injury under the individual chapters.

- *Save life before limb.* Follow standard Advanced Trauma Life Support (ATLS®) principles.
- Wash all wounds, and if possible, irrigate all wound tracks. Do **not** close wounds.
- Exclude venous/arterial injury.
- Watch for compartment syndrome in limb injuries.
- Apply damage control principles for all high-energy wounds.

Casualties do not arrive with labelled wounds. Treat the wound, not the weapon.

21.4 SHOTGUN INJURIES

Shotguns fire a cartridge full of steel, lead, or plastic balls (see **Figure 21.7**). These can spread out over a wide area. The spread of the wounds is generally inversely proportional to the distance from the weapon: the farther away, the wider the spread, and the less deep the penetration (see **Figure 21.8**).

Shotguns are widely used for hunting, and sometimes for crowd control. The shotgun fires multiple pellets at low velocity. Individual pellets should not be removed, as exploration will cause damage to previously normal tissue, and the pellets can safely be left untouched (**Figure 21.9**).

Pitfalls

- Do **not** try to retrieve pellets unless they are in a joint or close to a nerve or blood vessel. You will damage more normal tissue.

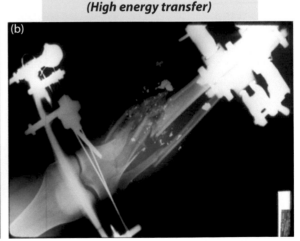

Figure 21.7 (a) Low-velocity but high-mass, high-energy injury from a shotgun. (b) High-velocity but lower-mass, high-energy long bone injuries from a rifle.

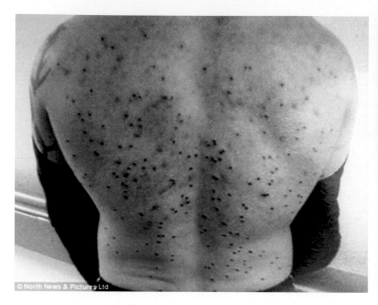

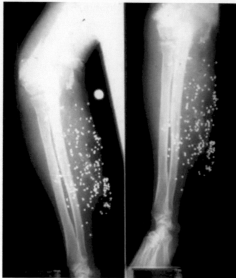

Figure 21.8 Shotgun injuries, showing multiple puncture wounds and closer-range injury of limbs.

- Pellets within a joint will react with synovial fluid and should be removed, preferably with an arthroscope.
- Injuries to the abdominal cavity should be explored – not for the pellets, but for hollow viscus holes which can be primarily repaired. It is helpful to pass the bowel through a bowl of water, and look for gas bubbles.
- Always exclude pellet emboli by X-ray of the entire body (preferable to computed tomography [CT] scan due to the 2 mm cuts necessary and consequent radiation dose). Look for a solitary pellet remote from the injury. For example, after a torso injury, a pellet in the leg implies arterial injury. A pellet in the chest implies a major venous injury – which can be treated non-operatively (**Figure 21.9**).

- If you see a 1–2 cm hole, it has been caused by the plastic pellet wad. The wad is radiolucent, but can be seen on ultrasound. **It must be removed.**

Pitfall

Although each individual pellet is low energy, the total mass of the pellets converts these wounds to a high-energy wound, and at close range, long bone fractures are common. A rifle bullet, though lower mass, can cause similar injuries due to its velocity. Bullet fragments may be left behind. It is easy to underestimate the injury. Management of both is external fixators until the wounds have stabilized.

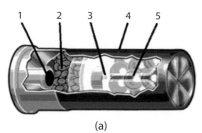

1) Primer
2) Gunpowder
3) Wad
4) Shell
5) Shot

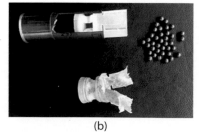

(a)

(b)

Figure 21.9 (a) Shotgun shell showing contents. (b) Note the plastic 'wad' which must be removed if in tissue.

21.5 **BLAST INJURY**

Blast injury is a physiological and anatomical insult to the human body caused by the physical properties of an explosion. The energy impulse that results from the explosion is referred to as the *blast wave*, its leading edge is the *blast front*, and the rush of hot gases caused by the explosion is the *blast wind*.

In open air, the force of a blast rapidly dissipates, but within confined spaces the blast wave is magnified by its reflection off walls, floors, and ceilings, increasing its destructive potential. Because water is less compressible than air, an underwater blast wave loses energy less quickly and so is transmitted over longer distances, being approximately three times greater in strength than that which is detonated in the air.

High-explosive blast is defined by the supersonic (1000 m/sec) blast wave it produces. Low-explosive blast waves only very rarely have sufficient energy to cause primary blast injury. Their blast wind does not energize

fragments over long distances. Survivors of low-explosive blast are commonly affected by burns. High-explosive blast survivors are rarely burnt, as if close enough to the explosion to suffer burns, the blast wave will have been fatal.

The exception is if wounded in an enclosed environment, such as a vehicle that has caught on fire, and this is the predominant wounding mechanism rather than the blast per se. The cause of injury in most survivors of high-explosive blast in an open environment is secondary (penetrating) blast.

Blast injuries are classified into five specific and distinct categories that reflect the mechanism of tissue injury. They are described in the remainder of this section (see also **Figure 21.10**).

21.5.1 **Primary Blast Injury**

The blast wave is a very highly compressed atmosphere layer driven by the blast itself and travelling at very

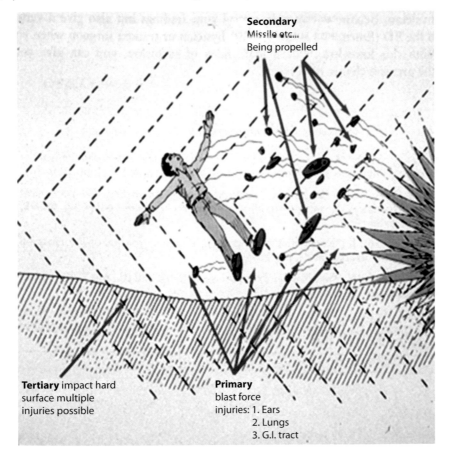

Secondary
Missile etc...
Being propelled

Tertiary impact hard surface multiple injuries possible

Primary blast force injuries: 1. Ears
2. Lungs
3. G.I. tract

Figure 21.10 Blast injuries.

high speed (> 1000 m/sec). This refers to the disruptive effects of the pressure wave as it passes from tissues of high to low density, a phenomenon known as *spalling*. Gas-enclosing organs, such as the lung, tympanic membrane (the most common injury), and bowel, are the most vulnerable.

- Generally low incidence in explosions and bombings in open spaces.
  - High overpressures required.
  - Fragments of the bomb and other debris are the principal threat.
- Higher incidence in very confined spaces.
  - Multiple high-frequency pressure loads.
- High incidence with blast weapons.
- The blast is always followed by **negative** pressure which sucks debris onto the victims; for example, falling glass from windows blown in, and then debris sucked out of the building and falling on the victims at ground level.

21.5.2 Secondary Blast Injury

These are penetrating injuries caused by projectiles energized by the blast wind.

- Fragments of the bomb itself
- Fragments and surrounding objects sucked into confined areas by the negative-pressure vacuum which follows

21.5.3 Tertiary Blast Injury

Tertiary blast injury causes blunt trauma from displacement injuries, resulting from persons or objects falling or being thrown because of the blast wave. Structural collapse or large airborne fragments lead to crush injury and extensive blunt trauma.

- Occurs when the victim is thrown out of a vehicle and strikes the ground or solid objects.
- Injuries are similar to those from blunt trauma or falls.
  - Fractures.
  - High incidence of skull fractures.
- Injuries by structural collapse.
- Crush syndrome (victims under debris).
- Hypothermia.

- Blood loss until rescued.
- Care follows blunt trauma guidelines.

21.5.4 Quaternary Blast Injury

This includes asphyxia, burns, and inhalation injuries.

- Mechanical
- Thermal
- Chemical/Biological

21.5.5 Quinary Blast Injury

This includes:

- Fragments from the bomber's or other victims' bodies transmitting human immunodeficiency virus (HIV), hepatitis C virus (HCV), and so on.
- Chemical agents (e.g., white phosphorus).
- Biologic agents.
- Radiation (radiation-enhanced explosives and 'dirty bombs').
- Fuel air explosives (FAEs).
- There is an early hyperinflammatory state defined by some texts, thought to be due to exposure to unconventional materials used in the manufacture of certain explosives.

21.5.6 Diagnosis and Management of Blast Injuries

21.5.6.1 RUPTURE OF THE TYMPANIC MEMBRANE

Eardrum rupture is a high risk, with low overpressures required (~35 kPa). There is sensorineural hearing loss with high-pitched tinnitus. Ossicular injury occurs with severe blast injury.

Pitfall

If you talk to a patient who does not respond to you, it may not be loss of awareness – it might be loss of hearing.

All explosion victims should be evaluated with an otoscopic examination (**Figure 21.11**). The orientation of the head to the blast is a major determinant of risk of tympanic membrane rupture. Small perforations

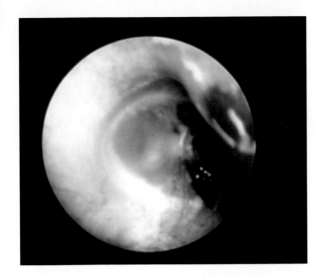

Figure 21.11 Rupture of eardrum after blast injury.

typically heal within 8 weeks, and treatment should be expectant, with topical antibiotics and steroids. Surgical repair can be considered if healing has not occurred after 8 weeks. Some studies have reported a high (30%) incidence of permanent high-frequency hearing loss 1 year after injury. Not a marker for lung injuries.

21.5.6.2 BLAST LUNG INJURY (BLI)

This may be immediately lethal or present a pattern like blunt trauma, with pulmonary contusion, often without rib fractures or chest wall injury. The earliest sign of blast lung injury is systemic arterial oxygen desaturation, often in the absence of other symptoms.

Radiological features can range from a typical 'butterfly pattern' in the capillary-dense hilar regions on the chest radiograph, to more extensive opacification of the entire lung fields (**Figure 21.12**). Management is principally supportive. Mechanical ventilation and effective chest drainage form the mainstay of treatment. High-peak inspiratory pressures should be avoided to decrease the chance of iatrogenic pulmonary barotrauma.

Use of steroids and pro-/anticoagulant medications has been attempted with no comparative evidence of benefit.

21.5.6.3 INTRA-ABDOMINAL INJURIES

Primary blast injury to the gastrointestinal tract is rare. The characteristic bowel lesion is a mural haematoma, ranging in severity from a minor submucosal haemorrhage to full-thickness disruption and perforation. The ileocaecal junction and colon are the most commonly affected sites, and delayed perforation can occur. Pneumoperitoneum alone may be a non-specific sign only associated with bowel perforation in less than 50% of the patients.

Rupture of solid organs has been observed in the absence of other mechanisms of injury. Management should be in accordance with the principles of damage control. Diagnostic peritoneal lavage can be difficult to interpret because of the high incidence of retroperitoneal and mesenteric haematoma. Patients can also develop haematemesis or melaena without obvious intraperitoneal involvement due to mucosal and submucosal haemorrhage.

Colonoscopy is not recommended because of the risk of perforation.

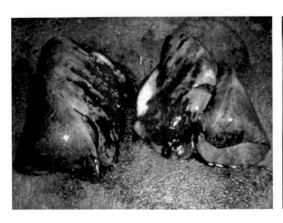

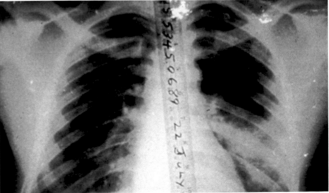

Figure 21.12 Blast lung.

21.5.6.4 OTHER INJURIES

- Transfer of kinetic energy from the blast wave to the eye can result in rupture of the globe, serous retinitis, and hyphaema. Ophthalmology consultation should be obtained.
- The most common blast-induced arrhythmias, in addition to bradycardia, are premature ventricular contractions and asystole. The treating physician should be aware that haemorrhaging, explosion-injured patients may not have the expected compensatory tachycardia and may become hypotensive without rapid resuscitation.
- Traumatic amputations from primary blast injury are uncommon. It is controversial as to whether the blast wave alone can be the cause.
- Primary blast injury can also result in cranial fractures around air-filled sinuses, and focal neurological deficits as a result of air embolism. There are data supporting the concept of blast-induced brain injury, with psychological as well as physical symptoms.
- Blast-related mild traumatic brain injury has been recognized as common in many survivors, with features including disorientation, impaired immediate memory, reduced concentration, and delayed recall. Several screening tests have been developed including the Military Acute Concussion Evaluation (MACE 2) Review – 2021. No treatment has been found effective in comparative trials; a key feature of management includes reducing the risk of repeat re-exposure to blast or other head injury.
- Blast injury is associated with apoptosis or programmed cell death. This results in delayed death of tissues and mandates recurrent debridement of tissue until there is no further necrosis. Apoptosis can result in delayed manifestation of brain injury and injury to other tissues.

21.5.6.5 EXTREMITY INJURIES

- **Initial casualty care by victim or buddies (Figure 21.13)**
  - Controlling catastrophic haemorrhage
  - Combat application tourniquet (CAT). More than one may be required.

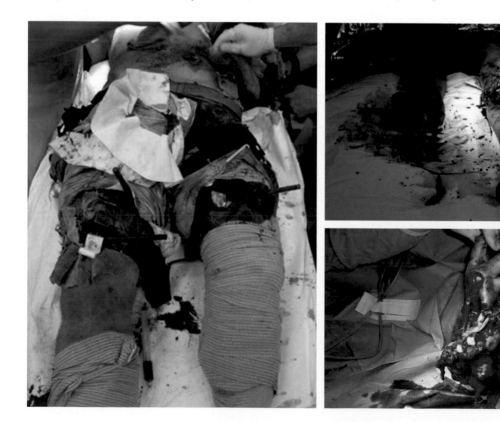

Figure 21.13 Blast injuries with amputation (note the combat application tourniquets).

Pitfall

It is critical to note the time of application of the CAT on the small white tab, because total ischaemic time is critical.

- Direct pressure
- Haemostatic agents
- Pelvic binder
- Vascular access/intraosseous (IO)
- Splint limbs
- Air evacuation
- **Communication, preparation, organization, and leadership**
- **Resuscitation (damage control resuscitation [DCR])**
  - Haemostatic resuscitation
  - Massive transfusion protocol (MTP)
  - Goal-directed stasis
  - Normothermia
- **Investigation**
  - Focussed assessment with sonography for trauma (FAST)
  - X-rays
- **Urgent surgery (damage control surgery [DCS])**
  - Damage control
  - Open wound care, delayed closure
  - Circulatory repair
  - Wide-spectrum antibiotics in therapeutic dosage
  - *Fractures*: Extra-focal immobilization, intra-focal antibiosis

- *Compartment syndrome*: Urgent fasciotomy
- Amputations

An amputation may be definitive treatment and is not an admission of failure or despair.

21.5.6.6 WHITE PHOSPHORUS

White phosphorus ignites spontaneously in oxygen. It produces white, dense, intense smoke (**Figure 21.14a**).

- Used in tracer ammunition or dropped as a weapon against civilians
- Asphyxiation in enclosed places
- Embeds in clothing/tissue (**Figure 21.14b**)
- Continues to burn in oxygen

21.5.6.6.1 Management

White phosphorus burns spontaneously in oxygen. Occlude oxygen with multiple layers of gauze, or by placing underwater. It dissolves in the fat of the skin, causing deep burns. Excise the phosphorus, and place in a sealed bottle for disposal. Treat the major burns caused in a conventional fashion.

21.5.7 Summary

- Work as a team (of surgeons and motivated allied professionals).
- Use damage control resuscitation and surgery.
- Provide optimal analgesia – **from the beginning**.

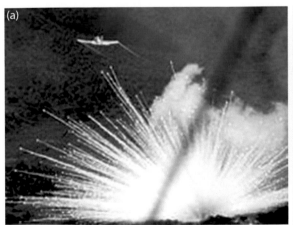
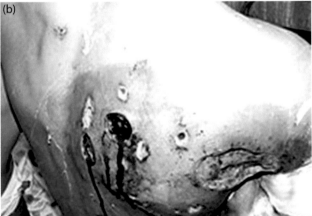

Figure 21.14 White phosphorus (a) explosion and (b) injuries.

- Leave the abdomen open – but close early.
- Use a binder and a plastic mesh.
- Do not hesitate to have early help if it is felt to be needed.

RECOMMENDED READING

Ballistics: History, mechanisms, ballistic protection, and casualty management

Mahoney PF, Ryan JM, Brooks AJ, Schwab CW. *Ballistic Trauma: A Practical Guide*. 2nd Edn. Springer Verlag, London. 2005.

Ryan J. *Ballistic Trauma: Clinical Relevance in Peace and War*. Arnold, London. 1997.

Volgas DA, Stannard JP, Alonso JE. Ballistics: a primer for the surgeon. *Injury*. 2005 Mar;**36(3)**:373–9. Review. doi: 10.1016/j.injury.2004.08.037.

Blast injury

Cannon JW, Hofmann LJ, Glasgow SC, et al. Dismounted complex blast injuries: a comprehensive review of the modern combat experience. *J Am Coll Surg*. 2016 Oct;**223(4)**:652–664.e8. doi: 10.1016/j.jamcollsurg.2016.07.009. Epub 2016 Jul 30. PMID: 27481095.

Champion HR, Holcomb JB, Young LA. Injuries from explosions: physics, biophysics, pathology, and required research focus. *J Trauma*. 2009 May;**66(5)**:1468–77; discussion 1477. doi: 10.1097/TA.0b013e3181a27e7f. Review.

Supplement on the management of blast injury. *J R Army Med Corps*. 2013;**159**.

DePalma RG, Burris DG, Champion HR, Hodgson MJ. Blast injuries. *N Engl J Med*. 2005 Mar 31;**352(13)**:1335–42. doi: 10.1056/NEJMra042083.

Ritenour AE, Baskin TW. Primary blast injury: update on diagnosis and treatment. *Crit Care Med*. 2008 Jul;**36(7 Suppl)**:S311–7. doi: 10.1097/CCM.0b013e31817e2a8c.

The Military Acute Concussion Evaluation, Revision 2 (MACE 2) available in PDF format can be downloaded from the Traumatic Brain Injury Center of Excellence (TBICoE). https://www.health.mil/Military-Health-Topics/Centers-of-Excellence/Traumatic-Brain-Injury-Center-of-Excellence www.health.mil/TBICoE (accessed online October 2023).

The MACE 2 in PDF format can be downloaded from the TBICoE website, www.health.mil/TBICoE (accessed online October 2023).

Psychology of Trauma **22**

> *And even in our sleep, pain which cannot forget, falls drop by drop upon the heart, until in our own despair, against our will, comes wisdom through the awful grace of God.*
>
> **Aeschylus (456 BC)**
>
> **The quotation was later inscribed on a memorial at the gravesite of Robert F. Kennedy.**[1]
>
> *Unless suffering is the direct and immediate object of life, our existence must entirely fail of its aim.*
>
> **Arthur Schopenhauer (1851)**
>
> *Was mich nicht umbringt, macht mich starker.*
> *What does not kill me makes me stronger.*
>
> **Friedrich Nietzsche (1888)**

22.1 DEFINITION

A definition of psychological trauma is provided by the *Diagnostic and Statistical Manual of Mental Health*, fifth edition (DSM-5):

> *Actual or threatened injury or death when the emotional response includes fear, helplessness, or horror.*

This results in an overwhelming amount of stress exceeding an individual's ability to cope.

With improved data and further study, in part from combat experience gained in modern conflicts, an emotional response is no longer required in the definition published in the DSM-5 (American Psychiatric Association, 2022) (2013), because it is recognized that emotions at the time of trauma are not predictive of later distress or of subsequent mental health pathologies.

The experience of a traumatic event will not only affect the patient, but also have an impact on all the individuals who are connected to the patient's ongoing experience. These individuals include the patient's support system (relatives, friends, and community), and the rescue workers and medical multidisciplinary team (MDT) in the hospital who are involved in the patient's care.

22.2 REACTIONS TO TRAUMA

Within 24 hours of the event, patients may begin to experience a number of common reactions affecting their thoughts (cognitive), feelings (emotional), body, and behaviour. However, over the next few days, weeks, or even months, the patient will continue to experience various reactions to the trauma. There is a bio-psycho-social impact on an individual following a trauma. Some of the responses in each of these areas include, but are not limited to, the following.

22.2.1 Biological: The Physiological Impact

- **Physical**
  - Irregularities in appetite and sleep patterns
  - Gastric issues

DOI: 10.1201/9781003258124-27

- Panic attacks
- Headaches
- Muscle tension
- Difficulty breathing
- Elevated heart rate

22.2.2 Psychological: The Mental, Emotional, and Behavioural Impact

- **Cognitive**
  - Difficulty concentrating
  - Difficulties with short-term memory loss/recall
  - Recurrent dreams, nightmares, or flashbacks
  - Mentally replaying/reconstructing the event
  - Questioning personal belief systems
  - Trying to make sense of the event
- **Emotional**
  - A sense of helplessness and/or hopelessness
  - Feeling numb or disconnected
  - Low mood/depression/guilt
  - Anger, frustration, or irritability
  - Experiencing fear
  - Negativity
  - Guilt
  - Anxiety
  - Blunted affect (no fluctuation in mood)
  - Anhedonia (inability to experience pleasure in normally pleasurable acts)

- **Behavioural**
  - Hypervigilance
  - Easily startled
  - Tearful
  - Aggressive or emotional outbursts
  - Avoidance of people, places, and discussions associated with the event
  - Disinhibited
  - Impulsivity
  - Endangering oneself or others

22.2.3 Social

This encompasses changes in relationships/interactions with the environment and other people.

Psychiatrist Elisabeth Kübler-Ross's well-known framework, originally describing the emotional grief response to bereavement, applies equally well to any form of personal crisis such as trauma (see **Figure 22.1**).[2]

Each person will experience a trauma in their own unique way; thus, how they react to that trauma will also be unique. Therefore, their reactions may vary in intensity and duration. It is important to note that these are normal reactions to the abnormal event. The following aspects influence how an individual will react to a trauma:

- Gender
- Age
- Culture

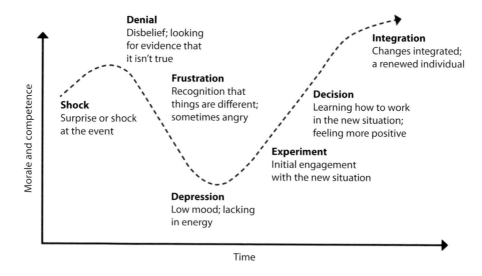

Figure 22.1 The Kübler-Ross grief cycle on death and dying.

Source: Kübler-Ross E. (1969). On Death and Dying. New York: McMillan.

- Religion
- Socioeconomic group
- Level of education
- Living conditions
- Access to resources
- Relationship dynamics
- Number of dependents
- Profession
- Level of knowledge about the situation
- Past trauma experiences
- Past psychiatric diagnoses
- Current life stressors
- Level of insight
- Coping mechanisms
- Availability of support systems

The large majority of individuals respond to a profound threat with normative activity and behaviour in an acute transient disturbance characterized in three domains:

- Reminders of the exposure, such as reliving the event, flashbacks, and intrusive thoughts
- Activation, such as hyperarousal, anger, impulsivity, and agitation
- Deactivation phenomena, such as avoidance, withdrawal, dissociation, and derealization

Responses in these three areas are self-limiting, and in general produce little functional impairment over time. A significant minority respond in a similar but more profound way through the three domains but with a longer-term outlook, often accompanied with significant functional impairment. This abnormal response has been validated and codified as post-traumatic stress disorder (PTSD), which is described as a persistent abnormal (or pathological) adaptation of the normal neurobiological systems in response to witnessed trauma.

Some of these aspects result in some individuals being at greater risk for developing sustained and long-term reactions to a traumatic event, such as depression and generalized anxiety.

If the trauma also involved loss, the above reactions will also be accompanied by grief reactions. Loss may include death of a loved one, or a person not connected to the patient but who was involved in the same traumatic event.

Loss also relates to changes in physical functionality, such as the amputation of any body part or loss of mobility (paraplegia or quadriplegia), sight, speech, and so on, including loss of an expected future: this means that, as a result of their injury or loss, there may be changes related to future life events/milestones, employment, financial circumstances, status, and so on.

The five stages of grief were outlined by Kübler-Ross; this model suggests that we go through five distinct stages of grief after experiencing a loss: denial, anger, bargaining, depression, and finally acceptance. These stages are not always experienced in this order and may be repeated; the duration of each stage is determined by the individual's ability to process the experience and move forward.

22.3 **POST-TRAUMATIC STRESS DISORDER**[3]

PTSD is a serious and potentially debilitating mental condition triggered by being exposed to a trauma. Symptoms are intense, invasive, and extreme, and may include distress, physical reactions (nausea, sweating, heart racing), flashbacks, nightmares, anxiety, and depression lasting for greater than one month following the traumatic event.

In order to diagnose PTSD, the patient needs to meet certain criteria outlined by the DSM-5.

The DSM-5 divides the symptoms experienced by the patient that are the result of the traumatic event into four categories. Each of these categories has a number of related symptoms:

- Intrusion of thoughts
- Avoidance of thoughts and behaviours
- Negative changes in thoughts and mood
- Changes in arousal and reactivity

According to the DSM-5, the following criteria must be met in order to diagnose a patient with PTSD:

- Exposure to a traumatic event
- One (or more) intrusion symptom(s)
- One (or more) symptom(s) of avoidance
- Two (or more) symptoms of negative changes in feelings and mood
- Two (or more) symptoms of changes in arousal or reactivity

These symptoms must:

- Last for longer than one month
- Bring about considerable distress and/or interfere greatly with a number of different areas of life
- Not be due to a medical condition or substance use

Healthcare professionals often look out for symptoms of PTSD, but as outlined in the DSM-5, the symptoms must include symptoms from each of the four categories and be present for more than a month for a diagnosis of PTSD to be made. However, acute stress disorder shares many of the same symptoms as PTSD, but not all of them, and not always one or more from each category; and these may only be present for 3 days to one month.

22.4 TRAUMA AND THE INTENSIVE CARE UNIT (ICU)[4]

Patients who were physically injured through a traumatic event and are thus admitted to hospital are experiencing psychological distress not only due to the initial event but also from the current environment and the medical treatment they are receiving. Being in the ICU, the patient will experience a number of things, such as undergoing medical procedures, sleep disturbance, delirium, pain, and the general chaos of an ICU environment (many people coming and going, seeing other patients suffering from their own injuries, distressed family members, resuscitation of patients, death, etc.). The patient is already psychologically vulnerable due to having experienced a trauma, so this environment could exacerbate or add to their current level of psychological distress. Some patients may not feel the impact of the ICU experience immediately, as they are too sick or heavily medicated, but as they begin to recover physically, they may become more distressed mentally and emotionally. The psychological impact of the ICU may only become apparent when the patient is in the ward, after being discharged from hospital, or even weeks, months, or years after discharge.

Contributing factors to the patients' psychological distress and frustration whilst in ICU may include: reduced physical functioning resulting from injuries, unforeseen complications in their recovery resulting in additional procedures or a longer recovery period than initially anticipated, the medication being administered having additional side effects, slow progress of healing, a long hospital stay, the prospect of many months of physical rehabilitation, the inability to remember the events of the initial trauma due to the injury, not knowing what has happened or is happening to the other people who were in the same incident, as well as seeing their distressed loved ones when they come to visit. Furthermore, the occurrence of bizarre hallucinations (which may be auditory, visual, or tactile) and delusions in ICU ('ICU psychosis') is a terrifying experience and can cause the patient to be extremely upset, aggressive, paranoid, and uncooperative, sometimes even violent. This may last for just 24 hours or for weeks. Not only does it impact the patient, but it has a significant impact on their loved ones and the medical team treating the patient.

22.5 THE CLINICAL PSYCHOLOGIST

22.5.1 The Role of the Clinical Psychologist in Trauma

The clinical psychologist will assist in identifying, treating, and where possible preventing the occurrence of the psychological aspects of trauma for the patient, their support system, and the medical team.

22.5.1.1 FOR THE PATIENT

The psychologist will:

- Identify/diagnose, treat, and potentially prevent psychological disorders.
- Identify other complications that may hinder the patient's ability to heal (substance abuse, family dynamics, personality traits, pre-existing psychiatric conditions).
- Offer psychological support (orientation, containment, acknowledgement, and normalization of situation).
- Debriefing of incident and ICU environment.
- Provide psycho-education on the ICU process, trauma, recovery, and the mental/emotional/social aspects of the experience.
- Teach and develop coping mechanisms/strategies to deal with the shock of waking up in ICU, being ventilated, processing the initial event, and managing ongoing trauma in ICU and throughout the recovery process, even after the patient is discharged from hospital/rehabilitation.
- Motivate patients to be compliant with other disciplines (physiotherapists, dietician, etc.).
- Help the patient to accept physical changes and process losses.
- Assist the patient to be able to contemplate their future and reintegration back into their life.
- Conduct grief counselling.
- If the patient is still ventilated or unable to speak due to the nature of their injury, the psychologist will establish a method of communication. This is often done in conjunction with the speech therapist and/or occupational therapist.

22.5.1.2 **FOR THE SUPPORT SYSTEM**

The patient has their own support system which consists of family, friends, and community. The psychologist will begin assisting the support system from day one of the patient's hospital admission. It is even more important to do so if the patient is unconscious. The psychologist will:

- Teach family-centred collaborative decision-making.
- Manage family dynamics.
- Debriefing of the incident, ICU environment, and appearance of the patient.
- Provide psycho-education on the ICU process, trauma, patient recovery, and the mental/emotional/social aspects of the experience.
- Teach coping mechanisms to deal with the many facets of this experience.
- Teach the family skills that help them to support the patient mentally and emotionally.
- Assist family self-care to ensure that they are also taking care of themselves through the stressful event and after discharge.
- Conduct grief counselling.

22.5.1.2.1 Visitors

Visitors are important for the patient's well-being; however, it is important to realize that the patient's support system experiences symptoms of compassion fatigue, anxiety, depression, and PTSD as well. This may at times have a negative influence on the patient, their recovery, and the MDT.

22.5.1.2.2 Relatives

The patients' relatives have experienced a shock and are seeing their loved one being so critically ill for days, weeks, or even months in ICU, with every day being an emotional struggle. The family members are scared, and they feel helpless and very overwhelmed; many of them do not have effective coping mechanisms to manage the enormity of this experience. They too are experiencing a trauma, as described in the definition of trauma in Section 22.1, even if they were not a part of the initial traumatic event.

The patient's support system will often experience symptoms of compassion fatigue, anxiety, depression, and PTSD. This can at times be extremely overprotective or overbearing to the point of disruption in the patient's care by the MDT and could be due to the need to help 'fix' the situation and make their loved one feel better and in so doing make themselves feel better.

The psychologist is sometimes needed to assist with mediation between the support system and the MDT or between the patient and their support system.

22.5.1.3 **FOR THE TEAM**

The psychologist will be available to assist all the members of the MDT.

- Promote development of skills so they can assist in psychological well-being of the patient.
- Provide training to reinforce the psychological support required.
- Encourage communication with patients and family members.
- Inspire a multidisciplinary approach to patient care.
- Offer debriefing, as team members are constantly exposed to trauma, death, and psychological stressors.
- Assist in helping them take care of themselves mentally/emotionally and socially.
- Provide mediation between team members, or with the patient or with the patient's support system.

22.6 **WHEN TO CALL THE CLINICAL PSYCHOLOGIST**

No matter what the physical injury, every patient admitted to the ICU should be referred to the clinical psychologist. Some of the interventions will overlap with the trauma counsellors and the social worker, all of whom are trained to assist the patient and their family through the trauma experience.

Based on their ongoing assessment of the patient and in consultation with the primary physician/surgeon, the psychologist will determine the length of therapy and type of intervention.

Early intervention can assist the patient to recover more quickly, both physically and emotionally, as well as limit new psychological disorders. **Patients should be referred within 48 hours of admission**.

For those patients who are ventilated and sedated, the psychologist will begin working with the family. Once the patient's sedation is lifted, the psychologist will begin assessing and subsequently treating the patient. It is not necessary to wait for the patient to be weaned from the ventilator, become distressed, or personally request psychological assistance before intervening. All trauma patients can benefit from some form of psychological intervention, as it assists them to manage the mental and emotional impacts of the situation, whilst also providing an outlet for their thoughts and feelings. Invariably, the patient is often more compliant when working with the MDT.

22.7 SUMMARY

There is no single approach that can improve teams and individuals to be resilient in the surgical setting, but a multidimensional approach is required which includes considerations of individual factors, organizational or work-related factors, and most importantly social and cultural factors.

In the absence of any formal curriculum for developing non-technical 'soft' skills in trauma team training (see Chapter 2 on non-technical skills), a distillation of the literature would suggest clinical and support staff alike should focus on developing protective factors in themselves and across teams which include personal individual factors, aspects of professional practice, and organizational and socio-cultural considerations. Designing formal workshops and informal engagements which draw together a strong cultural and team identity, and delivering organizationally and culturally appropriate post-deployment activities, would appear to be effective interventions.

REFERENCES AND RECOMMENDED READING

References

1. U.S. Senator Robert F. Kennedy used this quote on the night of the assassination of Rev. Martin Luther King, Jr. in 1968, remembering the assassination of his own brother President John F Kennedy in 1963. https://www.youtube.com/watch?v=3j2p6P5eSP0 (accessed September 2023). The quotation was later inscribed on a memorial at the gravesite of Robert F. Kennedy.
2. Kübler-Ross E. On Death & Dying – What the dying have to teach Doctors, Nurses, Clergy & Their Own Families. 1969. Scribner Classics.
3. Javidi H, Yadollahie M. Post-traumatic stress disorder. *Int J Occup Environ Med*. 2012 Jan;**3**(1):2–9.
4. Dannenfeldt G. The psychological aspects of intensive care units. *Curationis*. 2182;Sep;**5**(3):27–31. doi: 10.4102/curationis.v5i3.425.
5. Welker M. ICU Psychosis. 2022. https://www.medicinenet.com/icu_psychosis/article.htm (accessed September 2022).

Recommended Reading

American Psychiatric Association. Diagnostic And Statistical Manual Of Mental Disorders, Fifth Edition, Text Revision (DSM-5-TR). Published online March 2022 https://doi.org/10.1176/appi.books. 9780890425787; https://doi.org/10.1176/appi.books.9780890425596 (PDF)

American Psychological Association (APA) Handbooks in Psychology. https://www.apa.org/pubs/books/handbooks (accessed August 2023).

APA Handbook of Trauma Psychology: Cook JM, Gold SN Eds. Volume 1. Foundations in Knowledge; Volume 2. Trauma Practice (this two-volume handbook provides a survey of major areas and subtopics of empirical knowledge and practical applications in the field of trauma psychology.) Available from https://www.apa.org/pubs/books/4311531 (accessed August 2023).

Hibbert C. Understanding & Coping with Loss and Trauma. 2023. https://www.drchristinahibbert.com/understanding-and-coping-with-loss-and-trauma/ (accessed September 2023).

Kübler-Ross E. *Encountering Death and Dying*. Worth, Richard. Chelsea House Publishers, Philadelphia. 2005. ISBN0-7910-8027-7.

Physical and Rehabilitation **23**
Medicine (P&RM)

23.1 **DEFINITION**

This speciality is known as *physiatry* in the United States, or *P&RM* elsewhere. This is a medical speciality which treats the injured patient following acute trauma to restore function and work towards reintegration of the patient into all spheres of social and occupational life. The terms are often used to describe the whole medical team caring for the patient, not only the doctor.

23.2 **THE REHABILITATION 'TEAM'**

Just as the concept in trauma resuscitation of the 'team' is well established as per Advanced Trauma Life Support (ATLS®) principles, a similar concept applies to the rehabilitation process. The team members will include a doctor, physiotherapist, occupational therapist, speech therapist, social worker, dietician, psychologist, vocational therapist (a subspeciality of occupational therapy), and possibly recreational therapist. The type of therapy each patient receives is determined according to their injury and physical needs, and is a team decision following a full assessment.

23.3 **REHABILITATION STARTS IN THE ICU**

Ideally, the rehabilitation of all trauma patients should commence in the intensive care unit (ICU), especially once the patient is reasonably physiologically stable. *Physiotherapy* is critical in the ICU setting for respiratory function as well as joint mobility to prevent contractures. *Occupational therapy*, particularly for hand and upper limb function, should also commence, and is essential

in the management of burn patients. The *speech therapist* can assist in the ICU if the patient is unable to swallow, and can formally evaluate the swallowing to advise, for example, whether a percutaneous gastrostomy (PEG) is required if swallowing is neurologically impaired. A video swallow examination is the ideal investigation in a cooperative patient to fully assess the swallowing function. The *dietician* can work closely with the speech therapist, advising the type of diet to maintain optimal nutrition during the ICU stay. Within a few days post-injury, a patient will develop malnutrition, requiring anticipation by the clinician, as this will impact wound healing, raise the risk of pressure injury, and increase the risk of wound sepsis. Many trauma patients develop a paralytic ileus, and this will need prokinetics as well as careful nutritional support. *Social worker* intervention in the ICU is invaluable to identify premorbid social issues and liaise with the *psychologist* to provide support and treatment for both the patient and the family members. Many patients benefit from early intervention with antidepressant medication commenced in intensive care. The role of the *doctor* is to minimize secondary disability and guide the trauma team regarding specific functional impairments such as bladder and bowel function. Acidification of the urine, using ascorbic acid (vitamin C) or cranberry juice, may be helpful in minimizing urinary tract infections. In spinal cord injury (SCI), urodynamic studies will be performed only after the 'spinal shock' phase of the injury, and this will guide long-term management of bladder function. For SCI patients, it is critical to ensure regular functioning of the bowel with the use of laxatives, especially as higher spinal injuries (above T6) are prone to autonomic dysreflexia with constipation.

The doctor can advise as to where the patient should be transferred, post ICU, to continue rehabilitation. Traumatic brain injury (TBI) patients who are unable

DOI: 10.1201/9781003258124-28

to follow commands or respond to therapy may require initial treatment post ICU in a sub-acute unit and continual assessment to evaluate their readiness for acute rehabilitation therapy. Medical stability is important, although the need for subsequent surgery (e.g., orthopaedic, or reconstructive plastic surgery) should not delay the process of commencing rehabilitation. It is essential that the acute care surgeons communicate their future surgical plans to allow for preparation of the patient whilst in a rehabilitation facility.

Specific issues which require resolution prior to transfer for acute rehabilitation include establishment of a colostomy if required. If the patient is likely to be a long-term wheelchair user, consideration should include siting the colostomy higher up on the abdominal wall for ease of patient access and maintenance.

> **Nursing care in the ICU to prevent pressure injuries is critical, as they can delay the whole process of acute rehabilitation and result in extremely high costs for funders, patients, and their families.**

A restless patient is not usually the one at high risk, but rather the immobilized patient for example in traction or on a ventilator. An occipital injury is a scar for life, with no hair growth.

Medical management in the ICU will directly affect the medical care in the rehabilitation facility. For example, management of pain with drugs containing codeine results in dependency and chronic constipation. The use of a pain scale when administering analgesia is essential in the cooperative patient. Poorly controlled pain impacts the patient negatively and affects the ability of the patient to participate in the rehabilitation process. This includes post-concussion headaches which cause significant morbidity in TBI patients. SCI patients and amputees experience neuropathic pain, and many centres have clear guidelines for treatment of this common complication. Treatment and education of both the patient and the family should commence as soon as the patient develops symptoms.

23.4 OUTCOMES-BASED REHABILITATION (OBR)

OBR is the common method for continual monitoring and assessment of the progress of the rehabilitation patient and the setting of individualized goals for various aspects of the therapy as well as social and psychological goals which all aim to reintegrate the patient into their home, community, and work environment. The assessment covers physical as well as cognitive goals and is based on the anticipated outcomes of all the rehabilitation therapies.[1] OBR uses a variety of standardized tools to achieve this.

23.4.1 FIM/FAM Assessment[2,3]

One of the commonest tools used is the FIM/FAM assessment (Functional Independence Measure and Functional Assessment Measure). See Appendix B.5.1.

The 18-item Functional Independence Measure (FIM) is a global measure of disability that is widely used internationally to measure outcomes from rehabilitation. However, its predominant focus is on motor function, providing scant coverage of cognition and communication, which are often the main factors that limit function following severe brain injury.

The UK Functional Assessment Measure (FAM) was designed to address this shortcoming.

- It does not stand alone but adds 12 items to the FIM that primarily address cognitive and psychosocial function.
- Hence the acronym for the combined 30-item UK Function Assessment Measure is the 'UK FIM+FAM'.
- The FIM+FAM "Splat' Radar diagram provides a graphic representation and is used to compare progress between admission and discharge, **Figure 23.1**.
  - The 30 scale items are arranged as spokes of a wheel. Scoring levels from 1 (total dependence) to 7 (total independence) run from the centre outwards. Thus, a perfect score would be demonstrated as a large circle.
  - The yellow shaded portion represents the median scores on admission for each item.
  - The blue-shaded area represents the change in median score from admission to discharge. (See **Figure 23.1**).

23.4.2 Glasgow Outcome Scale[4]

Specific to TBI is the Glasgow Outcome Score (GOS). This divides patients into five categories and assists in the prediction of longer-term outcomes in rehabilitation. See **Table 23.1** and Appendix B.5.2.

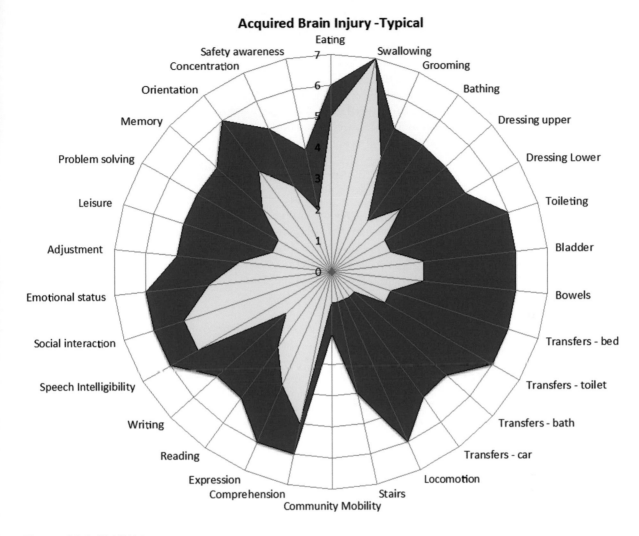

Figure 23.1 FIM/FAM

Table 23.1 Glasgow Outcome Scale (GOS)		
Outcome Parameters		
1. Low disability (Good recovery)	GR	Light damage with minor neurological and psychological deficits.
2. Moderate disability	MD	No need for assistance in everyday life, employment is possible but may require special equipment.
3. Permanent Severe disability	PVS	Severe injury with permanent help with daily living
4. Persistent vegetative state	SD	Severe damage with prolonged state of unresponsiveness and a lack of higher mental functions.
5. Death	D	Severe injury or death without recovery of consciousness

23.4.3 Rancho Los Amigos Scale[5]

The Rancho Los Amigos Scale of Cognitive Functioning,[4] developed in a rehabilitation centre of the same name in California, is a graded scale assessing TBI patients with closed injury on a score of 1 to 10, based on cognition and behaviour (see **Table 23.2**). This can be used in combination with the OBR assessment tools and assists the family members to understand the stages of recovery in TBI.

23.4.4 International Classification of Functioning, Disability and Health (ICF)[6]

The ICF is a classification of health and health-related domains. As the functioning and disability of an individual occur in a context, ICF also includes a list of environmental factors. ICF is the World Health Organisation (WHO) framework for measuring health and disability at both individual and population levels.

23.5 WORLD HEALTH ORGANISATION INITIATIVES

23.5.1 World Rehabilitation Alliance[7]

In May 2023, the World Health Assembly endorsed a resolution creating the World Rehabilitation Alliance, expanding and integrating rehabilitation in health systems as part of universal health coverage (UHC), emphasizing the importance of rehabilitation in primary care and as part of emergency preparedness and response.

The importance of rehabilitation as a strategy for healthy ageing was noted. There is a major unmet need for rehabilitation from a range of health conditions including from communicable and noncommunicable diseases and injuries. There was an overwhelming emphasis that rehabilitation should be available to the whole population and should be integrated into health planning and implementation.

23.5.2 Rehabilitation 2030[8]

The Rehabilitation 2030 initiative (started in 2017) draws attention to the profound unmet need for rehabilitation worldwide and highlights the importance of strengthening health systems to provide rehabilitation. The initiative marks a new strategic approach for the global rehabilitation community by emphasizing that:

- Rehabilitation should be available for all the population and through all stages of the life course.
- Efforts to strengthen rehabilitation should be directed towards supporting the health system as a whole and integrating rehabilitation into all levels of healthcare.
- Rehabilitation is an essential health service and crucial for achieving UHC.

With ageing populations, and an increase in the number of people living with chronic disease, rehabilitation is a priority health strategy for the 21st century that uniquely contributes to optimizing the functioning of the population.

Table 23.2 Rancho Los Amigos Scale

Level	Definitions	
Level I	*No response*:	Total assistance
Level II	*Generalized response*:	Total assistance
Level III	*Localized response*:	Total assistance
Level IV	*Confused/Agitated*:	Maximal assistance
Level V	*Confused/Inappropriately non-agitated*:	Maximal assistance
Level VI	*Confused/Appropriate*:	Moderate assistance
Level VII	*Automatic, appropriate*:	Minimal assistance for daily living skills
Level VIII	*Purposeful, appropriate*:	Stand-by assistance
Level IX	*Purposeful, appropriate*:	Stand-by assistance on request
Level X	*Purposeful, appropriate*:	Modified independent

23.6 **SUMMARY**

In general terms, following trauma, most patients admitted to an acute rehabilitation facility will be dependent for all or some of their needs. The goal of physical rehabilitation is to maximize independence for each patient in terms of activities of daily living (ADLs). Most acute rehabilitation facilities will accept patients with tracheostomy tubes, PEG tubes, and intravenous (IV) lines. Tracheostomy patients should be carefully reviewed prior to transfer for rehabilitation, and efforts made to replace with a fenestrated tube, to encourage communication. Ventilated patients are accepted by some units; however, the ability of the patient to follow an intensive therapy program may be curtailed if the patient is ventilator dependent.

Recent technological developments for use in the rehabilitation of patients, such as the Lokomat® (Hocoma, Zurich, Switzerland) and Exoskeleton, are becoming more widespread and available in rehabilitation facilities and are used in SCIs and TBIs.

Rehabilitation in a dedicated and suitable facility with access to a variety of supplies and equipment is the continuation of the acute trauma care for the patient and is essential for reintegration of each trauma patient into home, community, and workplace.

Pitfalls

- Failure to refer early, before muscle wasting or contractures develop.
- Failure to communicate on weight-bearing status.
- Early psychological counselling is an integral part of physical rehabilitation.
- Intensive care medication is not always congruent with good rehabilitation therapy.

REFERENCES AND RECOMMENDED READING

References

1. Landrum PK, Schmidt ND, McLean A. *Outcome-oriented Rehabilitation: Principles, Strategies, and Tools for Effective Program Management*. Aspen Publishers Inc., Gaithersburg, Maryland. 1995.

2. UK Functional Assessment Measure (UK FIM+FAM): Cicely Saunders Institute of Palliative Care, Policy & Rehabilitation, Florence Nightingale Faculty of Nursing, Midwifery & Palliative Care, Kings College London. https://www.kcl.ac.uk/cicelysaunders/resources/toolkits/fimfam-overview (accessed online January 2024).

3. Wright J. The Functional Assessment Measure. (2000). The Center for Outcome Measurement in Brain Injury. http://www.tbims.org/combi/FAM (accessed online August 2023).

4. Jennett B, Bond M. Assessment of outcome after severe brain damage. *Lancet*. 1975 Mar 1;**1**(**7905**):480–4. doi: 10.1016/s0140-6736(75)92830-5.

5. Rancho Los Amigos National Rehabilitation Center. The Rancho Levels of Cognitive Functioning Scale (revised 1997). Available from: http://www.neuroskills.com/resources/rancho-los-amigos-revised.php (accessed online August 2023).

6. https://www.who.int/standards/classifications/international-classification-of-functioning-disability-and-health (accessed online August 2023).

7. https://www.who.int/initiatives/world-rehabilitation-alliance (accessed August 2023).

8. https://www.who.int/initiatives/rehabilitation-2030 (accessed August 2023).

Recommended Reading

Braddon's Physical Medicine and Rehabilitation. 6th Edn. David C MD ed. Elsevier. 2020. ISBN-13: 978-0323625395.

De Lisa's Physical Medicine and Rehabilitation: Principles and Practice. Walter R F ed. Lippincott Williams Wilkins/Wolters Kluwer, Philadelphia PA, USA. 2010.

ISCoS Textbook on Comprehensive Management of Spinal Cord Injuries. Harvinder Singh C ed. Wolters Kluwer, Philadelphia PA, USA. 2015.

Trauma Rehabilitation. Robinson LR ed. Lippincott Williams Wilkins/Wolters Kluwer, Philadelphia PA, USA. 2005.

Appendix A
Trauma Systems

A.1 INTRODUCTION

Care of the injured patient has been fundamental to the practice of medicine since recorded history. The word *trauma* derives from the Greek, meaning 'bodily injury'. The first trauma centres were used to care for wounded soldiers in Napoleon's armies, and the first modern trauma centre was the Birmingham Accident Hospital in the United Kingdom, which opened in 1944 in what the Queen's Hospital was then. It is most unfortunate that many trauma cases are still managed within non-existing or poorly organized trauma systems.

The lessons learned in successive military conflicts have advanced our knowledge of care of the injured patient. The Korean conflict and the Vietnam War established the concept of minimizing the time from injury to definitive care. The extension of this concept to the management of civilian trauma led to the evolution from the 1970s onwards of today's trauma systems. The Middle East and Afghan conflicts in the past two decades resulted in massive progress in the sphere of military trauma care, with significant enhancement in civilian care as well. For the first time, prospective high-quality research has taken place in the conflict situation. In civilian practice, the concepts behind trauma systems have been expanded to systems from pre-hospital care, emergency medical care, stroke care, and cardiac emergency care.

A.2 THE INCLUSIVE TRAUMA SYSTEM

In principle, a hospital that provides acute care for the severely injured patient (a trauma centre) should be a key component of a system that encompasses all aspects and phases of care, from prevention and education to pre-hospital care, acute care, definitive surgical and medical care, and continuing through to rehabilitation (**Figure A.1**). The initial trauma systems did not consider the non–trauma centre hospitals (an 'exclusive' system), where advanced trauma surgery was not often practised, even though these centres cared for most patients, including those who were less severely injured (about 85% of the total load). These hospitals are the most likely to need skills in, for example, damage control surgery. A system must be fully integrated into the emergency medical services (EMS) system and must meet the needs of all the patients requiring acute care for injury, regardless of severity of injury, geographical location, and population density. The trauma centre remains an essential component, but the system recognizes the necessity for other healthcare facilities.

The goal of the system is to match the regional needs and facilities with the resources available, the patient care loads, and the needs of the patients.

A.3 COMPONENTS OF AN INCLUSIVE TRAUMA SYSTEM

The structure of a trauma care system involves several components and providers, each of which must be adapted to a specific environment. These components and providers, graphically represented in **Figure A.2**, are:

- **Administrative components**
  - Leadership
  - System development
  - Legislation
  - Finances
- **Operational and clinical components**
- **Injury prevention and control**
- **Human resources – workforce resources**
- **Education**
- **Pre-hospital care – EMS system**
- **Ambulance and non-transporting guidelines**
  - Communications systems
  - Emergency disaster preparedness plan
- **Definitive care facilities**
  - Interfacility transfer
  - Trauma care facilities (including care for burns, electrical injury, and drowning)

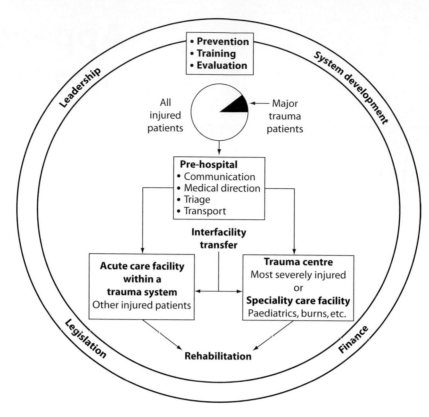

Figure A.1 The inclusive trauma system.

- Physical rehabilitation
- Long-term care for disabled patients
- **Information systems**
- **Evaluation**
- **Research**

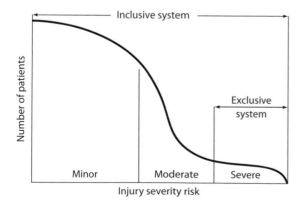

Figure A.2 The components of an inclusive trauma system.

A.3.1 **Administration**

The system requires administrative leadership, authority, planning and development, legislation, and finances. Together, these components form an outer sphere of stability that is vital for the continuation of activities directly related to patient care. The diversity of the population, as defined by the environment (urban or rural) or by special segments of the population (the young or the elderly), must be addressed by the system.

*Political will is essential to drive
the change, guided by public-health data
on outcome.*

A.3.2 **Prevention**

Prevention reduces the actual incidence of injury and is cost-efficient for the system and for society. Injury prevention is achieved through research, public education, legislation, and environmental modification.

A.3.3 **Public Education**

Public education leads to a change in behaviour (e.g., laws against driving under the influence of alcohol and, more recently, recreational drugs and drugs of abuse) to minimize injury exposure.

A.3.4 **The Healthcare System**

The system includes the proper recognition of injury as a healthcare problem, and efficient access to the EMS system. These components stimulate the necessary political and legislative activity to establish legal authority, leadership, and system changes.

The development of a system is a major challenge for any community. The concept of centralizing trauma care creates potential political and economic problems, since the normal flow of patients might be altered by trauma triage protocols. Trauma systems, by their nature, will direct the care of the most critically injured patients to a limited number of designated 'trauma centres'. The trauma system will only succeed if all parties are involved in the initial planning, development, and implementation, including those with a financial incentive (private healthcare/for-profit facilities), to avoid competition and supersession issues.

It is crucial that doctors, especially emergency physicians, surgeons, and anaesthesiologists, are involved in the system-planning process. They should help to establish standards of care for all clinical components, and participate in planning, verification, performance improvement, and system evaluation.

A.4 **MANAGEMENT OF THE INJURED PATIENT WITHIN A SYSTEM**

Once the injury has been identified, the system must ensure easy access and an appropriate response at the scene of injury. The system must assign responsibility and authority for care and triage decisions made prior to trauma centre access. Triage guidelines must be accepted by all providers and used to determine which patients require access to trauma centre care. This coordination requires direct communication between pre-hospital care providers, medical direction, and the trauma facility. Protocols at the primary care level should focus on early detection of severe injuries, initiation of resuscitation, and prompt transfer to an appropriate facility.

The trauma centre, which serves as the definitive specialized care facility, is a key component of the system, and is different from other hospitals within the system in that it acts as a lead agency and guarantees immediate availability of *all* the specialities necessary for the assessment and management of the patient with multiple injuries. These centres need to be integrated into the other components of the system to allow the best match of resources with patients' needs. The system coordinates care between all levels of the facility, so that prompt and efficient integration of hospital and resources can take place according to patient need.

Access to rehabilitation services, first in the acute care hospital and then in more specialized rehabilitation facilities, is an integral part of the total management of the patient. It is important that the patients be returned to their communities when appropriate. Community support and psychosocial services are an integral part of this overarching system.

A.5 **STEPS IN ORGANIZING A SYSTEM**

A.5.1 **Public Support**

Public support is necessary for the enabling and necessary legislation to take place. The process takes place as follows:

- Identification of the need
- Establishment of a patient database to assist with need and resource assessment
- Analysis to determine the resources available
- Resource assessment, formulated to identify the current capabilities of the system
- Highlighting of deficiencies, and formulation of solutions

A.5.2 **Legal Authority**

This is established once the need for a system has been demonstrated. Legislation will be required to establish a lead agency with strong oversight, or an advisory body composed of healthcare, public, and medical representatives. This agency will develop the criteria for the system, regulate and direct pre-hospital care, establish pre-hospital triage, ensure medical direction, designate the proper facilities to render care, establish a trauma registry, and establish performance improvement programmes.

A.5.3 Establish Criteria for Optimal Care

These must be established by the lead authority in conjunction with health and medical professionals. The adoption of system-wide standards is integral to the success of any system.

A.5.4 Designation of Trauma Centres

Development of a system requires that all the principal players be involved from the beginning. This takes place through a public process. Consideration must be given to the role of all acute care facilities within the region. Representatives from all these facilities must be involved in the planning process. There must be agreement about the minimal data that will be contributed by *all* acute care facilities. Without the data from the hospitals managing the less severely injured, the data will be incomplete, and skewed towards major injury.

The number of trauma centres should be limited to the number required (based on the established need) for the patient population at risk of major injury. Having too many trauma centres may weaken the system by diluting the workload, thus reducing the experience for training, and will unnecessarily consume resources that are not fully utilized. Having too few trauma centres will, however, overburden the system and prevent timely access. Systems in lower- and middle-income regions should be adapted to the realities of the local health systems, while aiming to increase access and level of care progressively.

A.5.5 System Evaluation

Trauma systems are complex organizational structures with evolving methods and standards of care. It is necessary to have a mechanism for ongoing evaluation, based on:

- Self-monitoring
- External evaluation

A.6 RESULTS AND STUDIES

The Skamania Conference was held in July 1998, with the purpose of evaluating the evidence regarding the efficacy of trauma systems. During the conference, the evidence was divided into three categories: that resulting from panel studies, registry comparisons, and population-based research.

A.6.1 Panel Review

An overview of panel studies was presented at the Skamania Conference. The critique of panel reviews is that they vary widely, and interrater reliability has been very low in some studies. Furthermore, autopsy results alone are inadequate, and panel studies vary regarding the process of review and the rules used to come to a final judgement. In general, all panel studies were classified as weak class III evidence. Nevertheless, MacKenzie et al.[1] concluded that when all panel studies are considered collectively, they do provide some face validity and support of the hypothesis that treatment at a trauma centre versus a non–trauma centre is associated with fewer inappropriate deaths and possibly disabilities.

A.6.2 Registry Study

Jurkovich and Mock[2] reported on the evidence provided by trauma registries in assessing overall effectiveness. They concluded that this was not class I evidence, but that it was probably better than a panel study. Their critique of trauma registries included the following six items: data are often missing, miscodings occur, there may be interrater reliability factors, the national norms are not population-based, there is less detail about the causes of death, and they do not consider pre-hospital deaths. A consensus of the participants at the Skamania Conference concluded that registry studies were better than panel studies but not as good as population studies.

A.6.3 Population-Based Studies

Populated-based studies probably also fall into class II evidence. They are not prospective randomized trials, but, because of the nature of the population-based evidence, they cover all aspects of trauma care, including pre-hospital, hospital, and rehabilitative. A critique of the population-based studies pointed out that there are a limited number of clinical variables, and it is difficult to adjust for severity of injury and physiological dysfunction. There are other problems, although these probably apply to all studies, including secular trends, observational issues, and problems with longitudinal population mortality studies. The Joanna Briggs Institute guidelines[3] suggest that, for health system research, certain interrupted time series studies are probably better than simple before–after or cohort studies, and yet these must follow pre-set rigorous guidelines.

A.7 SUMMARY

Although there are difficulties with all three types of study, each may also offer advantages to various communities and regions. All three types may also influence health policy, and all can be used pre- and post-trauma system start-up. There was consensus at the Skamania Conference that the evaluation of trauma systems should be extended to include an economic evaluation and assessment of quality-adjusted life-years. Two recent systematic reviews of the effect of trauma systems on outcome, however, could not show a clear benefit, with no studies in the lower- and middle-income regions meeting inclusion criteria when using the strict guidelines.[4,5]

REFERENCES AND RECOMMENDED READING

References

1. MacKenzie EJ, Rivara FP, Jurkovich GJ, Nathens AB, Frey KP, Egleston BL, et al. A national evaluation of the effect of trauma-center care on mortality. *N Engl J Med.* 2006 Jan;**354**(**4**):366–78. doi: 10.1056/NEJMsa052049.

2. Jurkovich GJ, Mock C. Systematic review of trauma system effectiveness based on registry comparisons. *J Trauma.* 1999 Sept;**47**(**3 Suppl**):S46–55. doi: 10.1097/00005373-199909001-00011.

3. Jordan Z, Lockwood C, Munn Z, Aromataris E. The updated Joanna Briggs Institute Model of Evidence-Based Healthcare. *Int J Evid Based Healthcare.* 2019 Mar;**17(1)**:58–71. doi: 10.1097/XEB.0000000000000155.

4. Moore L, Champion H, Tardif PA, Kuimi BL, O'Reilly G, Leppaniemi A, et al Impact of trauma system structure on injury outcomes: a systematic review and meta-analysis. *World J Surg.* 2018 May;**42(5)**:1327–39. doi: 10.1007/s00268-017-4292-0.

5. Mwandri M, Stewart B, Hardcastle TC, Rubiano AM, Gruen RL. Organized trauma systems and designated trauma centres for improving outcomes in injured patients. Cochrane Database of Systematic Reviews 2017, Issue 1. http://www.cochrane.org/CD012500/EPOC_organised-trauma-systems-and-designated-trauma-centres-improving-outcomes-injured-patients 19 January 2017. DOI: 10.1002/14651858.CD012500. (accessed online August 2023).

Recommended Reading

American College of Emergency Physicians: *Trauma Care Systems. 2018* Available from https://www.acep.org/globalas-sets/new-pdfs/policy-statements/trauma-care-systems.pdf (accessed online August 2023).

American College of Surgeons. *Resources for Optimal Care of the Injured Patient 2022.* Chicago: American College of Surgeons, https://www.facs.org/quality-programs/trauma/quality/verification-review-and-consultation-program/standards/ (accessed online August 2023).

Ciesla DJ, Kerwin AZ, Tepasa JJ III. Trauma systems, triage, and transport. In Feliciano DV, Mattox KL, Moore EE, eds. *Trauma,* 9th ed. New York, NY: McGraw Hill Education, 2022: 47–70.

Appendix B
Trauma Scores and Scoring Systems

B.1 INTRODUCTION

Estimates of the severity of injury or illness are fundamental to the practice of medicine. The earliest known medical text, the Smith Papyrus, classified injuries into three grades: treatable, contentious, and untreatable.

Modern trauma scoring methodology uses a combination of an assessment of the severity of anatomical injury with a quantification of the degree of physiological derangement to arrive at scores that correlate with clinical outcomes.

Trauma scoring systems facilitate pre-hospital triage, identify trauma patients suitable for quality assurance audit, allow an accurate comparison of different trauma populations, and organize and improve trauma systems.

In principle, scoring systems can be divided into:

- Physiological scoring systems, based on the body's response to injury
- Anatomical scoring systems, based on the physical injury that has occurred
- Scoring systems based on both anatomical injury description and physiological response
- Outcome analysis systems based on the result after recovery

B.2 PHYSIOLOGICAL SCORING SYSTEMS

B.2.1 Glasgow Coma Scale (GCS)

The GCS,[1] devised in 1974, was one of the first numerical scoring systems (**Table B.1**). The GCS has been incorporated into many later scoring systems, emphasizing the importance of head injury as a triage and prognostic indicator.

Table B.1 Glasgow Coma Scale

Parameter	Response	Score
Eye-opening	Nil	1
	To pain	2
	To speech	3
	Spontaneously	4
Motor response	Nil	1
	Extensor	2
	Flexor	3
	Withdrawal	4
	Localizing	5
	Obeys command	6
Verbal response	Nil	1
	Groans	2
	Words	3
	Confused	4
	Orientated	5

B.2.2 Paediatric Trauma Score (PTS)

The PTS (**Table B.2**)[2] has been designed to facilitate triage of children. The PTS is the sum of six scores, and values range from −6 to +12, with a PTS of 8 or less being recommended as the trigger to send the child to a trauma centre. The PTS has been shown to accurately predict risk for severe injury or mortality but is not significantly more accurate than the RTS (see Section B.2.3) and is a great deal more difficult to measure.

B.2.3 Revised Trauma Score (RTS)

Introduced by Champion et al., the RTS[3] evaluates blood pressure, the GCS, and the respiratory rate to provide a scored physiological assessment of the patient.

Table B.2 Paediatric Trauma Score (PTS)

Clinical Parameter	Category	Score
Size (kg)	> 20	2
	10–20	1
	< 10	−1
Airway	Normal	2
	Maintainable	1
	Unmaintainable	−1
Systolic blood pressure (mmHg)	> 90	2
	50–90	1
	< 50	−1
Central nervous system	Awake	2
	Obtunded/Decreased LOC	1
	Coma/decerebrate	−1
Open wound	None	2
	Minor	1
	Major/Penetrating	
Skeletal	None	2
	Closed fracture	1
	Open/Multiple fractures	−1

Note: The values for the six parameters are summed to give the overall PTS.

LOC, Level of consciousness.

Table B.3 Revised Trauma Score (RTS)

Clinical Parameter	Category	Score	× Weight
Respiratory rate (breaths per minute)	10–29	4	0.2908
	> 29	3	
	6–9	2	
	1–5	1	
	0	0	
Systolic blood pressure	> 89	4	0.7326
	76–89	3	
	50–75	2	
	1–49	1	
	0	0	
Glasgow Coma Scale score	13–15	4	0.9368
	9–12	3	
	6–8	2	
	4–5	1	
	3	0	

Note: The values for the three parameters are summed to give the triage-RTS. Weighted values are summed for the RTS.

to 7.8408 (best). The RTS is the most widely used physiological scoring system in the trauma literature.

B.2.4 Acute Physiologic and Chronic Health Evaluation II (APACHE II)[4]

The APACHE II score is used to evaluate mortality and prognosis in ICU patients.

Calculation is based on several physiological and clinical comorbidity parameters, as well as age.[5] Each parameter can score 0 points, considered as normal physiology, to a maximum of 4 points. See **Table B.4**.

Mortality interpretation is based on overall score. See **Table B.5**.

B.3 ANATOMICAL SCORING SYSTEMS

B.3.1 Abbreviated Injury Scale (AIS)

The AIS[6] is an anatomically based, consensus-derived, global severity–based scoring system that classifies each injury by body region according to its relative importance on a 6-point ordinal scale.

The RTS can be used for field triage and enables prehospital and emergency care personnel to decide which patients should receive the specialized care of a trauma unit. An RTS score of 11 or less is suggested as the triage point for patients requiring at least level 2 trauma centre status (surgical facilities, 24-hour X-ray, etc.). An RTS of 10 or less carries a mortality of up to 30%, and these patients should be moved to a level 1 institution.

The difference between a patient's RTS on arrival and best RTS after resuscitation will give a reasonably clear picture of the prognosis. By convention, the RTS on admission is the one documented.

The RTS (non-triage) is designed for retrospective outcome analysis. Weighted coefficients are used, which are derived from trauma patient populations and provide a more accurate outcome prediction than the raw RTS (**Table B.3**). Since a severe head injury carries a poorer prognosis than a severe respiratory injury, the weighting is therefore heavier. The RTS thus varies from 0 (worst)

Table B.4 APACHE II Score

Input	Measured	Measured	Points
Temperature (°C)	36–38 °C		0
	34.0–35.9 °C	38–38.5 °C	1
	32–33.9 °C	38.5–39 °C	2
	30–31.9 °C	39.0–40.9 °C	3
	≤ 29.9 °C	≥ 41 °C	4
Heart rate	70–109		0
	—	—	1
	55–69	110–139	2
	40–54	140–179	3
	< 40	≥ 180	4
Mean arterial pressure (mmHg)	70–109		0
			1
	50–69	110–129	2
		130–159	3
	≤ 49	≥ 159	4
Respiratory rate (bpm)	12 – 24		0
	10–11	25–34	1
	6–9	35–49	2
	—	—	3
	< 5	> 50	4
A-aPO$_2$ (FiO$_2$ > 50%) or PaO$_2$ (FiO$_2$ < 50%) (mmHg)	< 200 or PaO$_2$ > 70		0
	—	PaO$_2$ 61–70	1
	200–349	—	2
	350–499	PaO$_2$ 55–60	3
	> 500	PaO$_2$ < 55	4
Arterial pH or HCO$_3$ (mmol/L)	7.33–7.49/22–31.9		0
	—	7.5–7.59/32–40.9	1
	7.25–7.32/18–21.9	—	2
	7.15–7.24/15–17.9	7.6–7.69/41–51.9	3
	< 7.15 / < 15	≥ 7.7 / > 52	4
Serum Na+ (mmol/L)	130–149		0
	—	150–154	1
	120–129	155–159	2
	111–119	160–179	3
	< 110	> 180	4

(Continued)

Table B.4 (*Continued*) APACHE II Score

Input	Measured	Measured	Points
Serum K+ (mmol/L)	3.5–5.4		0
	3–3.4	5.5–5.9	1
	2.5–2.9	—	2
	—	6–6.9	3
	< 2.5	>7	4
Haematocrit (%)	30–45.9		0
	—	46–49.9	1
	20–29.9	50–59.9	2
	—	—	3
	< 20	> 60	4
White cell count (×10^3 cells / mm^3)	3–14.9		0
	—	15–19.9	1
	1–2.9	20–39.9	2
	—	—	3
	< 1	40	4
Glasgow Coma Scale	15		0
	Subtract actual GCS from 15 *Example:* GCS 9/15 = 6 points		0–15
Age (years)	≤ 44 years		0
	45–54		1
	55–64		2
	65–74		3
	> 75		4
			5
			6
Chronic health problems	None		0
	Acute renal failure		1
	Yes + elective surgery		+2
	Yes, but not postoperative		+5
	Yes + emergency surgery		+6

The AIS was developed in 1971 as a system to describe the severity of injury throughout the body. The 2015 revision (AIS 2015) is currently used.

In AIS 2015, each injury is assigned a six-digit unique numerical identifier, to the left of the decimal point. This is known as the 'pre-dot' code, and is based on:

- Body region (first digit)
- Type of anatomical structure (second digit)

Table B.5 Mortality Based on APACHE II Scores

APACHE II Score: Approximate Mortality Interpretation		
Score	Non-Operative	Postoperative
0–4	4%	1%
5–9	8%	3%
10–14	15%	7%
15–19	24%	12%
20–24	40%	30%
25–29	55%	35%
30–34	73%	73%
35–100	85%	88%

- Nature of injury (third and fourth digits)
- Level (fifth and sixth digits)
- There is an additional single digit to the right of the code (the 'post-dot' code), which is the AIS severity code. The AIS grades each injury by severity from 1 (least severe) to 5 (critical: survival uncertain). A score of 6 is given to certain injuries termed 'maximal (currently untreatable/unsurvivable)'.

The AIS manual is divided, for ease of reference, into nine different sections based on anatomy. All injuries therefore carry a unique code that can be used for classification, for indexing in trauma registry databases, and for severity.

B.3.2 **The Injury Severity Score (ISS)**

In 1974, Baker et al. created the ISS[7] to relate AIS scores to patient outcomes. ISS body regions are listed in **Table B.6**.

The ISS is calculated by summing the square of the highest AIS scores in the three most severely injured regions. ISS scores range from 1 to 75 (since the highest AIS score for any region is 5). By convention, an AIS score

Table B.6 Injury Severity Score

Number	Body Region
1	Head and neck
2	Face
3	Thorax
4	Abdomen/ Pelvic contents
5	Extremities
6	External/ Skin/ General

of 6 (defined as a non-survivable injury) for any region becomes an ISS of 75.

The ISS only considers the single most serious injury in each region, ignoring the contribution of injury to other organs within the same region. Diverse injuries may have identical ISS scores but markedly different survival probabilities (an ISS of 25 may be obtained with isolated severe head injury or by a combination of lesser injuries across different regions). In addition, the ISS does not have the power to discriminate between the impact of similarly scored injuries to different organs, and therefore cannot identify, for example, the different impact of cerebral injury over injury to other organ systems.

B.3.3 **The New Injury Severity Score (NISS)**

In response to these limitations, the ISS was modified in 1997 to become the NISS.[8] The NISS is calculated in the same way as the ISS, but takes the three most severe injuries (i.e. the three highest AIS scores, regardless of body region). The NISS is then the simple sum of the squares of these three body regions.

The NISS can predict survival outcomes better than the ISS. In a separate study, the NISS yielded better separation between patients with and without multiple organ failure and showed that the NISS is superior to the ISS in the prediction of multiple organ failure.[9] Although the proponents of the NISS proclaim its superiority, its use is not yet widespread.

B.3.4 **Anatomic Profile Score (APS)**

The APS[10] was introduced in 1990 to overcome some of the limitations of the ISS. In contrast to the ISS, the APS allows the inclusion of more than one serious body injury per region and considers the primacy of central nervous system and torso injury over other injuries. AIS scoring is used, but four values are used for injury characterization, roughly weighting the body regions. Serious trauma to the brain and spinal cord, anterior neck and chest, and all remaining injuries constitute three of the four values. The fourth value is a summary of all the remaining non-serious injuries. The APS score is the square root of the sum of the squares of all the AIS scores in a region, thus enabling the impact of multiple injuries within that region to be recognized. Component values for the four regions are summed to constitute the APS score.

A modified APS (mAPS) has recently been introduced, which is a four-number characterization of injury.

The four component scores are the maximum AIS score and the square root of the sum of the squares of all AIS values for serious injury (AIS ≥ 3) in specified body regions (**Table B.7**). This leads to an APS, the weighted sum of the four mAPS components. The coefficients are derived from logistic regression analysis of admissions to four level 1 trauma centres (the 'controlled sites') in the Major Trauma Outcome Study.

A limitation of the use of AIS-derived scores is their cost. International Classification of Disease (ICD) taxonomy is a standard used by most hospitals and other healthcare providers to classify clinical diagnoses. Computerized mapping of ICD-9CM rubrics into AIS body regions and severity values has been used to compute ISS, APS, and NISS scores. Despite limitations, ICD-to-AIS conversion has been useful in population-based evaluations when AIS scoring from medical records is not possible. Outside North America, the ICD-10 is most commonly used.

B.3.5 ICD-Based Injury Severity Score (ICISS)

Severity scoring systems also have been directly derived from ICD-coded discharge diagnoses. Most recently, the ICD-9 Severity Score (ICISS)[11] has been proposed, which is derived by multiplying survival risk ratios associated with individual ICD diagnoses. Neural networking has been employed to further improve ICISS accuracy. ICISS has been shown to be better than ISS and to outperform the Trauma and Injury Severity Score (TRISS) in identifying outcomes and resource utilization. However, mAPS, APS, and NISS appear to outperform ICISS in predicting hospital mortality.

There is some confusion over which anatomical scoring system should be used; however, currently,

NISS probably should be the system of choice for AIS-based scoring.

B.3.6 Organ Injury Scaling System[12]

Organ Injury Scaling (OIS) is a scale of anatomical injury within an organ system or body structure. The goal of OIS is to provide a common language between trauma surgeons and to facilitate research and continuing quality improvement. It is not designed to correlate with patient outcomes. The OIS tables can be found on the American Association for the Surgery of Trauma (AAST) website[12] or at the end of this appendix.

B.3.7 Penetrating Abdominal Trauma Index (PATI)

Moore and colleagues facilitated the identification of the patient at high risk of postoperative complications when they developed the PATI[13] scoring system for patients whose only source of injury was penetrating abdominal trauma. A complication risk factor was assigned to each organ system involved, and then multiplied by a severity-of-injury estimate. Each factor was given a value ranging from 1 to 5. The complication risk designation for each organ was based on the reported incidence of postoperative morbidity associated with that injury.

The severity of injury was estimated by a simple modification to the AIS, ranging from 1 = minimal injury to 5 = maximal injury. The sum of the individual organ score times the risk factor comprises the final PATI score. If the PATI score is 25 or less, the risk of complications is reduced (and where it is 10 or less, there are no complications), whereas if it is greater than 25, the risks are much higher.

In a group of 114 patients with gunshot wounds to the abdomen, Moore et al.[13] showed that a PATI score of more than 25 dramatically increased the risk of postoperative complications (46% of patients with a PATI score of over 25 developed serious postoperative complications, compared with 7% of patients with a PATI of less than 25). Further studies have validated the PATI scoring system.

B.3.8 Revised Injury Severity Classification (RISC) II

The first version of this score was derived from the German Trauma Registry DGU (TR-DGU®) in 2003,[14] and it was updated in 2014 to RISC II.[15]

Table B.7 Anatomic Profile Score

Component Definitions of the Modified Anatomic Profile Score		
Component	**Body Region**	**Abbreviated Injury Scale Severity**
mA	Head/Brain	3–6
	Spinal cord	3–6
mB	Thorax	3–6
	Front of neck	3–6
mC	All other	3–6

Note: mA, mB, and mC scores are derived by taking the square root of the sum of the squares for all injuries defined by each component.

The first version was developed and validated on 2000 patients documented between 1993 and 2000 in the TR-DGU. Eleven different data points were required from a trauma patient: NISS, head injury, pelvic injury, age, GCS, coagulation, base deficit, haemoglobin, cardiac arrest, shock, and mass transfusion. Similar as for the TRISS, the calculated score is transformed into a probability of survival $P(s)$ by the logistic function $P(s) = 1 / (1 + e^{-x})$. Comparative analyses showed that the predictive performance of the RISC was better than that of the TRISS, since it contained additional predictive variables, such as initial laboratory values on admission. The RISC has been used by the TR-DGU for outcome adjustment in interhospital comparisons and scientific analyses since 2003.

However, the original RISC also had some limitations. Missing values were partly replaced by a specific algorithm, but the number of patients who did not receive a RISC prognosis increased to more than 15% in the registry. Furthermore, observed mortality was about 2% lower than the predicted RISC prognosis. Finally, additional prognostic factors had been proposed, based on recent database analyses. Thus, in 2013, an enhanced version of the RISC was developed.[15]

The RISC II includes some well-known prognostic factors, like age and blood pressure; some variables already used in the original RISC, such as base deficit, haemoglobin, and cardiac arrest; but also new variables like gender, pre-injury ASA (American Society of Anesthesiologists) score, and pupil size and reactivity. It is also interesting to mention that the overall injury severity is no longer described as ISS or NISS, but as AIS severity level of the worst and the second worst injury (plus head injury). This also allows differentiation between isolated and multiple injuries. If the injury is an isolated one, the AIS level of the second worst injury is zero, which means that outcome prediction improves (the respective coefficient for the second worst injury is +0.2).

RISC II attempts a new concept of treating missing values, in that there is no attempt to impute a missing value; however, the values are included in the model. Thus, if a certain value is missing, it will not have any influence on the outcome prediction. This is seen in **Table B.8**, where all categories for missing values (indicated by '???') receive 0 points in the score. No missing values will be accepted for the variables which describe the injury pattern and age, because these elements were considered essential for any outcome estimation. Both variables (age and list of injuries as AIS codes) are also compulsory variables in the TR-DGU which means that

a prognostic score could be calculated for all patients in the registry.

The RISC II is based on data of 30,000 trauma cases documented in 2010 and 2011. Data from 2012 were used to validate the score. It is applied to patients with an injury of at least OIS grade 2 (thus, the ISS is at least 4 points). The components of the RISC II are listed in **Table B.8**.

Validation results and comparisons with existing scores (ISS, TRISS, and RISC) showed that RISC II not only could be applied to more patients but also has improved discrimination (area under the ROC [receiver operating characteristic] curve), precision (the predicted mortality better fits the observed one), and calibration (Hosmer–Lemeshow goodness-of-fit).[15]

B.4 COMORBIDITY SCORING SYSTEMS

There are several comorbidities which are known to affect trauma outcomes:

- Liver cirrhosis
- Chronic obstructive pulmonary disease
- Congenital coagulopathy
- Diabetes
- Congenital heart disease
- Morbid obesity

Specific comorbidity weighting is used in other disciplines (including the APACHE II); however, their use in trauma so far has not been validated.

- *Charlson comorbidity index*:[16] This is generally used in medical disciplines.
- *TRISSCOM*:[17] This adjusts the TRISS score with an age factor of 65 years, rather than the more common 55 years, and includes eight comorbidities.

B.5 OUTCOME ANALYSIS

B.5.1 Functional Independence Measure (FIM) and Functional Assessment Measure (FAM) (FIM + FAM)[18,19]

The FIM is an 18-item global measure of disability, and can be scored alone or with the additional 12 items that formulate the FAM. The FIM + FAM is designed to measure disability in the brain-injured population. It has an ordinal scoring

Table B.8 Components of RISC

Variable	Value	Coefficient	Variable	Value	Coefficient
Worst injury	AIS 3	−0.5	Sex	Female	+0.2
	AIS 4	−1.3		Male/???	0
	AIS 5	−1.7	ASA pre-trauma	1–2	+0.3
	AIS 6	−2.9		3/???	0
Second worst injury	AIS 0–2	+0.2		4	−0.3
	AIS 3	0	Mechanism	Blunt/???	0
	AIS 4	−0.6		Penetrating	−0.6
	AIS 5	−1.4	GCS motor function	Normal	+0.6
Head injury	AIS 0–2	0		Localizes/???	0
	AIS 3–4	−0.1		No localizing	−0.4
	AIS 5–6	−0.8		None	−0.8
Age	1–5	+1.4	Systolic BP on admission	< 90	−0.7
	6–10	+0.6		90–110/???	0
	11–54	0		111–150	+0.3
	55–59	−0.5		> 150	0
	60–64	−0.8	CPR	No	0
	65–69	−0.9		Yes	−1.8
	70–74	−1.2	Coagulation (INR)	< 1.2	+0.6
	75–79	−1.9		1.2–1.4	+0.2
	80–84	−2.4		1.4–2.4/???	0
	85+	−2.7		> 2.4	−0.4
Pupil reactivity	Brisk	+0.2	Blood haemoglobin (g/dL)	7.0–11.9/???	0
	Sluggish /???	0		< 7.0	−0.5
	Fixed	−1.0	Acidosis (base deficit)	< 6	+0.3
Pupil size	Normal	+0.2		6–9/???	0
	Unequal	0		9–15	−0.4
	Bilat dilated	−0.5		> 15	−1.5

Note: Coefficients of the RISC II Score: Starting with the constant value of 3.6, specific values (the coefficients) were added or subtracted, based on the observed findings, to finally give the score value. This value is then transformed into a probability of survival using the logistic function. Positive coefficients refer to an improved prognosis, while negative ones worsen the prognosis.

system of 1–7 for all 30 items, where 1 is complete dependence and 7 is complete independence. Scoring is completed at two time points, the first at 7–10 days after admission (admission score), and the second within 7 days of discharge (discharge score). See Section 23.4.1 and **Figure 23.1**.

B.5.2 **Glasgow Outcome Scale (GOS)**

For head-injured patients, the level of coma on admission or within 24 hours expressed by the GCS was found to correlate with outcome. The Glasgow Outcome Scale[20]

Table B.9 Glasgow Outcome Scale

Outcome Parameters		
1. Low disability (good recovery)	GR	Light damage with minor neurological and psychological deficits.
2. Moderate disability	MD	No need for assistance in everyday life; employment is possible but may require special equipment.
3. Severe disability	SD	Severe injury with permanent help with daily living.
4. Persistent vegetative state	PVS	Severe damage with a prolonged state of unresponsiveness and a lack of higher mental functions.
5. Death	D	Severe injury or death without recovery of consciousness.

was an attempt to quantify the outcome parameters for head-injured patients. A five-point scale was described. See **Table B.9**.

Duration as well as intensity of disability should be included in an index of ill health; this applies particularly after head injury, because many disabled survivors are young.

The grading of depth of coma and neurological signs was found to correlate strongly with outcome, but the low accuracy of individual signs limits their use in predicting outcomes for individuals (**Table B.10**).

Table B.10 Outcome Related to Signs in the First 24 Hours of Coma after Injury: Outcome Scale as Described by Glasgow Group

	Dead or Vegetative (%)	Moderate Disability or Good Recovery (%)
Pupils		
Reacting	39	50
Non-reacting	91	4
Eye movements		
Intact	33	56
Absent/bad	90	5
Motor response		
Normal	36	54
Abnormal	74	16

B.5.3 Major Trauma Outcome Study (MTOS)

In 1982, the American College of Surgeons Committee on Trauma began the ongoing Major Trauma Outcome Study, a retrospective, multicentre study of trauma epidemiology and outcomes.

The MTOS uses the TRISS methodology[21] to estimate the probability of survival, or $P(s)$, for a given trauma patient. $P(s)$ is derived according to the formula:

$$P(s) = 1/(1+e^{-b})$$

where e is Euler's constant (approximately 2.718282), and $b = b_0 + b_1(\text{RTS}) + b_2(\text{ISS}) + b_3(\text{age} > 55)$. The b coefficients are derived by regression analysis from the MTOS database (**Table B.11**).

The $P(s)$ values range from zero (survival not expected) to 1.000 for a patient with a 100% expectation of survival. Each patient's values can be plotted on a graph with ISS and RTS axes (**Figure B.1**).

The sloping line in **Figure B.1** represents patients with a probability of survival of 50%; these PRE-charts (from 'PREliminary') are provided for those with blunt versus penetrating injury, and for those above versus below 55 years of age. Survivors whose coordinates are above the $P(s)50$ isobar and non-survivors below the $P(s)50$ isobar are considered atypical (statistically unexpected), and such cases are suitable for focussed audit.

In addition to analysing individual patient outcomes, TRISS allows a comparison of a study population with the huge MTOS database. The Z-statistic identifies whether study group outcomes are significantly different from expected outcomes as predicted from the MTOS. Z is the ratio $(A - E)/S$, where A = actual number of survivors, E = expected number of survivors, and S = scale factor, to transform the value into a standard normal distribution. Z may be positive or negative, depending on whether the survival rate is greater or less than predicted by TRISS. Z-values of greater than 1.96 or less than –0.96 describe statistically significant deviation from prognosis ($P < 0.05$).

The so-called M-statistic is an injury severity match allowing a comparison of the range of injury severity in

Table B.11 Coefficients from the Major Trauma Outcome Study Database

	Blunt	Penetrating
$b_0 = -1.2470$		−0.6029
$b_1 = 0.9544$		1.1430
$b_2 = -0.0768$		−0.1516
$b_3 = -1.9052$		−2.6676

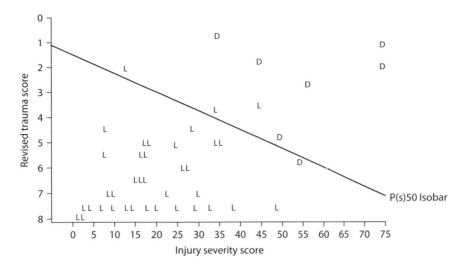

Figure B.1 PRE-chart. *Abbreviations*: D, dead; L, live; PRE, preliminary.

the sample population with that of the main database (i.e., the baseline group). The closer M is to 1, the better the match; the greater the disparity, the more biased Z will be. This bias can be misleading; for example, an institution with many patients with low-severity injuries can falsely appear to provide a better standard of care than another institution that treats a higher number of more severely injured patients.

The W-statistic, or relative outcome score, calculates the actual numbers of survivors greater (or fewer) than predicted by the MTOS, per 100 trauma patients treated. The relative outcome score can be used to compare W-values against a 'perfect outcome' of 100% survival. Thus, W could also be interpreted as the percentage of survivors above or below prediction. The relative outcome score may then be used to monitor improvements in trauma care delivery over time.

TRISS has been used in numerous studies. Its value as a predictor of survival or death has been shown to be from 75% to 90% as good as a perfect index, depending on the patient data set used.

B.5.4 **A Severity Characterization of Trauma (ASCOT)**[22,23]

ASCOT, introduced by Champion et al. in 1990, is a scoring system that uses the APS to characterize injury in place of the ISS. Different coefficients are used for blunt and penetrating injury, and the ASCOT score is derived from the formula $P(s) = 1 / (1 + e^{-k})$. The ASCOT model coefficients are shown in **Table B.12**. ASCOT

Table B.12 Coefficients Derived from Major Trauma Outcome Study Data for the ASCOT Probability of Survival, or $P(s)$

K Coefficients	Type of Injury	
	Blunt	Penetrating
K_1	−1.157	−1.135
K_2 (RTS GCS value)	0.7705	1.0626
K_3 (RTS SBP value)	0.6583	0.3638
K_4 (RTS RR value)	0.281	0.3332
K_5 (APS head region value)	−0.3002	−0.3702
K_6 (APS thoracic region value)	−0.1961	−0.2053
K_7 (APS other serious injury value)	−0.2086	−0.3188
K_8 (Age factor)	−0.6355	−0.8365

APS, Anatomic Profile Score
ASCOT, A Severity Characterization of Trauma
GCS, Glasgow Coma Scale
RR, respiratory rate
RTS, Revised Trauma Score
SBP, systolic blood pressure

has been shown to outperform TRISS, particularly for penetrating injury.

B.6 **COMPARISON OF TRAUMA SCORING SYSTEMS**

Table B.13 presents a comparison of trauma scoring systems.

Table B.13 Comparison of Trauma Scoring Systems

Scoring System	Year	Predicts What?	How Calculated?	Score Range/ Interpretation	Benefits	Limitations
Physiological Scoring Systems						
GCS	1977	Brain function and patient survival	Based on higher cerebral response to stimulation (eyes, motor, and verbal)	Range from 3/15 (no or minimal neurological function) to 15/15 (normal or near-normal neurological function)	Simple and easy to calculate	The best available score needs to be used; otherwise, scale is inaccurate.
PTS	1988	Facilitates triage Measure of mortality risk	Sum of six physiological scores	Range from 2 (best) to –1 (worst)	Used as a trigger to refer a child to a trauma centre	Not widely used
RTS	1989	Patient survival		Range from 0 (severe physiological derangement) to 7.84 (no physiological derangement)	Provides physiological assessment of the patient High association with mortality. Superior to TRISS and ISS in predicting mortality in the ICU.	Incubation and sedation prior to arrival alter accuracy.
APACHE-II	1985	Patient survival and disease severity	Based on the worst 12 routine physiological measurements in the first 24 hours of ICU admission, as well as age and chronic health conditions	Range from 0 (very low risk of mortality) to 71 (very high risk of mortality). Scores of greater than 15 are considered moderate to severe risk.	Superior to TRISS and ISS in predicting mortality in the ICU. Generally, now web-based entry and calculation.	ICU specific. Use limited by missing data. Time-consuming and complex to calculate.
Anatomical Scoring Systems						
AIS	1971	Patient survival			Developed to classify severity of injury, but validated to measure probability of death.	Does not predict functional impairment.

(Continued)

Table B.13 (*Continued*) Comparison of Trauma Scoring Systems

Scoring System	Year	Predicts What?	How Calculated?	Score Range/ Interpretation	Benefits	Limitations
ISS	1974	Patient survival	Body divided into six anatomical regions, each of which is given a score. Highest three scores are squared and summed.	44 possible scores, ranging from 1 (less severe) to 75 (unsurvivable).	Most widely used trauma severity score. Relates AIS to patient outcomes.	No physiological predictors. Does not account for more than one injury in the same region. Complex.
NISS	1997	Patient survival	Sum of the squares of the three most severe AIS severities, regardless of body region.	Same as for ISS.	Addresses multiple occurrences of serious injury within body region. Slight predictive advantage over ISS and ICISS.	Not widely used. Complex.
APS	1990	Patient survival	Three 'modified components' are scored based on AIS and weighted to form a single APS.	Range varies. Higher numbers have worse prognosis.	Based on location and severity of trauma.	Not widely used. Complex.
ICISS	1996	Patient survival	Computed directly from ICD-9 codes into a survival risk ratio (SRR).	Range from 0 (unsurvivable) to 1 (high chance of survival).	Not based on AIS/ISS. No specialized training required. Outperforms ISS.	Not widely used. Based on ICD-9 codes only. May reflect hospital rather than injury survival.
ICDMAP-90	1997	Injury severity	Translates ICD-9 discharge diagnosis codes into an ISS and APS.	Variability in ICD/AIS scores.	Like ICISS. Conservative estimates of injury severity.	Not widely used. Based on ICD-9 codes only.
TRAIS	2003	Patient survival	Same as ICISS, but uses AIS descriptor codes.	Range from 0 (unsurvivable) to 1 (high chance of survival)	Like ICISS. Outpredicts ISS, NISS, and APS.	Not widely used.

(*Continued*)

Table B.13 (*Continued*) Comparison of Trauma Scoring Systems

Scoring System	Year	Predicts What?	How Calculated?	Score Range/ Interpretation	Benefits	Limitations
OIS	1987	Anatomic injury	Anatomic injury.	Ranges from grade 1 (minor injury) to grade 5 (major injury) and grade 6 (fatal injury).	Standardized severity of injury. Widely used.	No predictability of mortality when used in isolation.
RISC II	2014	Patient survival	German Trauma Registry based.	Uses multiple coefficients based on injury, age, and physiology.	Validation results and comparisons with existing scores showed that RISC II had improved discrimination, predicted mortality, and calibration.	Not widely used outside Germany.
Comorbidity Scoring Systems						
Charlson	1987	Patient survival	Score consists of 19 possible comorbid conditions, each allocated a weight of 1–6 based on the relative risk of 1-year mortality. Values are summed.	Range from 0 (low chance of death) to 37 (high chance of death).	Validated in internal medicine patients only.	Not trauma specific, and not generally used for the trauma patient. Adapted for ICD-9 codes only.
TRISSCOM	2004	Patient survival	Like TRISS, but with adjustments for age (dichotomized to 65 rather than 55) and with the addition of 8 comorbidity variables.	Scores range from 0 (unsurvivable) to 1 (high likelihood of survival).	Reflects the ageing population.	Not widely used. No severity weighting on comorbidities.
Combination Scoring Systems						
TRISS	1987	Patient survival	Combines ISS, RTS, and age; regression coefficients derived from MTOS database.	Scores run from 0 (unsurvivable) to 1 (high likelihood of survival).	Separate coefficients/ probabilities for patients with blunt and penetrating injuries.	Requires multiple variables.

(*Continued*)

Table B.13 (Continued) Comparison of Trauma Scoring Systems

Scoring System	Year	Predicts What?	How Calculated?	Score Range/ Interpretation	Benefits	Limitations
ASCOT	1990	Patient survival	Uses APS to define injury severity.	Range varies.	Same as for TRISS, but with better predictive values for penetrating trauma.	Requires multiple variables.
Outcome-Based Analysis						
FIM + FAM	2000	Outcome following brain injury	Two scores – an admission score and a discharge score.	30 data points, each of which can be scored from 1 (fully dependent) to 7 (fully independent).	Allows objective assessment of recovery, and the setting of goals.	Proprietary score, therefore expensive. Widely used in rehabilitation centres.
GOS	1975	For outcome following head injury	The level of coma on admission correlates with outcome. The GOS attempts to quantify this.	Grading is made between a good recovery to death.	Grading of coma correlates strongly with outcome.	Low accuracy of individual signs.
MTOS	1982	Probability of survival	ISS methodology for a given trauma patient using coefficients representing RTS, ISS, and age.	The predictability of survival can be calculated.	Allows a comparison of the study population by a huge database, with individuals or hospitals.	Complex to calculate.

Source: Table modified from Champion H, Moore L, Vickers R. Injury Severity Scoring and Outcomes Research. In: Moore EE, Feliciano DV, Mattox KL, Eds. *Trauma* 8th Ed. New York, NY: McGraw Hill Education; 2017. 75–77.

AIS, Abbreviated Injury Score
APACHE-II, Acute Physiologic and Chronic Health Evaluation II
APS, Anatomic Profile Score
ASCOT, A Severity Characterization of Trauma
CCI, Charlson, Charlson Comorbidity Index
FAM, Functional Assessment Measure
FIM, Functional Independence Measure
GCS, Glasgow Coma Scale
GOS, Glasgow Outcome Scale
ICDMAP-90, International Classification of Disease 'map' – 1990
ICISS, International Classification of Disease Injury Severity Score

ISS, Injury Severity Score
MTOS, Major Trauma Outcome Study
NISS, New Injury Severity Score
OIS, American Association for the Surgery of Trauma Organ Injury Scale
PTS, Paediatric Trauma Score
RISC II, Revised Injury Severity Classification II
RTS, Revised Trauma Score
TRAIS, Trauma Registry Abbreviated Injury Score
TRISS, Trauma and injury Severity Score
TRISSCOM, Trauma and Injury Severity Score Comorbidity

B.7 **SCALING SYSTEM FOR ORGAN-SPECIFIC INJURIES**[12,26–32]

In all of the tables in this section (**Tables B.14–B.45**), *ICD* refers to the International Classification of Diseases (ICD-9CM[24] and ICD-10 [2015 edition][25]), and *AIS* to the Abbreviated Injury Scale, 2015 revision, of the American Association for the Advancement of Automotive Medicine.[6]

ICD-11 was released in June 2018 and was to be implemented in January 2022.[25] However, this was left by the World Health Organisation (WHO) to the discretion of individual countries.

When necessary, in the ICD-10 system, a *fifth* digit is used as follows:

Closed injury	0
Open injury	1

Table B.14 Cervical Vascular Organ Injury Scale

Grade*	Description of Injury	ICD-9	ICD-10	AIS-2005
I	Thyroid vein	900.8	S15.8	
	Common facial vein	900.8	S15.8	
	External jugular vein	900.81	S15.2	1–3
	Non-named arterial/Venous branches	900.9	S15.9	
II	External carotid arterial branches (ascending pharyngeal, superior thyroid, lingual, facial, maxillary, occipital, posterior auricular)	900.8	S15.0	1–3
	Thyrocervical trunk or primary branches	900.8	S15.8	1–3
	Internal jugular vein	900.1	S15.3	1–3
III	External carotid artery	900.02	S15.0	2–3
	Subclavian vein	901.3	S25.3	3–4
	Vertebral artery	900.8	S15.1	2–4
IV	Common carotid artery	900.01	S15.0	3–5
	Subclavian artery	901.1	S25.1	3–4
V	Internal carotid artery (extracranial)	900.03	S15.0	3–5

Source: From Moore et al.[26]

*Increase one grade for multiple grade III or IV injuries involving more than 50% of the vessel circumference. Decrease one grade for less than 25% vessel circumference disruption for grade IV or V.

Table B.15 Chest Wall Injury Scale

Grade*	Injury Type	Description of Injury	ICD-9	ICD-10	AIS-2005
I	Contusion	Any size	911.0/922.1	S20.2	1
	Laceration	Skin and subcutaneous	875.0	S20.4	1
	Fracture	< 3 ribs, closed	807.01/807.02	S22.3	1–2
		Non-displaced, clavicle closed	810.00/810.03	S42.0	2
II	Laceration	Skin, subcutaneous, and muscle	875.1	S20.4	2
	Fracture	> 3 adjacent ribs, closed	807.03/807.08	S22.4	1
		Open or displaced clavicle	810.10/810.13	S42.0	2–3
		Non-displaced sternum, closed	807.2	S22.2	2
		Scapular body, open or closed	811.00/811.18	S42.1	2
III	Laceration	Full-thickness including pleural penetration – front	862.29	S21.1	2
		Full-thickness including pleural penetration – back	862.29	S21.2	2
	Fracture	Open or displaced sternum	807.2	S22.2	2
		Flail sternum	807.3	S22.2	2
		Unilateral flail segment (< 3 ribs)	807.4	S22.5	3–4
IV	Laceration	Avulsion of chest wall tissues with underlying rib fractures	807.10/807.18	S22.8	4
	Fracture	Unilateral flail chest (≥ 3 ribs)	807.4	S22.5	3–4
V	Fracture	Bilateral flail chest (≥ 3 ribs on both sides)	807.4	S22.5	5

Source: From Moore et al.[27]

Note: This scale is confined to the chest wall alone and does not reflect associated internal or abdominal injuries. Therefore, further delineation of upper versus lower or anterior versus posterior chest wall was not considered, and a grade VI was not warranted. Specifically, thoracic crush was not used as a descriptive term; instead, the geography and extent of fractures and soft tissue injury were used to define the grade.

*Upgrade by one grade for bilateral injuries.

Table B.16 Heart Injury Scale

Grade*	Description of Injury	ICD-9	ICD-10	AIS-2005
I	Blunt cardiac injury with minor ECG abnormality (non-specific ST or T wave changes, premature arterial or ventricular contraction, or persistent sinus tachycardia)	861.01	S26.0	3
	Blunt or penetrating pericardial wound without cardiac injury, cardiac tamponade, or cardiac herniation			
II	Blunt cardiac injury with heart block (right or left bundle branch, left anterior fascicular or atrioventricular) or ischaemic changes (ST depression or T wave inversion) without cardiac failure	861.01	S26.0	3
	Penetrating tangential myocardial wound up to, but not extending through, endocardium, without tamponade	861.12	S26.0	3
III	Blunt cardiac injury with sustained (≥ 6 beats/min) or multifocal ventricular contractions	861.01	S26.0	3–4
	Blunt or penetrating cardiac injury with septal rupture, pulmonary or tricuspid valvular incompetence, papillary muscle dysfunction, or distal coronary arterial occlusion without cardiac failure	861.01	S26.0	3–4
	Blunt pericardial laceration with cardiac herniation	861.01	S26.0	3–4
	Blunt cardiac injury with cardiac failure	861.01	S26.0	3–4
	Penetrating tangential myocardial wound up to, but extending through, endocardium, with tamponade	861.12	S26.0	3
IV	Blunt or penetrating cardiac injury with septal rupture, pulmonary or tricuspid valvular incompetence, papillary muscle dysfunction, or distal coronary arterial occlusion producing cardiac failure	861.12	S26.0	3
	Blunt or penetrating cardiac injury with aortic mitral valve incompetence	861.03	S26.0	5
	Blunt or penetrating cardiac injury of the right ventricle, right atrium, or left atrium	861.03	S26.0	5
V	Blunt or penetrating cardiac injury with proximal coronary arterial occlusion	861.03	S26.0	5
	Blunt or penetrating left ventricular perforation	861.13	S26.0	5
	Stellate wound with < 50% tissue loss of the right ventricle, right atrium, or left atrium	861.03	S26.0	5
VI	Blunt avulsion of the heart; penetrating wound producing > 50% tissue loss of a chamber	861.13	S26.0	6

Source: From Moore et al.[28]

Note: With ICD-10, use the following supplementary characters: 0 = without an open wound into the thoracic cavity; 1 = with an open wound into the thoracic cavity.

*Advance one grade for multiple wounds to a single chamber or multiple-chamber involvement.

ICD-10, International Classification of Disease, 2015 edition

Table B.17 Lung Injury Scale

Grade*	Injury Type	Description of Injury	ICD-9	ICD-10	AIS-2005
I	Contusion	Unilateral, < 1 lobe	861.12/861.31	S27.3	3
II	Contusion	Unilateral, single lobe	861.20/861.30	S27.3	3
	Laceration	Simple pneumothorax	860.0/1/4/5	S27.0	3–5
III	Contusion	Unilateral, > 1 lobe	861.20/861.30	S27.3	3
	Laceration	Persistent (> 72-hour) air leak from distal airway	860.0/1/4/5	S27.3	3–4
	Haematoma	Non-expanding intraparenchymal	862.0/861.30	S27.3	
IV	Laceration	Major (segmental or lobar) air leak	862.21/861.31	S27.4	4–5
	Haematoma	Expanding intraparenchymal		S25.4	
	Vascular	Primary branch intrapulmonary vessel disruption	901.40	S25.4	3–5
V	Vascular	Hilar vessel disruption	901.41/901.42	S25.4	4
VI	Vascular	Total uncontained transection of pulmonary hilum	901.41/901.42	S25.4	4

Source: From Moore et al.[28]
Note: Haemothorax is scored under the thoracic vascular injury scale. With ICD-10, use the following supplementary characters: 0 = Without an open wound into the thoracic cavity; 1 = with an open wound into the thoracic cavity.
*Advance one grade for bilateral injuries up to grade III.

Table B.18 Thoracic Vascular Injury Scale

Grade*	Description of Injury	ICD-9	ICD-10	AIS-2005
I	Intercostal artery/vein	901.81	S25.5	2–3
	Internal mammary artery/vein	901.82	S25.8	2–3
	Bronchial artery/vein	901.89	S25.4	1–3
	Oesophageal artery/vein	901.9	S25.8	2–3
	Hemiazygos vein	901.89	S25.8	2–3
	Unnamed artery/vein	901.9	S25.9	2–3
II	Azygos vein	901.89	S25.8	2–3
	Internal jugular vein	900.1	S15.3	2–3
	Subclavian vein	901.3	S25.3	3–4
	Innominate vein	901.3	S25.3	3–4
III	Carotid artery	900.01	S15.0	3–5
	Innominate artery	901.1	S25.1	3–4
	Subclavian artery	901.1	S25.1	3–4
IV	Thoracic aorta, descending	901.0	S25.0	4–5
	Inferior vena cava (intrathoracic)	902.10	S35.1	3–4
	Pulmonary artery, primary intraparenchymal branch	901.41	S25.4	3
	Pulmonary vein, primary intraparenchymal branch	901.42	S25.4	3
V	Thoracic aorta, ascending and arch	901.0	S25.0	5
	Superior vena cava	901.2	S25.2	3–4
	Pulmonary artery, main trunk	901.41	S25.4	4
	Pulmonary vein, main trunk	901.42	S25.4	4
VI	Uncontained total transection of thoracic aorta or pulmonary hilum	901.0	S25.0	5
	Uncontained total transection of pulmonary hilum	901.41/901.42	S25.4	5

Source: From Moore et al.[28]
*Increase one grade for multiple grade III or IV injuries if more than 50% of the circumference. Decrease one grade for grade IV injuries if less than 25% of the circumference.

Table B.19 Diaphragm Injury Scale

Grade*	Description of Injury	ICD-9	ICD-10	AIS-2005
I	Contusion	862.0	S27.8	2
II	Laceration < 2 cm	862.1	S27.8	3
III	Laceration 2–10 cm	862.1	S27.8	3
IV	Laceration > 10 cm with tissue loss ≤ 25 cm²	862.1	S27.8	3
V	Laceration with tissue loss > 25 cm²	862.1	S27.8	3

Source: From Moore et al.[28]
*Advance one grade for bilateral injuries up to grade III.

Table B.20 Spleen Injury Scale (1994 Revision)

Grade*	Injury Type	Description of Injury	ICD-9	ICD-10	AIS-2005
I	Haematoma	Subcapsular, < 10% surface area	865.01/865.11	S36.0	2
	Laceration	Capsular tear, < 1 cm parenchymal depth	865.02/865.12	S36.0	2
II	Haematoma	Subcapsular, 10%–50% surface area; intraparenchymal, < 5 cm in diameter	865.01/865.11	S36.0	2
	Laceration	Capsular tear, 1–3 cm parenchymal depth that does not involve a trabecular vessel	865.02/865.12	S36.0	2
III	Haematoma	Subcapsular, > 50% surface area or expanding; ruptured subcapsular or parenchymal haematoma; intraparenchymal haematoma > 5 cm or expanding	865.03	S36.0	3
	Laceration	> 3 cm parenchymal depth or involving trabecular vessels	865.03	S36.0	3
IV	Laceration	Laceration involving segmental or hilar vessels producing major devascularization (>25% of spleen)	865.13	S36.0	4
V	Laceration	Completely shattered spleen	865.04	S36.0	5
	Vascular	Hilar vascular injury with devascularized spleen	865.14	S36.0	5

Source: From Moore et al.[29]
Note: With ICD-10, use the following supplementary characters: 0 = Without an open wound into the abdominal cavity; 1 = with an open wound into the abdominal cavity.
*Advance one grade for multiple injuries up to grade III.

Table B.21 Liver Injury Scale (1994 Revision)

Grade*	Type of Injury	Description of Injury	ICD-9	ICD-10	AIS-2005
I	Haematoma	Subcapsular, < 10% surface area	864.01/864.11	S36.1	2
	Laceration	Capsular tear, < 1 cm parenchymal depth	864.02/864.12	S36.1	2
II	Haematoma	Subcapsular, 10%–50% surface area: intraparenchymal < 10 cm in diameter	864.01/864.11	S36.1	2
	Laceration	Capsular tear, 1–3 cm parenchymal depth, < 10 cm in length	864.03/864.13	S36.1	2
III	Haematoma	Subcapsular, > 50% surface area or ruptured subcapsular or parenchymal haematoma; intraparenchymal haematoma > 10 cm or expanding	864.04/864.14	S36.1	3
	Laceration	3 cm parenchymal depth	864.04/864.14	S36.1	3
IV	Laceration	Parenchymal disruption involving 25%–75% hepatic lobe or 1–3 Couinaud's segments within a single lobe	864.04/864.14	S36.1	4
V	Laceration	Parenchymal disruption involving > 75% of hepatic lobe or > 3 Couinaud's segments within a single lobe	864.04/864.14	S36.1	5
	Vascular	Juxtahepatic venous injuries; i.e. retrohepatic vena cava/ central major hepatic veins	864.04/864.14	S36.1	5
VI	Vascular	Hepatic avulsion	864.04/864.14	S36.1	5

Source: From Moore et al.[29]
Note: With ICD-10, use the following supplementary characters: 0 = Without an open wound into the abdominal cavity; 1 = with an open wound into the abdominal cavity.
*Advance one grade for multiple injuries up to grade III.

Table B.22 Extrahepatic Biliary Tree Injury Scale

Grade*	Description of Injury	ICD-9	ICD-10	AIS-2005
I	Gallbladder contusion/haematoma	868.02	S36.1	2
	Portal triad contusion	868.02	S36.1	2
II	Partial gallbladder avulsion from liver bed; cystic duct intact	868.02	S36.1	2
	Laceration or perforation of the gallbladder	868.12	S36.1	2
III	Complete gallbladder avulsion from liver bed	868.02	S36.1	3
	Cystic duct laceration	868.12	S36.1	3
IV	Partial or complete right hepatic duct laceration	868.12	S36.1	3
	Partial or complete left hepatic duct laceration	868.12	S36.1	3
	Partial common hepatic duct laceration (< 50%)	868.12	S36.1	3
	Partial common bile duct laceration (< 50%)	868.12	S36.1	3
V	> 50% transection of common hepatic duct	868.12	S36.1	3–4
	> 50% transection of common bile duct	868.12	S36.1	3–4
	Combined right and left hepatic duct injuries	868.12	S36.1	3–4
	Intraduodenal or intrapancreatic bile duct injuries	868.12	S36.1	3–4

Source: From Moore et al.[30]
Note: With ICD-10, use the following supplementary characters: 0 = Without an open wound into the abdominal cavity; 1 = with an open wound into the abdominal cavity.
*Advance one grade for multiple injuries up to grade III.

Table B.23 Pancreas Injury Scale

Grade*	Type of Injury	Description of Injury	ICD-9	ICD-10	AIS-2005
I	Haematoma	Minor contusion without duct injury	863.81/863.84	S36.2	2
	Laceration	Superficial laceration without duct injury		S36.2	2
II	Haematoma	Major contusion without duct injury or tissue loss	863.81/863.84	S36.2	2
	Laceration	Major laceration without duct injury or tissue loss	863.81/863.84	S36.2	3
III	Laceration	Distal transection or parenchymal injury with duct injury	863.92/863.94	S36.2	3
IV	Laceration	Proximal transection or parenchymal injury involving ampulla	863.91	S36.2	4
V	Laceration	Massive disruption of pancreatic head	863.91	S36.2	5

Source: From Moore et al.[31]

Note: Head, 863.51, 863.91; body, 863.99, 862.92; tail, 863.83, 863.93. The proximal pancreas is to the patient's right of the superior mesenteric vein. With ICD-10, use the following supplementary characters: 0 = Without an open wound into the abdominal cavity; 1 = with an open wound into the abdominal cavity.

*Advance one grade for multiple injuries up to grade III.

Table B.24 Oesophagus Injury Scale

Grade*	Type of Injury	Description of Injury	ICD-9	ICD-10	AIS-2005
I	Contusion	Contusion/haematoma: Cervical oesophagus	862.22/826.32	S10.0	2
		Contusion/haematoma: Thoracic oesophagus	862.22/826.32	S27.8	3
		Contusion/haematoma: Abdominal oesophagus	862.22/862.32	S36.8	3
II	Laceration	Partial-thickness laceration	862.22/826.32	S10.0/S27.8/S36.8	4
III	Laceration	Laceration < 50% circumference	862.22/826.32	S10.0/S27.8/S36.8	4
IV	Laceration	Laceration > 50% circumference	862.22/826.32	S10.0/S27.8/S36.8	5
V	Tissue loss	Segmental loss or devascularization < 2 cm	862.22/826.32	S10.0/S27.8/S36.8	5
	Tissue loss	Segmental loss or devascularization > 2 cm	862.22/826.32	S10.0/S27.8/S36.8	

Source: From Moore et al.[30]

Note: With ICD-10, use as a fifth character the following supplementary characters: 0 = without an open wound into the abdominal or thoracic cavity; 1 = with an open wound into the abdominal or thoracic cavity.

*Advance one grade for multiple lesions up to grade III.

AIS, Abbreviated Injury Scale
ICD, International Classification of Diseases
S10.0, cervical oesophagus
S27.8, thoracic oesophagus
S36.8, abdominal oesophagus

Table B.25 Stomach Injury Scale

Grade*		Description of Injury	ICD-9	ICD-10	AIS-2005
I	Contusion	Contusion/haematoma	863.0/863.1	S36.3	2
	Laceration	Partial-thickness laceration	863.0/863.1	S36.3	2
II	Laceration	< 2 cm in gastro-oesophageal junction or pylorus	863.0/863.1	S36.3	3
		< 5 cm in proximal one-third stomach	863.0/863.1	S36.3	3
		< 10 cm in distal two-thirds stomach	863.0/863.1	S36.3	3
III	Laceration	> 2 cm in gastro-oesophageal junction or pylorus	863.0/863.1	S36.3	3
		> 5 cm in proximal one-third stomach	863.0/863.1	S36.3	3
		> 10 cm in distal two-thirds stomach	863.0/863.1	S36.3	3
IV	Tissue loss	Tissue loss or devascularization < two-thirds stomach	863.0/863.1	S36.3	4
V	Tissue loss	Tissue loss or devascularization > two-thirds stomach	863.0/863.1	S36.3	4

Source: From Moore et al.[30]
Note: With ICD-10, use the following supplementary characters: 0 = Without an open wound into the abdominal cavity; 1 = with an open wound into the abdominal cavity.
*Advance one grade for multiple lesions up to grade III.

Table B.26 Duodenum Injury Scale

Grade*	Type of Injury	Description of Injury	ICD-9	ICD-10	AIS-2005
I	Haematoma	Involving single portion of duodenum	863.21	S36.4	2
	Laceration	Partial thickness, no perforation	863.21	S36.4	3
II	Haematoma	Involving more than one portion	863.21	S36.4	2
		Disruption of < 50% of circumference	863.31	S36.4	3
III	Laceration	Disruption of 50%–75% of circumference of D2	863.31	S36.4	4
		Disruption of 50%–100% of circumference of D1, D3, or D4	863.31	S36.4	4
IV	Laceration	Disruption of > 75% of circumference of D2	863.31	S36.4	5
		Involving ampulla or distal common bile duct	863.31	S36.4	5
V	Laceration	Massive disruption of duodenopancreatic complex	863.31	S36.4	5
	Vascular	Devascularization of duodenum	863.31	S36.4	5

Source: From Moore et al.[31]
Note: With ICD-10, use the following supplementary characters: 0 = without an open wound into the abdominal cavity; 1 = with an open wound into the abdominal cavity.
*Advance one grade for multiple injuries up to grade III.

Table B.27 Small Bowel Injury Scale

Grade*	Type of Injury	Description of Injury	ICD-9	ICD-10	AIS-2005
I	Haematoma	Contusion or haematoma without devascularization	863.20	S36.4	2
	Laceration	Partial thickness, no perforation	863.20	S36.4	2
II	Laceration	Laceration < 50% of circumference	863.30	S36.4	3
III	Laceration	Laceration ≥ 50% of circumference without transection	863.30	S36.4	3
IV	Laceration	Transection of the small bowel	863.30	S36.4	4
V	Laceration	Transection of the small bowel with segmental tissue loss	863.30	S36.4	4
	Vascular	Devascularized segment	863.30	S36.4	4

Source: From Moore et al.[31]
Note: With ICD-10, use the following supplementary characters: 0 = Without an open wound into the abdominal cavity; 1 = with an open wound into the abdominal cavity.
*Advance one grade for multiple injuries up to grade III.

Table B.28 Colon Injury Scale

Grade*	Type of Injury	Description of Injury	ICD-9	ICD-10	AIS-2005
I	Haematoma	Contusion or haematoma without devascularization	863.40–863.44	S36.5	2
	Laceration	Partial thickness, no perforation	863.40–863.44	S36.5	2
II	Laceration	Laceration < 50% of circumference	863.50–863.54	S36.5	3
III	Laceration	Laceration ≥ 50% of circumference without transection	863.50–863.54	S36.5	3
IV	Laceration	Transection of the colon	863.50–863.54	S36.5	4
V	Laceration	Transection of the colon with segmental tissue loss	863.50–863.54	S36.5	4

Source: From Moore et al.[31]
Note: With ICD-9, 863.40/863.50 = non-specific site in colon; 863.41/863.51 = ascending colon; 863.42/863.52 = transverse colon; 863.43/863.53 = descending colon; 863.44/863.54 = sigmoid colon. With ICD-10, use the following supplementary characters: 0 = without an open wound into the abdominal cavity; 1 = with an open wound into the abdominal cavity.
*Advance one grade for multiple injuries up to grade III.

Table B.29 Rectum Injury Scale

Grade*	Type of Injury	Description of Injury	ICD-9	ICD-10	AIS-2005
I	Haematoma	Contusion or haematoma without devascularization	863.45	S36.6	2
	Laceration	Partial-thickness laceration	863.45	S36.6	2
II	Laceration	Laceration < 50% of circumference	863.55	S36.6	3
III	Laceration	Laceration ≥ 50% of circumference	863.55	S36.6	4
IV	Laceration	Full-thickness laceration with extension into the perineum	863.55	S36.6	5
V	Vascular	Devascularized segment	863.55	S36.6	5

Source: From Moore et al.[31]
Note: With ICD-10, use the following supplementary characters: 0 = Without an open wound into the abdominal cavity; 1 = with an open wound into the abdominal cavity.
*Advance one grade for multiple injuries up to grade III.

Table B.30 Abdominal Vascular Injury Scale

Grade*	Description of Injury	ICD-9	ICD-10	AIS-2005
I	Non-named superior mesenteric artery or superior mesenteric vein branches	902.20/902.39	S35.2	NS
	Non-named inferior mesenteric artery or inferior mesenteric vein branches	902.27/902.32	S35.2	NS
	Phrenic artery or vein	902.89	S35.8	NS
	Lumbar artery or vein	902.89	S35.8	NS
	Gonadal artery or vein	902.89	S35.8	NS
	Ovarian artery or vein	902.81/902.82	S35.8	NS
	Other non-named small arterial or venous structures requiring ligation	902.80	S35.9	NS
II	Right, left, or common hepatic artery	902.22	S35.2	3
	Splenic artery or vein	902.23/902.34	S35.2	3
	Right or left gastric arteries	902.21	S35.2	3
	Gastroduodenal artery	902.24	S35.2	3
	Inferior mesenteric artery/Trunk or inferior mesenteric vein/trunk	902.27/902.32	S35.2	3
	Primary named branches of mesenteric artery (e.g., ileocolic artery) or mesenteric vein	902.26 / 902.31	S35.2	3
	Other named abdominal vessels requiring ligation or repair	902.89	S35.8	3
III	Superior mesenteric vein, trunk, and primary subdivisions	902.31	S35.3	3
	Renal artery or vein	902.41 / 902.42	S35.4	3
	Iliac artery or vein	902.53 / 902.54	S35.5	3
	Hypogastric artery or vein	902.51 / 902.52	S35.5	3
	Vena cava, infrarenal	902.10	S35.1	3
IV	Superior mesenteric artery, trunk	902.25	S35.2	3
	Coeliac axis proper	902.24	S35.2	3
	Vena cava, suprarenal and infrahepatic	902.10	S35.1	3
	Aorta, infrarenal	902.00	S35.0	4
V	Portal vein	902.33	S35.3	3
	Extraparenchymal hepatic vein only	902.11	S35.1	3
	Extraparenchymal hepatic veins and liver	902.11	S35.1	5
	Vena cava, retrohepatic or suprahepatic	902.19	S35.1	5
	Aorta suprarenal, subdiaphragmatic	902.00	S35.0	4

Source: From Moore et al.[27]

Note: With ICD-10, use the following supplementary characters: 0 = Without an open wound into the abdominal cavity; 1 = with an open wound into the abdominal cavity.

*Advance one grade for multiple injuries up to grade III.

*This classification system is applicable to extraparenchymal vascular injuries. If the vessel injury is within 2 cm of the organ parenchyma, refer to the specific organ injury scale. Increase one grade for multiple grade III or IV injuries involving > 50% of the vessel circumference. Downgrade one grade if < 25% of the vessel circumference laceration is grade IV or V.

Table B.31 Adrenal Organ Injury Scale

Grade*	Description of Injury	ICD-9	ICD-10	AIS-2005
I	Contusion	868.01/868.11	S37.9	1
II	Laceration involving only cortex (< 2 cm)	868.01/868.11	S37.8	1
III	Laceration extending into medulla (≥ 2 cm)	868.01/868.11	S37.8	2
IV	> 50% Parenchymal destruction	868.01/868.11	S37.8	2
V	Total parenchymal destruction (including massive intraparenchymal haemorrhage)	868.01/868.11	S37.8	3
	Avulsion from blood supply			

Source: From Moore et al.[1]
Note: With ICD-10, use the following supplementary characters: 0 = Without an open wound into the abdominal cavity; 1 = with an open wound into the abdominal cavity.
*Advance one grade for bilateral lesions up to grade V.

Table B.32 Kidney Injury Scale

Grade*	Type of Injury	Description of Injury	ICD-9	ICD-10	AIS-2005
I	Contusion	Microscopic or gross haematuria, urological studies normal	866.00/866.01	S37.0	2
	Haematoma	Subcapsular, non-expanding without parenchymal laceration	866.01	S37.0	2
II	Haematoma	Non-expanding perirenal haematoma confined to renal retroperitoneum	866.01	S37.0	2
	Laceration	< 1.0 cm parenchymal depth of renal cortex without urinary extravasation	866.11	S37.0	2
III	Laceration	> 1.0 cm parenchymal depth of renal cortex without collecting system rupture or urinary extravasation	866.11	S37.0	3
IV	Laceration	Parenchymal laceration extending through renal cortex, medulla, and collecting system	866.02/866.12	S37.0	4
	Vascular	Main renal artery or vein injury with contained haemorrhage	866.03/866.11	S37.0	4
V	Laceration	Completely shattered kidney	866.04/866.14	S37.0	5
	Vascular	Avulsion of renal hilum that devascularizes kidney	866.13	S37.0	5

Source: From Moore et al.[32]
Note: With ICD-10, use the following supplementary characters: 0 = Without an open wound into the abdominal cavity; 1 = with an open wound into the abdominal cavity.
*Advance one grade for bilateral injuries up to grade III.

Table B.33 Ureter Injury Scale

Grade*	Type of Injury	Description of Injury	ICD-9	ICD-10	AIS-2005
I	Haematoma	Contusion or haematoma without devascularization	867.2/867.3	S37.1	2
II	Laceration	< 50% transection	867.2/867.3	S37.1	2
III	Laceration	≥ 50% transection	867.2/867.3	S37.1	3
IV	Laceration	Complete transection with < 2 cm devascularization	867.2/867.3	S37.1	3
V	Laceration	Avulsion with > 2 cm devascularization	867.2/867.3	S37.1	3

Source: From Moore et al.[27]

Note: With ICD-10, use the following supplementary characters: 0 – Without an open wound into the abdominal cavity; 1 = with an open wound into the abdominal cavity.

*Advance one grade for bilateral up to grade III.

Table B.34 Bladder Injury Scale

Grade*	Injury Type	Description of Injury	ICD-9	ICD-10	AIS-2005
I	Haematoma	Contusion, intramural haematoma	867.0/867.1	S37.2	2
	Laceration	Partial thickness	867.0/867.1	S37.2	3
II	Laceration	Extraperitoneal bladder wall laceration < 2 cm	867.0/867.1	S37.2	4
III	Laceration	Extraperitoneal (≥ 2 cm) or intraperitoneal (< 2 cm) bladder wall laceration	867.0/867.1	S37.2	4
IV	Laceration	Intraperitoneal bladder wall laceration ≥ 2 cm	867.0/867.1	S37.2	4
V	Laceration	Intraperitoneal or extraperitoneal bladder wall laceration extending into the bladder neck or ureteral orifice (trigone)	867.0/867.1	S37.2	4

Source: From Moore et al.[27]

Note: With ICD-10, use the following supplementary characters: 0 = Without an open wound into the pelvic cavity; 1 = with an open wound into the pelvic cavity.

*Advance one grade for multiple lesions up to grade III.

Table B.35 Urethra Injury Scale

Grade*	Injury Type	Description of Injury	ICD-9	ICD-10	AIS-2005
I	Contusion	Blood at urethral meatus; urethrography normal	867.0/867.1	S37.3	2
II	Stretch injury	Elongation of urethra without extravasation on urethrography	867.0/867.1	S37.3	2
III	Partial disruption	Extravasation of urethrography contrast at injury site with visualization in the bladder	867.0/867.1	S37.3	2
IV	Complete disruption	Extravasation of urethrography contrast at injury site without visualization in the bladder; < 2 cm of urethra separation	867.0/867.1	S37.3	3
V	Complete disruption	Complete transection with ≥ 2 cm urethral separation, or extension into the prostate or vagina	867.0/867.1	S37.3	4

Source: From Moore et al.[27]

Note: With ICD-10, use the following supplementary characters: 0 = Without an open wound into the pelvic cavity; 1 = with an open wound into the pelvic cavity.

*Advance one grade for bilateral injuries up to grade III.

Table B.36 Uterus (Non-Pregnant) Injury Scale

Grade*	Description of Injury	ICD-9	ICD-10	AIS-2005
I	Contusion/haematoma	867.4/867.5	S37.6	2
II	Superficial laceration (< 1 cm)	867.4/867.5	S37.6	2
III	Deep laceration (≥ 1 cm)	867.4/867.5	S37.6	3
IV	Laceration involving the uterine artery	902.55	S37.6	3
V	Avulsion/devascularization	867.4/867.5	S37.6	3

Source: From Moore et al.[30]
Note: With ICD-10, use the following supplementary characters: 0 = Without an open wound into the pelvic cavity; 1 = with an open wound into the pelvic cavity.
*Advance one grade for multiple injuries up to grade III.

Table B.37 Uterus (Pregnant) Injury Scale

Grade*	Description of Injury	ICD-9	ICD-10	AIS-2005
I	Contusion or haematoma (without placental abruption)	867.4/867.5	S37.6	2
II	Superficial laceration (< 1 cm) or partial placental abruption < 25%	867.4/ 867.5	S37.6	3
III	Deep laceration (≥ 1 cm) occurring in second trimester, or placental abruption > 25% but < 50%	867.4/867.5	S37.6	3
	Deep laceration (≥ 1 cm) in third trimester	867.4/867.5	S37.6	4
IV	Laceration involving uterine artery	902.55	S37.6	4
	Deep laceration (≥ 1 cm) with > 50% placental abruption	867.4/867.5	S37.6	4
V	Uterine rupture			
	• Second trimester	867.4/867.5	S37.6	4
	• Third trimester	867.4/867.5	S37.6	5
	Complete placental abruption	867.4/867.5	S37.6	4–5

Source: From Moore et al.[30]
Note: With ICD-10, use the following supplementary characters: 0 = Without an open wound into the pelvic cavity; 1 = with an open wound into the pelvic cavity.
*Advance one grade for multiple injuries up to grade III.

Table B.38 Fallopian Tube Injury Scale

Grade*	Description of Injury	ICD-9	ICD-10	AIS-2005
I	Haematoma or contusion	867.6/867.7	S37.5	2
II	Laceration < 50% circumference	867.6/867.7	S37.5	2
III	Laceration ≥ 50% circumference	867.6/867.7	S37.5	2
IV	Transection	867.6/867.7	S37.5	2
V	Vascular injury; devascularized segment	902.89	S35.8	2

Source: From Moore et al.[30]
Note: With ICD-10, use the following supplementary characters: 0 = Without an open wound into the pelvic cavity; 1 = with an open wound into the pelvic cavity.
*Advance one grade for multiple injuries up to grade III.

Table B.39 Ovary Injury Scale

Grade*	Description of Injury	ICD-9	ICD-10	AIS-2005
I	Contusion or haematoma	867.6/867.7	S37.4	1
II	Superficial laceration (depth < 0.5 cm)	867.6/867.7	S37.4	2
III	Deep laceration (depth ≥ 0.5 cm)	867.8/867.7	S37.4	3
IV	Partial disruption or blood supply	902.81	S35.8	3
V	Avulsion or complete parenchymal destruction	902.81	S37.4	3

Source: From Moore et al.[30]
Note: With ICD-10, use the following supplementary characters: 0 = without an open wound into the pelvic cavity; 1 = with an open wound into the pelvic cavity.
*Advance one grade for multiple injuries up to grade III.

Table B.40 Vagina Injury Scale

Grade*	Description of Injury	ICD-9	ICD-10	AIS-2005
I	Contusion or haematoma	922.4	S30.2	1
II	Laceration, superficial (mucosa only)	878.6	S31.4	1
III	Laceration, deep into fat or muscle	878.6	S31.4	2
IV	Laceration, complex, into cervix or peritoneum	868.7	S31.4	3
V	Injury into adjacent organs (anus, rectum, urethra, bladder)	878.7	S39.7	3

Source: From Moore et al.[30]
Note: With ICD-10, use the following supplementary characters: 0 = Without an open wound into the pelvic cavity; 1 = with an open wound into the pelvic cavity.
*Advance one grade for multiple injuries up to grade III.

Table B.41 Vulva Injury Scale

Grade*	Description of Injury	ICD-9	ICD-10	AIS-2005
I	Contusion or haematoma	922.4	S30.2	1
II	Laceration, superficial (skin only)	878.4	S31.4	1
III	Laceration, deep (into fat or muscle)	878.4	S31.4	2
IV	Avulsion; skin, fat, or muscle	878.5	S38.2	3
V	Injury into adjacent organs (anus, rectum, urethra, bladder)	878.5	S39.7	3

Source: From Moore et al.[30]
*Advance one grade for multiple injuries up to grade III.

Table B.42 Testis Injury Scale

Grade*	Description of Injury	ICD-9	ICD-10	AIS-2005
I	Contusion/haematoma	911.0–922.4	S30.2	1
II	Subclinical laceration of tunica albuginea	922.4	S31.3	1
III	Laceration of tunica albuginea with < 50% parenchymal loss	878.2	S31.3	2
IV	Major laceration of tunica albuginea with ≥ 50% parenchymal loss	878.3	S31.3	2
V	Total testicular destruction or avulsion	878.3	S38.2	2

Source: From Moore et al.[26]
*Advance one grade for bilateral lesions up to grade V.

Table B.43 Scrotum Injury Scale

Grade	Description of Injury	ICD-9	ICD-10	AIS-2005
I	Contusion	922.4	S30.2	1
II	Laceration < 25% of scrotal diameter	878.2	S31.2	1
III	Laceration ≥ 25% of scrotal diameter	878.3	S31.3	2
IV	Avulsion < 50%	878.3	S38.2	2
V	Avulsion ≥ 50%	878.3	S38.2	2

Source: From Moore et al.[26]

Table B.44 Penis Injury Scale

Grade*	Description of Injury	ICD-9	ICD-10	AIS-2005
I	Cutaneous laceration/contusion	911.0/922.4	S30.2/31/2	1
II	Buck's fascia (cavernosum) laceration without tissue loss	878.0	S37.8	1
III	Cutaneous avulsion	878.1	S38.2	3
	Laceration through glans/meatus			
	Cavernosal or urethral defect < 2 cm			
IV	Partial penectomy	878.1	S38.2	3
	Cavernosal or urethral defect ≥ 2 cm			
V	Total penectomy	876.1	S38.2	3

Source: From Moore et al.[26]
*Advance one grade for multiple injuries up to grade III.

Table B.45 Peripheral Vascular Organ Injury Scale

Grade*	Description of Injury	ICD-9	ICD-10	AIS-2005
I	Digital artery/vein	903.5	S65.5	1–3
	Palmar artery/vein	903.4	S65.3	1–3
	Deep palmar artery/vein	904.6	S65.3	1–3
	Dorsalis pedis artery	904.7	S95.0	1–3
	Plantar artery/vein	904.5	S95.1	1–3
	Non-named arterial/venous branches	903.8/904.7	S55.9/S85.9	1–3
II	Basilic/cephalic vein	903.8	S45.8/S55.8	1–3
	Saphenous vein	904.3	S75.2	1–3
	Radial artery	903.2	S55.1	1–3
	Ulnar artery	903.3	S55.0	1–3
III	Axillary vein	903.02	S45.1	2–3
	Superficial/deep femoral vein	903.02	S75.1	2–3
	Popliteal vein	904.42	S85.5	2–3
	Brachial artery	903.1	S45.1	2–3
	Anterior tibial artery	904.51/904.52	S85.1	1–3
	Posterior tibial artery	904.53/904.54	S85.1	1–3
	Peroneal artery	904.7	S85.2	1–3
	Tibioperoneal trunk	904.7	S85.2	2–3
IV	Superficial/deep femoral artery	904.1/904.7	S75.0	2–3
	Popliteal artery	904.41	S85.0	2–3
V	Axillary artery	903.01	S45.0	3–4
	Common femoral artery	904.0	S75.0	3–4

Source: From Moore et al.[26]

*Increase one grade for multiple grade III or IV injuries involving > 50% of the vessel circumference. Decrease one grade for < 25% disruption of the vessel circumference for grade IV or V.

B.8 SUMMARY

Trauma scoring systems are designed to facilitate pre-hospital triage, identify trauma patients whose outcomes are statistically unexpected for quality assurance analysis, allow an accurate comparison of different trauma populations, and organize and improve trauma systems. They are vital for the scientific study of the epidemiology and the treatment of trauma and may even be used to define resource allocation and reimbursement in the future.

Trauma scoring systems that measure outcome solely in terms of death or survival are at best blunt instruments. Despite the existence of several scales (Quality of Well-Being Scale, Sickness Impact Profile, etc.), further efforts are needed to develop outcome measures that evaluate the multiplicity of outcomes across the full range of diverse trauma populations.

Despite the profusion of acronyms, scoring systems are a vital component of trauma care delivery systems. The effectiveness of well-organized, centralized, multidisciplinary trauma centres in reducing the mortality and morbidity of injured patients is well documented, and trauma scoring systems play a central role in the provision of trauma care today and for the future.

REFERENCES

1. Teasdale G, Jennet B. Assessment of coma and impaired consciousness: a practical scale. *Lancet.* 1974;**ii**:81–4.
2. Tepas JJ 3rd, Ramenofsky ML, Mollitt DL, Gans BM, DiScala C. The Paediatric Trauma Score as a predictor of injury severity: an objective assessment. *J Trauma.* 1988 April;**28**(**4**):425–9.
3. Champion HR, Sacco WJ, Copes WS, Gann DS, Gennarelli TA, Flanagan ME. A revision of the Trauma Score. *J Trauma.* 1989 May;**29**(**5**):623–9.
4. Knaus WA, Draper EA, Wagner DP, Zimmerman JE. APACHE II: A severity of disease classification system. *Crit Care Med.* 1985 Oct;**13**(**10**):818–29.

5. Calculation of the APACHE II Score. Available from htpp://https://www.mdcalc.com/apache-ii-score (accessed online December 2018).

6. American Association for the Advancement of Automotive Medicine. *The Abbreviated Injury Scale: 2015 Revision.* Chicago, IL: AAAM, 2015. Available from: www.AAAM.org.

7. Baker SP, O'Neill B, Haddon W, Long WB. The Injury Severity Score: a method for describing patients with multiple injuries and evaluating emergency care. *J Trauma.* 1974 Mar;**14**(**3**):187–96.

8. Osler T, Baker SP, Long W. A modification of the Injury Severity Score that both improves accuracy and simplifies scoring. *J Trauma* 1997 Dec;**43**(**6**):922–5; discussion 925–6.

9. Balogh Z, Offner PJ, Moore EE, Biffl WL. NISS predicts postinjury Multiple Organ Failure better than the ISS. *J Trauma.* 2000 Apr;**48**(**4**):624–7; discussion 627–8.

10. Copes WS, Champion HR, Sacco WJ, Lawnick MM, Gann DS, Gennarelli T, et al. Progress in characterising anatomical injury. *J Trauma.* 1990 Oct; **30**(**10**):1200–1207

11. Osler T, Rutledge R, Deis J, Bedrick E. ICISS: An International Classification of Disease-9 based injury severity score. *J Trauma.* 1997 Sep;**41**(**3**):380–6; discussion 386–8.

12. Organ Injury Scale of the American Association for the Surgery of Trauma (OIS-AAST). Available from www.aast.org (accessed December 2018).

13. Moore EE, Dunn EL, Moore JB, Thompson JS. Penetrating Abdominal Trauma Index. *J Trauma.* 1981 Jun;**21**(**6**):439–45.

14. Lefering R. Development and validation of the Revised Injury Severity Classification (RISC) score for severely injured patients. *Europ. J. Trauma Emerg. Surg.* 2009 Oct;35(5):437–47. doi: 10.1007/s00068-009-9122-0.

15. Lefering R, Huber-Wagner S, Nienaber U, Maegele M, Bouillon B. Update of the trauma risk adjustment model of the Trauma Register DGU: the Revised Injury Severity Classification, version II. *Crit Care.* 2014 Sep 5;18(5):476. doi: 10.1186/s13054-014-0476-2.

16. Gabbe BJ, Magtengaard K, Hannaford AP, Cameron PA. Is the Charlson Comorbidity Index (CCI) useful for predicting trauma outcomes? *Acad Emerg Med.* 2005;**12**(**4**);318–21.

17. Bergeron E, Rossignol M, Osler T, Clas D, Lavoie A. Improving the TRISS methodology by restructuring age categories and adding comorbidities. *J Trauma.* 2004 April;**56**(**4**):760–67.

18. Turner-Stokes L, Nyein K, Turner-Stokes, Gatehouse C. The UK FIM+FAM Functional Assessment Measure. *Clin Rehabil.* 1999 Aug;**13**(**4**):277–87.

19. Wright J. The Functional Assessment Measure. *The Center for Outcome Measurement in Brain Injury.* http://www.tbims.org/combi/FAM (accessed December 2018).

20. Jennet B, Bond M. Assessment of outcome: a practical scale. *Lancet*; 1975 Mar;**i**(**9705**):480–4.

21. Boyd CR, Tolson MA, Copes WS. Evaluating trauma care: the TRISS model. *J Trauma.* 1987 April;**27**(**4**):370–8.

22. Champion HR, Copes WS, Sacco WJ, Lawnick MM, Bain LW, Gann DS, et al. A new characterisation of injury severity. *J Trauma.* 1990 May;**30**(**5**):539–46.

23. Champion HR, Copes WS, Sacco WJ, Frey CF, Holcroft JW, Hoyt DB, et al. Improved predictions from A Severity Characterization of Trauma (ASCOT) over Trauma and Injury Severity Score (TRISS): results of an independent evaluation. *J Trauma.* 1996 Jan;**40**(**1**):42–8; discussion 48–9.

24. World Health Organization. ICD-9CM. International classification of diseases, ninth revision, clinical modification. Center for Diseases Control and Prevention, Hyattsville MD. Available from https://www.cdc.gov/nchs/icd/index.htm (accessed online December 2018).

25. World Health Organization. ICD-10 Codes. 2015 version online. Available from www.who.int/classifications/icd/en/ (accessed online December 2018).

26. Moore EE, Malangoni MA, Cogbill TH, Peterson NE, Champion HR, Shackford SR. Organ injury scaling VII: cervical vascular, peripheral vascular, adrenal, penis, testis and scrotum. *J Trauma.* 1996 Sept;**41**(**3**):523–4.

27. Moore EE, Cogbill TH, Jurkovich GJ. Organ injury scaling III: chest wall, abdominal vascular, ureter, bladder and urethra. *J Trauma.* 1992 Sept;**33**(**3**):337–8.

28. Moore EE, Malangoni MA, Cogbill TH, Shackford SR, Champion HR, Jurkovich GJ, et al. Organ injury scaling IV: thoracic, vascular, lung, cardiac and diaphragm. *J Trauma.* 1994 Mar;**36**(**3**):299–300.

29. Moore EE, Cogbill TH, Jurkovich GJ, Shackford SR, Malangoni MA, Champion HR. Organ injury scaling: spleen and liver (1994 Revision). *J Trauma.* 1995 Mar;**38**(**3**):323–4.

30. Moore EE, Jurkovich GJ, Knudson MM, Cogbill TH, Malangoni MA, Champion HR, et al. Organ injury scaling VI: extrahepatic biliary, oesophagus, stomach, vulva, vagina, uterus (non-pregnant), uterus (pregnant), fallopian tube, and ovary. *J Trauma.* 1995 Dec;**39**(**6**):1069–70.

31. Moore EE, Cogbill TH, Malangoni MA, Jurkovich GJ, Champion HR, Gennarelli TA, et al. Organ injury scaling II: pancreas, duodenum, small bowel, colon and rectum. *J Trauma.* 1990 Nov;**30**(**11**):1427–9.

32. Moore EE, Shackford SR, Pachter HL, McAninch JW, Browner BD, Champion HR, et al. Organ injury scaling: spleen, liver and kidney. *J Trauma.* 1989 Dec;**29**(**12**):1664–6.

Appendix C
Trauma Guidelines

Below is a list of currently published and generally accepted trauma guidelines. This is an always expanding and dynamic list. Failure to include any others is not a reflection on any guideline itself, but rather the sheer density of what is available.

C.1 EASTERN ASSOCIATION FOR THE SURGERY OF TRAUMA (EAST)

https://www.east.org/education-resources/practice-management-guidelines
Listed alphabetically.

C.1.1 Archived Guidelines

EAST Practice Management Guidelines (PMGs) are reviewed every 5 years and assessed for content and relevance. The PMGs below were reviewed and determined to be no longer relevant to practice today and/or outdated and were therefore archived.

- Abdominal Penetrating Trauma, Non-Operative Management 2007
- Blunt Abdominal Trauma, Evaluation of 2002
- Blunt Aortic Injury 2000
- Blunt Aortic Injury, Diagnosis and Management of 2000
- Blunt Cardiac Injury, Screening for 1998
- Blunt Cerebrovascular Injury 2010
- Blunt Cerebrovascular Injury, Diagnosis and Management of 2007
- Blunt Liver and Spleen Injuries, Non-Operative Management 2003
- Cervical Spine Injuries Following Trauma 2009
- Cervical Spine Injuries Following Trauma, Identification of (1998) 1998
- Colon Injuries, Penetrating 1998
- Geriatric Trauma, Evaluation and Management of 2012

- Geriatric Trauma: Parameters for Resuscitation 2001
- Geriatric Trauma (Update) 2010
- Long Bone Fracture Stabilization in Polytrauma Patients 2001
- Long Bone Fracture Stabilization in Polytrauma Patients 2000
- Mild Traumatic Brain Injury, Management of 2001
- NEW Geriatric Trauma: Triage 2003
- Open Fractures Prophylactic Antibiotics 1998
- Pancreatic Trauma, Diagnosis and Management of 2009
- Pelvic Hemorrhage in Pelvic Fracture, Management of 2001
- Penetrating Abdominal Trauma, Prophylactic Antibiotics in 1998
- Penetrating Arterial Extremity Trauma, Management of 2002
- Penetrating Combined Arterial and Skeletal Extremity Trauma, Management of 2002
- Primer: Utilizing Evidence-Based Outcomes Measures to Develop Practice Management Guidelines 2001
- Pulmonary Contusion and Flail Chest Management 2006
- Small Bowel Obstruction 2007
- Thoracolumbar Spine Injuries Following Trauma, Identification of 2006
- Tracheal Intubation Following Traumatic Injury 2002
- Trauma in Pregnancy 2005
- Tube Thoracostomy for Traumatic Hemopneumothorax Prophylactic Antibiotic Use 1998
- Venous Thromboembolism: A-V Foot Pumps in the Prophylaxis of DVT/PE–old 1998
- Venous Thromboembolism: Low Dose Heparin (LDH) for DVT/PE Prophylaxis–old 1998
- Venous Thromboembolism: Risk Factors after Injury 2002
- Venous Thromboembolism: Risk Factors after Injury–old 1998

- Venous Thromboembolism: Sequential Compression Devices (SCD) in the Prevention of DVT/PE–old 1998
- Venous Thromboembolism: Ultrasound in Diagnostic Imaging–old 1998
- Venous Thromboembolism: Vena Cava Filter in the Prophylaxis and Treatment of PE–old 1998
- Venous Thromboembolism: Venography in the Diagnosis of DVT–old 1998

C.1.2 **Current Guidelines: Trauma**

- Antibiotic Prophylaxis for Tube Thoracostomy Placement in Trauma: A Practice Management Guideline from the Eastern Association for the Surgery of Trauma 2022
- Blunt Aortic Injury, Evaluation and Management of 2015
- Blunt Cardiac Injury, Screening for 2012
- Blunt Cerebrovascular Injury 2010
- Blunt Cerebrovascular Injury, Evaluation and Management of 2020
- Blunt Force Bladder Injuries, Management of 2019
- Cervical Spine Collar Clearance in the Obtunded Adult Blunt Trauma Patient (UPDATE IN PROCESS) 2015
- Cervical Spine Injuries Following Trauma 2009
- Damage Control Resuscitation in Patients with Severe Traumatic Hemorrhage 2017
- Diaphragmatic Injury, Evaluation and Management of 2018
- Efficacy and Safety of Non-Steroidal Anti-Inflammatory Drugs (NSAIDs) for the Treatment of Acute Pain after Orthopaedic Trauma 2022
- Elderly Adults with Isolated Hip Fractures – Orthogeriatric Care versus Standard Care 2020
- Emergency Department Thoracotomy 2015
- Emergency Department Thoracotomy in Children: A PTS, WTA, and EAST Systematic Review and Practice Management Guideline 2023
- Endotracheal Intubation Following Trauma 2012
- Femur Fractures, Open Reduction and Internal Fixation, Timing of – Update 2014
- Genitourinary Trauma, Diagnostic Evaluation of 2003
- Genitourinary Trauma, Management of 2004
- Geriatric Trauma: Parameters for Resuscitation 2003
- Geriatric Trauma, Triage of 2003
- Haemothorax and Occult Pneumothorax, Management of 2011

- Hepatic Injury, Blunt, Selective Nonoperative Management of 2012
- Identifying Maltreatment in Infants and Young Children Presenting with Fractures: Does Age Matter? 2020
- Management of Rhabdomyolysis 2021
- Management of Simple and Retained Haemothorax: A Practice Management Guideline from the Eastern Association for the Surgery of Trauma 2020
- Management of the Open Abdomen: A Systematic Review with Meta-Analysis and Practice Management Guideline from the Eastern Association for the Surgery of Trauma 2022
- Neck Trauma, Penetrating Zone II 2008
- Non-Surgical Management and Analgesia Strategies for Older Adults with Multiple Rib Fractures: A Systematic Review, Meta-Analysis, and Practice Management Guideline 2022
- Open Abdomen in Trauma and Emergency General Surgery, Management of: Part 1 2010
- Open Abdomen Management, A Review: Part 2 2011
- Open Abdomen Management, Review of Abdominal Wall Reconstruction: Part 3 2013
- Open Fractures, Prophylactic Antibiotic Use in – Update 2011
- Pancreatic Injuries 2017
- Pediatric Blunt Renal Trauma 2019
- Pelvic Fracture Hemorrhage, Update and Systematic Review (UPDATE IN PROCESS) 2011
- Penetrating Abdominal Trauma, Prophylactic Antibiotic Use in 2012
- Penetrating Abdominal Trauma, Selective Non-Operative Management of 2010
- Penetrating Combined Arterial and Skeletal Extremity Trauma, Management of 2002
- Penetrating Intraperitoneal Colon Injuries, Management of 2019
- Penetrating Lower Extremity Arterial Trauma, Evaluation and Management of 2012
- Penetrating Neck Injuries, Management of 2008
- Penetrating Venous Extremity Trauma, Management of 2002
- Pregnancy and Trauma 2010
- Prehospital Spine Immobilization/Spinal Motion Restriction in Penetrating Trauma 2018
- Rectal Injuries, Penetrating Extraperitoneal (UPDATE IN PROCESS) 2016
- Rib Fractures, Open Reduction, and Internal Fixation of (UPDATE IN PROCESS) 2017
- Splenic Injury, Blunt, Selective Nonoperative Management of 2012

- Thoracolumbar Spinal Injuries in Blunt Trauma, Screening for 2012
- Thromboelastography and Rotational Thromboelastometry in Bleeding Patients with Coagulopathy 2020
- Traumatic Brain Injury, Mild 2012
- Triage of the Trauma Patient 2010
- Tube Thoracostomy, Presumptive Antibiotics in 2012
- Vaccination after Spleen Embolization: A Practice Management Guideline from the Eastern Association for the Surgery of Trauma 2022

C.1.3 **Current Guidelines: Critical Care**

- Antimotility Agents for the Treatment of Acute Non-Infectious Diarrhoea in Critically Ill Patients 2019
- Beta Blockers after Traumatic Brain Injury 2017
- Blunt Thoracic Trauma (BTT), Pain Management in 2004
- Monitoring Modalities, Assessment of Volume Status, and Endpoints of Resuscitation 2018
- Nutritional Support in Trauma Patients (UPDATE IN PROCESS) 2004
- Nutritional Support: Macronutrient Formulation (Assessment of Energy and Substrate Requirements) (UPDATE IN PROCESS) 2003
- Nutritional Support: Monitoring (Which Tests and How Often?) (UPDATE IN PROCESS) 2004
- Nutritional Support: Route (Total Parenteral versus Total Enteral) (UPDATE IN PROCESS) 2004
- Nutritional Support: Site of Enteral Support (Gastric versus Jejunal) (UPDATE IN PROCESS) 2004
- Nutritional Support: Timing (Early versus Delayed Enteral Feedings) (UPDATE IN PROCESS) 2004
- Nutritional Support: Type (Standard versus Enhanced) (UPDATE IN PROCESS) 2003
- Prehospital Fluid Resuscitation in the Injured Patient 2009
- Promotility Agents for the Treatment of Ileus in Adult Surgical Patients 2019
- Pulmonary Contusion and Flail Chest, Management of 2012
- Red Blood Cell Transfusion (Converted) 2011
- Red Blood Cell Transfusion in Adult Trauma and Critical Care 2009
- Resuscitation Endpoints 2004

- Stress Ulcer Prophylaxis 2008
- Thoracic Trauma, Blunt, Pain Management of 2016
- Tracheostomy Timing in Trauma Patients (UPDATE IN PROCESS) 2009
- Venous Thromboembolism, Adult Trauma Patients 2002
- Venous Thromboembolism: Low Dose Heparin for DVT/PE Prophylaxis 2002
- Venous Thromboembolism: Pneumatic Compression Devices in the Prevention of DVT/PE 2002
- Venous Thromboembolism Prophylaxis, Pediatric Trauma Patients – Joint between EAST and PTS 2017
- Venous Thromboembolism: Risk Factors after Injury 2002
- Venous Thromboembolism: Role of Low-Molecular-Weight Heparin in VTE Prophylaxis 2002
- Venous Thromboembolism: Role of Ultrasound in Diagnostic Imaging for DVT in Trauma 2002
- Venous Thromboembolism: Role of Vena Cava Filter in the Prophylaxis and Treatment of PE (UPDATE IN PROCESS) 2002
- Venous Thromboembolism: Venography in the Diagnosis of DVT 2002

C.1.4 **Injury Prevention**

- Alcohol-Related Trauma Reinjury Prevention with Hospital-Based Screening in Adult Populations 2020
- All-Terrain Vehicle Injuries, Prevention of 2018
- Child Passenger Safety: An Evidence-Based Review 2010
- Contact Sports-Related Concussion in Amateur Athletes, Primary Prevention of 2018
- Distracted Driver: An Evidence-Based Review 2015
- Fall-Related Injuries in the Elderly, Prevention of 2016
- Full-Face Motorcycle Helmets to Reduce Injury and Death 2022
- Helmet Efficacy to Reduce Head Injury and Mortality in Motorcycle Crashes 2010
- Hospital-Based Violence Intervention Programs Targeting Adult Populations 2016
- Motor Vehicle Collision-Related Injuries in the Elderly, Prevention of 2015
- Palliative Care for Geriatric Trauma Patients, Trauma Center Care and Routine Processes for Care – Evidence-Based Review 2019

- Prevention of Firearm Injuries with Gun Safety Devices and Safe Storage 2018
- Prevention of Firearm-Related Injuries with Restrictive Licensing and Concealed Carry Laws 2016
- Prevention of Firearm Violence through Specific Types of Community-Based Programming: An Eastern Association for the Surgery of Trauma Evidence-Based Review 2021
- Safety Helmets, Efficacy of in Reduction of Head Injuries in Recreational Skiers and Snowboarders 2011

C.2 WESTERN TRAUMA ASSOCIATION (WTA) ALGORITHMS

https://www.westerntrauma.org/western-trauma-association-algorithms/published-algorithms/
https://www.westerntrauma.org/western-trauma-association-algorithms/
Algorithms listed chronologically.

1. McIntyre RC, Jr., Moore FA, Davis JW, Cocanour CS, West MA, Moore EE, Jr. Western Trauma Association Critical Decisions in Trauma: Foreword. J Trauma 2008;65(5):1005-6. doi: 10.1097/TA.0b013e31818a93bf.
2. Davis JW, Moore FA, McIntyre RC, Jr., Cocanour CS, Moore EE, West MA. Western **Trauma Association Critical Decisions in Trauma: Management of Pelvic Fracture** with Hemodynamic Instability. J Trauma 2008;65(5):1012-5. doi: 10.1097/TA.0b013e318189a836.
3. Moore FA, Davis JW, Moore EE, Jr., Cocanour CS, West MA, McIntyre RC, Jr. Western Trauma Association (WTA) Critical Decisions in Trauma: **Management of Adult Blunt Splenic Trauma.** J Trauma 2008;65(5):1007-11. doi: 10.1097/TA.0b013e31818a93bf.
4. Biffl WL, Cothren CC, Moore EE, Kozar R, Cocanour C, Davis JW, et al. Western Trauma Association Critical Decisions in Trauma: **Screening for And Treatment of Blunt Cerebrovascular Injuries.** J Trauma 2009;67(6):1150-3. doi: 10.1097/TA.0b013e3181c1c1d6.
5. Kozar RA, Moore FA, Moore EE, West M, Cocanour CS, Davis J, et al. Western Trauma Association Critical Decisions in Trauma: **Nonoperative Management of Adult Blunt Hepatic Trauma**. J Trauma 2009;67(6):1144-8; discussion 8-9. doi: 10.1097/TA.0b013e3181ba361f.
6. Feliciano DV, Moore FA, Moore EE, West MA, Davis JW, Cocanour CS, et al. **Evaluation and Management of Peripheral Vascular Injury. Part 1.** Western Trauma Association Critical Decisions in Trauma. J Trauma 2011;70(6):1551-6. doi: 10.1097/TA.0b013e31821b5bdd.
7. Kozar RA, Feliciano DV, Moore EE, Moore FA, Cocanour CS, West MA, et al. Western Trauma Association Critical Decisions in Trauma: **Operative Management of Adult Blunt Hepatic Trauma.** J Trauma 2011;71(1):1-5. doi: 10.1097/TA.0b013e318220b192.
8. Burlew CC, Moore EE, Moore FA, Coimbra R, McIntyre RC, Jr., Davis JW, et al. Western Trauma Association Critical Decisions in Trauma: **Resuscitative Thoracotomy**. J Trauma Acute Care Surg 2012;73(6):1359-63. doi: 10.1097/TA.0b013e318270d2df.
9. Moore FA, Moore EE, Burlew CC, Coimbra R, McIntyre RC, Jr., Davis JW, et al. Western Trauma Association Critical Decisions in Trauma: **Management of Complicated Diverticulitis.** J Trauma Acute Care Surg 2012;73(6):1365-71. doi: 10.1097/TA.0b013e31827826d8.
10. Moore HB, Moore EE, Burlew CC, Moore FA, Coimbra R, Davis JW, et al. Western Trauma Association Critical Decisions in Trauma: **Management of Parapneumonic Effusion**. J Trauma Acute Care Surg 2012;73(6):1372-9. doi: 10.1097/TA.0b013e31825ff7e4.
11. Scalea TM, DuBose J, Moore EE, West M, Moore FA, McIntyre R, et al. Western Trauma Association Critical Decisions in Trauma: **Management of the Mangled Extremity**. J Trauma Acute Care Surg 2012;72(1):86-93. doi: 10.1097/TA.0b013e318241ed70.
12. Biffl WL, Moore EE, Croce M, Davis JW, Coimbra R, Karmy-Jones R, et al. Western Trauma Association Critical Decisions in Trauma: **Management of Pancreatic Injuries**. J Trauma Acute Care Surg 2013;75(6):941-6. doi: 10.1097/TA.0b013e3182a96572.
13. Feliciano DV, Moore EE, West MA, Moore FA, Davis JW, Cocanour CS, et al. Western Trauma Association Critical Decisions in Trauma: **Evaluation and Management of Peripheral Vascular Injury, Part II.** J Trauma Acute Care Surg 2013;75(3):391-7. doi: 10.1097/TA.0b013e3182994b48.

14. Sperry JL, Moore EE, Coimbra R, Croce M, Davis JW, Karmy-Jones R, et al. Western Trauma Association Critical Decisions in Trauma: **Penetrating Neck Trauma.** J Trauma Acute Care Surg 2013;75(6):936-40. doi: 10.1097/TA.0b013e31829e20e3.

15. Karmy-Jones R, Namias N, Coimbra R, Moore EE, Schreiber M, McIntyre R, Jr., et al. Western Trauma Association Critical Decisions in Trauma: **Penetrating Chest Trauma.** J Trauma Acute Care Surg 2014;77(6):994-1002. doi: 10.1097/TA.0000000000000426.

16. Biffl WL, Moore EE, Feliciano DV, Albrecht RA, Croce M, Karmy-Jones R, et al. Western Trauma Association Critical Decisions in Trauma: **Diagnosis and Management of Esophageal Injuries**. J Trauma Acute Care Surg 2015;79(6):1089-95. doi: 10.1097/TA.0000000000000772.

17. Feliciano DV, Moore EE, Biffl WL. Western Trauma Association Critical Decisions in Trauma: **Management of Abdominal Vascular Trauma**. J Trauma Acute Care Surg 2015;79(6):1079-88. doi: 10.1097/TA.0000000000000869.

18. Malhotra A, Biffl WL, Moore EE, Schreiber M, Albrecht RA, Cohen M, et al. Western Trauma Association Critical Decisions in Trauma: **Diagnosis and Management of Duodenal Injuries.** J Trauma Acute Care Surg 2015;79(6):1096-101. doi: 10.1097/TA.0000000000000870.

19. Tran TL, Brasel KJ, Karmy-Jones R, Rowell S, Schreiber MA, Shatz DV, et al. Western Trauma Association Critical Decisions in Trauma: **Management of Pelvic Fracture with Hemodynamic Instability-2016 Updates**. J Trauma Acute Care Surg 2016;81(6):1171-4. doi: 10.1097/TA.0000000000001230.

20. Brasel KJ, Moore EE, Albrecht RA, deMoya M, Schreiber M, Karmy-Jones R, et al. Western Trauma Association Critical Decisions in Trauma: **Management of Rib Fractures**. J Trauma Acute Care Surg 2017;82(1):200-3. doi: 10.1097/TA.0000000000001301.

21. Rowell SE, Biffl WL, Brasel K, Moore EE, Albrecht RA, DeMoya M, et al. Western Trauma Association Critical Decisions in Trauma: **Management of Adult Blunt Splenic Trauma-2016 Updates**. J Trauma Acute Care Surg 2017;82(4):787-93. doi: 10.1097/TA.0000000000001323.

22. Biffl WL, Moore EE, Feliciano DV, Albrecht RM, Croce MA, Karmy-Jones R, et al. **Management of Colorectal Injuries:** A Western Trauma Association Critical Decisions Algorithm. J Trauma Acute Care Surg 2018;85(5):1016-20. doi: 10.1097/TA.0000000000001929.

23. Brown CVR, Alam HB, Brasel K, Hauser CJ, de Moya M, Martin M, et al. Western Trauma Association Critical Decisions in Trauma: **Management of Renal Trauma.** J Trauma Acute Care Surg 2018;85(5):1021-5. doi: 10.1097/TA.0000000000001960.

24. Martin MJ, Brown CVR, Shatz DV, Alam HB, Brasel KJ, Hauser CJ, et al. **Evaluation and Management of Abdominal Stab Wounds**: A Western Trauma Association Critical Decisions Algorithm. J Trauma Acute Care Surg 2018;85(5):1007-15. doi: 10.1097/TA.0000000000001930.

25. Martin MJ, Brown CVR, Shatz DV, Alam H, Brasel K, Hauser CJ, et al. **Evaluation and Management of Abdominal Gunshot Wounds:** A Western Trauma Association Critical Decisions Algorithm. J Trauma Acute Care Surg 2019;87(5):1220-7. doi: 10.1097/TA.0000000000002410.

26. Sava J, Alam HB, Vercruysse G, Martin M, Brown CVR, Brasel K, et al. Western Trauma Association Critical Decisions in Trauma: **Management of the Open Abdomen After Damage Control Surgery.** J Trauma Acute Care Surg 2019;87(5):1232-8. doi: 10.1097/TA.0000000000002389.

27. Sperry JL, Martin MJ, Moore EE, Sava JA, Ciesla D, Rizzo AG, et al. Prehospital **Resuscitation in Adult Patients Following Injury:** A Western Trauma Association Critical Decisions Algorithm. J Trauma Acute Care Surg 2019;87(5):1228-31. doi: 10.1097/TA.0000000000002488.

28. Vercruysse GA, Alam HB, Martin MJ, Brasel K, Moore EE, Brown CV, et al. Western Trauma Association Critical Decisions in Trauma: **Preferred Triage and Initial Management of the Burned Patient.** J Trauma Acute Care Surg 2019;87(5):1239-43. doi: 10.1097/TA.0000000000002520.

29. Alam H, Vercruysse G, Martin M, Brown C, Brasel K, Moore EE, et al. Western Trauma Association Critical Decisions in Trauma: **Management of Intracranial Hypertension in Patients with Severe Traumatic Brain Injuries.** J Trauma Acute Care Surg 2020;epub ahead of print: doi: 10.1097/TA.0000000000002555.

30. Ciesla DJ, Shatz DV, Moore EE, Sava J, Martin M, Brown CVR, et al. Western Trauma Association Critical Decisions in Trauma: **Cervical Spine Clearance in Trauma Patients**. J Trauma Acute Care Surg 2020;epub ahead of print: doi: 10.1097/TA.0000000000002520x.

31. Ley EJ, Brown CFV Moore EE, Sava JA, Peck5 KA, Ciesla DJ, Sperry JL, Rizzo AG, Rosen NG, Brasel KJ, Kozar R, Inaba K, Martin MJ. **Updated Guidelines to Reduce Venous Thromboembolism in Trauma Patients**: A Western Trauma Association Critical Decisions Algorithm. Journal of Trauma and Acute Care Surgery, Publish Ahead of Print. doi: 10.1097/TA.0000000000002830.

32. Inaba K, Alam HB, Brasel KJ, Brenner M, Brown CVR, Ciesla DJ, et al. A Western Trauma Association critical decisions algorithm: **Resuscitative endovascular balloon occlusion of the aorta.** *J Trauma Acute Care Surg.* 2022 Apr 1;**92(4):**748-753. doi: 10.1097/TA.0000000000003438.

33. Peck KA, Ley EJ, Brown CV, Moore EE, Sava JA, Ciesla DJ, et al. Early anticoagulant reversal after trauma: A Western Trauma Association critical decisions algorithm. *J Trauma Acute Care Surg.* 2021 Feb 1;**90(2):**331-336. doi: 10.1097/TA.0000000000002979.

34. Rosen NG, Escobar MA Jr, Brown CV, **Moore EE**, **Sava JA**, Peck K, et al. Child physical abuse trauma evaluation and management: A Western Trauma Association and Pediatric Trauma Society critical decisions algorithm. *J Trauma Acute Care Surg.* 2021 Apr 1;**90(4):**641-651. doi: 10.1097/TA.0000000000003076.

C.2.1 **Additional Algorithms**

WTA Algorithm for Blunt Thoracic Aortic Injury Management:
   https://custom.cvent.com/2A7C589629FA4A7181E1D1A892311435/files/a4eaeb3baa984ad181747f704a1108fa.pdf
   WTA Algorithm for Blunt Abdominal Trauma:
   https://custom.cvent.com/2A7C589629FA4A7181E1D1A892311435/files/603730a847af494fa170694b778b703a.pdf
   WTA Algorithm for Blunt Pancreatic Injury:
   https://custom.cvent.com/2A7C589629FA4A7181E1D1A892311435/files/7ae053a528cb4a7281b734f0a19fe660.pdf

WTA Algorithm for Paediatric Resuscitative Thoracotomy:
   https://custom.cvent.com/2A7C589629FA4A7181E1D1A892311435/files/1343f0f563a64002ac64c1afce2c9877.pdf

C.3 **SURGICAL CRITICAL CARE.NET**

https://surgicalcriticalcare.net/guidelines.html

Listed alphabetically by system.	*mm/dd/yyyy*
CARDIOVASCULAR	
EBM Guideline	**Revised**
Acute Atrial Fibrillation in the Surgical Patient	12/12/2017
Axillary Artery and Vein Cannulation	11/18/2022
Blunt Cardiac Injury	3/23/2021
Blunt Thoracic Aortic Injury	3/24/2021
Free Flap Management	3/4/2018
Hypertension Management	11/25/2015
Non-Invasive Hemodynamic Monitoring	9/28/2016
Resuscitative Balloon Occlusion of the Aorta (REBOA)	5/29/2023
Ultrasound Guided Peripheral IV Insertion	5/27/2020
Vasopressors and Inotropes in Shock	9/11/2019
ENDOCRINE	
EBM Guideline	**Revised**
Critical Illness-Related Corticosteroid Insufficiency	6/21/2022
Hyperglycaemia Control in the Critically Ill	12/6/2011
Thyroid Management in the ICU	4/1/2019
FLUIDS, ELECTROLYTES, AND NUTRITION	
EBM Guideline	**Revised**
Burn Patient Nutrition	7/2/2023
Electrolyte Replacement	9/27/2019
Fluid Resuscitation	11/2/2017
Nasogastric/Enteric Tube Placement in Traumatic Craniofacial Fractures	1/25/2017
Rhabdomyolysis: Prevention and Treatment	7/2/2023

GASTROINTESTINAL	
EBM Guideline	**Revised**
Acute Cholecystitis	1/7/2015
Acute Gastrointestinal Hemorrhage: Pharmacologic Management	12/12/2017
Blunt Splenic Injury	9/30/2015
Cirrhotic Management	2/24/2016
Clostridium difficile Infection	9/7/2022
Diverticulitis	9/30/2015
Enteral Feeding Guidelines	4/9/2017
Intra-Abdominal Pressure Monitoring	3/2/2015
Octreotide in the Prevention and Treatment of Gastrointestinal and Pancreatic Fistulas	1/2/2017
Percutaneous Endoscopic Gastrostomy	6/8/2020
Post-Splenectomy Vaccine Prophylaxis	12/27/2022
Premature Gastrostomy/Jejunostomy Removal	10/20/2009
Small Bowel Obstruction	6/3/2014
Stress Ulcer Prophylaxis	2/22/2023

HEMATOLOGIC	
EBM Guideline	**Revised**
Blood Conservation and Transfusion Avoidance Strategies in the Surgical Patient	6/26/2019
Deep Venous Thrombosis Prophylaxis in Surgery and Trauma Patients	7/2/2023
Disseminated Intravascular Coagulation	4/9/2017
Erythropoietin Use in the Critically Ill	2/5/2008
Heparin Induced Thrombocytopenia	9/13/2019
Inferior Vena Caval Filter Use in Patients at High Risk for Pulmonary Embolism	10/27/2009
Massive Transfusion Protocol for Haemorrhagic Shock	5/7/2020
Non-Vitamin K Anticoagulation Reversal	7/25/2018
Thromboelastography (TEG) in Trauma	11/7/2021
Warfarin Dosing	8/31/2009
Warfarin Reversal	11/29/2017

INFECTIOUS DISEASE	
EBM Guideline	**Revised**
Aerosolized Antibiotic Therapy in the ICU	3/29/2016
Antibiotic Administration in Facial and Skull Fractures	2/24/2021
Antibiotic Prophylaxis in Surgery	11/29/2013
Candida Infections in Surgical Patients	4/9/2017
Continuous Antibiotic Infusions	7/2/2023
Empiric Antibiotic Use in Critically Ill Patients	5/8/2007
Presumptive Chest Tube Antibiotics	3/6/2013

MISCELLANEOUS	
EBM Guideline	**Revised**
Alcohol Withdrawal	4/25/2023
Central Venous Catheterization	12/3/2009
Fever Assessment	1/30/2013
Gabapentin in Post-Operative Pain Management	7/2/2023
Ketamine for Analgesia	3/11/2021
Laparoscopy in Trauma	2/24/2016
Mangled Extremity	4/27/2016
Muscle Relaxants in Multimodal Pain Management	1/25/2017
Necrotizing Soft Tissues Infections	9/27/2018
Negative Pressure Wound Therapy	2/5/2014
Neuromuscular Blocking Agents in the Adult ICU	8/1/2018

NEUROLOGIC	
EBM Guideline	**Revised**
Acute Spinal Cord Injury	9/10/2018
Antiplatelet Agent Reversal in Adults – Traumatic Intracranial Hemorrhage	4/9/2017
Blunt Cerebrovascular Injury	3/31/2021
Brain Death Determination/Apnoea Test Procedure	9/30/2015
Cervical Spine Clearance	12/12/2017
Delirium Management in the ICU	7/2/2023
Hypertonic Saline Solution Instructions	5/6/2008
Management of Status Epilepticus in Adults	7/27/2022
Methylprednisolone (Solumedrol) in Acute Spinal Cord Injury	8/1/2014

Pain Management in Surgery	9/30/2015
Sedation and Agitation Management in the ICU	6/21/2022
Seizure Prophylaxis in Traumatic Brain Injury	7/2/2023
Syncope Evaluation in the Trauma Patient	9/28/2016
Therapeutic Hypothermia Following Cardiac Arrest	9/2/2020
Traumatic Brain Injury Management	1/16/2023

PULMONARY	
EBM Guideline	**Revised**
Air Travel Following Traumatic Pneumothorax	11/18/2022
Chest Tube Management	9/28/2016
Extubating the Trauma Patient with an Open Abdomen	6/21/2022
High-Frequency Oscillatory Ventilation in the Surgical Patient	3/3/2009
Independent Lung Ventilation	12/3/2014
Multi-Modality Rib Fracture Management	3/5/2020
Paracostal Infusion of Bupivacaine for Management of Rib Fracture Pain	4/20/2010
Peri-Procedural Tracheostomy Complications	1/3/2013
Post-Extubation Stridor	6/28/2017
Post-Tracheostomy Hemorrhage	1/3/2013
Pulmonary Blast Injury	9/28/2016
Rescue Ventilation	8/21/2018
Retained Haemothorax	4/27/2016
Surgical Fixation of Rib Fractures	9/4/2020
Thrombolytics for Pulmonary Embolism	9/28/2016
Timing of Tracheostomy	9/30/2015
Tissue Plasminogen Activator in Traumatic Haemothorax	3/31/2018
Tracheostomy Dislodgement	2/20/2020
Ventilator-Associated Pneumonia	2/24/2016

SKIN	
EBM Guideline	**Revised**
Acute Burn Resuscitation	11/26/2019
Perioperative Hypothermia Prevention in Burn Patients	3/29/2018
Snakebite/Crotalid Envenomation	7/2/2023

C.4 AMERICAN COLLEGE OF SURGEONS (ACS)

Listed alphabetically.

ACS TQP Best Practices Guidelines:
https://www.facs.org/quality-programs/trauma/quality/best-practices-guidelines/

Acute Pain Management in Trauma Patients:
https://www.facs.org/media/exob3dwk/acute_pain_guidelines.pdf

Child Abuse, Elder Abuse, and Intimate Partner Violence:
https://www.facs.org/media/o0wdimys/abuse_guide-lines.pdf

Geriatric Trauma Management:
https://www.facs.org/for-medical-professionals/news-publications/news-and-articles/press-releases/2023/american-college-of-surgeons-releases-the-revised-best-practices-guidelines-in-geriatric-trauma-management/

Imaging Guidelines:
https://www.facs.org/media/oxdjw5zj/imaging_guidelines.pdf

Management of Orthopaedic Trauma:
https://www.facs.org/media/mkbnhqtw/ortho_guidelines.pdf

Management of Traumatic Brain Injury:
https://www.facs.org/media/mkej5u3b/tbi_guide-lines.pdf

Massive Transfusion in Trauma:
https://www.facs.org/media/zcjdtrd1/transfusion_guildelines.pdf

Mental Health and Substance Use Guidelines:
https://www.facs.org/media/nrcj31ku/mental-health-guidelines.pdf

Palliative Care:
https://www.facs.org/media/g3rfegcn/palliative_guidelines.pdf

Spine Injury:
https://www.facs.org/media/k45gikqv/spine_injury_guidelines.pdf

C.5 AMERICAN ASSOCIATION FOR THE SURGERY OF TRAUMA (AAST)

CDC Guidelines for the Field Triage of Injured Patients:
https://www.cdc.gov/mmwr/preview/mmwrhtml/rr6101a1.htm

EAST Guidelines:
https://www.east.org/education-career-development/practice-management-guidelines

National Guidelines Clearing House:
http://www.guideline.gov/
Agency for Healthcare Research and Quality:
http://www.ahrq.gov/clinic/epcix.htm
Antithrombotic Therapy and Prevention of Thrombosis, 9th ed.: American College of Chest Physicians Evidence-Based Clinical Practice Guidelines:
https://journal.chestnet.org/article/S0012-3692(12)60115-9/fulltext

C.6 BRAIN TRAUMA FOUNDATION GUIDELINES

Guidelines for the Management of Pediatric Severe TBI, 3rd edition:
https://braintrauma.org/coma/guidelines/pediatric
Guidelines for the Management of Severe TBI, 4th edition:
https://braintrauma.org/coma/guidelines-for-the-management-of-severe-tbi-4th-ed
Early Indicators of Prognosis in Severe TBI:
https://braintrauma.org/coma/guidelines/prognosis
Guidelines for Pre-Hospital Management of TBI:
https://braintrauma.org/coma/guidelines/pre-hospital
Guidelines for the Surgical Management of TBI:
https://braintrauma.org/coma/guidelines/guidelines-for-the-surgical-management-of-tbi
Guidelines for Field Management of Combat-Related Trauma:
https://braintrauma.org/coma/guidelines/combat-related
The Seattle International Severe Traumatic Brain Injury Consensus Conference (SIBICC) Severe TBI Algorithm for Patients with ICP Monitoring:
https://braintrauma.org/coma/guidelines/sibicc-severe-tbi-algorithm-for-patients-with-icp-monitoring

C.7 EUROPEAN SOCIETY OF TRAUMA AND EMERGENCY SURGERY (ESTES)

https://www.estesonline.org/?s=guidelines

C.8 WORLD SOCIETY OF EMERGENCY SURGERY (WSES) GUIDELINES

https://www.wses.org.uk/guidelines
Listed chronologically. Trauma guidelines only.

2013
Management of Hemodynamically Unstable Pelvic Trauma:
https://www.wses.org.uk/guidelines#collapse7141
Emergency Repair of Complicated Abdominal Wall Hernias:
https://www.wses.org.uk/guidelines#collapse7144
Position Paper: Oesophageal Injuries:
https://www.wses.org.uk/guidelines#collapse7144
2015
Clostridium difficile Infection in Surgical Patients:
https://www.wses.org.uk/wp-content/uploads/2018/07/Clostridium-difficile-infection-in-surgical-patients.pdf
2016
Liver Trauma Guidelines:
https://www.wses.org.uk/wp-content/uploads/2019/09/liver-trauma-guidelines.pdf
Acute Cholecystitis Guidelines:
https://www.wses.org.uk/wp-content/uploads/2018/07/acute-cholecystitis-guidelines.pdf
Acute Appendicitis Guidelines:
https://www.wses.org.uk/wp-content/uploads/2018/07/acute-appendicitis-guidelines.pdf
2017
Splenic Trauma: WSES Classification and Guidelines for Adult and Pediatric Patients:
https://wjes.biomedcentral.com/articles/10.1186/s13017-017-0151-4
Pelvic Trauma Guidelines:
https://www.wses.org.uk/wp-content/uploads/2018/07/Clostridium-difficile-infection-in-surgical-patients.pdf
2017 Update of the WSES Guidelines for Emergency Repair of Complicated Abdominal Wall Hernias:
https://wjes.biomedcentral.com/articles/10.1186/s13017-017-0149-y
2018
Adhesive Small Bowel Obstruction (ASBO) 2017 Update of the Evidence-Based Guidelines from the World Society of Emergency Surgery ASBO Working Group:
ten Broek T, Krielen P), Di Saverio S, Coccolini F, Biffl WL, Ansaloni L, et al. World Journal of Emergency Surgery (2018) 13:24 https://doi.org/10.1186/s13017-018-0185-2
https://www.wses.org.uk/wp-content/uploads/2018/02/GL-iatrogenic-colonoscopy-perforations.pdf
Acute Mesenteric Ischemia:
https://www.wses.org.uk/wp-content/uploads/2018/01/Acute-Mesenteric-Ischemia.pdf
2019
Oesophageal Emergencies:

https://www.wses.org.uk/wp-content/uploads/2019/06/esophageal-emergencies.pdf

Clostridium Guidelines:

https://www.wses.org.uk/wp-content/uploads/2019/03/clostridium-GL.pdf

2020

WSES Guidelines on Blunt and Penetrating Bowel Injury: Diagnosis, Investigations, and Treatment:

https://www.wses.org.uk/wp-content/uploads/2022/03/972-WSES-guidelines-on-blunt-and-penetrating-bowel-injury_-diagnosis-investigations-and-treatment.pdf

American Association for the Surgery of Trauma–World Society of Emergency Surgery Guidelines on Diagnosis and Management of Abdominal Vascular Injuries:

No link available

American Association for the Surgery of Trauma–World Society of Emergency Surgery Guidelines on Diagnosis and Management of Peripheral Vascular Injuries:

No link available

Liver Trauma Guidelines:

https://www.wses.org.uk/wp-content/uploads/2020/04/2020-liver-guidelines.pdf

2022

WSES Guidelines on Blunt and Penetrating Bowel Injury: Diagnosis, Investigations, and Treatment:

https://www.wses.org.uk/wp-content/uploads/2022/03/972-WSES-guidelines-on-blunt-and-penetrating-bowel-injury_-diagnosis-investigations-and-treatment.pdf

Appendix D
The Definitive Surgical Trauma Care Course: The Definitive Anaesthetic Trauma Care Course: Course Requirements and Syllabus

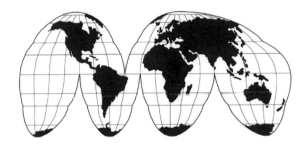

International Association for Trauma Surgery and Intensive Care

IATSIC Secretariat
International Society of Surgery
Seefeldstrasse
CH-8008 Zurich
Switzerland

D.1 BACKGROUND

Injury (trauma) remains a major healthcare problem throughout the world. In addition to improving awareness of trauma prevention and management, improved application of surgical skills is expected to save further lives and contribute to minimizing disability. It is widely recognized that training of surgeons and anaesthesiologists in the management of trauma is substantially deficient because of:

- Limited exposure within individual training programmes to the types of patients required to develop the appropriate level of skills.
- Traditional trauma training, which has been organ-specific.

Consequently, surgeons can finish their training with suboptimal skills in this field, where there is often little time to contemplate an appropriate course of action.

Through the early 1990s, it became apparent to several surgeons familiar with trauma management around the world that there was a specific need for surgical training in the technical aspects of the operative care of trauma patients, with emphasis on those who were close to completing, or had recently completed, their training. This course had its origins during a meeting in October 1993 between Howard Champion (United States), David Mulder (Canada), Donald Trunkey (United States), Stephen Deane (Australia), and Abe Fingerhut (France).

This postgraduate surgical course, developed in collaboration with professional educators, assumes competence with assessment and resuscitative measures that have become standardized through the Advanced Trauma Life Support® (ATLS) course of the American College of Surgeons. It draws on the specialist training of all course participants, and reviews, strengthens, and organizes the performance of established and new procedures specially required in trauma surgery. The course has special relevance for surgeons and anaesthesiologists in countries where major trauma rates are high. It is also likely to be valuable in developing countries where education and physical resources are limited, and particularly in those countries with humanitarian or military peacekeeping roles, where use is made of healthcare professionals who have limited experience in trauma.

D.2 COURSE DEVELOPMENT AND TESTING

There have been many attempts to test the concept:

- There was a Swedish Trauma Surgery Course which Drs Trunkey, Fingerhut, and Champion attended in Sweden in November 1994. This was run by Dr Sten Lennquist. The course was 4 days of didactic teaching and 1 day of practical work.
- In Sydney in May 1996, a very successful pilot course was organized at Prince Henry Hospital. The international faculty at that course included Don Trunkey, Abe Fingerhut, and Howard Champion. The course was a tremendous success, and successful courses have since been held worldwide.
- From 1999, following courses in Australia, Austria, and South Africa, a standardized manual and slide set were developed.
- The course is revised every 4 years, with updated material, in order to stay current and to recognize the rapid improvements in trauma care globally.

D.3 COURSE DETAILS

D.3.1 Ownership

The Definitive Surgical Trauma Care™ (DSTC™) and Definitive Anaesthetic Trauma Care™ (DATC™) courses are registered trademarks of the International Association for Trauma Surgery and Intensive Care (IATSIC). IATSIC is an Integrated Society of the International Society of Surgery/Société Internationale de Chirugie (ISS–SIC), based in Zurich, Switzerland. Only courses recognized by IATSIC may be called DSTC courses, and a unique course number will be issued for each course held. The DATC course is a registered module included within the DSTC course.

D.3.2 Mission Statement

The course is designed to train participants in the techniques required for the overall care of the injured trauma patient. This is done by a combination of lectures, demonstrations, case discussions, and practical sessions, utilizing live tissue and human (cadaver or prosected) tissue if available.

D.3.3 Application to Hold a Course

Application can be made to IATSIC for recognition of a course. Provided the minimum requirements for the course have been met, as laid down below, IATSIC will recognize the course, which will then be entitled to be called a DSTC course and carry the IATSIC logo.

DATC is a specific module within the DSTC course. The initial course to be presented will be the course prescribed by IATSIC, and no changes may be made to the course material or syllabus.

D.3.4 Eligibility to Present

D.3.4.1 LOCAL ORGANIZATIONS

The DSTC course can be presented by any tertiary academic institution or recognized surgical organization.

D.3.4.2 NATIONAL ORGANIZATIONS

National organizations can present the course in their own country on behalf of IATSIC. A memorandum of understanding will be signed with IATSIC. Following the presentation of the first two courses, the national organization shall have the right to modify the course to enhance its relevance to local conditions, although still respecting the core curriculum.

D.3.5 Course Materials and Overview

The course takes place over 3 days with the following course materials:

- The administrative details of running the course are contained in the *Course Director's Manual*, available from the IATSIC office.

- The content of the course will, at a minimum, contain the core curriculum, as laid down in the IATSIC DSTC/DATC manual (see Appendix D). Additional material and modules may be included at the discretion of the local organizers, provided such material is not in conflict with the core curriculum.
- Additional 'add-on' modules may be presented at the discretion of the local organizers.
- The course will use a specific set of slides and the DSTC course manual.
- IATSIC is able to furnish the IATSIC course manual, and course materials (including slides on PowerPoint) if requested, at a substantial discount.

D.3.6 **Course Director**

In addition to the requirements below, the course director must be a full, current member of IATSIC. For an inaugural course, the course director must be a member of the IATSIC Executive Committee.

D.3.7 **Course Faculty**

- Course faculty will be divided into:
- Local faculty
- International faculty
- Guest lecturers
- Course faculty members must have themselves attended a DSTC course.
- Course faculty members must have completed an ATLS® Instructor course, Royal College of Surgeons 'Train the Trainers' course, or an equivalent instructor training course.
- Course international faculty must be members of IATSIC.
- Additional guest lecturers with particular expertise in a subject are permitted.
- Details of all faculty members with confirmation of the above, and full Ethics Committee approval, must be lodged with IATSIC at least 3 months prior to commencement of the course.
- The recommended student:instructor ratio should ideally be 4:1, not including the course director.

D.3.8 **Course Participants**

- All course participants must be licensed medical practitioners.

- Attendance at the entire course is mandatory.
- The level of applicants can be decided locally, provided that the participants are licensed medical practitioners and are *actively involved in the surgical decision-making and surgical care* of the trauma patient.
- An entrance examination can be used if needed. An exit examination is not mandatory.

D.3.9 **Practical Skill Stations**

Practical skills may take place on different material, depending on the local constraints. The practical component of the course *must* include a live tissue training laboratory. However, the use of cadavers is optional and dependent on local conditions. Full local ethical committee certificates of approval for all animal and other tissue work, and any other necessary legal approvals, *must* be obtained and must be submitted to IATSIC *before* a course can be approved or held.

D.3.10 **Course Syllabus**

In order for IATSIC to recognize the course as a valid DSTC course, the course must meet or exceed the minimum requirements of the core curriculum. The core curriculum and 'modules' are contained in this manual, and the course consists of:

- Core knowledge.
- Surgical skills (see Appendix D).
- Additional modules, which may be added as required, at the discretion of the local organizing committee and as required for local needs.
- Where human material is available for dissection, the course is often enhanced by presentation, in association with the American College of Surgeons (ACS), of the ACS Course in Advanced Surgical Skills for Exposure in Trauma (ASSET®).

D.3.11 **Course Certification**

- Participants are required to attend the entire course.
- Certification of attendance and completion of the course can be issued.
- The certificates of the courses will be numbered.
- Details of the course, final faculty, and participants, as well as a course evaluation, must be submitted to IATSIC after the course.

D.4 IATSIC RECOGNITION

Application for recognition of individual courses should be made to IATSIC. IATSIC-recognized courses may carry the endorsement logos of IATSIC and the ISS–SIC and will be entitled to be called DSTC courses.

As mentioned above, the DSTC course is the intellectual property and a registered trademark of IATSIC, and IATSIC is an Integrated Society of the ISS–SIC based in Zurich, Switzerland. Although it may carry the endorsement (support) of other bodies, this does not imply that other organizations may operate or control the DSTC course in any way.

The DSTC course is designed to train medical practitioners in the techniques required for the definitive surgical care of the trauma patient. This is done by a combination of lectures, demonstrations, case discussions, and practical sessions.

The registration and control of the DSTC courses will be controlled by the DSTC Sub-Committee on behalf of IATSIC. Whilst it is desirable that national courses be controlled by a national organization, there will be no restriction on local courses provided that international DSTC criteria are met. Application to hold a course must be made through IATSIC.

Only courses recognized by IATSIC may be called DSTC courses.

D.5 COURSE INFORMATION

Course information is obtainable from IATSIC.

D.5.1 The DSTC Course

D.5.1.1 COURSE OBJECTIVES

By the end of the course, the student has:

- Enhanced knowledge of the surgical physiology of the trauma patient
- Enhanced resuscitation and surgical decision-making capabilities in trauma
- Enhanced surgical expertise in the techniques for the management of major trauma
- A more comprehensive awareness of the treatment possibilities in major trauma and their evidence base

D.5.2 The DATC Course

D.5.2.1 COURSE OBJECTIVES

By the end of the course, the student has:

- An enhanced knowledge of trauma surgery decision-making and the procedures involved.
- An enhanced knowledge of the physiological abnormalities associated with trauma and their management before, during, and after surgery.
- An enhanced knowledge of trauma-induced coagulopathy and its management.
- Enhanced technical skills needed to expedite the surgical and critical care process.

D.5.2.2 DESCRIPTION OF THE COURSE

A prerequisite of the DSTC and DATC courses is a complete understanding of all the principles outlined in general surgical and anaesthesiology training, and the ATLS® course. For this reason, there are no presentations on the basic principles of trauma surgery, nor the initial resuscitation of the patient with major injuries.

The course consists of a core curriculum, designed to be an activity lasting at least two and one-half days. In addition to the core curriculum, there are a variety of add-on modules that can be used to enhance the course, thereby adapting to local needs.

The course consists of several core components:

- *Interactive presentations*: Designed to introduce and cover the key concepts of surgical resuscitation, the endpoints, and an overview of the best access to organ systems.
- *Cadaver sessions (optional session)*: In which use is made of fresh or preserved human cadavers and dissected tissue. These are used to reinforce the vital knowledge of human anatomy related to access in major trauma. Other alternatives are available if local custom or legislation does not permit the use of such laboratories.
- *Skills laboratories with use of live tissue*: The instructor introduces various injuries. The objects of the exercise are to both improve psychomotor skills and teach new techniques for the preservation of organs and the control of haemorrhage. This re-creates the real-world scenario of managing a severely injured patient in the operating room.
- *Case presentations*: This component is a strategic thinking session illustrated by case presentations. Different cases are presented that allow free

discussion between the students and the instructors. These cases are designed to put the didactic and psychomotor skills that have been learned into the context of real patient management scenarios.

D.5.1.3 **Summary**

The DSTC course is designed to prepare the already well-trained surgeon to manage difficult injuries and to apply trauma care–specific knowledge in their practice. The combined DSTC and DATC courses provide a higher level of trauma understanding by focussing on the multidisciplinary nature of the decision-making processes and the core concepts of teamwork in managing patients with severely compromised physiology. The course fulfils the educational, cognitive, and psychomotor needs for surgeons and anaesthetists, be they specialist or trainee, civilian or military, or a mix, all of whom need to be comfortable in dealing with life-threatening penetrating and blunt injury, irrespective of the nature of the injury.

Appendix E
Definitive Surgical Trauma Care™ Course: Core Surgical Skills

E.1 THE NECK

E.1.1 Standard neck (pre-sternomastoid) incision
E.1.2 Control and repair of the carotid vessels
    E.1.2.1 Zone II
    E.1.2.2 Extension into zone III
    E.1.2.3 Division of the digastric muscle and subluxation or division of the mandible
    E.1.2.4 Extension into zone I
E.1.3 Extension by supraclavicular incision
    E.1.3.1 Ligation of the proximal internal carotid artery
    E.1.3.2 Repair with a divided external carotid artery
    E.1.3.3 Access to, control of and ligation of the internal jugular vein
E.1.4 Access to and repair of the trachea
E.1.5 Access to and repair of the cervical oesophagus

E.2 THE CHEST

E.2.1 Incisions
    E.2.1.1 Anterolateral thoracotomy
    E.2.1.2 Sternotomy
    E.2.1.3 'Clamshell' bilateral thoracotomy incision
E.2.2 Thoracotomy
    E.2.2.1 Exploration of the thorax
    E.2.2.2 Ligation of the intercostal and internal mammary vessels
    E.2.2.3 Emergency department (resuscitative) thoracotomy
        E.2.2.3.1 Supradiaphragmatic control of the aorta
        E.2.2.3.2 Control of the pulmonary hilum
        E.2.2.3.3 Internal cardiac massage
E.2.3 Pericardiotomy
    E.2.3.1 Preservation of the phrenic nerve
    E.2.3.2 Access to the pulmonary veins
E.2.4 Access to and repair of the thoracic aorta
    E.2.4.1 Cross-clamping of the aorta
E.2.5 Lung wounds
    E.2.5.1 Oversewing
    E.2.5.2 Stapling
    E.2.5.3 Partial lung resection
    E.2.5.4 Tractectomy
    E.2.5.5 Lobectomy
E.2.6 Access to and repair of the thoracic oesophagus
E.2.7 Access to and repair of the diaphragm
E.2.8 Compression of the left subclavian vessels from below
E.2.9 Left anterior thoracotomy
    E.2.9.1 Visualization of the supra-aortic vessels
E.2.10 Heart repair
    E.2.10.1 Finger control
    E.2.10.2 Involvement of the coronary vessels
E.2.11 Insertion of a shunt

E.3 THE ABDOMINAL CAVITY

E.3.1 Midline laparotomy
    E.3.1.1 How to explore (priorities)
    E.3.1.2 Packing
    E.3.1.3 Localization of retroperitoneal haematomas – when to explore?
    E.3.1.4 Damage control
        E.3.1.4.1 Techniques
        E.3.1.4.2 Abdominal closure
    E.3.1.5 Extension of laparotomy incision
        E.3.1.5.1 Lateral extension
        E.3.1.5.2 Sternotomy
    E.3.1.6 Cross-clamping of the aorta at the diaphragm (division at the left crus)

E.3.2 Left visceral medial rotation
    E.3.2.1 Reflection of the left (descending) colon medially
    E.3.2.2 Reflection of the pancreas and spleen towards the midline
E.3.3 Right visceral medial rotation
    E.3.3.1 Kocher's manoeuvre
    E.3.3.2 Reflection of the right (ascending) colon medially
E.3.4 Abdominal oesophagus
    E.3.4.1 Mobilization
    E.3.4.2 Repair
        E.3.4.2.1 Simple
        E.3.4.2.2 Mobilization of the fundus to reinforce sutures
E.3.5 Stomach
    E.3.5.1 Mobilization
    E.3.5.2 Access to vascular control
    E.3.5.3 Repair of anterior and posterior wounds
E.3.6 Bowel
    E.3.6.1 Resection
    E.3.6.2 Small and large bowel anastomosis
    E.3.6.3 Staple colostomy
    E.3.6.4 Ileostomy technique

E.4 THE LIVER

E.4.1 Mobilization (falciform, suspensory, triangular and coronary ligaments)
E.4.2 Liver packing
E.4.3 Hepatic isolation
    E.4.3.1 Control of the infrahepatic inferior vena cava
    E.4.3.2 Control of the suprahepatic superior vena cava
    E.4.3.3 Pringle's manoeuvre
E.4.4 Repair of parenchymal laceration
E.4.5 Technique of finger fracture
E.4.6 Tractotomy
E.4.7 Packing for injury to hepatic veins
E.4.8 Hepatic resection
E.4.9 Non-anatomical partial resection
E.4.10 Use of tissue adhesives
E.4.11 Tamponade for penetrating injury (Foley/Penrose drains, Sengstaken tube)

E.5 THE SPLEEN

E.5.1 Mobilization
E.5.2 Suture

E.5.3 Use of tissue adhesives
E.5.4 Partial splenectomy
    E.5.4.1 Sutures
    E.5.4.2 Staples
E.5.5 Total splenectomy

E.6 THE PANCREAS

E.6.1 Mobilization of the tail of the pancreas
E.6.2 Mobilization of the head of the pancreas
E.6.3 Localization of the main duct and its repair
E.6.4 Distal pancreatic resection
    E.6.4.1 Stapler
    E.6.4.2 Oversewing
E.6.5 Use of tissue adhesives
E.6.6 Access to the mesenteric vessels (division of the pancreas)

F.7 THE DUODENUM

E.7.1 Mobilization of the duodenum
    E.7.1.1 Kocher's manoeuvre (rotation of the duodenum)
    E.7.1.2 Division of the ligament of Treitz
    E.7.1.3 Repair of the duodenum

E.8 THE GENITOURINARY SYSTEM

E.8.1 Kidney
    E.8.1.1 Mobilization
    E.8.1.2 Vascular control
    E.8.1.3 Repair
    E.8.1.4 Partial nephrectomy
    E.8.1.5 Nephrectomy
E.8.2 Ureter
    E.8.2.1 Mobilization
    E.8.2.2 Stenting
    E.8.2.3 Repair
E.8.3 Bladder
    E.8.3.1 Repair of intraperitoneal rupture
    E.8.3.2 Repair of extraperitoneal rupture

E.9 ABDOMINAL VASCULAR INJURIES

E.9.1 Exposure and control
    E.9.1.1 Aorta and its branches
        E.9.1.1.1 Exposure

E.9.1.1.2 Repair

E.9.1.1.3 Shunt

E.9.1.2 Inferior vena cava

E.9.1.2.1 Suprahepatic inferior vena cava

E.9.1.2.2 Infrahepatic inferior vena cava

E.9.1.2.3 Control of haemorrhage with swabs

E.9.1.2.4 Repair both anteriorly and posteriorly, through an anterior wound

E.9.1.2.5 Shunting

E.9.2 Pelvis

E.9.2.1 Control of the pelvic vessels

E.9.2.1.1 Extraperitoneal packing

E.9.2.1.2 Suture of artery and vein

E.9.2.1.3 Ligation of artery and vein

E.9.2.1.4 Packing/anchor ligation of the sacral vessels

E.10 PERIPHERAL VASCULAR INJURIES

E.10.1 Extremities: vascular access

E.10.1.1 Axillary

E.10.1.2 Brachial

E.10.1.3 Femoral

E.10.1.4 Popliteal

E.10.2 Fasciotomy

E.10.2.1 Upper limb

E.10.2.2 Lower limb

E.11 INSERTION OF RESUSCITATIVE BALLOON CATHETER (REBOA)

E.11.1 Groin insertion, using ultrasound

E.12 INSERTION AND USE OF VACUUM WOUND DRESSING

E.12.1

Appendix F
Briefing for Operating Room Scrub Nurses

F.1 INTRODUCTION

Damage control techniques for the management of the major trauma patient are now accepted concepts, and include temporizing measures to prevent a cold, acidotic, and coagulopathic patient from further deterioration and eventual death. Some personnel working in the operation room/theatre (OR/OT) environment may not have had previous exposure to these techniques, especially in countries where trauma volumes are limited, and major trauma is a stressful rarity. This appendix is intended to help prepare the team for the imminent arrival and intraoperative management of the major trauma patient. Good communication is the key to success. Anticipate and think laterally.

Refer also to Chapter 9.1: 'The Trauma Laparotomy'.

The aspects of care referred to in this section are as follows:

- Preparation
- Cleaning and draping
- Instruments and issues of technique
- Special tools and equipment – including improvised gadgets
- Medicolegal aspects
- Communication

F.2 PREPARING THE OPERATING ROOM

Patients with major trauma are complex; they have deranged physiology and may have complex injuries with competing priorities for treatment. Optimizing the OR before the patient arrives and planning for every eventuality are what will make the difference between a stressful, chaotic experience for all concerned and a planned environment where every member of the team has a role and acknowledges the strength of all the members of the team.

A perioperative checklist is important, even if specifically modified for the trauma scenario.

F.2.1 Environment

Because of the underlying coagulopathy and hypothermia, the patient needs to be prevented from further heat loss at all costs to maximize haemostasis.

- The internal temperature of the OR should be set to at least 27 °C and maintained at this level.[1]
- Fluid and blood should be warmed before and during administration, using devices such as a Level 1® (Smiths Medical, St. Paul, MN, USA) or Ranger® (3M Medical, St. Paul, MN, USA) device, which allow for rapid infusion without sacrificing adequate heat transmission to the fluid. Ideally, the temperature should be set at 41 °C.
- Patient-warming devices should be present and readied for use. These can include a circulating warm fluid underlay or warm air circulation device (e.g., a Bair Hugger®, 3M Medical), which must be directly in contact with the skin and not over a bedsheet.

F.2.2 Blood Loss

Because of the propensity for massive blood loss, one should consider activating and priming a cell-saving device of some description. Blood from the chest drain need not be washed and can be autotransfused directly, provided that normal saline (0.9%) has been used in the collection device (plus 1000 IU of calcium heparin) and not water.

F.2.3 Instruments

- Now is the time to request extra instrument packs and obtain packs of sponges and swabs, as these will be rapidly required in large numbers.
- A trolley with multiple drawers with pre-packed equipment may be a useful option.[2]
- Equipment for thoracotomy and vascular access/repair should be mandatory, and a large selection of sutures, staplers, and drains should be available including items for unusual uses, such as a Sengstaken–Blakemore tube.
- The World Health Organisation recently released standardized equipment set lists that can guide the development of local resources.

F.2.4 Cleaning

With damage control surgery, there is less time than usual to provide a truly sterile field, and alternate methods should be used to achieve the same result. It is often said that 'sterility is a luxury in trauma'.

- Typically, either an iodophore- or a chlorhexidine-based skin preparation is utilized, and this applies equally to the trauma patient. One should not use both types, as they may inactivate each other. Chlorhexidine-based solutions are the current solution of choice.[3]
- The method of application may, however, vary. One option, utilized in several prominent North American centres, is the use of a spray bottle to apply the preparation solution. This has been shown to be as effective as traditional circular sponging techniques.[3,4]
- Cleaning should be extended widely beyond the expected bounds of the operative field, and the recommendation is to clean from neck to knees, as this allows for extension from abdomen to chest or for vein harvesting from the saphenous veins.
    - Laparotomy cleaning should extend to the chest and the knees to allow for extension into the chest or control of vessels in the thigh.
    - Cleaning the chest for vascular injury to the subclavian or axillary injury must extend into free draping of the affected limb and the thigh for possible saphenous vein harvesting.
    - Laparotomy cleaning should be extended as laterally as possible to accommodate drains.

F.2.5 Draping

Draping is also along unconventional lines, and this ensures that the surgeons can have ready access to more than just the area of single focus, which is usual for when elective surgery is performed.

- Drape widely using drapes that attach to the skin, or fix them with skin staples, laterally from the neck, lateral to the chest at the mid-axillary lines, and along the same plane to the knees. The genitalia are covered with a small drape or an opened swab (**Figure F.1**).
- Prevent further heat loss by covering the areas not initially needed for surgical access with sterile drapes. For example, if the abdomen is the default operation, cover the chest and legs with drapes that are easily removed if access to those regions is required.

F.2.6 Adjuncts

As far as pre-planning for the actual procedure is concerned, one can only recommend that the OR team

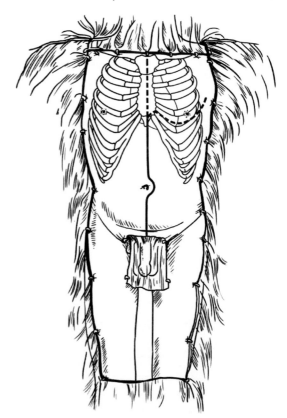

Figure F.1 Draping required for a trauma laparotomy.

'anticipate' all eventualities. Remember, too, that as there is little time to spare, the risk of injury to operative team members is high, and that all precautions should be taken to ensure maximal protection.

Meticulous 'sharps' handling is required in this relatively uncontrolled situation.

Never hand or receive sharps, except in a bowl.

- Although there is no good evidence that masks, overshoes, and caps protect the patient from infection during surgery, standard precautions should be maintained to protect the team members. The OR nurse should ensure that all staff in the 'sterile area' are appropriately attired.
- Place the scalpel in a receiver (kidney bowl) for the surgeon to take and replace. The body cavities should be opened primarily with a scalpel and heavy (Mayo) scissors.
- Have 20–30 large *dry* swabs or sponges ready for the surgeon to perform rapid packing. These are best passed 'folded' initially, unless the surgeon specifies otherwise, because for definitive packing, swabs should be used *folded* in layers.
- Do *not* use wet swabs. They rapidly become cold wet swabs!
- The suction devices should be ready and should preferably be routed to the cell-saver device. It is useful for there to be *two* suction devices at the table.
- An electrocautery machine should be available, but there is no time for small vessel haemostasis at this point, and this will most likely be used later.

F.3 SURGICAL PROCEDURE

F.3.1 Instruments

The instrument sets one should have at the ready are as follows:

- A thoracotomy tray ready in the room, but not open unless the chest is the primary operative focus. A sternal saw or Lebsche knife should also be available.
- A standard laparotomy set, open and ready, including a bowel resection set.
- Vascular instruments, including large aortic clamps (Crawford and Satinsky) open on the set-up trolley.

- Extra small, medium, and large crushing clamps (e.g., Halstead, Crile, Roberts, and mosquito), as there may be many bleeding vessels to clamp.
- Several Babcock forceps for holding or marking a bowel injury.
- A right-angled dissecting forceps such as is used for bile ducts (Lahey, Heiss, Mixter, etc.).
- A full selection of retractors (e.g., Morris, Army-Navy, Langenbeck, Deaver, and copper malleables), as well as some form of a self-retaining system such as a Bookwalter, Omni-Tract, or Gray system.
- At least one pair of forceps should be rubber-shod, as retrieval of a bullet will otherwise result in scratching the round, rendering it inadmissible for forensic evidence should the case come to court.

Since most major trauma (especially penetrating trauma) affects the abdomen, one must prepare for bowel and solid organ injury.

- Skin staplers can temporize small holes from bullets and lacerations in the stomach (and may be useful on the heart).
- GIA-type linear cutting staplers are handy for the rapid closure of bowel ends during non-reconstructive resection of small bowel or colon.
- Transverse anastomosis (TA)-type non-cutting staplers can be used to fashion a pyloric exclusion, or for distal pancreas resection when the need for rapid resection is present.
- Umbilical tapes or the tapes on large sponges can be used to ligate segments of bowel to control effluent.
- Ligaclips can be useful for controlling bleeding vessels on the liver or spleen or in the mesentery.
- It is useful to keep handy a Sengstaken–Blakemore tube for placing in a bleeding hepatic tract to attempt to tamponade the deep bleeding. A Penrose drain, inflated over a 16G nasogastric tube, can achieve a similar effect.
- For suspected vascular injury or to control bleeding from non-ligatable vessels, various forms of temporary arterial shunts and similar devices are required.
- The Rumel tourniquet is a useful device made by simply placing a cylindrical plastic tube over a vascular loop and using this to compress a friable vessel once it has been isolated and looped. It may also be used to hold a shunt in place proximally and distally in an injured artery. The tourniquets can be kept in place with either Ligaclips or small artery clamps.
- Proprietary shunts (such as Javid or Barker shunts) should be available; alternatively, one can manufacture

them using intravenous tubing, nasogastric tubing, or chest drain tubing, depending on the vessel size.

- A selection of vascular grafts should be close at hand. A selection of plastic drapes for damage control closure are as follows:
  - Opsite® (Smith and Nephew, London, UK)
  - Ioban® or Steridrape® (3M Medical)
- Proprietary vacuum closures include the following:
  - VAC® (Kinetic Concepts Inc. [KCI], San Antonio, TX, USA, Renasys® (Smith and Nephew, London UK etc.)

F.3.2 Special Instruments and Improvised Gadgets

The first goal of the damage control procedure is to stop the bleeding and then control contamination, whilst maintaining tissue perfusion. This may require the use of other specific instruments and some improvised or 'home-made' gadgets to achieve the desired result. Again, a useful option is to have this equipment 'pre-selected' and placed for use in a dedicated mobile, multiple-drawer trolley.

A suitable damage control surgery storage cupboard will contain a selection such as is shown in **Table F.1** and **Figure F.2**.

Table F.1 Damage Control Equipment

Top	Sutures
Tray 1	Surgical drapes
Tray 2	Disposable gowns
Tray 3	Universal instrument set: Babcocks
	Right-angled forceps, Satinsky clamp
Tray 4	Thoracic instrument set
Tray 5	Abdominal instrument set
Tray 6	Vascular instrument set
Tray 7	Disinfection material
	Drapes (Steridrape, Opsite, Ioban)
Tray 8	Large gauze, abdominal swabs
Tray 9	Mesh grafts, pledgets
	Shunts: Carotid, Javid
	Tubes: Nasogastric, urinary, chest
	Silicone loops, Rumel tourniquets
Tray 10	Staplers: Skin stapler, GIA, TA, vascular
Side	Fogarty catheters
	List of contents

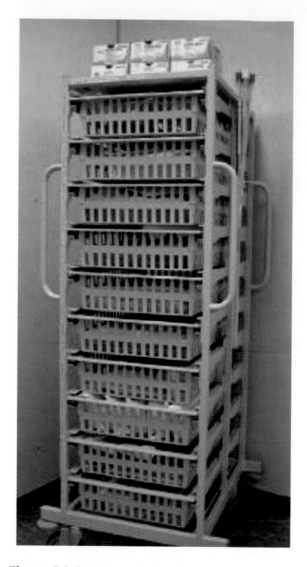

Figure F.2 Damage control trolley.

F.4 ABDOMINAL CLOSURE

Closure of the abdomen may be final and definitive, but more likely will involve some form of temporary closure device. The options include a vacuum-assisted closure (VAC) sandwich (best option), or plastic silo bags sutured to the skin (Bogota bag) or towel-clip closures (neither of the latter are recommended). Recently, a 'whipstitch' skin-only closure technique has been described that is associated with less long-term open abdomen.[5] Equipment for the vacuum sandwich is described below. The commercial vacuum dressings are not appropriate until definitive closure.

- One sterile adhesive drape (Opsite or Ioban) is placed sticky side up, and one or two sterile towels or swabs are placed on the sticky surface. Note that only one side of the swab is covered in plastic membrane. Placing plastic on *both* sides allows the drape to slide somewhat inside the abdomen, and prevents the gauze swabs from effectively 'wicking' any intra-abdominal fluid away into the suction drains, but traps the fluid inside the abdominal cavity.
  - Do **not** make slits in the plastic.
  - Do **not** have suction of greater than 24 mmHg, as this predisposes to fistulae in the hypotensive, cold, damage control patient.
- This is tucked under the fascia over the bowel, with the smooth plastic protecting the bowel, whilst the sponges and swabs prevent evisceration by adhering to the parietal peritoneal surface.
- Two large drains or nasogastric tubes are laid inside the gap between the sheath and the skin and are tunnelled cranially for about 5–8 cm under the skin to enable an adequate seal of the other adhesive drape over the entire abdomen.
- A second large, sterile adhesive drape is then used to close the wound.
- The drains are connected with a Y-connector and may be placed on *low-pressure* wall suction (maximum suction < 25 mmHg). This controls effluent and creates a good seal. It is also easiest to nurse in the ward or intensive care unit.

A commercial VAC device is available, but due to expense and, often, the higher suction used, it is **not** recommended for *initial* closure. It is, however, the device of choice for subsequent wound management of the open abdomen.

F.5 INSTRUMENT AND SWAB COUNT

As usual, counts are performed before closure.

However, after *damage control*, a second count is performed *after* the abdominal vacuum dressing has been completed. This allows a count of how many swabs have been left in the abdomen. (Don't forget to count the swabs in the vacuum sandwich!)

An accurate record should be kept of any retained instruments and swabs, as there may be a different scrub team at the time of the re-look laparotomy.

An abdominal X-ray before final closure is advisable, as an extra safeguard to avoid retained swabs or instruments.

F.6 MEDICOLEGAL ASPECTS AND COMMUNICATION SKILLS

- Failing to plan and failing to communicate efficiently are the two major instigators of error, and error avoidance is an important aspect of medicine. The common medicolegal areas of dispute in trauma relate to aspects of consent and management of foreign bodies.
- Consent in emergency in most countries is based on the clinician doing what is in the best interest of the patient, and as such the surgery to save a life takes precedence over a piece of paper. Family assent is useful and is of importance with small children, but must not influence against needed surgery unless there is an advanced directive. Surgical checklists are also of benefit in reducing error prior to surgery.
- Foreign bodies are often present in penetrating trauma. There is a need to remove these, and the local procedure for forensic analysis should be well-known to the operation suite staff. Bullets should be removed without metal-to-metal instrument contact, to prevent damage to the markings used for identification of the bullet. Rubber- or plastic-shod instruments should be used for removal if they are removed at all, as there are clear indications to leave alone those that are unlikely to cause further harm.[6]
- Forensic evidence is also essential in cases of major trauma due to sexual and paediatric abuse. Try to preserve all the evidence as best as possible. Never handle bullets or metal fragments with metal instruments. Use mosquito forceps, the jaws of which are plastic or rubber covered. Wrap the fragment in gauze. Place each fragment in a separate container, marked with the exact site of removal.
- Communication is enhanced by all the members of the trauma team addressing the following aspects:
  - Information-sharing allows for optimal preparation.
  - Assign roles to each member, and ensure each prepares their aspect of the care pathway.

- Think ahead to ensure all possible equipment and patient care aspects are addressed.
- Closed-loop communication, with feedback to the initial person asking the question or giving the instruction and assignment of actions to named persons, reduces the risk of error (see Chapter 2 on non-technical skills).

F.7 CRITICAL INCIDENT STRESS ISSUES

The trauma environment is stressful for all concerned, and time is of the essence – tempers often flare, and one must not take the issues personally.

Occasionally, the patient will not survive, and the risk is that staff may develop post-traumatic stress disorder, especially if major trauma is a rare occurrence for them. The best method for dealing with this situation is via a debriefing session as soon as everyone has cleaned up or first thing the next morning. (See Chapter 22, 'Psychology of Trauma'.)

F.8 CONCLUSION

The success of trauma surgery depends on a team performing at its peak with effective communication, willing to work outside of the traditional norms, and yet with maximal concern for patient safety.

REFERENCES AND RECOMMENDED READING

References

1. Hardcastle TC, M Stander, N Kalafatis, E Hodgson, D Gopalan. External patient temperature control in emergency centres, trauma centres, intensive care units and operating theatres: a multi-society literature review. *S Afr Med J.* 2013 Aug 6;**103**(**9**):609–11. doi: 10.7196/samj.7327.

2. Goslings JC, Haverlag R, Ponsen KJ, Luitse JSK. Facilitating damage control surgery with a dedicated DCS equipment trolley. *Injury.* 2006 May;**37**(**5**):466–7. doi: 10.1016/j.injury.2005.09.010. Epub 2005 Dec 20.

3. Woodhead K, Taylor EW, Bannister G, Chesworth T, Hoffman P, Humphreys H. Behaviours and rituals in the operating theatre: a report from the Hospital Infection Society Working Group on Infection Control in the Operating Theatres. *J Hosp Infect.* 2002 Aug;**51**(**4**):241–55. doi: 10.1053/jhin.2002.1220.

4. Ritter MA, French ML, Eitzen HE, Gioe TJ. The antimicrobial effectiveness of operative-site preparative agents: a microbiological and clinical study. *J Bone Joint Surg Am.* 1980;**62**:826–8.

5. Collins R, Dhanasekara CS, Morris E, Marschke B, Dissanaike S. Simple suture whipstitch closure is a reasonable option for many patients requiring temporary abdominal closure for blunt or penetrating trauma. *Trauma Surg Acute Care Open.* 2022 Oct 21;**7**(**1**):e000980. doi: 10.1136/tsaco-2022-000980.

6. Dienstknecht T, Horst K, Sellei R, Berner A, Nerlich N, Hardcastle T. Indications for bullet removal: a literature overview and clinical practice guideline for European Trauma Surgeons. *Eur J Trauma and Emerg Surg.* 2012;38(2):89–93. doi: 10.1007/s00068-011-0170-x.

Recommended Reading

Emergency Exploratory Laparotomy. In: Phillips N. ed. Berry and Kohn's Operating Room Technique, 11th Edn. Mosby, St Louis MO. 2007.

Firth-Cozens J. Why communication fails in the operating room. Qual Saf Health Care. 2004;13:327.

Goldman MA. Pocket Guide to the Operating Room, 3rd Edn. F A Davis, Philadelphia, PA. 2008.

Saullo DC. Trauma surgery. In: Rothrock JC. ed. Alexander's Care of the Patient in Surgery, 14th Edn. Mosby, St Louis. 2003:1182–223.

*Wick JM. Don't destroy the evidence. AORN J. 2000 Nov;**72**(**5**):807–18, 820–7; quiz 828–30, 833–6. doi: 10.1016/s0001-2092(06)62013-9.*

Index

A

AA, *see* Arachidonic acid
AAST, *see* American Association for Surgery of T; Association
      for the Surgery of Trauma
Abbreviated Injury Scale (AIS), 458–460, 466
Abdominal/abdomen
   bowel, rectum, and diaphragm, 172–178
   cavity, 503–504
   closure, 158–159, 510–511
   compliance, 373
   duodenum, 179–184
   injury complexes, 148
   injury, 307–308
   liver and biliary system, 185–203
   pancreas, 204–214
   spleen, 215–222
   trauma, 76, 153
   trauma laparotomy, 147–163
   urogenital system, 223–236
   vascular injury, 165–172
Abdominal compartment syndrome (ACS), 87, 372–377, 391
   cardiovascular system, 372
   consensus definitions of World society of, 373
   intracranial pressure, 374
   management, 375
   management algorithm, 375
   measurement of IAP, 376
   medical management algorithm, 377
   pathophysiology, 372
   prevention, 375
   effect of raised IAP on individual organ function,
      372–374
   renal system, 374
   respiratory system, 374
   reversible factors, 375
   surgery for raised IAP, 375
   treatment, 375
   visceral perfusion, 374
Abdominal perfusion pressure (APP), 373
   measurement, 374
Abdominal vascular injury, 165, 504–505
   retroperitoneal haematoma, 166–167
   scale, 479
   shunting, 171–172
   surgical approach to major abdominal vessels,
      167–171

Abdominal wall closure, 91
   delayed primary abdominal closure, 91
   planned hernia, 92
   secondary abdominal closure, 91–92
   secondary closure, 91
Abscess formation, 212
Absorbable material, 160
Acetabular fractures, 241
Acetabulum, 239
Acetyl coenzyme A (acetyl CoA), 30
Acidosis, 38, 115, 353, 392
ACoT, *see* Acute coagulopathy of trauma
ACS, *see* Abdominal compartment syndrome; American
      College of Surgeons
ACTH, *see* Adrenocorticotrophic hormone
Activated protein C (APC), 29, 353
Active bleeding, 48
Acute coagulopathy of trauma (ACoT), 391
Acute kidney injury (AKI), 378
Acute lung injury (ALI), 391
Acute phase, 255
Acute Physiologic and Chronic Health Evaluation II score
      (APACHE II score), 458, 466
Acute presentation, 206
Acute respiratory distress syndrome (ARDS), 347, 391
Adenosine triphosphate (ATP), 30
ADH, *see* Antidiuretic hormone
Adjuncts, 177, 211, 508–509
   antibiotics, 298
   in burn care, 297–299
   to care, 278–279
   nutrition in burned patient, 297–299
   ulcer prophylaxis, 298
   venous thromboembolism prophylaxis, 298
   vitamin C, 298
Adrenal hormones, 30
Adrenaline, 42, 124
Adrenal organ injury scale, 480
Adrenocorticotrophic hormone (ACTH), 29
Adult respiratory distress syndrome (ARDS), 31, 282, 290
Advanced Surgical Skills for Exposure in Trauma (ASSET), 499
Advanced Trauma Life Support® (ATLS), 67, 99, 127, 343, 497
Afferent block, 312
Ageing, 310
Aggressive crystalloid resuscitation, consequences of, 391
Aggressive initial resuscitation, 314
Agitation, 351

'Air-Man', 7
Air embolism, 70, 124, 139
Airway, 68, 288, 302–303, 392–393
  burns, 296
  indications for intubation, 40
AIS, *see* Abbreviated Injury Scale
AKI, *see* Acute kidney injury
ALARA, *see* As low as reasonably achievable
Albumin, 46
Aldosterone, 30–31
  secretion, 30
ALI, *see* Acute lung injury
Alpha angle (α angle), 55
'Alveolar' burn, 296
American Association for Surgery of Trauma (AAST), 461
American College of Surgeons (ACS), 8, 494
Amino acids, 32
Amputations, 404
Anabolic steroid, 298
Anaemia, 46
Anaesthetic/anaesthesia, 127, 163, 405
  blunt thoracic injury, 141–142
  considerations, 142–144, 202–203, 280, 313
  drugs for, 396–398
  effects of anaesthetic induction agents, 396
  in hypovolaemic shock, 395–396
  management of thoracic injury, 142
  penetrating thoracic injury, 140
  for thoracic trauma, 140
Analgesia, 289, 308–309
Anastomosis, 175
Anatomical scoring systems, 457, 458
  AIS, 458–460
  APS, 460–461
  ICISS, 461
  ISS, 460
  NISS, 460
  OIS system, 461
  PATI, 461
  RISC II, 461–462
  TRISS, 461
Anatomic Profile Score (APS), 460–461, 467
ANF, *see* Atrial natriuretic factor
Angioembolization, 245
Angiography, 102
  embolization, 216
Anorectal injuries, 250–251
ANP, *see* Atrial natriuretic peptide
Ansa cervicalis, 108
Anteroposterior compression (APC), 243
Anterior urethra, 235
Anterolateral thoracotomy, 131–132
Antibiotics, 150, 177, 259, 298, 370–372
Anticoagulants, 312
Antidiuretic hormone (ADH), 26, 282
Antimicrobial therapy, 362
Aortic/aorta, 167–168
  cross-clamping, 139
  and great vessels, 118
  hiatus, 116

  injury, 140
  occlusion, 326
  and vena caval injuries, 148
APACHE II score, *see* Acute Physiologic and Chronic Health Evaluation II score
APC, *see* Activated protein C; Anterior posterior compression
AP imaging, *see* Anteroposterior imaging
APP, *see* Abdominal perfusion pressure
APS, *see* Anatomic Profile Score
ARDS, *see* Acute respiratory distress syndrome; Adult respiratory distress syndrome
Arousal, 72
Arteriovenous ECMO (AV-ECMO), 352
ASCOT, *see* A Severity Characterization of Trauma
A Severity Characterization of Trauma (ASCOT), 465, 469
As low as reasonably achievable (ALARA), 307
Aspiration, 371
Aspirin, 52
ASSET, *see* Advanced Surgical Skills for Exposure in Trauma
Associated injuries, 250–251, 290
Association for the Surgery of Trauma (AAST), 207
(AT)MIST, *see* Mechanism of injury, Injuries sustained, Signs and symptoms, Treatment
ATLS, *see* Advanced Trauma Life Support®
ATP, *see* Adenosine triphosphate
Atrial natriuretic factor (ANF), 30
Atrial natriuretic peptide (ANP), 30
Austere environments, 401; *see also* Military environments
  health protection of deployed surgical team, 403
  hospital structures, 402–403
  infrastructure, 402–403
  location of field hospital, 402
  patterns of injury for non-survivors in, 415
  postoperative care and documentation, 405
  surgical techniques, 403–405
Autoregulation, 274
Autotransfusion, 57–58, 120, 151
AV-ECMO, *see* Arteriovenous ECMO
Awareness, 72

B

Barbiturates, 275–276
Barker shunts, 509
Base deficit (BD), 348
BATLS™, *see* UK Battlefield Advanced Life Support course
Battlefield anaesthesia, 398–399, 420
  induction, 421–422
  maintenance, 422
Battlefield analgesia, 420
BD, *see* Base deficit
Behavioural Pain Scale (BPS), 351
Behavioural theme, potential errors related to, 19–20
Benzodiazepines, 396
β-endorphin, 29
Bicarbonate therapy, 58–59, 369
Bilateral trans-sternal thoracotomy, 133
Bile ducts, 202
Biliary fistulae, 201

Biobrane®, 296–297
Bispectral index (BIS index), 397
Bladder injuries, 162, 234–235, 250
    scale, 481
Blast lung injury (BLI), 435–436
Blast wave, 434
Bleeding control, 404
Blood pressure, pharmacologic support of, 41–42
BLI, *see* Blast lung injury
Blood, 47–48
    bank, 403
    collection, 151
    components, 71
    effects of transfusing blood and blood products, 49–51
    flow, 36
    loss, 507–508
    product administration, 366
    purification, 366
    volume, 60
Bloody vicious cycle, 390
Blunt
    abdominal trauma, 337
    chest, 153
    compression injury, 239
    head trauma, 271
    pancreatic trauma, 208
    thoracic trauma, 337
    trauma, 141, 147, 205, 179, 224, 238, 255
Blunt thoracic injury, 141
    contained large vessel rupture/aneurysm, 141
    diaphragmatic injury, 142
    flail chest, 142
    large airway disruption, 141
    pulmonary contusion, 141
BNP, *see* B-type natriuretic peptide
Body temperature restoration, 89–90
Bowel, 173–178
    injury, 323
BPS, *see* Behavioural Pain Scale
Breathing, 69, 393–394
    indications for intubation, 40
    indications for ventilation, 40
Bronchoscopy, 102
B-type natriuretic peptide (BNP), 30
Burns, 282
    adjuncts in burn care, 297–299
    anatomy, 283–285
    assessing and managing airway, 296
    chemical burns, 284–285
    closing burn wound, 291–292
    definitive management, 291–292
    depth of, 286
    DPT, 287
    electrical injury, 285–286
    escharotomy and fasciotomy, 290–291
    feet, 297
    first aid, 288
    full-thickness, 287
    indeterminate partial thickness, 287
    initial management, 288–290

management, 288
    pathophysiology, 282
    safe retrieval, 288
    special types, 284, 296
    SPT, 286
    superficial, 286
    TBSA, 287–288
    technique of excision and split skin grafting, 292
    tracheostomy, 296
    tumescent technique, 292
    wound coverage, 292, 295
    wound excision and closure, 295–296
Burr holes and emergency craniotomy, 276
    decompressive craniectomy, 278
    emergency burr hole craniotomy, 276–277
    emergency craniotomy, 278

C

Cadavers, 7
CAM-ICU, *see* Confusion Assessment Method for Intensive Care Unit
Carbohydrates, 31, 298
Carbon dioxide (CO_2), 37, 297
Carboxyhaemoglobin (COHb), 288
Cardiac
    arrest, 304
    arrhythmias, 285
    compressive shock, 35
    function, 34
    injury, 124–126, 138–139
    output, 33, 36–37
    tamponade, 35
Cardiac index (CI), 39
Cardiogenic shock, 34–35
Cardiopulmonary resuscitation (CPR), 328
Cardiovascular system, 311
Carotid artery, 108–109
CAT, *see* Combat applied tourniquet
Catastrophic external bleeding, 254
Catecholamines, 31, 39
Catheterization, 297
CBD, *see* Common bile duct
CBF, *see* Cerebral blood flow
CCPOT, *see* Critical-Care Pain Observation Tool
Cell salvage techniques, 58
Cell-washing and centrifugation techniques, 58
Central haematoma, 166
Centralizing trauma care, 453
Central retroperitoneal haematoma, 168
Central venous pressure, 37
Central venous saturation ($ScvO_2$), 348
Cerebral blood flow (CBF), 274, 393
Cerebral perfusion pressure (CPP), 272–274
    threshold, 274–275
Cervical spine immobilization techniques, 99
Cervical vascular organ injury scale, 470
CEUS, *see* Contrast-enhanced US
CFA, *see* Common femoral artery

Charitable organizations, 7
Charlson comorbidity index, 462, 469
Chemical burns, 484–485
Chemical pneumonitis, 288
Chemical vascular injuries, 258
Chest, 503
    air embolism, 124
    anaesthesia for thoracic trauma, 140–142
    aortic injury, 140
    cardiac injury, 124–126, 138–139
    chest drainage, 127–130
    damage control in, 119
    diagnosis, 118–119
    diaphragmatic injuries, 122
    emergency department thoracotomy, 134–137
    fixation of multiple fractures of ribs,
            123–124, 125
    flail chest, 122–123
    floor, 116
    injuries to great vessels, 126–127
    lobectomy or pneumonectomy, 139
    management of specific injuries, 119
    massive haemothorax, 120–121
    oesophageal injury, 121–122, 140
    open pneumothorax, 119–120
    pathophysiology of thoracic injuries, 115–116
    pericardial tamponade, 138
    pulmonary contusion, 122
    pulmonary haemorrhage, 139
    pulmonary laceration, 124
    pulmonary tractotomy, 139
    spectrum of thoracic injury, 114–115
    surgical anatomy of chest, 116–118
    surgical approaches to thorax, 130–134
    surgical procedures, 138
    tension pneumothorax, 120
    thoracotomy with aortic cross-clamping, 139
    tracheobronchial injuries, 121, 140
    trauma, 75–76
    X-ray, 173
Chest contents, 116, 117
    aorta and great vessels, 118
    heart and pericardium, 118
    left hemithorax and mediastinum, 117
    lungs and pleurae, 117–118
    oesophagus, 118
    right hemithorax and mediastinum, 117
    thoracic duct, 118
    tracheobronchial tree, 117
Chest drainage, 127
    drain insertion, 127–130
    drain removal, 130
Chest wall, 116
    injury scale, 471
Children, pancreatic injury in, 211
Chimney effect, 238
Chitosan (HemCon®), 62, 419
CI, see Cardiac index
Circulation, 68, 304, 394
    indication for intubation, 40

Clamshell thoracotomy, 133
Clinical psychologist, 442–443
Clopidogrel, 52
Closed-loop communication, 5
CM, see Combined mechanism
Coagulation status monitoring, 53
    personalized medicine, 53
    traditional assays, 53
    VHA, 54–57
Coagulopathy, 85, 200
    of major trauma, 353–354
Cochrane review, 380
Coeliac axis, 168
Cognitive biases, 8
COHb, see Carboxyhaemoglobin
Collagen fleece, 62
Collar incisions, 109–110
Colloids, 46
Colon injury scale, 478
Colostomy, 251
Combat applied tourniquet (CAT), 254
Combined mechanism (CM), 241–243
Command, 412
Common bile duct (CBD), 202
Common femoral artery (CFA), 329
Communication, 413
    skills, 511
    and teamwork, 14
    in trauma setting, 11–14
Comorbid conditions, 176, 311, 384
Comorbidity scoring systems, 462
Compartment syndrome, 262–263, 282
Component therapy, 48–49
Computed tomography (CT), 68, 99, 118, 147, 180, 205–206,
            216, 243, 270, 276, 303, 334, 349, 411
Computed tomography angiogram (CTA), 102, 119, 334
Confirm, Clear, Cordon, Control of Incident Management
            (4 Cs of Incident Management), 412
Confusion Assessment Method for Intensive Care Unit
            (CAM-ICU), 351
Consciousness, 72
Contained large vessel rupture/aneurysm, 141
Contamination control, 87, 404
Continuous positive airway pressure (CPAP), 142
Continuous RRT (CRRT), 378
Contrast-enhanced US (CEUS), 338
Control, 412
Contusion, 141
    injuries, 208–209
Coronary arteries, 138
Corticosteroids, 366
Cortisol, 32
Costochondral junction, 132
CPAP, see Continuous positive airway pressure
CPP, see Cerebral perfusion pressure
CPR, see Cardiopulmonary resuscitation
CRASH-2 trial, 52, 392
C reactive protein (CRP), 370
Crew resource management (CRM), 4, 5, 10
    communication in trauma setting, 11–14

leadership in trauma care, 12–17
    Swiss Cheese theory, 11
Cricoid cartilage, 117
Cricothyroidotomies, 100
Critical care, 347, 422
    ACS, 372–377
    AKI, 378
    antibiotics, 370–372
    coagulopathy of major trauma, 353–354
    ECMO, 351–352
    family contact and support, 384
    hypothermia, 354–355
    ICU tertiary survey, 384
    metabolic disturbances, 379–380
    MODS, 355
    nutritional support, 380–381
    pain control, 383–384
    phases of ICU care, 347–351
    prophylaxis in ICU, 381–383
    sepsis, 355–370
    SIRS, 355
Critical-Care Pain Observation Tool (CCPOT), 351
Critical decision-making process, 12
Critical incident stress issues, 512
CRM, see Crew resource management
CRP, see C reactive protein
CRRT, see Continuous RRT
Crush syndrome, 258
Cryoprecipitate, 48–49
CRYOSTAT trials, 49
CSF drainage, 275
CT, see Computed tomography
CTA, see Computed tomography angiogram
Cumulative act effect, 11
Cyclic adenosine monophosphate (cAMP), 31
Cyclo-oxygenase, 26
Cysterna chyli, 118
Cytokine
    cytokine-mediated inflammatory response, 282
Cytoprotective agents, 382

D

DAI, see Diffuse axonal injury
Damage-associated molecular patterns (DAMPs), 26
Damage control
    anaesthesia in military setting, 398
    DCO, 92–93
    DCR, 81–83
    DCS, 83–93
        equipment, 510
        principles, 80
        techniques, 42
        trolley, 511
Damage control laparotomy (DCL), 177
Damage control orthopaedics (DCO), 82, 92
Damage control resuscitation (DCR), 82–83, 147, 270, 390, 416, 419–420
    limited fluid administration, 390–391

    preventing and treating hypothermia, 392
    targeting coagulopathy, 391
Damage control surgery (DCS), 12–14, 80–83, 147, 246, 392, 411, 416; see also Minimal access surgery in trauma
    abdominal wall closure, 91–92
    anaesthetic procedures, 392–395
    definitive surgery, 90–91
    evidence-based guidelines for, 149
    in military setting, 419–420
    monitoring, 395
    operative haemorrhage and contamination control, 86–90
    outcomes, 92
    patient selection, 85–86
    physiological restoration in ICU, 89–90
DAMPs, see Damage-associated molecular patterns
DATC™, see Definitive Anaesthetic Trauma Care™
DCL, see Damage control laparotomy
DCO, see Damage control orthopaedics
DCR, see Damage control resuscitation
DCS, see Damage control surgery
D-dimer values, 53
Decision-making, 12
Decompressive craniectomy, 278
Dedicated trauma service, 5
Deep partial thickness (DPT), 286–287
Deep vein thrombosis prophylaxis, 279
Deep venous thrombosis (DVT), 350, 382–383
Definitive Anaesthetic Trauma Care™ (DATC™), 498
Definitive Surgical Trauma Care™ course (DSTC™ course), 498, 503–505
    application to holding course, 498
    certification, 500
    course details, 498
    development and testing, 498
    director, 499
    eligibility to present, 498
    faculty, 499
    IATSIC recognition, 500
    information, 500–501
    materials and overview, 499
    mission statement, 498
    ownership, 498
    participants, 499
    practical skill stations, 499
    syllabus, 499–500
    trauma management, 497–498
Delayed presentation, 206
Delayed primary abdominal closure, 91
Delirium, 351, 384
Depressed fractures, 278
Desmopressin, 52–53
Deteriorating neurological status, 276
Diagnostic laparoscopy, 180, 321
Diagnostic peritoneal lavage (DPL), 74, 205, 180, 247
Diaphragm, 173–175
    injury scale, 474
Diaphragmatic injury, 122, 142, 323
Diathermy, 404
DIC, see Disseminated intravascular coagulation
Dietician, 445

Dietitian, 297
Diffuse axonal injury (DAI), 270
Diffuse brain injuries, 270, 303
Dilutional thrombocytopenia, 353
Dimethyl sulfoxide (DMSO), 285
Direct measurements of shock, 37–38
Disability, 72, 303–304
  indications for intubation, 40
Discretionary non-intervention, 416
Disseminated intravascular coagulation (DIC), 353–354
Distal aorta, 168
Distal pancreatectomy, 209
Distal pulse, 255
Distributive shock, 36
DLT, *see* Double lumen tube
DMSO, *see* Dimethyl sulfoxide
Dobutamine, 42
Dopamine, 42
Doppler ultrasound, 255
Doppler monitoring, 77
Double jeopardy, 3
Double lumen tube (DLT), 140
DPL, *see* Diagnostic peritoneal lavage
DPT, *see* Deep partial thickness
Drainage, 221, 209
Drains, 161, 232
  insertion, 127–130
  removal, 130
Draping, 151, 508
DSTC™ course, *see* Definitive Surgical Trauma Care™ course
Dual-energy imaging, 338
Ductal injuries, 209–210
Duodenal diversion, 184
Duodenal diverticulation, 184
Duodenal injuries, 179, 308
  scale, 180–181
Duodenal laceration, 183
Duodenal rotation, 208
Duodenum, 154, 156, 175, 209–201, 179, 504
  complete transection, 183–184
  diagnosis, 179–180
  duodenal injury scale, 180–181
  injury scale, 477
  management, 180–181
  mechanism of injury, 179
  surgical approach, 181–184
DVT, *see* Deep venous thrombosis
Dysfunctional teams, 5

E

Early life support phase, 349
Early tracheostomy, 162–163
Eastern Association for the Surgery of Trauma (EAST), 164, 173
  evidence-based guidelines for pancreatic trauma, 213–214
ECCO$_2$R system, *see* Extracorporeal carbon dioxide removal system
ECG, *see* Electrocardiographic

Echelons of medical care, 411–412
ECMO, *see* Extracorporeal membrane oxygenation
ED, *see* Emergency department
EDT, *see* Emergency department thoracotomy
eFAST, *see* Extended focused abdominal sonography for trauma
Elderly, trauma in, 310
  access to trauma care, 310
  anaesthetic considerations in elderly, 313
  analgesia, 312
  decision to operate, 312
  multiple medications–polypharmacy, 311–312
  older and susceptibility to trauma, 310
  physiology, 310–311
Electrical burn, 290
Electrical injury, 285
Electrocardiographic (ECG), 59
Electrolytes, 283–284
Emergency
  burr hole craniotomy, 276–277
  craniotomy, 278
  management of burn wound, 289
  emergency department (ED), 5, 66, 92
  chest X-ray, 116
  resuscitation in, 68
Emergency department surgery, 74–75; *see also* Damage control surgery
  abdominal trauma, 76
  chest trauma, 75–76
  head trauma, 75
  long bone fractures, 77
  pelvic trauma, 76–77
  peripheral vascular injuries, 77
Emergency department thoracotomy (EDT), 114, 133–134, 137, 165
  EDT, 137
  history, 134–135
  indications and contraindications, 134–135
  objectives, 134
  results, 135
  technique, 135–136
Emergency medical services system (EMS system), 411, 451
Echelons of medical care, 411–412
  incident management and multiple casualties, 412–413
  medical management and support, 412
Emergency room (ER), 334, 389
EMS system, *see* Emergency medical services system
Endocrine deficiency, 212
Endogenous DAMPs, 39
Endoscopic retrograde cholangiopancreatography (ERCP), 201, 206, 323
End-tidal CO$_2$ (ETCO$_2$), 395
Endotoxin, 39, 51
Endourological techniques, 250
Endovascular resuscitation and trauma management (EVTM), 324
Energy, 402
Enteral nutrition, 380
  access for, 381
Enteric illness, 403

Environment
  indication for intubation, 40
  in primary survey, 72
Epidermis, 286
Epidural anaesthesia, 422
Epidural catheter, 275
Epigastrium, 153
Epinephrine, *see* Adrenaline
EPP, *see* Extraperitoneal pelvic packing
ER, *see* Emergency room
ERCP, *see* Endoscopic retrograde cholangiopancreatography
Erythema, 283–284, 284
Escharotomy, 290–291, 296–297
Essential Trauma Care (EsTC), 7
EsTC, *see* Essential Trauma Care
Etomidate, 397–398
Evacuation, 417
EVD, *see* External ventricular drain
EVTM, *see* Endovascular resuscitation and trauma
      management
Excision technique, 292
Exclusions, 352
'Exclusive' trauma systems, 83
Exocrine deficiency, 212
Exploration, 208
Extended focused abdominal sonography for trauma (eFAST),
      71, 244, 334
External compression devices, 245
External fixation of pelvis, 245–247
External ventricular drain (EVD), 275
Extracorporeal carbon dioxide removal system (ECCO$_2$R
      system), 352
Extracorporeal membrane oxygenation (ECMO), 141, 348,
      350–351
Extrahepatic biliary tree injury scale, 475
Extraperitoneal pelvic packing (EPP), 167, 244–246
Extremity arterial injury, 255
Extremity injury severity scoring systems, 260
Extremity trauma
  compartment syndrome, 262–263
  complications of major limb injury, 267
  Crush syndrome, 258
  fasciotomy, 263–266
  management of open fractures, 258–260
  management of severe injury to extremity, 254–255
  management of vascular injury of extremity, 255–256, 257
  massive limb trauma, 260–262
Extubation criteria, 350

F

Face (burn), 296–297
Fallopian tube injury scale, 482
FAM, *see* Functional Assessment Measure
Family contact and support, 384–385
Fasciotomy, 263–264, 290–291
  lower leg, 264–265
  upper and lower arm, 266–267
  upper leg, 266

FAST, *see* Focused abdominal sonography for trauma
Fat, 31–32, 298
FATE, *see* Focus assessed transthoracic echocardiography
Feet, 297
Fentanyl, 422
Fever, non-infectious causes of, 350
FFP, *see* Fresh frozen plasma
FG, *see* French gauge
Fibreoptic bronchoscopy, 121
Fibrin, 59, 62
  glue, 59, 62
Fibrinogen concentrate, 49
Fibrinolysis, 392
Fibulectomy, 265–266
FIM, *see* Functional Independence Measure
FIM/FAM, *see* Functional Independence Measure and
      Functional Assessment Measure
Finger fracture, 198
Finochietto retractor, 132
First aid (burn), 288
Fistula, 212
Fixation of multiple fractures of ribs, 123, 125
Flail chest, 122–123, 141–142
  evidence-based guidelines, 123
Fluid
  resuscitation, 289
  therapy, 357–358
  volume expansion, therapy for, 40
FMT, *see* Forward Medical Team
Focal brain injuries, 270
Focus-assessed transthoracic echocardiography (FATE), 395
FAST HUGS BID (medical mnemonic for surgical patient), 384
Forward Medical Team (FMT), 401
Forward surgical team(s), 415
  decision-making, 415–416
Fraction of inspired oxygen (FiO$_2$), 289
Fracture, 254
  combinations, 241
  complications, 267
Frank–Starling principle, 36
Free fatty acids, 32
Free radicals, 274
French gauge (FG), 70, 326
Fresh frozen plasma (FFP), 48–49, 82, 357–358
Fresh whole blood (FWB), 46
Front-end processes, 422–423
Full-thickness burns, 287
Functional Assessment Measure (FAM), 462–463, 469
Functional Independence Measure (FIM), 462–463, 469
Functional Independence Measure and Functional Assessment
      Measure (FIM/FAM), 446
FWB, *see* Fresh whole blood

G

Gallbladder, 202
Gastric bypass, 210
Gastric residual volumes (GRVs), 183
Gastro-oesophageal junction, 168

Gastrointestinal anastomosis, 176
Gastrointestinal bleeding (GI bleeding), 358
Gastrojejunostomy, 184
GCS, *see* Glasgow Coma Scale
Genitourinary system, 504
Gerota's fascia, 157, 231
GFR, *see* Glomerular filtration rate
GI bleeding, *see* Gastrointestinal bleeding
GI-type linear cutting staplers, 509
Glasgow Coma Scale (GCS), 72, 270, 398, 457, 465
Glasgow Outcome Scale (GOS), 446, 463–464, 465–466
Glomerular filtration rate (GFR), 282
Glucagon, 29
Glucose control, 31
Glycerol, 31
Goal-directed therapy, 53
GOS, *see* Glasgow Outcome Scale
Governance, 423
Greater sac, 155
GRVs, *see* Gastric residual volumes
Guildford technique, 160
Gunshot wounds (GSW), 254
Gustilo classification of injury, 259
Gut, 32
Gynaecological injury and sexual assault, 236

H

Haematomas, 256
Haematuria, 233
Haemobilia, 201
Haemodilution, 353
Haemodynamically normal patients, 73, 244
Haemodynamically stable patients, 73, 187–188, 244–245
Haemodynamically unstable patients, 74, 187–188, 244–245
Haemodynamic monitoring, 395
Haemoglobin (Hb), 46
Haemophilus influenza type B, 383
Haemo/pneumothorax, 119–120
Haemorrhage control, 86, 100–101
Haemostasis, 53
Haemostatic adjuncts in trauma, 59–63
Haemostats, 166
Haemothorax, 119
Hands (burn), 296–299
Harsh (definition), 401
Head injury, 250, 259, 304–305
Headlight, 160
Head trauma, 75
    adjuncts to care, 278–279
    anaesthetic considerations, 280
    CPP threshold, 274–275
    ICP monitoring and threshold, 275
    imaging, 276
    indications for surgery, 276–278
    injury patterns and classification, 270–272
    management of TBI, 225

    measurable physiological parameters in TBI, 224–225
    paediatric considerations, 279
    pathophysiology of TBI, 272
Healing process, 297
Heart, 118
    injury scale, 472
Helicopter Emergency Services (HEMS), 40
HemoPatch®, 62
HEMS, *see* Helicopter Emergency Services
Heparinization, 256
Hepatic
    anatomy, 185
    injury, 158, 192–193, 197
    isolation, 199
    resection, 198
    shunts, 198
    suture, 198
    tourniquet, 197
    vein, 186–187
Herniation, 173
HESs, *see* Hydroxyethyl starches
Heterologous fibrin, 59–60
Hierarchical-but-fluid model, 5
High-voltage electrical injuries, 285
Histamine-2 receptor antagonist (H2RAs), 382
HIV, *see* Human immunodeficiency virus
Hollow viscus organs, 87
Hormonal
    mediators, 29–30
Human immunodeficiency virus (HIV), 134, 236
Humeral placement, 338
Hydrodissector, 295
Hydrofluoric acid, 285
Hydroxyethyl starches (HESs), 46, 373
Hyperdynamic state, 30–31
Hypermetabolic/hyperdynamic phase of burn, 282, 284
Hypertonic saline, 275
Hyperventilation, 34, 275
Hypocalcaemia, 51
Hypocarbia, 394
Hypotension, 29, 303
Hypotensive resuscitation, 40–41, 270
Hypothalamus, 29
Hypothermia, 48, 81, 354–355
    preventing and treating, 392
Hypoventilation, 303
Hypovolaemia, 26, 29, 36, 114, 254
Hypovolaemic shock, 33–34
    anaesthesia induction in, 395–398
Hypoxia, 114

I

IAH, *see* Intra-abdominal hypertension
IAP, *see* Intra-abdominal pressure
Iatrogenic injuries, 256
IATSIC, *see* International Association for Trauma Surgery and Intensive Care
ICD, *see* International Classification of Disease

ICD-based Injury Severity Score (ICISS), 481, 465
ICDMAP-90 scoring system, 465
ICE, *see* Imaging and clinical examination
ICISS, *see* ICD-based Injury Severity Score
ICP, *see* Intracranial pressure
ICRC, *see* International Committee of the Red Cross
ICU, *see* Intensive care unit
IEDs, *see* Improvised explosive devices
IFN-γ, *see* Interferon gamma
IGF-1, *see* Insulin-like growth factor
IL, *see* Interleukins
Iliac-crest route, 246
Iliac vessels, 169, 238–239
IMA, *see* Inferior mesenteric artery
Imaging and clinical examination (ICE), 274
Imaging in trauma, 334
    pitfalls and pearls, 238
    principles, 335–336
    radiation doses and protection from radiation, 334–335
    ultrasound, 337–338
Immediate haemorrhage control, 416
Immediately life-threatening injuries, 114
Immune response to trauma, 26
    inflammatory pathway, 26–28
    PAMPs and DAMPs, 26
Immunoglobulin administration, 358
Improvised explosive devices (IEDs), 410
Incision, 151, 166–167, 194–195, 208, 291
Inclusive trauma system, 66, 451
    administration, 452
    components, 451–452
    prevention, 452
    public education, 452–453
Increased venous oxygen saturation (↑SvO$_2$), 282
Indeterminate partial-thickness burns, 287
Indirect measurement of flow, 37
Infection prophylaxis, 278
Infectious complications, 349–350
Inferior cava, 313
Inferior mesenteric artery (IMA), 166, 169
Inferior vena cava (IVC), 152, 169–171, 199–200, 230, 279
Inflammatory pathway, 26–28
Inflammatory shock, *see* Distributive shock
Infracolic portion, 166
Infrahepatic IVC, 169–170
Inhalational toxicity, 288
Injury, 497
    classification, 270–271
    location, 101–102
    patterns, 270–271, 301, 408–411
    prevention, 452–453
Injury Severity Score (ISS), 66, 30, 460, 467
INR, *see* International normalized ratio
Institutional performance improvement, 6
Integrated Society of International Society of Surgery/Société
    Internationale de Chirurgie (ISS-SIC), 498
Intensive Care Delirium Screening Checklist, 351
Intensive care unit (ICU), 68, 31, 47, 88, 260, 347, 384, 394,
        442, 445
    correction of clotting profiles, 90

improvement of physiological endpoints, 90
liberation ABCDEF bundle, 351
monitoring for and minimizing incidence of IAH
        and ACS, 90
optimization of oxygen delivery, 90
phases of ICU care, 347–351
physiological restoration in, 89
prophylaxis in, 381–382
recognition of additional injuries, 90
rehabilitation in, 445–446
restoration of body temperature, 89
tertiary survey, 384
trauma and, 439–440
Intercostal neurovascular bundle, 127
Interleukins (IL), 26
IL-1, 26–27
IL-6, 26
IL-8, 27
IL-10, 27
IL-12, 26
Intermittent occlusion resuscitative endovascular balloon
        occlusion of aorta (iREBOA), 327–328
Intermittent RRT, 366
Internal jugular route, 37
International Association for Trauma Surgery and Intensive
        Care (IATSIC), 498
    recognition of DSTC course, 500
International Classification of Disease (ICD), 461
International Committee of the Red Cross (ICRC), 402
International normalized ratio (INR), 53
Interventional radiology (IR), 166–167, 334
Intra-abdominal hypertension (IAH), 372–373, 375–377
Intra-abdominal injuries, 250, 435
Intra-abdominal pressure (IAP), 90, 372, 373
    causes of raised, 374
    measurement, 374–375
    surgery for raised, 373–374
Intraoperative normothermia, 395
Intraoperative pancreatography, 206
Intraosseous needle (IO needle), 338
Intracranial haematoma, 276
Intracranial pressure (ICP), 272–273, 331, 348, 374, 392–393
    monitoring and threshold, 275–276
Intraluminal shunts, 256
Intramural haematoma, 181–182
Intraosseous devices, 41
Intraosseous infusion, 41
Intraparenchymal catheter, 275
Intrapericardial control of inferior vena cava, 199
Intravascular
    obstructive shock, 34
    shunt, 86
    volume restoration, 419
Intravenous access, 289
Intravenous cannulas (IV cannulas), 394
Intravenous devices, 41–42
Intravenous H2-receptor blockade therapy, 382
Intravenous pyelogram (IVP), 224
Intraventricular catheter, 275
Intubation, 40

IO needle, *see* Intraosseous needle
IR, *see* Interventional radiology
iREBOA, *see* Intermittent occlusion resuscitative endovascular balloon occlusion of aorta
Ischaemia, 263
ISS, *see* Injury Severity Score
ISS–SIC, *see* Integrated Society of International Society of Surgery/Société Internationale de Chirugie
IVC, *see* Inferior vena cava
IV cannulas, *see* Intravenous cannulas
IVP, *see* Intravenous pyelogram

J

Javid shunts, 509–510
Jejunostomy, 381
Jugular vein oxygen saturation (SjO$_2$), 275
Jumper's fracture, 241–242

K

Ketamine, 397
Kidney injury scale, 480
Kinetic time (K time), 55
Kocher manoeuvre, 156–157, 208

L

Laceration, 173
Lacertus fibrosis, 266
Lactic acidosis, 30
Langenbeck retractor, 109
Laparoscopy, 118–19, 321–322
    applications, 323–324
    diagnostic, 321
    non-therapeutic, 322
    risks, 322–323
    screening, 321
    technique, 322
    therapeutic, 322
Laparotomy, 224, 246
Large airway disruption, 141
Large bowel, 176–177
Large mesenteric haematoma, 154–155
Laryngoscopy, 102
Lateral compression (LC), 241–242
Lateral haematoma, 134
Lateral incision, 218
Lateralization of abdominal wall, 293
Lateral retroperitoneal haematomas, 118
Latissimus dorsi, 96
LC, *see* Lateral compression
Leadership, 12, 342
    function, 4
    in trauma care, 14–17
Left anterolateral thoracotomy, 138
Left medial visceral rotation, 168, 208
Lesser sac, 155

Life-threatening thoracic injuries, 114
Life, 260–262
    saving, 254
Ligaclips, 509
Ligamentum arteriosum, 141
Lignocaine, 127
Limb, 260–262
    saving, 254
Limb injury complications, 267
Line sepsis, 383
Lipids, 31
Lithotomy position, 160
Liver, 155, 504
    bile ducts and gallbladder, injury to, 202–203
    and biliary system, 185
    complications, 200–201
    diagnosis, 187
    injury, 323
    injury scale, 332–333, 475
    management, 190–193
    perihepatic drainage, 200–201
    porta hepatis, injury to, 201–202
    resuscitation, 332
    retrohepatic vena cava, injury to, 201
    surgical approach, 193–200
LMICs, *see* Low-and middle-income countries
LMWH, *see* Low-molecular-weight heparin
Lobectomy, 139
Long bone fractures, 77
Low-molecular-weight heparin (LMWH), 279, 366
Low-and middle-income countries (LMICs), 270
Lower airway, 296
Lower leg fasciotomy, 264–265
LPV, *see* Lung protective ventilation
LT, *see* Leucotrienes
Lung protective ventilation (LPV), 349
Lungs, 114, 116
    injury scale, 473
    rescue, *see* Extracorporeal membrane oxygenation (ECMO)
Ly30, 52, 55

M

MA, *see* Maximum amplitude
Magnetic resonance cholangiopancreatography (MRCP), 206
Major abdominal vessels
    iliac vessels, 169
    incision, 167
    inferior mesenteric artery, 169
    IVC, 169–171
    medial visceral rotation, 167–168
    portal vein, 171
    renal arteries, 169
    superior mesenteric artery, 168–169
    surgical approach to, 167
Major limb injury, 267
Major liver injuries, 147
Major trauma centre (MTC), 6

Major trauma management, 66–74
  resuscitation, 68–74
Major Trauma Outcome Study (MTOS), 464–465, 469
Mandatory neck exploration, 104
Mangled Extremity Severity Score (MESS), 261
Mangled Extremity Syndrome Index (MESI), 260–261
Mangled limbs, 260
Mannitol, 275
MAP, *see* Mean arterial pressure
mAPS, *see* Modified APS
MASH, *see* Mobile army surgical hospitals
Mass casualties, 401, 416–417
Massive haemorrhage, 58–60, 139
Massive haemothorax, 120–121
Massive limb trauma, 260
  scoring systems, 260–262
Massive retroperitoneal haemorrhage, 375
Massive transfusion protocols (MTPs), 71, 59, 82, 391
Maximum amplitude (MA), 55
MDCT, *see* Multidetector computed tomography
Mean arterial pressure (MAP), 40, 81, 272, 359, 373, 393; *see also*
    Intra-abdominal pressure
Mechanical ventilation, 393
Mechanism of injury, Injuries sustained, Signs and symptoms,
    Treatment (MIST), 13, 66
  Handover, 67
Medial incision, 265
Medial visceral rotation, 167–168
Median sternotomy, 132–133
Mediastinum, 238
Medical text, 457
Medical treatment facilities (MTFs), 411–412
Medicolegal aspects, 511
Membranous urethra, 235
Mental health, 403
MERT, *see* UK Medical Emergency Response Team
Mesentery, 152–153, 177
Mesh
  graft technique, 295
MESI, *see* Mangled Extremity Syndrome Index
MESS, *see* Mangled Extremity Severity Score
Metabolic
  disturbances, 379
  response to trauma, 25–32
MIC, *see* Minimum inhibitory concentration
Midazolam, 398, 422
Midline visceral structures, 109
Mild TBI, 270
Military environments, 408; *see also* Austere environments
  battlefield anaesthesia, 420–422
  battlefield analgesia, 420
  blast injury, 433–434
  common training, 423
  critical care, 422
  evacuation, 417
  front-end processes, 422–423
  governance, 423
  injury patterns, 409–411
  leadership, 422
  mass casualties, 416–417

percent casualties arriving to casualty reception, 416
  rehabilitation services, 423
  resuscitation, 417–419
  translating military experience to civilian trauma care,
      422–423
  translational research, 423
  triage, 416–418
Military experience for shock, 42–43
MilliSieverts (mSv), 335
Mineral zeolyte, 63
Minimal access surgery in trauma, 321
  laparoscopy, 321–324
  REBOA, 324–329
  VATS, 324
Minimum inhibitory concentration (MIC), 150
Minor lacerations, 220
MIST, *see* Mechanism of injury, Injuries sustained, Signs
      and symptoms, Treatment
Mobile army surgical hospitals (MASH), 417
Mobility, 404
Mobilization
  of ascending colon, 156–157
  of liver, 199
Moderate TBI, 270
Modern autotransfusion devices, 58
Modern CT scanners, 162
Modern trauma scoring methodology, 457
Modified APS (mAPS), 460
MODS, *see* Multiple organ dysfunction syndrome
MOF, *see* Multiple organ failure
Motor vehicle crashes (MVC), 141
MRCP, *see* Magnetic resonance cholangiopancreatography
M-statistic, 464–465
mSv, *see* MilliSieverts
MTC, *see* Major trauma centre
MTFs, *see* Medical treatment facilities
MTOS, *see* Major Trauma Outcome Study
MTPs, *see* Massive transfusion protocols
Multidetector computed tomography (MDCT), 334
Multiple casualties, 401
Multiple medications–polypharmacy, 311–312
Multiple organ dysfunction syndrome (MODS), 28, 200,
      349, 355
Multiple organ failure (MOF), 28, 347
  syndromes, 39
Musculature, 116
Musculoskeletal system, 311
MVC, *see* Motor vehicle crashes
Myocardial
  contusion, 69
  infarction, 69
  injuries, 126–127
Myocutaneous flaps, 119

N

National Emergency X-Radiography Utilization Study
      (NEXUS), 302
National Trauma Database (NTDB), 6

National Trauma Management Course (NTMC™), 7
National trauma registries, 6
Neck, 503
    access to, 104
    collar incisions, 109–110
    incision, 105
    management based on anatomical zones, 104
    mandatory vs. selective neck exploration, 104
    midline visceral structures, 109
    penetrating cervical injury, 99–101
    position, 105
    priorities, 108–109
    root of, 109
    surgical access, 106–108
    trauma, 99
    vertebral arteries, 109
Nervous system, 311
Neurogenic shock, 36
Neuropathic pain, 285
New Injury Severity Score (NISS), 460, 469
NEXUS, *see* National Emergency X-Radiography
        Utilization Study
NIBP, *see* Non-invasive blood pressure
NISS, *see* New Injury Severity Score
NISSSA scoring system, 261–262
Nitric oxide (NO), 26
Nitrous oxide, 142
NOM, *see* Non-operative management
Non-absorbable material, 160
Non-anatomical lung preservation, 139
Non-beneficial (futile) care, 314–315
Non-discretionary intervention, 416
Non-invasive blood pressure (NIBP), 421
Non-operative management (NOM), 76, 119, 190, 193,
        215–216, 219, 207, 230, 232, 234, 323
    of penetrating abdominal injury, 148–149
Non-responders, 244–246
Non-Technical Skills for Surgeons (NOTSS), 5, 14
Non-therapeutic laparoscopy, 322
Noradrenaline, 42
Norepinephrine, *see* Noradrenaline
NOTSS, *see* Non-Technical Skills for Surgeons
NRS, *see* Numeric Rating Scale
NTDB, *see* National Trauma Database
NTMC™, *see* National Trauma Management Course
Numeric Rating Scale (NRS), 351
Nutrition(al), 279, 369
    in burned patient, 297–298
    support, 211, 380–382

O

OBR, *see* Outcomes-based rehabilitation
Obstetrics, 404
Obstructive shock, 34
Occult hypoperfusion, 347
Occult injuries, evaluation for, 384
Occupational therapy, 445
Oedema, 296

Oesophageal blow-out injury, 173
Oesophageal injuries, 109, 121–122, 140
Oesophagus, 116, 118, 140
    injury scale, 476
Ohm's law, 36
OIS system, *see* Organ Injury Scaling system
Oliguria, 34
Omnipaque, 102
Omohyoid muscle, 105
'One-hit' model, 355
Open abdomen, 373
Open fracture management, 258–260
Open pelvic fractures, 251
Open pneumothorax, 114
Operating room (OR), 392, 402–403, 507
    abdominal closure, 510–511
    adjuncts, 508–509
    blood loss, 507
    cleaning, 508
    critical incident stress issues, 512
    draping, 508
    environment, 507
    instruments, 508–511
    medicolegal aspects and communication skills, 511
    preparing, 507–509
    special instruments and improvised gadgets, 510
    surgical procedure, 509–510
    swab count, 511
Operation room/theatre (OR/OT), 507
Operations Desert Shield/Desert Storm, 417
Operative haemorrhage, 86
    contamination control, 87
    control, 86–87
    copious washout, 87
    initial incision, 86
    TAC, 87–89
Operative management, 215, 207
Operative (surgical) management, 193
Opiates, 308
Opportunistic post-splenectomy infection
        (OPSI), 222
OPSI, *see* Opportunistic post-splenectomy infection
Optimal method of closure, 158–159
OR, *see* Operating room
Organ Injury Scaling system (OIS system), 461, 466
Organ injury, specific, 304–305
    scaling system for, 470–485
Organ perfusion, 390
OR/OT, *see* Operation room/theatre
Orotracheal intubation, 302
Orthopaedic injuries, 290
Osmotherapy, 275
Outcome analysis, 457, 462–465
Outcomes-based rehabilitation (OBR), 448
Ovary injury scale, 483
Overtriage, 414
Overwhelming post-splenectomy infection
        (OPSI), 383
Oxandrolone, 298
Oxidative stress, 310

Oxygen
consumption, 297
debt, 38
oxygen-carrying capacity, 46
Oxygenation, 40
Oxygen delivery (DO$_2$), 39
optimization, 90
Oxygen delivery index (DO$_2$I), 39
Oxyhaemoglobin, 38–39

P

P&RM, *see* Physical and rehabilitation medicine
Packed red blood cells (pRBCs), 46–47, 60, 81, 193
Paediatric airway management, 302
Paediatric burn nutrition, 298
Paediatric chest trauma, 116
Paediatric considerations, 115–116, 179, 279
Paediatric trauma, 301
analgesia, 308–309
injury patterns, 301
pre-hospital, 301
resuscitation room, 301–302
specific organ injury, 302–303
Paediatric Trauma Score (PTS), 457, 466
Pain, 351
control, 383 384
Pain, paraesthesia, paralysis, pallor, and pulselessness
(5Ps), 263
PAMPs, *see* Pathogen-associated molecular patterns
Pancreas, 204, 504
adjuncts, 211
anatomy, 204–205
complications, 211–212
diagnosis, 205–207
evidence-based guidelines, 212–213
injury scale, 207, 476
management, 207–208
mechanisms of injury, 206
operative evaluation, 208
pancreatic injury in children, 211
surgical approach, 208–211
Pancreatic hormones, 30
Pancreatic injury, 158, 208–209, 308
in children, 211
contusion and parenchymal injuries, 208–209
damage control, 209–210
distal pancreatectomy, 209
drainage alone, 209
ductal injuries, 209
pancreaticoduodenectomy, 210–211
pyloric exclusion, 210
splenic salvage in distal pancreatectomy, 29
T-tube drainage, 210
Pancreaticoduodenal injuries, 148, 209
Pancreaticoduodenectomy, 183, 184
Pancreatic trauma, 204
Pancreatitis, 211
Paraplegia, 127

Parenchymal injuries, 208–209
Parietal pleura, 132
Partial occlusion resuscitative endovascular balloon occlusion
of aorta (pREBOA), 326–327
Partial pressure of carbon dioxide (PaCO$_2$), 348, 355
Partial pressure of oxygen (PaO$_2$), 38, 348, 356
Partial splenectomy, 220
Partial thromboplastin time (PTT), 53, 85
Pathogen-associated molecular patterns (PAMPs), 26
PATI, *see* Penetrating Abdominal Trauma Index
Patient-controlled analgesia (PCA), 383
PAWP, *see* Pulmonary arterial wedge pressure
PBW, *see* Predicted body weight
PCA, *see* Patient-controlled analgesia
PC-FC, *see* Pulmonary contusion-flail chest
PCT level, *see* Procalcitonin level
PE, *see* Pulmonary embolus
PEA, *see* Pulseless electrical activity
Pectoralis, 119
Pedestrian-vehicle crash (PVC), 301
PEEP, *see* Positive end expiratory pressure
PEG, *see* Percutaneous endoscopic gastrostomy; Percutaneous
gastrostomy
Pelvic/pelvis, 155, 238
anatomy, 238–239
associated injuries, 250–251
Pelvic/pelvis
C-clamp, 246
classification, 239
clinical examination and diagnosis, 243–244
external fixation, 245–246
extraperitoneal pelvic packing, 246–249
fractures, 238, 310
haematomas, 157, 166–167
injury, 76–77, 238, 301, 337
inlet, 238
laparotomy, 247
open pelvic fractures, 250
resuscitation, 245–246
Tile's classification, 239–241
Young and Burgess classification, 241–243
Penetrating abdominal injury, 148–149
Penetrating abdominal trauma, 337–338
Penetrating Abdominal Trauma Index (PATI), 461
Penetrating cervical injury, 99–100
diagnostic studies, 102
frequency of injury, 102
haemorrhage control, 100–101
initial assessment and definitive airway, 99–100
location, 101–102
mechanism, 102
Penetrating cranial injury, 278
Penetrating extraperitoneal rectal injuries, 178
Penetrating head trauma, 271
Penetrating thoracic injury, 140–141, 337–338
Penetrating trauma, 205, 179, 224
management, 74
Penis injury scale, 484
Percutaneous endoscopic gastrostomy (PEG), 381
Percutaneous gastrostomy (PEG), 445

Percutaneous suprapubic catheterization, 234
Percutaneous tracheostomy, 350
Perfluorocarbon (PFC), 58–59
Performance improvement activities, 6
Pericardial tamponade, 85, 138
Pericardial window, 161
Pericardiocentesis, 7, 418
Pericardium, 118
Perihepatic
    drainage, 200
    infections, 200
    packing, 195–196
Perineum (burn), 297
Peripheral vascular injuries, 485
Peripheral vascular organ injury scale, 485
Peritoneum, 321
Peritonitis, 179
Permissive hypertension, 68
Permissive hypotension, 81
Personal protective equipment (PPE), 410
PFC, see Perfluorocarbon
PG, see Prostaglandins
PGI, see Prostacyclins
Pharyngeal injuries, 108
Phrenic nerves, 116
Physical and rehabilitation medicine (P&RM), 445
    OBR, 446
    rehabilitation starts in ICU, 445–446
    rehabilitation team, 445
Physical health, 403
Physical injury, 25
Physiological scoring systems, 457–458
Physiotherapy, 445
PICO format, 123, 164
Pituitary gland, 29
Planned hernia, 92
Platelets (PLT), 47
Platysma, 120
Pledgets, 232
Pleurae, 117
Pleural cavities, 117
PLT, see Platelets
PMN, see Polymorphonucleocyte
Pneumonectomy, 139
Pneumothorax, 119–120
Polycompartment syndrome, 373
Polyglycolic acid, 92
Polymorphonucleocyte (PMN), 374–375
Polytetrafluoroethylene (PTFE), 92, 173, 175
Polytrauma patients, timing of skeletal fixation in, 260
Population
    ageing, 310
    population-based studies, 454–455
Porta hepatis, 185, 197, 201–202
Portal vein, 171
Portocaval shunting, 171
Positive end expiratory pressure (PEEP), 99, 348, 390–391
Posterior pelvic integrity, 239
Posterior urethra, 234
Posterolateral thoracotomy, 133

Postoperative care, 232
Post-shock, 36
Post-splenectomy vaccination guidelines, 221
Post-traumatic acute lung injury, 348–349
Post-traumatic amnesia (PTA), 270
Post-traumatic seizures (PTS), 278–279
Post-traumatic stress disorder (PTSD), 441
Potentially life-threatening injuries, 114–115
PPE, see Personal protective equipment
PPIs, see Proton pump inhibitors
Prasugerl, 52–53
pRBCs, see Packed red blood cells
Pre-hospital
    interventions, 302
    resuscitation in pre-hospital setting, 81
Pre-operative adjuncts, 150–151
Pre-surgery platelet count, 48
pREBOA, see Partial occlusion resuscitative endovascular
        balloon occlusion of aorta
Predicted body weight (PBW), 258
Predictive salvage index system, 261
Pregnancy, trauma in, 313–314
Pregnant uterus, injury of, 236
Pressure support ventilation (PSV), 348
Primary ACS, 372–373
Primary blast injury, 433–434
Primary brain injury, 270
Primary closure, 159–160
Primary hypothermia, 354
Primary survey of resuscitation, 83
    airway, 83
    breathing, 84
    circulation, 84–87
    environment, 87–88
    neurological status, 87
Pringle's manoeuvre, 171
Procalcitonin level (PCT level), 373
Professionalism, 4
Prolonged life support phase, 349–350
Prophylaxis, 48
    in ICU, 381–382
    infection, 278
    seizure, 278–279
Propofol, 275, 397
Proprietary shunts, 509–510
Protein, 283–284, 297
Proton pump inhibitors (PPIs), 382
5Ps, see Pain, paraesthesia, paralysis, pallor, and pulselessness
Pseudocyst, 212
PSV, see Pressure support ventilation
Psychologist, 442–443
Psychology of trauma, 439
    clinical psychologist, 442–443
    and ICU, 442
    psychological trauma, 439–440
PTSD, 441–442
    reactions to trauma, 439
PTA, see Post-traumatic amnesia
PTFE, see Polytetrafluoroethylene
PTS, see Paediatric Trauma Score; Post-traumatic seizures

PTSD, *see* Post-traumatic stress disorder
PTT, *see* Partial thromboplastin time
Public education, 453
Public support, 453
Pulmonary
  arteries, 117
  contusion, 122, 141, 307
  haemorrhage, 139
  laceration, 124
  tractotomy, 139
Pulmonary arterial wedge pressure (PAWP), 31
Pulmonary contusion-flail chest (PC-FC), 125
Pulmonary embolus (PE), 350, 382–383
Pulmonary vascular resistance (PVR), 282
Pulseless electrical activity (PEA), 422
PVC, *see* Pedestrian–vehicle crash
PVR, *see* Pulmonary vascular resistance
Pyloric exclusion, 184, 210

Q

Quaternary blast injury, 434
Quinary blast injury, 434

R

Radiation doses and protection, 334–335
Radiological
  contrast studies, 180
  investigation, 180
Rancho Los Amigos Scale, 448
Rapid sequence induction (RSI), 99, 398–399, 421–422
RASS, *see* Richmond Agitation-Sedation Scale
RBCs, *see* Red blood cells
Re-look laparotomy, 90
Reaction time (R time), 54
REBOA, *see* Resuscitative endovascular balloon occlusion
    of the aorta; Retrograde endovascular balloon
    occlusion of aorta
Recombinant activated factor VII (rFVIIa), 53
Recovery phase, 297
Rectum, 177
  injury scale, 478
Recurrent ACS, 373
Red blood cells (RBCs), 47, 195–196
Rehabilitation, 255–256
  in ICU, 445–446
  services, 423
  team, 445
Relative Outcome Score, 465
Relief of pain, 399
Renal arteries, 169
Renal function, 34
Renal hormones, 30
Renal injuries, 223
  diagnosis, 224
  injury scale, 224–226
  management, 224, 226
  surgical approach, 226–228

Renal replacement therapy (RRT), 367
Renal system, 312
Repair of perforation, 183
Respiratory
  assessment and monitoring, 348
  failure, 349
  insufficiency, 259
  system, 310
Respiratory rate (RR), 69
Resuscitation, 13, 68, 187–188, 244, 417
  civilian pre-hospital tourniquet uses, 68
  clinical considerations in penetrating injury, 418
  DCR, 418–419
  DCS in military setting, 419–420
  in emergency department and pre-hospital setting, 66
  emergency department surgery, 74–75
  initial, 46
  management of penetrating trauma, 74
  metabolic response to trauma, 25–32
  physiology, 25
  primary survey, 68–73
  room, 249–250
  secondary survey, 73–74
  shock, 32–42
  'traditional' endpoints, 347
Resuscitative endovascular balloon occlusion of the aorta
    (REBOA), 77, 86, 134, 165, 245, 325
  anaesthetic considerations, 331
  anatomy, 325
  complications, 329
  contraindications, 329
  evidence-based recommendations, 329
  indications, 328–329
  insertion, 327, 505
  landing zones, 326
  monitoring, 327–328
  perioperative and postoperative care, 328
  physiology, 326–327
  puncture of femoral artery, 328
  total, partial, and intermittent occlusion, and targeted
      blood pressure, 328
Resuscitative phase, 347–348
Retrograde cystography, 234
Retrograde endovascular balloon occlusion of aorta
    (REBOA), 151
Retrohepatic anatomy of liver, 186
Retrohepatic IVC injury, 186
Retrohepatic vena cava, 201
Retroperitoneal haematoma, 158, 166–167
Retroperitoneum, 148
Revised Injury Severity Classification II (RISC II),
    461–462, 468
Revised Trauma Score (RTS), 457–458, 466
  rFVIIa, *see* Recombinant activated factor VII Ribs
    fixation of multiple fractures of, 123
    PICO format, 123
Richmond Agitation-Sedation Scale (RASS), 351
Right hemicolon, 156–157
Right medial visceral rotation, 156–157, 208
RISC II, *see* Revised Injury Severity Classification II

Road trauma, 403
Role 1 MTF, 411
Role 2E, *see* Role 2 Enhanced MTF
Role 2 Enhanced MTF (Role 2E), 411
Role 2 Light Manoeuvre (Role 2LM), 411
Role 2LM, *see* Role 2 Light Manoeuvre
Role 2 MTF, 411
Role 3 MTFs, 411
Role 4 MTFs, 412
Rotary thromboelastomerography (RoTEM), 54–57, 90
Rotational thromboelastometry, (RoTEM), 71
Routine antibiotics, 130
Roux-en-Y limb, 202
RR, *see* Respiratory rate
RRT, *see* Renal replacement therapy
RSI, *see* Rapid sequence induction
RTS, *see* Revised Trauma Score
Rumel tourniquet, 509
Rupture(d)
  of tympanic membrane, 434
  urethra, 228–229

S

SA, *see* Situational awareness
Sacroiliac joint, 238–239
SAFE, *see* Saline versus Albumin Fluid Evaluation
Safe retrieval, 288
Safe Surgery 2020, 7
Safe trauma care, 4; *see also* Trauma care
  global activities, 6–7
  individual factors, 4–5
  institutional factors, 5
  national activities, 6
  performance improvement activities, 6
  regional activities, 6
Saline versus Albumin Fluid Evaluation (SAFE), 46
Salt retention, 31
Saphenous veins, 264–265
SAS, *see* Sedation-Agitation Scale
SAT, *see* Spontaneous Awakening Trials
SBP, *see* Systolic blood pressure
SBT, *see* Spontaneous Breathing Trials
Scaling system for organ-specific injuries, 470
  abdominal vascular injury scale, 479
  adrenal organ injury scale, 480
  bladder injury scale, 481
  cervical vascular organ injury scale, 470
  chest wall injury scale, 371
  colon injury scale, 478
  diaphragm injury scale, 474
  duodenum injury scale, 477
  extrahepatic biliary tree injury scale, 475
  fallopian tube injury scale, 482
  heart injury scale, 472
  kidney injury scale, 480
  liver injury scale, 475
  lung injury scale, 473
  oesophagus injury scale, 476
  ovary injury scale, 483

pancreas injury scale, 476
  penis injury scale, 484
  peripheral vascular organ injury scale, 485
  rectum injury scale, 478
  scrotum injury scale, 484
  small bowel injury scale, 478
  spleen injury scale, 474
  stomach injury scale, 477
  testis injury scale, 484
  thoracic vascular injury scale, 473
  ureter injury scale, 481
  urethra injury scale, 481
  uterus (non-pregnant and pregnant) injury scale, 482
  vagina injury scale, 483
  vulva injury scale, 483
SCI, *see* Spinal cord injury
Scoring systems, 260–262, 457
Screening laparoscopy, 321
Scrotum
  injury scale, 484
  injury to, 236
Sealants, 232
Secondary abdominal closure, 91
Secondary ACS, 372
Secondary blast injury, 434
Secondary brain injury, 271
Secondary hypothermia, 354
Secondary survey of resuscitation, 73–74
Secretions, oxygenation, alert, airway, pressures or parameters (SOA2P), 350
Sedation-Agitation Scale (SAS), 351
Sedation, 280
Seizure prophylaxis, 278–279
Selective neck exploration, 104
Selective non-operative management (SNOM), 414
Self-retaining retractor, 199
Sepsis, 28–29, 184, 213–214, 284, 300
  mechanical ventilation of sepsis-induced ARDS, 365–366
  sepsis-induced hypoperfusion, 357
Septic shock, 355–357
Sequential Trauma Education Programme (STEPS), 7
Serum amylase, 180, 205
Serum lipase, 180, 205
Severe injury management to extremity, 254–255
Severe sepsis, 356
Sexual
  assault, 236
  health, 403
Shock, 69, 32–33
  cardiac compressive, 35
  cardiogenic, 34–35
  distributive, 36
  endpoints in shock resuscitation, 38–43
  fluid therapy for volume expansion, 44
  hypovolaemic, 33–34
  measurements in, 36–38
  neurogenic, 36
  obstructive, 33
  oxygenation, 40
  pharmacologic support of blood pressure, 41–42

post-shock and multiple organ failure syndromes, 39
    prognosis in, 42
    recommended protocol for, 42–43
    route of administration, 41
    shocked patient management, 39–40
Shunting, 171–172
Siewert (Sv), 335
Sigmoidoscopy, 177
Simulation, 7
    training, 5
Single incision fasciotomy, 265–266
SIRS, *see* Systemic inflammatory response syndrome
Situational awareness (SA), 5, 14
Skeletal fixation timing in polytrauma patients, 259–260
Skin
    skin-only closure, 91
    staplers, 509
Skull X-rays, 276
Sliding lung, 336
SMA, *see* Superior mesenteric artery
Small bowel, 175–176
    injury scale, 478
SNOM, *see* Selective non-operative management
SOA2P, *see* Secretions, oxygenation, alert, airway, pressures
    or parameters
Social worker, 445
Sodium bicarbonate, 59
Somatostatin and analogues, 211
Special patient situations
    non-beneficial (futile) care, 314–315
    paediatric trauma, 301–310
    trauma in elderly, 310–313
    trauma in pregnancy, 313–314
Specific organ
    injury, 304–308
    techniques, 158
Spectrum of thoracic injury, 114–115
Speech therapist, 445
Spinal anaesthesia, 422
Spinal cord injury (SCI), 446; *see also* Traumatic brain injury
Spinopelvic dissociation, 241
Spleen, 197, 216, 504
    anatomy, 216
    diagnosis, 216
    injury scale, 474
    management, 218
    OPSI, 222
    outcome, 221
    splenic injury scale, 216, 218
    surgical approach, 219, 220
Splenectomy, 220
Splenic artery, 205
Splenic injury, 158, 323–324
    scale, 216–217
Splenic salvage in distal pancreatectomy, 209
Splenic surface bleed, 220
Splenic suspensory ligaments, 216
Splenic tears, 220
Split-skin grafting (SSG), 286, 292
Spontaneous Awakening Trials (SAT), 351

Spontaneous Breathing Trials (SBT), 351
SPT, *see* Superficial partial thickness
SSG, *see* Split-skin grafting
Stability, 404
Stabilization of fractures, 404
Stable patients of small bowel, 175–176
Staphylococcus aureus, 259
Stapling devices, 198
STEPS, *see* Sequential Trauma Education Programme
Sterilization department, 402
Steroids, 276, 279
Stirrups position, 160
Stomach, 175
    injury scale, 477
Stomas, 161–2
Stress
    ulceration, 381
    ulcer prophylaxis, 366
Stroke volume, 33, 41
Subarachnoid catheter, 275
Subcapsular haematoma, 193–195
Subclavian route, 37
Subcutaneous fasciotomy, 266
Subdural catheter, 275
Substrate metabolism, mediators effects on, 31–32
Sucralfate, 382
Superficial burn, 286
Superficial partial thickness (SPT), 286–287
Superior mesenteric artery (SMA), 166, 168–169
Supra-acetabular route, 246
Supracolic portion, 16
Suprahepatic IVC, 169–170
Suprapubic cystostomy, 235
Suprarenal aorta, 166
Surgery
    burr holes and emergency craniotomy, 276–279
    indications for, 276
Surgical anatomy of chest, 116
    chest contents, 116–118
    chest floor, 116
    chest wall, 116
Surgical approach(es)
    duodenum, 181–183
    liver and biliary system, 193–200
    to major abdominal vessels, 167–170
    pancreas, 208–210
    to thorax, 130–135
Surgical decision-making algorithm in major hepatic
    trauma, 208
Surgical equipment, 324
Surgical triage, 414
Surviving sepsis guidelines, 357–370
Suspected non-accidental injury, 308
Sv, *see* Siewert
SVR, *see* Systemic vascular resistance
Swedish Trauma Surgery Course, 498
Swiss cheese model, 11
Symphyseolysis, 203
Syncope, 36
Synman, 7

Systemic arterial pressure, 37
Systemic inflammatory response syndrome (SIRS), 26–28,
    69, 98, 233, 239, 278, 283; *see also* Abdominal
    compartment syndrome
Systemic vascular resistance (SVR), 282
Systolic blood pressure (SBP), 255, 270, 347

T

Table tilt, 160
TAC, *see* Temporary abdominal closure
TachoSil®, 62
Tachycardia, 36
TAFI, *see* Thrombin-activated fibrinolysis inhibitor
TARN, *see* Trauma Audit and Research Network
TASC, *see* Temporary abbreviated surgical control
Task management, 14
TA-type non-cutting staplers, 509
TBI, *see* Traumatic brain injury
TBSA, *see* Total body surface area; Total burn surface area
Team STEPPS programme, 5
Team training, 5
TEG, *see* Thromboelastography
Temperature control, 150–151
Temporary abbreviated surgical control (TASC), 420
Temporary abdominal closure (TAC), 87
Temporary closure, 87, 91, 159, 246
Temporary control of haemorrhage, techniques for, 195–198
Tension pneumothorax, 69, 75
Tensor fascia lata flap (TFL flap), 92
Tertiary blast injury, 434
Testis injury scale, 484
Tetanus prophylaxis, 383
TFL flap, *see* Tensor fascia lata flap
TGF-β, *see* Transforming growth factor beta
Theatre teams, 14
Therapeutic laparoscopy, 322
Thiopental, 398
Thoracic aorta, 139
Thoracic duct, 118
Thoracic injury, 114, 307
    anaesthetic management of, 142
    paediatric considerations, 115–116
    pathophysiology, 115
    spectrum, 114–115
Thoracic trauma, anaesthesia for, 140
Thoracic vascular injury scale, 473
Thoracoscopy, 119
Thoracotomy
    with aortic cross-clamping, 139
    tray, 509
Thorax, surgical approaches to, 130–134
3D trauma surgeon, 5
Thrombin-activated fibrinolysis inhibitor (TAFI), 353
Thrombin–thrombomodulin complex, 353
Thromboelastography (TEG), 71, 54–56, 90, 152
    abnormal appearances of, 55
Thrombophlebitis, 383
Thromboxanes (TX), 26

Thymus, 116
TIC, *see* Trauma-induced coagulopathy
Ticegrelor, 52
Tile's classification, 239
    acetabular fractures, 241
    completely stable, 239
    fracture combinations, 241
    jumper's fracture, 241
    vertically stable, 239
    wholly unstable in rotational and vertical planes, 239
Tissue
    adhesives, 59, 62
    hypoperfusion, 26
    hypoxia, 290
TIVA, *see* Total intravenous anaesthesia
TLRs, *see* Toll-like receptors
TNF, *see* Tumour necrosis factor
TOE, *see* Transoesophageal echo
Toll-like receptors (TLRs), 26
Total body surface area (TBSA), 287–288
Total burn surface area (TBSA), 286
Total intravenous anaesthesia (TIVA), 422
Total occlusion resuscitative endovascular balloon occlusion
    of aorta (tREBOA), 328
Toxins, 282, 411
T-piece bladder pressure device, 374
T-POD, *see* Traumatic pelvic orthotic device
Trachea, 117
Tracheal injuries, 109
Tracheobronchial
    injuries, 121, 140
    tree, 117
Tracheostomy, 100, 296
Traction, 404
Tract tamponade balloons, 197
TRAIS scoring system, 467
Tranexamic acid (TXA), 52, 353, 392
Transoesophageal echo (TOE), 141
Transthoracic echo (TTE), 141
Transfusion
    adjuncts to clotting enhancement, 51
    autotransfusion, 57–58
    blood, 47–48
    colloids, 46
    component therapy, 48–49
    effects of transfusing blood and blood products, 49–51
    fluids, 46–49
    haemostatic adjuncts in trauma, 59, 62
    indications for, 46
    initial response, 51
    massive haemorrhage/massive, 58–59
    monitoring coagulation status, 53–57
    oxygen-carrying capacity, 46
    ratios, 51
    red blood cell substitutes, 58–59
Transient responders, 244
Translational research, 423
Transoesophageal echocardiography, 118
Transverse process, 105
Trapdoor thoracotomy, 133–134

Trauma, 25, 263, 451
  anabolic phase, 32
  anaesthesiologists, 389
  clinical and therapeutic relevance, 32
  communication in trauma setting, 11–14
  designation of trauma centres, 453
  effects of mediators, 30–32
  in elderly, 310–313
  establishment criteria for optimal care, 454
  evaluation, 454
  haemostatic adjuncts in, 58, 62
  hormonal mediators, 29–30
  immune response, 26
  inclusive, 451–453
  initiating factors, 25–26
  injured patient management within system, 453
  legal authority, 453
  metabolic response to, 25
  panel review, 454
  population-based studies, 454–455
  in pregnancy, 313
  public support, 453
  registry study, 454
  results and studies, 454
  steps in organizing system, 453
  systems, 451
  team, 5
  trauma care facilities, 6
Trauma anaesthesia, 329; *see also* Battlefield anaesthesia
  anaesthesia induction in hypovolaemic shock, 395–398
  DCR, 390–392
  DCS, 392–395
  planning and communicating, 389
Trauma and Injury Severity Score (TRISS), 6, 461, 464–465,
      468
Trauma and Injury Severity Score Comorbidity (TRISSCOM),
      462, 468
Trauma Audit and Research Network (TARN), 6
Trauma care; *see also* Safe trauma care
  access to, 310
  leadership in, 14–17
Trauma-induced coagulopathy (TIC), 43, 47
Trauma laparotomy, 147, 149
  abdominal injury complexes, 147–148
  aortic compression spoon, 161
  bladder injury, 159
  closure of abdomen, 158–159
  definitive packing, 155
  drains, 161
  draping, 151
  early tracheostomy, 162–163
  headlight, 160
  incision, 151–152
  initial procedure, 152
  non-operative management of penetrating abdominal
      injury, 148–149
  operating room scrub nurses, 163
  perform, 153–155
  pericardial window, 161
  pre-operative adjuncts, 150–151

  retroperitoneum, 148
  specific routes of access, 155–158
  stirrups and lithotomy position, 160
  stomas, 161–162
  table tilt, 160–161
  temporary closure, 159
  washout, 161
'Trauma Man', 8
Trauma Registry DGU (TR-DGU®), 461–462
Trauma scores and scoring systems
  anatomical scoring systems, 458–462
  comorbidity scoring systems, 462–465
  comparison, 465–469
  outcome analysis, 462–464
  physiological scoring systems, 457–458
  scaling system for organ specific injuries, 470–485
Traumatic aortic rupture, 257
Traumatic brain injury (TBI), 41, 46, 270, 378, 446
  management, 274
  measurable physiological parameters in, 272–274
  pathophysiology, 274
  severity of, 258
Traumatic pelvic orthotic device (T-POD), 244
Trauma US, 335–336
  applications, 337–338
  eFAST, 336–337
  indications and results, 337
  training, 338
TR-DGU®, *see* Trauma Registry DGU
tREBOA, *see* Total occlusion resuscitative endovascular
      balloon occlusion of aorta
Triage, 414
  factors affecting, 415
  forward surgical team decision-making, 415
  forward surgical teams and, 415–416
  selection of patients for surgery, 416
  source and aim, 414–415
Trial-without-catheter (TWoC), 162
Tri-Service Anaesthetic Apparatus (TSAA), 422
TRISS, *see* Trauma and Injury Severity Score
TRISSCOM, *see* Trauma and Injury Severity Score
      Comorbidity
TSAA, *see* Tri-Service Anaesthetic Apparatus
TTE, *see* Transthoracic echo
T-tube drainage, 210
Tumescent technique, 292
Tumour necrosis factor (TNF), 26–29
'Two-hit' model, 355
TWoC, *see* Trial-without-catheter
Two incision–four compartment fasciotomy, 264–265
TX, *see* Thromboxanes
TXA, *see* Tranexamic acid

U

UFH, *see* Unfractionated heparin
UK Battlefield Advanced Life Support course (BATLS™), 419
UK Damage Control Resuscitation Protocol, 419
UK Medical Emergency Response Team (MERT), 417

Ulcer prophylaxis, 298
UltraSim, 7
Ultrasound (US), 91–92, 118, 216, 205, 235, 335–336; *see also*
    Trauma US
Umbilical tapes, 154, 509
Unfractionated heparin (UFH), 366
Unintentional injury, 301
Unstable patients of small bowel, 175–176
Upper airway, 296
Upper and lower arm, 266
Upper leg, 266
Ureters, 169
  injury scale, 482
Urethra(l)
  catheter, 162
  injuries, 235–236, 250
  injury scale, 481
  repair, 236
Urogenital system, 223
  adjuncts, 233
  bladder injuries, 234–235
  gynaecological injury and sexual assault, 236
  injury to scrotum, 236
  postoperative care, 233
  renal injuries, 224–232
  ureteric injuries, 233–234
  urethral injuries, 235–236
Urogenital trauma, 223
Urological tract, 243
US, *see* Ultrasound
Uterus (non-pregnant and pregnant) injury scale, 482

V

VAC, *see* Vacuum-assisted closure
Vacuum-assisted closure (VAC), 91, 510
VA-ECMO, *see* Veno-arterial ECMO
Vagina injury scale, 483
Vagus nerves, 116
VAP, *see* Ventilator-associated pneumonia
Vascular access, 394
Vascular injuries, 107
  EAST, 257
  management of extremity, 255–256
Vascular repair, 263
Vasoactive medications, 360
VATS, *see* Video-assisted thoracoscopy
Vector-borne disease, 403
Veno-arterial ECMO (VA-ECMO), 351–352
Veno-venous bypass, 201
Veno-venous ECMO (VV-ECMO), 351
Venous thromboembolism prophylaxis (VTE prophylaxis), 6,
    259, 298, 361
Ventilation, 39, 303
Ventilator-associated pneumonia (VAP), 123, 298, 284
Vertebral arteries, 107
Vertical shear (VS), 242–243

VHA, *see* Viscoelastic haemostatic assays
Video-assisted thoracoscopy (VATS), 121, 173, 323–324
VILI, *see* Ventilator-induced lung injury
VIRGIL, 7
Visceral perfusion, 375, 374
Viscoelastic assays, 84
Viscoelastic haemostatic assays (VHA), 54–57, 85, 244, 353
Viscohaemostatic assays, *see* Viscoelastic haemostatic assays
'Vision Zero' campaign, 6
Vitamin C, 298
Volume-dependent markers, 46
Volume expansion, fluid therapy for, 40
VS, *see* Vertical shear
VTE prophylaxis, *see* Venous thromboembolism prophylaxis
Vulva injury scale, 483
VV-ECMO, *see* Veno-venous ECMO

W

War wounds, treatment of, 404
Washout, 161
Waste disposal, 402
Water
  retention, 31
  supply, 402
WBCT, *see* Whole body CT scan
Weaning from ventilatory support, 350
Whipple's procedure, 184, 210–211
WHO, *see* World Health Organisation
Whole body CT scan (WBCT), 335
WISH, *see* World Innovation Summit for Health
Workforce development, 7
World Health Organisation (WHO), 7
World Innovation Summit for Health (WISH), 7
World Society of Emergency Surgery (WSES), 247
Wound(ing)
  coverage, 292–293
  factors, 30
  patterns, 410
WSES, *see* World Society of Emergency Surgery
'W-statistic', 465

X

Xiphoid cartilage, 132

Y

Young and Burgess classification, 241–243

Z

Zeolite (QuikClot®), 419
Zone III injuries of neck, 107–108
Zone II injuries of neck, 107
Zone I vascular injuries of neck, 107